An Updated View on an Emerging Target: Selected Papers from the 8th International Conference on Protein Kinase CK2

Special Issue Editors

Joachim Jose
Marc Le Borgne
Lorenzo A. Pinna
Mathias Montenarh

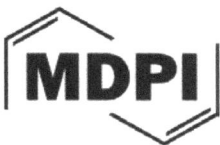

MDPI

Special Issue Editors

Joachim Jose
Westfälische Wilhelms-Universität
Germany

Marc Le Borgne
Université de Lyon
France

Lorenzo A. Pinna
University of Padova
Italy

Mathias Montenarh
Saarland University
Germany

Editorial Office
MDPI AG
St. Alban-Anlage 66
Basel, Switzerland

This edition is a reprint of the Special Issue published online in the open access journal *Pharmaceuticals* (ISSN 1424-8247) from 2016–2017 (available at: http://www.mdpi.com/journal/pharmaceuticals/special_issues/protein_kinase_CK2)

For citation purposes, cite each article independently as indicated on the article page online and as indicated below:

Author 1; Author 2; Author 3 etc. Article title. *Journal Name*. **Year**. Article number/page range.

ISBN 978-3-03842-412-3 (Pbk)
ISBN 978-3-03842-413-0 (PDF)

Table of Contents

Chapter 1: New horizons in the understanding of CK2 function

Chapter 2: CK2 as a therapeutic target

Chapter 3: Structural insights

Chapter 4: New inhibitors of human protein kinase CK2

Chapter 5: New insights into the physiological role of CK2: the clue to therapeutic intervention

About the Guest Editors

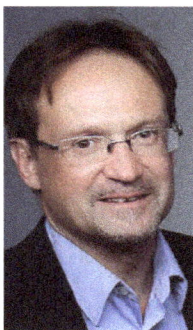

Joachim Jose graduated from the University Saarbrücken in 1994 with a thesis on the structure and reaction mechanism of bacterial ureases. He was a Post-Doc at the Max Planck Institute (MPI) for Biology, Tübingen, and the MPI for Infection Biology, Berlin, where he was mainly involved in the discovery of a new family of secreted proteins: the autotransporters. After his Habilitation at the Institute of Pharmaceutical and Medicinal Chemistry University Saarbrücken (1997–2003), he accepted an offer from the Heinrich-Heine-University, Düsseldorf, to be an Associate Professor in Bioanalytics in 2004. Since 2011, he is a full professor (W3) and Chair for Pharmaceutical and Medicinal Chemistry at the PharmaCampus of the Westfälische Wilhelms-Universität, Münster, as well as being the director of the institute. His research mainly focusses on the application of "autodisplay", a surface display technology for drug discovery purposes, including evolutive drug design, expression of challenging enzymes and new inhibitors for targeting protein–protein interactions.

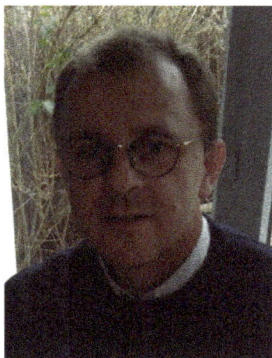

Marc Le Borgne completed his PhD at the Nantes Atlantic University after studying Pharmacy for six years. He started his career as an associate professor in the Faculty of Pharmacy of Nantes (1999–2008) and moved to Lyon as a professor of medicinal chemistry. In 2011, he became the director of EA 4446 Bioactive Molecules and Medicinal Chemistry (B2MC), a research group dedicated to drug design, synthesis and structural optimization. He has published more than 65 papers in reputed journals and is serving as an editorial board member of *Pharmaceuticals* (since 2016). He has given some invited lectures abroad (Duesseldorf, Saarbruecken, Oslo, Tromsø, Bergen, Debrecen, Helsinki, Oulu, Sacramento, La Jolla...). He is developing bioactive small molecules as anticancer agents (CYP19, protein kinase CK2, Dyrks), efflux pump inhibitors (Pg-p, BCRP) and anti-infective agents (CYP51). His other studies are focused on glycoconjugate vaccines such as depolymerisation of carbohydrates. The main scaffolds that he studies are indole, naphthyridine, indeno[1,2-b]indole, carbazole and oxazinocarbazoles, steroids, peptidomimetics, and polysialic acid.

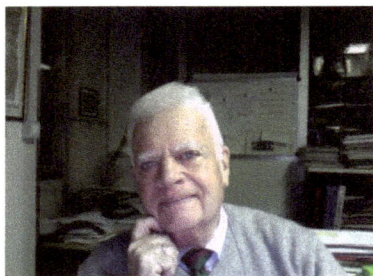

Lorenzo A. Pinna is Professor Emeritus at the department of Biomedical Sciences of the University of Padova, after having served as Director of the department of Biological Chemistry, of the Excellence Centre on Signal Transduction and of the PhD school of Biochemistry and Biotechnology at the same university. He became a full professor of biochemistry and medical chemistry at the University of Padova in 1975, after having been a postdoctoral fellow at the Department of Physiological Chemistry, the Johns Hopkins University Medical School in Baltimore. His research interests encompass many aspects of protein phosphorylation with special reference to the definition of the substrate specificity of protein kinases, the development of kinase inhibitors with therapeutic potential and the understanding of the biological role of "casein kinases".

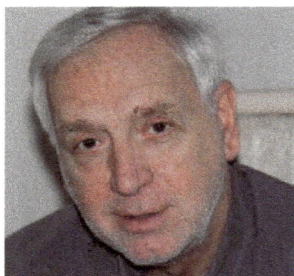

Matthias Montenarh graduated in Inorganic Chemistry from the Rheinische Friedrich Wilhelms University Bonn in 1976 with a thesis on the synthesis and characterisation of new sulfur–nitrogen compounds. He was a Post-Doc at the Department of Biochemistry at the University of Ulm, where he was mainly involved in the analysis of the structure and function of SV40 large T antigen. After his habilitation in 1985, he declined a professorship for Microbiology at the University of Bochum. In the same year, he accepted a professorship at the Department of Biochemistry at the University of Ulm. His main research focus was on p53 in both normal and cancer cells. In 1992, he accepted an offer from the Saarland University to be a chair in Medical Biochemistry and Molecular Biology. From 1996 to 2006, he was the head of a graduate school for "Cellular regulation and growth" at the Medical Faculty of the Saarland University funded by the German Research Foundation (DFG). From 2000 to 2002, he was the Dean for research and from 2004 to 2006 he was the Dean of the Medical Faculty of Saarland University. Over the last 25 years, his research has mainly focussed on the phosphorylation of proteins and in particular on protein kinase CK2, its function and regulation. Furthermore, he has analysed natural polysulfanes from garlic and their influence on cellular signalling pathways.

pharmaceuticals

MDPI

Editorial

An Updated View on an Emerging Target: Selected Papers from the 8th International Conference on Protein Kinase CK2

Joachim Jose [1,*], Marc Le-Borgne [2], Lorenzo A. Pinna [3] and Mathias Montenarh [4]

[1] PharmaCampus, Institute of Pharmaceutical and Medicinal Chemistry, Westfälische Wilhelms-Universität Münster, Corrensstr. 48, 48149 Münster, Germany

[2] EA 4446 Bioactive Molecules and Medicinal Chemistry, Faculté de Pharmacie—ISPB, Université Lyon 1, Université de Lyon, SFR Santé Lyon-Est CNRS UMS3453—INSERM US7, 69373 Lyon cedex 8, France; marc.le-borgne@univ-lyon1.fr

[3] Department of Biomedical Sciences, University of Padova, Via Ugo Bassi 58B, 35131 Padova, Italy; lorenzo.pinna@unipd.it

[4] Medizinische Biochemie und Molekularbiologie, Faculty of Medicine, Saarland University Geb. 44/45, D-66424 Homburg, Germany; Mathias.Montenarh@uks.eu

[*] Correspondence: joachim.jose@uni-muenster.de; Tel.: +49-251-8332200

Academic Editor: Jean Jacques Vanden Eynde

Received: 20 March 2017; Accepted: 21 March 2017; Published: 23 March 2017

The 8th International Conference on Protein Kinase CK2 took place in Homburg, Germany, from 6 September to 9 September 2016. Over 80 scientists from Australia, China, Japan, USA, Canada, Denmark, France, Italy, Spain, Poland and Germany participated. After the opening lecture by Lorenzo A. Pinna, Padova, Italy, entitled Exploring the CK2 Paradox: Restless, Dangerous, Dispensable, the scientists reported their latest research on the structural characterization of CK2, hence leading directly to the development of CK2 inhibitors. The driving force behind the development of inhibitors is their use in the treatment of various diseases, which was the next topic of the conference. New findings on protein kinase CK2 were addressed in the following session. The final topic of the conference addressed the role of CK2 in differentiation and development.

Lorenzo A. Pinna reminded everybody that the original name "casein kinase" was changed to protein kinase CK2 nearly 20 years ago, because casein did not appear to be among the natural substrates of CK2 [1]. Furthermore, CK2 has now been validated as a "druggable" kinase, which is targeted, in particular, in cancer cells. The most exciting news in this field was the establishment of viable $CK2\alpha^{-/-},\alpha'^{-/-}$ cells by CRISPR/cas9 technology and the subsequent phosphoproteome analysis of these non-neoplastic $CK2\alpha^{-/-},\alpha'^{-/-}$ cells.

Various crystallographic structures of the full-length as well as truncated version of $CK2\alpha$ are already published. The group of Karsten Niefind analysed $CK2\alpha$ and $CK2\alpha'$ in complex with ATP-competitive inhibitors [2]. This structural information not only provided further information about the ATP binding pocket, the interaction of individual residues in the polypeptide chain of both catalytic subunits with the inhibitors, and structural deformation of the enzymes, but also offered new elements for the design of more selective and potent inhibitors.

Starting approximately at the beginning of this century, there is an increasing list of inhibitors of CK2 comprising different chemical entities. Some of these are natural products, or compounds identified in drug libraries as well as molecules identified by an in silico approach, followed by chemical synthesis. Georgio Cozza compiled these different approaches to find more potent inhibitors of human CK2 [3]. Some of these approaches are based on crystallographic information about CK2 alone or in complex with an inhibiting compound. History has shown that inhibitors, which were considered initially to be CK2 specific, later on turned out to target multiple kinases. It is now clear that they need to be tested on a large scale of different kinases, before selectivity and specificity can be evaluated. Moreover, there is an increasing need for the analysis of off-target effects. Most of the inhibitors of CK2 known so far are indeed ATP-competitive inhibitors.

Samer Haidar reported on the development of new inhibitors based on an indeno[1,2-*b*]indole scaffold which was already known as a lead structure for the development of human CK2 inhibitors [4]. By using a pharmacophore model, which was developed on the inhibition data obtained with CK2 and more than 50 indeno[1,2-*b*]indoles, for mining the ZINC compound database, the natural compound bikaverin was identified and turned out to be a new potent CK2 inhibitor.

The group of Emilio Itarte used the inhibitor CX-4945, which is orally available, either alone or in combination with other cytostatic drugs for the treatment of cancer [5]. They used CX-4945 in combination with temozolomide to treat mice affected by glioblastoma. The best survival rates were obtained with a metronomic therapy comprising a combination of temozolomide and CX-4945 every 6 days. The group of Barbara Guerra used 1,3-dichloro-6-[(*E*)-((4-methoxyphenyl) imino)methyl]dibenzo(b,d)furan-2,7-diol (D11) also as a CK2 inhibitor for the treatment of glioblastoma cells [6]. They found that D11 led to a destabilization of HIF-1α under hypoxic conditions. They conclude from their results that D11 treatment deprives glioblastoma cells of oxygen and nutrient supply. These properties may improve the therapy of glioblastoma in combination with other cytostatic components.

The group of Joachim Jose established a bacterial surface display 12mer peptide library and screened it with fluorescence labelled human CK2 [7]. By this strategy, new non-ATP competitive CK2 inhibitors were identified. The most potent inhibitor identified, B2, not only inhibited CK2 kinase activity by binding to an allosteric pocket, but also disturbed the interaction of CK2α with CK2β.

Some years ago, the group of Claude Cochet and Odile Filhol published findings on a cyclic peptide interfering with the CK2 subunits interaction [8]. As a further development, a cell-permeable version of this peptide was analysed. This construct turned out to inhibit the cellular association of CK2α and CK2β, and consequently led to a shift in the phosphorylation efficiencies, in particular of CK2β-depending substrates. Moreover, they could show that the peptide led to a dissociation of already formed CK2 holoenzymes.

It is still an enigma how CK2 can regulate multiple functions and pathways in a cell without being itself regulated. By systematic analyses of published literature and proteomics databases together with the computational assembly of networks of CK2, the Litchfield group found that by phosphorylating its substrates [9], CK2 can modulate other post-translational modifications and, vice versa, that post-translational modifications affect CK2 phosphorylation of substrates.

Besides inhibitors, another approach was exploited for the study of CK2 functions, namely knock-down of expression of CK2 subunits. By this approach, the group of Hashemolhosseini found reduced activity of nicotinamide adenine dinucleotide dehydrogenase and succinate dehydrogenase in CK2β-deficient muscle fibres [10]. This result indicates a role of CK2β in the regulation of the oxidative capacity of skeletal muscle fibres.

Full or conditional CK2 knock-out mice were used for the elucidation of the role of CK2 in brain development, neuronal activity and behaviour, which was summarised by the group of Heike Rebholz [11]. They further described brain-specific substrates and the role of CK2 in various brain diseases such as glioblastoma, Parkinson's disease, Huntington's disease, Amyotrophic Lateral Sclerosis (ALS) and Alzheimer's disease.

The role of CK2 in the development of Drosophila was addressed by the group of Ashok Bidwai [12]. This article focuses on the structure, subunit diversity and mutations in the CK2 subunits and in particular on the role of CK2 in eye development.

The role of CK2 in the adipogenic differentiation of mesenchymal stem cells was addressed by Lisa Schwind and her colleagues [13]. CK2 seems to be essential at early time points after the start of differentiation, where it influences cell proliferation and the expression of different transcriptional factors such as C/EBPα and PPARγ2.

Adam Johnson and Ming Wu reported on the role of CK2 in the regulation of metal ion transport in *Saccharomyces cerevesia* and in mammalian cells [14]. On one hand, divalent metal ions such as Mg^{2+}, Mn^{2+} and Co^{2+} are required for CK2 activity. On the other hand, CK2 seems to be responsible for the toxicity of Al^{3+} and As^{3+} ions. Furthermore, CK2 subunits are implicated in metal ion transport. In the case of Zn^{2+} ions, it was shown that CK2 phosphorylates the Zinc ion channel ZIP7, the epithelial Na^+ channel and the chloride channel CFTR.

Another topic of the CK2 meeting was the search for new substrates and new functions of CK2. One of the substrates of CK2, particularly in pancreatic β-cells, is the transcription factor PDX-1. The group of Claudia Götz showed that the CK2 phosphorylation sites on the polypeptide chain of PDX-1 interfere with the binding site for PCIF1, which is an E3 ubiquitin ligase adaptor protein [15]. Binding of PCIF1 to CK2-phosphorylated PDX-1 promotes the degradation of PDX-1.

The group of Kubinski and Maslyk reported on the interaction of CK2 with an atypical kinase, Rio1, which plays a role in cellular proliferation and ribosome biosynthesis [16]. Rio1 is not only a substrate for CK2 but also a binding partner. At least in yeast, Rio1 is one of the very few binding partners of CK2α, as shown by an immunoprecipitation. A number of benzimidazole-derived compounds inhibited both, CK2 and Rio1. Molecular docking approaches indicated that the inhibitor tetrabromobenzimidazole (TBB) binds to the ATP-pocket of both kinases in quite a similar manner.

A topic addressed in two reviews was the role of CK2 as a target for the treatment of cancer cells. The group of Khalil Ahmed summarized their strategy for the delivery of RNAis down-regulating CK2 in cancer cells using nano-capsules [17]. In order to target cancer cells specifically, tenfibgen was used as a ligand of tenascin-C receptors, which are particularly numerous on the surface of cancer cells. This strategy proved successful with cancer cell lines and in animal models, opening the window for its use in the therapy of various tumours.

The group of Isabel Dominguez used a more general approach to analyze the implications of CK2 in cancer, its influence on cellular signalling pathways and its potential as a target in anti-cancer cells therapy [18]. The general conclusion is that CK2 is overexpressed in many cancers and this overexpression is accompanied by elevated protein kinase activity. Knock-down of individual subunits of CK2 resulted in the perturbation of diverse signalling pathways, including the SMAD2/3, β-catenin, PI3K-Akt-mTOR, and IκB-NFκB pathways and signalling pathways regulating apoptosis. The influence of CK2 on these pathways is qualitatively and quantitatively different in diverse tumours.

This 2016 CK2 conference emphasized once more that protein kinase Ck2 is an enticing enzyme with a broad range of physiological functions. The most unexpected new finding was that life without CK2—at least for non-neoplastic animal cells in culture—seems to be possible under special conditions. Furthermore, the role of CK2 in controlling cell proliferation, development and differentiation has been further elucidated. Because it appears to influence a variety of different cellular signalling pathways, the effects of CK2 inhibitors need to be considered under this light and careful use of such compounds is mandatory. In summary, the results presented during the 8th International Conference on Protein Kinase CK2 in Homburg underlined CK2's status as an emerging drug target and strengthened the view that pharmacological down-regulation of human CK2 with small molecules is a promising approach, not only in cancer.

Acknowledgments: The authors are grateful to their colleagues for contributing to the intense 8th International Conference on Protein Kinase CK2 in Homburg, in particular to those who could not be mentioned in this editorial.

Conflicts of Interest: The authors declare no conflict of interest.

References

1. Franchin, C.; Borgo, C.; Zaramella, S.; Cesaro, L.; Arrigoni, G.; Salvi, M.; Pinna, L.A. Exploring the CK2 Paradox: Restless, Dangerous, Dispensable. *Pharmaceuticals* **2017**, *10*, 11. [CrossRef] [PubMed]
2. Niefind, K.; Bischoff, N.; Golub, A.G.; Bdzhola, V.G.; Balanda, A.O.; Prykhod'ko, A.O.; Yarmoluk, S.M. Structural Hypervariability of the Two Human Protein Kinase CK2 Catalytic Subunit Paralogs Revealed by Complex Structures with a Flavonol- and a Thieno[2,3-d]pyrimidine-Based Inhibitor. *Pharmaceuticals* **2017**, *10*, 9. [CrossRef] [PubMed]
3. Cozza, G. The Development of CK2 Inhibitors: From Traditional Pharmacology to in Silico Rational Drug Design. *Pharmaceuticals* **2017**, *10*, 26. [CrossRef] [PubMed]
4. Haidar, S.; Bouaziz, Z.; Marminon, C.; Laitinen, T.; Poso, A.; Le Borgne, M.; Jose, J. Development of Pharmacophore Model for Indeno[1,2-b]indoles as Human Protein Kinase CK2 Inhibitors and Database Mining. *Pharmaceuticals* **2017**, *10*, 8. [CrossRef] [PubMed]
5. Ferrer-Font, L.; Villamañan, L.; Arias-Ramos, N.; Vilardell, J.; Plana, M.; Ruzzene, M.; Pinna, L.A.; Itarte, E.; Arús, C.; Candiota, A.P. Targeting Protein Kinase CK2: Evaluating CX-4945 Potential for GL261 Glioblastoma Therapy in Immunocompetent Mice. *Pharmaceuticals* **2017**, *10*, 24. [CrossRef] [PubMed]
6. Schaefer, S.; Svenstrup, T.H.; Fischer, M.; Guerra, B. D11-Mediated Inhibition of Protein Kinase CK2 Impairs HIF-1α-Mediated Signaling in Human Glioblastoma Cells. *Pharmaceuticals* **2017**, *10*, 5. [CrossRef] [PubMed]
7. Nienberg, C.; Garmann, C.; Gratz, A.; Bollacke, A.; Götz, C.; Jose, J. Identification of a Potent Allosteric Inhibitor of Human Protein Kinase CK2 by Bacterial Surface Display Library Screening. *Pharmaceuticals* **2017**, *10*, 6. [CrossRef] [PubMed]
8. Bestgen, B.; Belaid-Choucair, Z.; Lomberget, T.; Le Borgne, M.; Filhol, O.; Cochet, C. In Search of Small Molecule Inhibitors Targeting the Flexible CK2 Subunit Interface. *Pharmaceuticals* **2017**, *10*, 16. [CrossRef] [PubMed]
9. Nuñez de Villavicencio-Diaz, T.; Rabalski, A.J.; Litchfield, D.W. Protein Kinase CK2: Intricate Relationships within Regulatory Cellular Networks. *Pharmaceuticals* **2017**, *10*, 27. [CrossRef] [PubMed]
10. Eiber, N.; Simeone, L.; Hashemolhosseini, S. Ablation of Protein Kinase CK2β in Skeletal Muscle Fibers Interferes with Their Oxidative Capacity. *Pharmaceuticals* **2017**, *10*, 13. [CrossRef] [PubMed]
11. Castello, J.; Ragnauth, A.; Friedman, E.; Rebholz, H. CK2—An Emerging Target for Neurological and Psychiatric Disorders. *Pharmaceuticals* **2017**, *10*, 7. [CrossRef] [PubMed]
12. Bandyopadhyay, M.; Arbet, S.; Bishop, C.P.; Bidwai, A.P. Drosophila Protein Kinase CK2: Genetics, Regulatory Complexity and Emerging Roles during Development. *Pharmaceuticals* **2017**, *10*, 4. [CrossRef] [PubMed]
13. Schwind, L.; Schetting, S.; Montenarh, M. Inhibition of Protein Kinase CK2 Prevents Adipogenic Differentiation of Mesenchymal Stem Cells Like C3H/10T1/2 Cells. *Pharmaceuticals* **2017**, *10*, 22. [CrossRef] [PubMed]
14. Johnson, A.J.; Wu, M.J. The New Role for an Old Kinase: Protein Kinase CK2 Regulates Metal Ion Transport. *Pharmaceuticals* **2016**, *9*, 80. [CrossRef] [PubMed]
15. Klein, S.; Meng, R.; Montenarh, M.; Götz, C. The Phosphorylation of PDX-1 by Protein Kinase CK2 Is Crucial for Its Stability. *Pharmaceuticals* **2017**, *10*, 2. [CrossRef] [PubMed]
16. Kubiński, K.; Masłyk, M. The Link between Protein Kinase CK2 and Atypical Kinase Rio1. *Pharmaceuticals* **2017**, *10*, 21. [CrossRef] [PubMed]
17. Trembley, J.H.; Kren, B.T.; Abedin, M.J.; Vogel, R.I.; Cannon, C.M.; Unger, G.M.; Ahmed, K. CK2 Molecular Targeting—Tumor Cell-Specific Delivery of RNAi in Various Models of Cancer. *Pharmaceuticals* **2017**, *10*, 25. [CrossRef] [PubMed]
18. Chua, M.M.; Ortega, C.E.; Sheikh, A.; Lee, M.; Abdul-Rassoul, H.; Hartshorn, K.L.; Dominguez, I. CK2 in Cancer: Cellular and Biochemical Mechanisms and Potential Therapeutic Target. *Pharmaceuticals* **2017**, *10*, 18. [CrossRef] [PubMed]

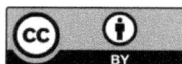

Chapter 1:
New horizons in the understanding of CK2 function

pharmaceuticals

MDPI

Review

Exploring the CK2 Paradox: Restless, Dangerous, Dispensable

Cinzia Franchin [1,2], Christian Borgo [1], Silvia Zaramella [2], Luca Cesaro [1], Giorgio Arrigoni [1,2], Mauro Salvi [1] and Lorenzo A. Pinna [1,3,*]

[1] Department of Biomedical Sciences, University of Padova, via U. Bassi, 58/B, 35131 Padova, Italy; cinzia.franchin@unipd.it (C.F.); christian.borgo@unipd.it (C.B.); luca.cesaro.1@unipd.it (L.C.); giorgio.arrigoni@unipd.it (G.A.); mauro.salvi@unipd.it (M.S.)

[2] Proteomics Center, University of Padova and Azienda Ospedaliera di Padova, via G. Orus, 2/B, 35129 Padova, Italy; silviazaramella7@gmail.com

[3] CNR Neurosciences Institute, via U. Bassi, 58/B, 35131 Padova, Italy

* Correspondence: lorenzo.pinna@unipd.it; Tel.: +39-049-8276108

Academic Editor: Marc Le Borgne
Received: 28 November 2016; Accepted: 16 January 2017; Published: 20 January 2017

Abstract: The history of protein kinase CK2 is crowded with paradoxes and unanticipated findings. Named after a protein (casein) that is not among its physiological substrates, CK2 remained in search of its targets for more than two decades after its discovery in 1954, but it later came to be one of the most pleiotropic protein kinases. Being active in the absence of phosphorylation and/or specific stimuli, it looks unsuitable to participate in signaling cascades, but its "lateral" implication in a variety of signaling pathways is now soundly documented. At variance with many "onco-kinases", CK2 is constitutively active, and no oncogenic CK2 mutant is known; still high CK2 activity correlates to neoplasia. Its pleiotropy and essential role may cast doubts on the actual "druggability" of CK2; however, a CK2 inhibitor is now in Phase II clinical trials for the treatment of cancer, and cell clones viable in the absence of CK2 are providing information about the mechanism by which cancer becomes addicted to high CK2 levels. A phosphoproteomics analysis of these CK2 null cells suggests that CK2 pleiotropy may be less pronounced than expected and supports the idea that the phosphoproteome generated by this kinase is flexible and not rigidly pre-determined.

Keywords: protein kinase CK2; casein kinase 2; cancer; signal transduction; non oncogene addiction; phosphoproteomics; CRISPR/Cas9 technology

1. Background

The discovery of the first phosphoprotein dates back to 1883 when Olof Hammarsten demonstrated that the milk protein casein contains almost 1% of tightly bound phosphorous [1]. In retrospect, this finding gave rise to one of the most teasing "cold cases" of biochemistry, considering that the enzyme(s) responsible for casein phosphorylation remained unknown for 130 years. In fact, none of the hundreds of protein kinases detected in the second half of the past century and forming the so-called "kinome" is responsible for the physiological phosphorylation of casein. The "genuine" casein kinase ("G-CK") remained an orphan enzyme until 2012 when it was identified with Fam20C, an atypical protein kinase responsible for the generation of a large proportion of the phosphosecretome [2–4].

In the meantime, however, casein had been successfully used as an artificial substrate for the characterization of many other protein kinases, with special reference to those denoted by the acronyms CK1 (with several isoforms) and CK2, reminiscent of the misnomers "casein kinase" -1 and -2. These two were responsible for the first "protein phospho kinase" activity ever described, isolated in 1954 from rat liver [5] and later shown to be ubiquitously present in many other organisms and tissues. CK2, in particular, is the subject of this special issue.

The rising interest for this unique kinase, as predicted by the Nobel laureate Edwin Krebs in a 1999 paper entitled "CK2, a protein kinase of the next millennium" [6], is largely accounted for by two features of this enzyme: outstanding pleiotropy and pathogenic potential. The former implies that an increasing number of researchers are "coming across" CK2 in the course of their investigations, the latter justifying the numerous efforts to dissect signaling pathways perturbed by abnormal CK2 activity and to develop therapeutic strategies aimed at its downregulation. Both aspects are amply documented by the multi-author contributions [7] and are dealt with in this special issue. Here, we present evidence that our current view about CK2 pleiotropy and indispensability may need to be reconsidered.

2. Pleiotropy

The paradox of CK2 pleiotropy is illustrated in Figure 1, illustrating that CK2 remained a kinase in search of its substrates for two decades after its discovery; the first were detected in the 1980s, followed by a snowball effect. Today, there are almost 600 phosphosites generated by CK2 according to PhosphoSitePlus, making it the second most pleiotropic member of the kinome (see also Table 1). This may be just the tip of the iceberg if we trust bioinformatics approaches based on the WebLogo of the whole phosphoproteome, where the features of typical CK2 sites are so remarkable that its contribution can reach 20% of all phosphosites [8,9].

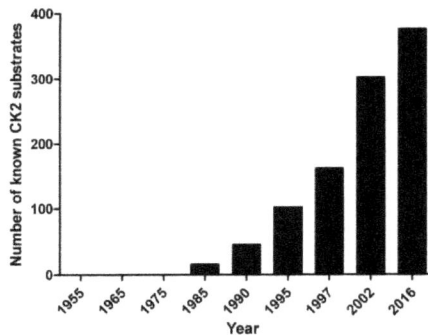

Figure 1. The growing number of proteins phosphorylated by CK2 since its discovery in 1954. Constructed with data from [10–13]. According to PhosphoSitePlus [10], the number of phosphosites known to be generated by CK2 is presently 640, which belong to almost 400 proteins altogether.

This figure is probably an overestimate, as we will see later, but we must consider that CK2 pleiotropy does not mean only many substrates, but also a plethora of interactors as reviewed in [14], and implication in many signaling pathways [15].

In this respect, it should be borne in mind that the mode of implication of CK2 in these pathways is unusual: not being activated by either phosphorylation or specific stimuli, its hierarchical participation in cascades, like other kinases, is hardly conceivable; in fact, its role is that of a lateral player, impinging "horizontally" on a variety of "vertical" signaling cascades, as discussed elsewhere [16,17].

3. Pathogenic Potential

Coincidental evidence of the oncogenic potential of CK2 was provided in the 1980s, as documented in a 1993 review quoting 11 reports where CK2 was invariably higher in a variety of tumors as compared to normal tissues/cells [18]. This repertoire was further implemented at later times [19,20].

In the meantime, work in David Seldin's lab demonstrated a cause–effect link between CK2 upregulation and transformation induced by oncogenes or by deficiency of tumor suppressor genes [21–23]. More recently, an analysis in the oncomine database revealed that the main CK2 catalytic subunit α is overexpressed in 5 out of the 6 most important types of cancer in the US [24].

The oncogenic potential of CK2 is challenged by the observation that, unlike other onco-kinases generated by gain of function mutation conferring constitutive/unscheduled activity, CK2 is constitutively active by itself, and no gain of function CK2 mutations are known to be responsible for neoplastic transformation. Thus, the rising concept is that elevated CK2 level makes the cellular environment more favorable to malignant transformation by the mechanism known as "non-oncogene addiction" [16]. Indeed, many of the effects of abnormally high CK2 are expected to potentiate the cancer phenotype, with special reference to its strong pro-survival and anti-apoptotic efficacy [25].

Addiction can therefore be simplistically depicted as a process by which cells stochastically enriched in CK2 are selected by the tumor itself, because they escape apoptosis offering a kind of "sanctuary" to malignancy. The term "oncophilic" has been coined to denote these cells particularly susceptible to malignant transformation [9]. CK2 blockage can therefore revert or even eradicate the cancer phenotype relying on abnormally high CK2.

Consistently, in many cases, cancer cells have been shown to be more sensitive to the cytotoxic efficacy of CK2 inhibitors than their normal counterparts, thus giving rise to a long and continuously increasing list of cells that are known to critically rely on CK2 for their survival.

CK2 is not only implicated in neoplasia but also in several other human diseases [15]. Of note in particular, recent reports have highlighted the role of CK2 in ischemia [26,27], thrombosis [28–30], diabetes [31], and inflammation induced by TNF-alpha [32].

4. Druggability

The pathogenic potential of CK2 accounts for many efforts done during the past two decades to develop cell permeable inhibitors of this kinase. Hundreds of these compounds have been described in the literature, mostly, but not exclusively, competitive with respect to ATP. A recent repertoire of these compounds is available in [33], and some of these are dealt with in this special issue. The amount of work done in this field is further documented by the more than 70 structures of CK2 in complex with its inhibitors deposited in PDB and by the observation that some of these have been already tested for their tolerability in animal models.

Despite considerable efforts to develop CK2 inhibitors, pharmaceutical companies have been reluctant to invest on CK2 druggability due to a number of properties of this kinase. One was the lack of any clear-cut connection between CK2 and individual pathways whose dysregulation specifically promotes malignancy. The other two were the striking pleiotropy of CK2, suggesting that its inhibition is likely to cause too many collateral effects, and its purported essential role, documented by lethality during embryogenesis of animals where its subunits had been knocked out [34,35]. The first caveat has been slowly overcome by the rising concept that, although CK2 may be not a *sensu stricto* oncogene, causative of malignancy by itself, many tumors are addicted to its abnormally high activity, rendering its downregulation a valuable multi-purpose anticancer strategy. On the other hand, it is conceivable that, although reliance on CK2 is critical during embryogenesis, CK2 reduction might be tolerated in adult cells. Consistent with this suspicion, a breakthrough was made in 2010 by the CK2 inhibitor CX-4945 (also known as Silmitasertib) that entered clinical trials for the treatment of different kinds of cancer [36] and is now in Phase II [37].

5. Dispensability

More recently, the proof of concept that CK2 may be dispensable for life has been provided by the generation of viable cell clones where both its catalytic subunits were knocked out by CRISPR(clustered regularly interspaced short palindromic repeats)/Cas9 technology [38,39]. A quantitative MS analysis indicates that these CK2 null cells cope with the lack of CK2 by undergoing proteomics alterations that reflect a functional rewiring expectedly adverse to malignant transformation.

Interestingly, the proteomics alteration induced by a pharmacological inhibition of CK2 is only partially overlapping the perturbation observed in CK2 null cells [39], thus corroborating the view that transient suppression of CK2 catalytic activity does not entirely account for the functional and metabolic rewiring underwent by cells deprived of this pleiotropic kinase. In other words, it is clear from the data available that cellular adaptation to CK2 suppression implies deep and complex re-adjustments, where failure to phosphorylate individual targets represents only one side of the coin.

From a practical standpoint, CK2 null cells will provide a valuable tool to address the crucial issue of off-target effects displayed by CK2 inhibitors. None of these in fact is endowed with absolute specificity, and even the first-in-class of these compounds, CX-4945, already in clinical trials, has been shown to affect splicing in a CK2-independent manner [40]. Therefore, viable CK2 null cells represent an excellent model where to dissect biological functions whose pharmacological alteration is either mediated or not by CK2.

The outcome of a parallel phosphoproteomics analysis reveals that, although a large proportion of quantified phosphosites conform to the consensus sequence of CK2 (s/t-X-X-E/D/s), only less than one third of these are significantly decreased in the CK2 null cells, while the majority are unaffected and a few are even increased (Figure 2).

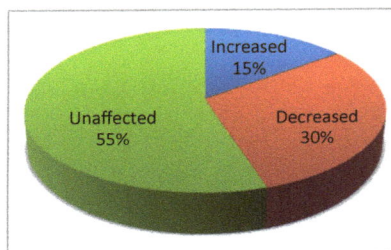

Figure 2. Only a minor proportion of the phosphosites, conforming to the CK2 consensus quantified in C2C12 myoblasts devoid of both CK2 catalytic subunits, is drastically reduced (>50%), as compared to the wild type. A SILAC experiment has been conducted on C2C12 cell lines where both the catalytic CK2 α subunits have been knocked out by the CRISPR/Cas9 technology, as described in Borgo et al. [39]. CK2 null cells have been compared with wild type, both from the proteomics [39] and the phosphoproteomics side (unpublished data). To determine which phosphosites are affected by the absence of CK2, phosphopeptide enrichment has been performed, as already described in [41], and only peptides with alterations in the phosphorylation state of at least 50% have been considered as significantly varied.

This apparent paradox is accounted for by a couple of considerations. Firstly, the CK2 consensus is present in more than 3000 phosphosites (out of almost 15,000) generated by kinases other than CK2, according to the PhosphoSitePlus database [13]. In fact, as shown in Table 1, where only the most pleiotropic kinases are considered, the CK2 consensus is invariably present in some of the phosphosites generated by all of these, with a frequency sometimes higher than 20%. Secondly, the proteomics analysis of CK2 null cells [39] has led to the quantification of 26 protein kinases: although these make up just about 5% of the whole kinome, they are sufficient to account for the indirect effects of CK2 knock out mediated by other kinases. Six kinases in fact are over-expressed in CK2 null cells. Among these, Aurora B is especially noteworthy as it is over-expressed 27-fold in CK2 null cells, while a considerable number of its phosphosites also conform to the CK2 consensus (see Table 1), thus providing an example of how the absence of CK2 can promote the paradoxical effect of increasing rather than decreasing the occupancy of some phosphosites displaying the CK2 consensus.

Table 1. Presence of the CK2 consensus S/T-x-x-E/D/pS/pT at the phosphosites generated by the most pleiotropic protein kinases. Calculated from the PhosphoSitePlus database [13]. Only the 24 most pleiotropic kinases have been considered. "%" expresses the percentage of phosphosites generated by each individual kinase where the CK2 consensus is present.

Kinase	p-Sites	p-Sites with CK2 Consensus	%
PKACA	834	201	24.10
CK2A1	640	483	75.46
PKCA	637	115	18.05
CDK2	588	94	15.98
CDK1	569	86	15.11
ERK2	497	78	15.69
ERK1	375	65	17.33
Akt1	325	73	22.46
GSK3B	322	89	27.63
ATM	232	64	27.58
PLK1	229	70	30.56
P38A	226	45	19.91
CAMK2A	216	50	23.14
Chk1	205	74	36.09
CDK5	190	20	10.52
JNK1	187	43	22.99
PKCD	156	24	15.38
AurB	153	35	22.87
AMPKA1	145	36	24.82
PKCB	145	27	18.62
CK1A	139	60	43.16
DNAPK	117	38	32.47
PKCE	104	20	19.23
mTOR	99	26	26.26

On the other hand, it is remarkable that even two well established bona fide CK2 phosphosites, pS13 of CDC37 and pS129 of AKT, often used as reliable reporters of endogenous CK2 activity, do not disappear, as one would expect, in CK2 null cells, the former being only modestly reduced (Figure 3). This means that other kinases can partially replace CK2 to ensure the phosphorylation of crucial residues that are normally targeted by this kinase.

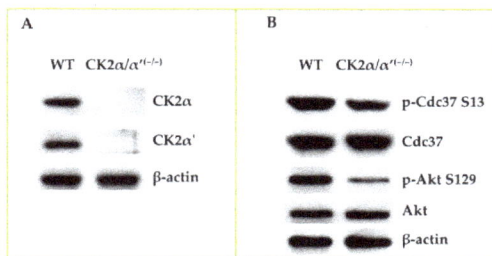

Figure 3. The phosphorylation of bona fide CK2 sites is not entirely abrogated in CK2 null cells. Wild-type (WT) and CK2 null (CK2α/α'(−/−)) cells were lysed in a buffer containing 20 mM Tris-HCl (pH 7.5), 1% Triton X-100, 10% glycerol, 1 mM EDTA, 150 mM NaCl, and protease and phosphatase inhibitor cocktails. Thirty micrograms of lysate proteins were subjected to 11% SDS-PAGE and analyzed by Western blot with the indicated antibodies. Panel **A** shows that both the CK2 catalytic subunits are absent in the CK2 null cells. In panel **B**, the significant residual phosphorylation of two bona fide CK2 sites in these cells can be appreciated. The figure is representative of three independent experiments.

6. Conclusions

The data presented support two unanticipated conclusions. Firstly, the pleiotropy of CK2 appears to be less pronounced than expected since many phosphosites conforming to the CK2 consensus are in reality generated by kinases different from CK2 as their occupancy is unaffected in CK2 null cells. Secondly, it seems likely that CK2 can be replaced by other kinases to perform the phosphorylation of critical sites whenever CK2 activity is abrogated. In other words, the rising concept is that the phosphoproteome generated by CK2 is not as ample as suspected before—and more importantly, it is not rigidly pre-determined.

Acknowledgments: The work was supported by the Associazione Italiana per la Ricerca sul Cancro (AIRC), grant IG 14180 to Lorenzo A. Pinna. Cinzia Franchin was supported by a grant from "Collegio Ghislieri," Pavia, Italy.

Author Contributions: Lorenzo A. Pinna conceived the review and wrote the manuscript with the contribution of Cinzia Franchin and of the other authors; Mauro Salvi and Giorgio Arrigoni designed the research; Cinzia Franchin, Christian Borgo, and Silvia Zaramella performed the experiments; Luca Cesaro. performed bioinformatics analyses.

Conflicts of Interest: The authors declare no conflict of interest.

References

1. Hammarsten, O. Zur Frage ob Caseín ein einheitlicher Stoff sei. *Hoppe-Seyler Z. Physiol. Chem.* **1883**, *7*, 227–273.
2. Tagliabracci, V.S.; Engel, J.L.; Wen, J.; Wiley, S.E.; Worby, C.A.; Kinch, L.N.; Xiao, J.; Grishin, N.V.; Dixon, J.E. Secreted kinase phosphorylates extracellular proteins that regulate biomineralization. *Science* **2012**, *336*, 1150–1153. [CrossRef] [PubMed]
3. Tagliabracci, V.S.; Pinna, L.A.; Dixon, J.E. Secreted protein kinase. *Trends Biochem. Sci.* **2013**, *38*, 121–130. [CrossRef] [PubMed]
4. Tagliabracci, V.S.; Wiley, S.E.; Guo, X.; Kinch, L.N.; Durrant, E.; Wen, J.; Xiao, J.; Cui, J.; Nguyen, K.B.; Engel, J.L.; et al. A single kinase generates the majority of the secreted phosphoproteome. *Cell* **2015**, *161*, 1619–1632. [CrossRef] [PubMed]
5. Burnett, G.; Kennedy, E.P. The enzymatic phosphorylation of proteins. *JBC* **1954**, *211*, 969–980.
6. Dobrowolska, G.; Lozeman, F.J.; Li, D.; Krebs, E.G. CK2, a protein kinase of the next millennium. *Mol. Cell. Biochem.* **1999**, *191*, 3–12. [CrossRef] [PubMed]
7. Pinna, L.A. (Ed.) *Protein Kinase CK2*; The Wiley-IUBMB Series on Biochemistry and Molecular Biology; John Wiley & Sons: New York, NJ, USA, 2013.
8. Salvi, M.; Sarno, S.; Cesaro, L.; Nakamura, H.; Pinna, L.A. Extraordinary pleiotropy of protein kinase CK2 revealed by weblogo phosphoproteome analysis. *Biochim. Biophys. Acta* **2009**, *1793*, 847–859. [CrossRef] [PubMed]
9. Ruzzene, M.; Tosoni, K.; Zanin, S.; Cesaro, L.; Pinna, L.A. Protein kinase CK2 accumulation in "oncophilic" cells: Causes and effects. *Mol. Cell. Biochem.* **2011**, *356*, 5–10. [CrossRef] [PubMed]
10. Pinna, L.A. Casein kinase 2: An "eminence grise" in cellular regulation? *Biochim. Biophys. Acta* **1990**, *1054*, 267–284. [CrossRef]
11. Pinna, L.A.; Meggio, F. Protein kinase CK2 ("casein kinase-2") and its implication in cell division and proliferation. *Prog. Cell. Cycle Res.* **1997**, *3*, 77–97. [PubMed]
12. Meggio, F.; Pinna, L.A. One-thousand-and-one substrates of protein kinase CK2? *FASEB J.* **2003**, *17*, 349–368. [CrossRef] [PubMed]
13. PhosphoSitePlus. Available online: http://www.phosphosite.org (accessed on 17 November 2016).
14. Montenarh, M.; Goetz, C. The interactome of Protein kinase CK2. In *Protein Kinase CK2*; Pinna, L.A., Ed.; John Wiley & Sons: New York, NJ, USA, 2013.
15. Guerra, B.; Issinger, O.G. Protein kinase CK2 in human diseases. *Curr. Med. Chem.* **2008**, *15*, 1870–1886. [CrossRef] [PubMed]
16. Ruzzene, M.; Pinna, L.A. Addiction to protein kinase CK2: A common denominator of diverse cancer cells? *Biochim. Biophys. Acta* **2010**, *1804*, 499–504. [CrossRef] [PubMed]

17. Venerando, A.; Ruzzene, M.; Pinna, L.A. Casein kinase: The triple meaning of a misnomer. *Biochem. J.* **2014**, *460*, 141–156. [CrossRef] [PubMed]
18. Issinger, O.G. Casein kinase: Pleiotropic mediators of cellular regulation. *Pharmacol. Ther.* **1993**, *59*, 1–30. [CrossRef]
19. Tawfic, S.; Yu, S.; Wang, H.; Faust, R.; Davis, A.; Ahmed, K. Protein kinase CK2 signal in neoplasia. *Histol. Histopathol.* **2001**, *16*, 573–582. [PubMed]
20. Trembley, J.H.; Chen, Z.; Unger, G.; Slaton, J.; Kren, B.T.; Van Waes, C.; Ahmed, K. Emergence of protein kinase CK2 as a key target in cancer therapy. *Biofactors* **2010**, *36*, 187–195. [CrossRef] [PubMed]
21. Seldin, D.C.; Leder, P. Casein kinase II alpha transgene-induced murine lymphoma: Relation to theileriosis in cattle. *Science* **1995**, *10*, 894–897. [CrossRef]
22. Kelliher, M.A.; Seldin, D.C.; Leder, P. Tal-1 induces T cell acute lymphoblastic leukemia accelerated by casein kinase IIalpha. *EMBO J.* **1996**, *15*, 5160–5166. [PubMed]
23. Landesman-Bollag, E.; Channavajhala, P.L.; Cardiff, R.D.; Seldin, D.C. p53 deficiency and misexpression of protein kinase CK2α collaborate in the development of thymic lymphomas in mice. *Oncogene* **1998**, *16*, 2965–2974. [CrossRef] [PubMed]
24. Ortega, C.E.; Seidner, Y.; Dominguez, I. Mining CK2 in cancer. *PLoS ONE* **2014**, *9*, e115609. [CrossRef] [PubMed]
25. Ahmad, K.A.; Wang, G.; Unger, G.; Slaton, J.; Ahmed, K. Protein kinase CK2—A key suppressor of apoptosis. *Adv. Enzyme Regul.* **2008**, *48*, 179–187. [CrossRef] [PubMed]
26. Ampofo, E.; Widmaier, D.; Montenarh, M.; Menger, M.D.; Laschke, M.W. Protein kinase CK2 regulates Leukocyte-endothelial cell interactions during ischemia and reperfusion in striated skin muscle. *Eur. Surg. Res.* **2016**, *57*, 111–124. [CrossRef] [PubMed]
27. Ka, S.O.; Hwang, H.P.; Jang, J.H.; Hyuk Bang, I.; Bae, U.J.; Yu, H.C.; Cho, B.H.; Park, B.H. The protein kinase 2 inhibitor tetrabromobenzotriazole protects against renal ischemia reperfusion injury. *Sci. Rep.* **2015**, *5*, 14816. [CrossRef] [PubMed]
28. Ampofo, E.; Müller, I.; Dahmke, I.N.; Eichler, H.; Montenarh, M.; Menger, M.D.; Laschke, M.W. Role of protein kinase CK2 in the dynamic interaction of platelets, leukocytes and endothelial cells during thrombus formation. *Thromb. Res.* **2015**, *136*, 996–1006. [CrossRef] [PubMed]
29. Nakanishi, K.; Komada, Y.; Hayashi, T.; Suzuki, K.; Ido, M. Protease activated receptor 1 activation of platelet is associated with an increase in protein kinase CK2 activity. *J. Thromb. Haemost.* **2008**, *6*, 1046–1048. [CrossRef] [PubMed]
30. Nakanishi, K.; Toyoda, H.; Tanaka, S.; Yamamoto, H.; Komada, Y.; Gabazza, E.C.; Hayashi, T.; Suzuki, K.; Ido, M. Phosphoinositide 3-kinase induced activation and cytoskeletal translocation of protein kinase CK2 in protease activated receptor 1-stimulated platelets. *Thromb. Res.* **2010**, *126*, 511–516. [CrossRef] [PubMed]
31. Rossi, M.; Ruiz de Azua, I.; Barella, L.F.; Sakamoto, W.; Zhu, L.; Cui, Y.; Lu, H.; Rebholz, H.; Matschinsky, F.M.; Doliba, N.M.; et al. CK2 acts as a potent negative regulator of receptor-mediated insulin release in vitro and in vivo. *Proc. Natl. Acad. Sci. USA* **2015**, *112*, E6818–E6824. [CrossRef] [PubMed]
32. Ampofo, E.; Rudzitis-Auth, J.; Dahmke, I.N.; Rössler, O.G.; Thiel, G.; Montenarh, M.; Menger, M.D.; Laschke, M.W. Inhibition of protein kinase CK2 suppresses tumor necrosis factor (TNF)-α-induced leukocyte-endothelial cell interaction. *Biochim. Biophys. Acta* **2015**, *1852*, 2123–2136. [CrossRef] [PubMed]
33. Cozza, G.; Pinna, L.A. Casein kinase as potential therapeutic targets. *Expert Opin. Ther. Targets* **2016**, *20*, 319–340. [CrossRef] [PubMed]
34. Buchou, T.; Vernet, M.; Blond, O.; Jensen, H.H.; Pointu, H.; Olsen, B.B.; Cochet, C.; Issinger, O.G.; Boldyreff, B. Disruption of the regulatory beta subunit of protein kinase CK2 in mice leads to a cell-autonomous defect and early embryonic lethality. *Mol. Cell. Biol.* **2003**, *23*, 908–915. [CrossRef] [PubMed]
35. Lou, D.Y.; Dominguez, I.; Toselli, P.; Landesman-Bollag, E.; O'Brien, C.; Seldin, D.C. The alpha catalytic subunit of protein kinase CK2 is required for mouse embryonic development. *Mol. Cell. Biol.* **2008**, *28*, 131–139. [CrossRef] [PubMed]
36. Siddiqui-Jain, A.; Drygin, D.; Streiner, N.; Chua, P.; Pierre, F.; O'Brien, S.E.; Bliesath, J.; Omori, M.; Huser, N.; Ho, C.; et al. CX-4945, an orally bioavailable selective inhibitor of protein kinase CK2, inhibits prosurvival and angiogenic signaling and exhibits antitumor efficacy. *Cancer Res.* **2010**, *70*, 10288–10298. [CrossRef] [PubMed]

37. Chon, H.J.; Bae, K.J.; Lee, Y.; Kim, J. The casein kinase 2 inhibitor, CX-4945, as an anti-cancer drug in treatment of human hematological malignancies. *Front. Pharmacol.* **2015**, *6*, 70. [CrossRef] [PubMed]
38. Salvi, M.; Borgo, C.; Franchin, C.; Donella-Deana, A.; Arrigoni, G.; Pinna, L.A. Life without CK2: Generation of the first viable mammalian cell line deprived of CK2 catalytic activity. In Proceedings of the 8th International Conference on Protein Kinase CK2, Homburg, Germany, 6–9 September 2016; p. 92.
39. Borgo, C.; Franchin, C.; Scalco, S.; Donella-Deana, A.; Arrigoni, G.; Salvi, M.; Pinna, L.A. Generation and quantitative proteomics analysis of CK2α/$\alpha'^{(-/-)}$ cells. *Sci. Rep.* **2017**, *7*, 42409. [CrossRef]
40. Kim, H.; Choi, K.; Kang, H.; Lee, S.Y.; Chi, S.W.; Lee, M.S.; Song, J.; Im, D.; Choi, Y.; Cho, S. Identification of a novel function of CX-4945 as a splicing regulator. *PLoS ONE* **2014**, *9*, e94978. [CrossRef] [PubMed]
41. Franchin, C.; Cesaro, L.; Salvi, M.; Millioni, R.; Iori, E.; Cifani, P.; James, P.; Arrigoni, G.; Pinna, L.A. Quantitative analysis of a phosphoproteome readily altered by the protein kinase CK2 inhibitor quinalizarin in HEK-293T cells. *Biochim. Biophys. Acta* **2015**, *1854*, 609–623. [CrossRef] [PubMed]

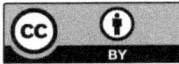

pharmaceuticals

MDPI

Review

Protein Kinase CK2: Intricate Relationships within Regulatory Cellular Networks

Teresa Nuñez de Villavicencio-Diaz [1], Adam J. Rabalski [1] and David W. Litchfield [1,2,*]

[1] Department of Biochemistry, Schulich School of Medicine & Dentistry, University of Western Ontario, London, ON N6A 5C1, Canada; tnunezde@uwo.ca (T.N.d.V.D.); arabalsk@uwo.ca (A.J.R.)
[2] Department of Oncology, Schulich School of Medicine & Dentistry, University of Western Ontario, London, ON N6A 5C1, Canada
* Correspondence: litchfi@uwo.ca; Tel.: +1-519-661-4186

Academic Editor: Joachim Jose
Received: 14 January 2017; Accepted: 2 March 2017; Published: 5 March 2017

Abstract: Protein kinase CK2 is a small family of protein kinases that has been implicated in an expanding array of biological processes. While it is widely accepted that CK2 is a regulatory participant in a multitude of fundamental cellular processes, CK2 is often considered to be a constitutively active enzyme which raises questions about how it can be a regulatory participant in intricately controlled cellular processes. To resolve this apparent paradox, we have performed a systematic analysis of the published literature using text mining as well as mining of proteomic databases together with computational assembly of networks that involve CK2. These analyses reinforce the notion that CK2 is involved in a broad variety of biological processes and also reveal an extensive interplay between CK2 phosphorylation and other post-translational modifications. The interplay between CK2 and other post-translational modifications suggests that CK2 does have intricate roles in orchestrating cellular events. In this respect, phosphorylation of specific substrates by CK2 could be regulated by other post-translational modifications and CK2 could also have roles in modulating other post-translational modifications. Collectively, these observations suggest that the actions of CK2 are precisely coordinated with other constituents of regulatory cellular networks.

Keywords: protein kinase CK2; post-translational modification; regulatory networks; protein–protein interaction networks; hierarchical phosphorylation; post-translational modification interplay

---

1. Introduction

Since its original discovery more than 50 years ago, protein kinase CK2 has been implicated in a continually expanding array of biological processes [1]. In this respect, CK2 has been shown to be a participant in the regulation of cellular processes such as transcription [2,3] and translation [4–7], control of protein stability [8–10] and degradation [11,12], cell cycle progression [13], cell survival [14–16], and circadian rhythms [17]. CK2 has also been linked to various aspects of tumor progression and suppression and has been shown to be elevated in many forms of cancer [18,19] as well as in virally infected cells [20–22]. Consequently, CK2 has recently emerged as a potential therapeutic target with two CK2 inhibitors, namely CX-4945 [23,24] and CIGB-300 [25,26], currently in clinical trials [27–29] for cancer treatment.

In humans, CK2 is typically considered to be a tetrameric enzyme comprised of two catalytic subunits (CK2α and/or CK2α' subunits that are encoded by the CSNK2A1 and CSNK2A2 genes, respectively) and two regulatory CK2β subunits [1,30] (encoded by the CSNK2B gene). Although typically classified as a protein serine/threonine kinase based on sequence relationships to other members of the protein kinase superfamily, CK2 has also been shown to exhibit protein tyrosine kinase activity [31–34]. Biochemical characterization of its enzymatic activity has demonstrated that CK2 is an acidophilic kinase with a consensus recognition motif that features aspartic acid and glutamic acid residues as well as some phosphorylated residues as its dominant specificity determinants [35–37]. Characterization of its specificity determinants has contributed to the identification of many CK2 substrates that have been shown to be directly phosphorylated by CK2 [38,39]. Phosphoproteomic profiling has also revealed many putative substrates that have been shown to be phosphorylated in cells at sites that match the consensus for phosphorylation by CK2 [40,41]. In fact, analysis of phosphoproteomic datasets typically suggests that CK2 could be responsible for more than 10% of the phosphoproteome [42].

While there is ample evidence that CK2 is an important constituent in the regulation of many fundamental biological processes, there are unresolved issues regarding its regulation in cells. In this respect, questions regarding its regulation arise because the catalytic subunits of CK2 are enzymatically active in the presence or absence of the regulatory CK2β subunit. Furthermore, the activity of CK2 is generally unaffected by second messengers, and unlike many kinases that are regulated by phosphorylation within an activation loop, the activation loop of CK2 is devoid of regulatory phosphorylation sites [43,44]. The fact that the catalytic subunits of CK2 are fully active when expressed as recombinant proteins in bacteria further suggests that the enzyme may be constitutively active [45–47]. Consequently, it is unclear how a constitutively active enzyme can be a key regulatory participant in tightly regulated cellular processes. To investigate this apparent paradox, we have examined the relationship between CK2 and other constituents of the regulatory networks within cells by performing text mining of the published literature and mining of proteomic databases. Furthermore, motivated by our demonstration that CK2 phosphorylation sites overlap with other post-translational modifications to enable CK2 to modulate caspase cleavage [48–50] and to participate in hierarchical phosphorylation relationships, we have analyzed proteomic databases to identify post-translational modifications that may regulate, or be regulated by, CK2 phosphorylation.

In this review, we explore database and literature information available in the context of CK2-dependent signaling with the objective of highlighting and discussing the extensive interplay of CK2 with regulatory networks in the cell. The analysis that we have provided is also intended to provide functional perspectives to the data available in the databases since these data are often isolated from the information regarding CK2 that exists within the literature; especially for non-experts in the field and for interpreting data related to CK2 emerging from high-throughput studies.

2. CK2 Networks

2.1. Functional Networks Involving CK2

The impact of CK2 in the cell can be, to some extent, predicted by considering the number of biological processes in which it has been implicated and the number of substrates that have been reported to date [39]. Furthermore, it is anticipated that the published literature will represent an important resource for deciphering and validating information that is emerging from genome- and proteome-wide analyses. Consequently, we performed text mining to identify publications that highlight CK2 and aspects of its function or regulation. To this point, CK2 substrate information remains "sparse" in the published literature that is represented by more than 2600 papers (PubMed [51] search: "Casein Kinase II" [Mesh]) directly describing CK2 function and more than 5000 papers mentioning the kinase (GoPubMed [52] search). Nevertheless, assembling this information to obtain a global but detailed view of CK2-dependent networks is one step towards deciphering genome and proteome scale analyses of CK2.

An initial evaluation of the functional relationship of CK2 with other cellular proteins can be obtained by querying STRING v10.0 [53], a database with known and predicted functional associations between proteins (see Figure 1A for a representation of the top 50 proteins functionally associated to CK2, Table S1). According to this analysis, CK2 regulates the activity of at least 15 cancer-related proteins such as the tumor suppressor TP53, the histone deacetylases HDAC1 and HDAC2, and the NFKB subunit RELA (Figure 1B,C, Table S1). CK2-dependent phosphorylation of these proteins has been reported either in vitro or in vivo [54–57] with the majority of the target sites identified conforming to the minimum CK2 consensus sequence: [ST]xx[DEpS]. The CK2 functional relationship to these substrates places the kinase in a central position in human protein–protein interaction networks since such proteins are considered "information hubs" [58]. For instance, the proteins TP53, HDAC1, HDAC2, and RELA bind to at least 997, 554, 323, and 271 unique interactors based on the BioGRID protein–protein interaction repository [59] (accessed 30 November 2016). In fact, in a human protein–protein interaction network (built from the BioGRID database in Cytoscape [60,61] v3.4.0, self-loops and duplicated edges removed) CK2 can "influence" approximately 23% of the established interactions (63,988 interaction pairs out of 270,000) if we assume a 'guilt by association' approach considering CK2 direct interactions (meaning step 1 interactors: 629 proteins, Table S2) and that of its indirect interactors (meaning step 2 interactors: 11,869 proteins, Table S2). A summary of the number of CK2 interactors for each human CK2 subunit is presented in Table 1. Based on this analysis and a search using the "find a gene" functionality of the Enrichr tool [62], further hub interactors of CK2 that can be identified include CDK1, XRCC6, CREB1, HNRNPA1, LYN, YWHAQ, FOS, and MAPK1 (Table S3).

Table 1. CK2 subunits interactors extracted from a human protein–protein interaction network built by retrieving the human interactome from BioGRID database build 3.4.129 using Cytoscape v3.4.0.

Direct (Step 1) Interactors of	Number of Interactors
CSNK2A1 (Gene ID: 1457)	398 unique direct interactors; 435 interaction pairs.
CSNK2A2 (Gene ID: 1459)	155 unique direct interactors; 171 interaction pairs.
CSNK2B (Gene ID: 1460)	247 unique direct interactors; 270 interaction pairs.
All CK2 subunits	632 unique direct interactors from which 36 are shared by the three subunits and 95 by two.
All CK2 subunits and their direct interactors	12,502 unique direct interactors (632 step 1 and 11,875 step 2); 63,988 interaction pairs.

Figure 1. *Cont.*

C)

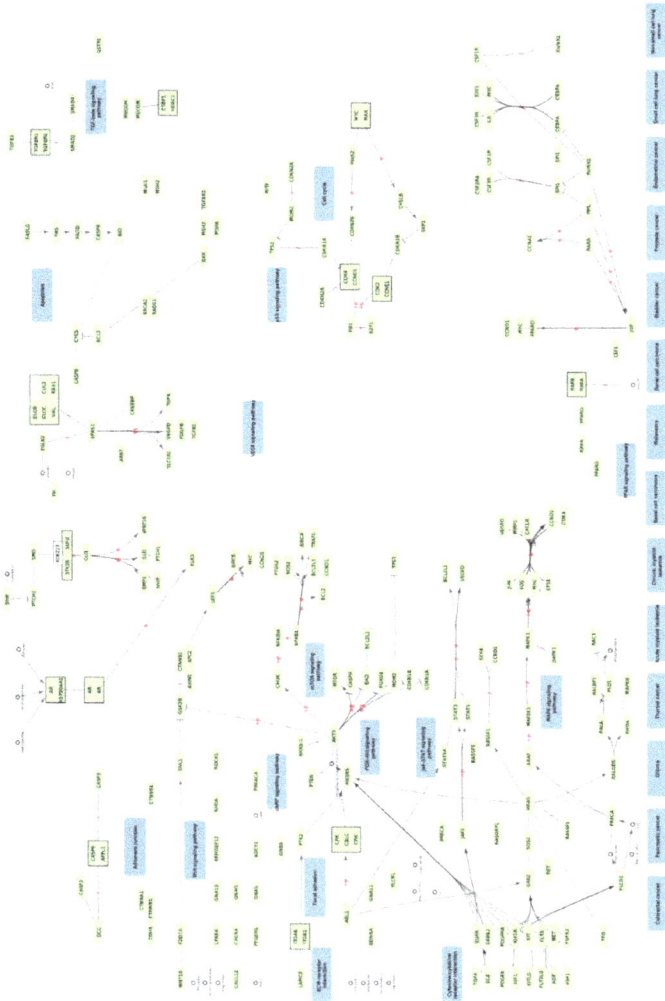

Figure 1. CK2-centered functional association network represented with the database STRING v10.0. (**A**) The network shows the top 50 human genes related to CK2 subunits CSNK2A1, CSNK2A2, and CSNK2B (number of nodes and edges: 53 and 369, respectively) based on neighborhood, experiments, text mining, and database sources. Briefly, the human CK2 subunits were searched in STRING by gene name using the multiple protein search functionality. The functional association network was then retrieved by selecting 50 as the maximum number of interactors to show from the first shell (step 1) and checking the mentioned interaction sources (these options are found within the "data settings" drop down menu); (**B**) A clone of network A with the red nodes representing proteins connected to deregulated pathways (KEGG pathway: hsa05200); (**C**) A network representation of the map: Pathways in cancer (KEGG pathway: hsa05200). The map was downloaded from the KEGG PATHWAY [63] database (accessed 30 November 2016) and imported to Cytoscape with the CyKEGGParser v1.2.7 plugin [64]. A high-resolution image of this figure is also available in the Supplementary Materials.

2.2. Protein–Protein Interaction Networks Involving CK2

In a complementary analysis, the direct interactors of CK2 subunits were represented in a protein–protein interaction network (Figure 2, Table S4) using BisoGenet [65] v3.0.0 Cytoscape plugin for the retrieval of physical interaction information. As expected from Table 1, differences in the number and identity of the panel of interactors can be observed for each CK2 subunit which suggests a certain degree of functional divergence as previously highlighted in the literature [66–70], and encourages the development of tools that allow us to differentiate the contributions of the endogenous catalytic subunits to the phosphoproteome. In addition, it points to CSNK2B as a hub itself, suggesting that it may have a role in coordinating interactions with the catalytic subunits of CK2 to modulate phosphorylation of certain substrates. Furthermore, since the interaction network for CSNK2B does not completely overlap that of the catalytic CK2 subunits (Figure 2, Table S4), this analysis reinforces the prospect that CSNK2B has CK2-independent roles within cells [67]. In fact, the CSNK2B-dependent interactome has been previously profiled using mouse brain homogenates [71] where CSNK2B is thought to have a crucial role since its mRNA expression levels are 2–3-fold higher compared with other organs, except the testis [72]. In this setting, CSNK2B was found to interact with both cytoplasmic and nuclear localized proteins involved in protein synthesis, RNA and DNA processing, the cytoskeleton, cell signaling, and transport [71]. Although not included among the references retrieved by BisoGenet, the functional classification of the proteins identified as part of the CSNK2B-dependent interactome is in agreement with the network generated by BisoGenet.

2.3. CK2 Networks Derived from Text Mining of the Published Literature

A way of summarizing and systematizing CK2 knowledge relies on the use of text mining to access literature information. In this regard, the analysis of GO cellular component annotations using GoPubMed revealed more than 200 subcellular locations and protein complexes studied in the context of CK2 (summarized in Figure 3, Table S5). This analysis also reflects the functional pleiotropy of CK2, which can associate with molecular machinery such as the ribosome, spliceosome, proteasome, and chromatin remodeling complexes, and to other smaller more dynamic complexes such as TRAIL-death inducing complex and the Ikappa-NFkB complex. Directly interrogating the literature followed by data extraction can provide information that otherwise may be missed if we only consider specialized databases such as the mammalian protein complexes database CORUM [73] where CSNK2A1, CSNK2A2 and CSNK2B (Table S5) are listed only as members of the "PDGF treated Ksr1-CK2-MEK-14-3-3 complex", the "MKP3-CK2alpha complex", the "Casein kinase II-HMG1 complex", and the "UV-activated FACT complex" with CSNK2B also listed as a member of the "Fgf2-Ck2 complex" (accessed 30 November 2016). However, protein complex data extracted from the CORUM database has been manually curated whereas the data extracted from the literature needs to be critically analyzed since the extraction process may be ambiguous and biased towards the algorithm used by the tool [74], in this case GoPubMed. A similar analysis can be made for the GO biological processes. The retrieval of CK2 related GO biological process from literature highlights frequently studied core processes such as cell cycle, cell proliferation, DNA damage, cell death, and viral infectious cycle, as well as other hot topics in the field (Figure 3B, Table S5). The later includes the involvement of CK2 in embryogenic development [75–78], T cell-mediated immunity [79,80], inflammation [81], glucose homeostasis [82–85], ion transport [86], bone remodeling [78,87], neurogenesis [88,89], neurological system process [90], response to misfolded and unfolded protein [90], stem cell differentiation and maintenance [91], and response to muscle activity [92,93].

Figure 2. *Cont.*

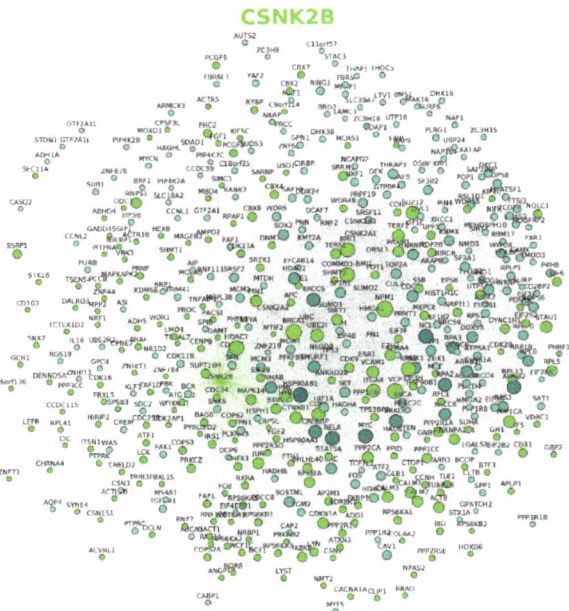

Figure 2. Protein–protein interaction network of human CK2 subunits generated using Cytoscape v3.4.0 and the BisoGenet v3.0.0 plugin. The three networks are clones, each of which highlights the interactors of CSNK2A1 (red nodes), CSNK2A2 (orange nodes), and CSNK2B (green nodes) subunits, respectively. Briefly, the network was represented by querying SysBiomics (BisoGenet's interaction database) through the plugin's interface using the human CK2 subunit gene names and selecting "protein–protein interaction" as the biorelation type and the input nodes and neighbors to step 1 method as the criteria for building the network. A high resolution image of this figure is also available in the Supplementary Materials.

Text mining of the CK2-related literature can also provide insights regarding holoenzyme-dependent regulation, which relates to the events where CK2-mediated phosphorylation of a given substrate is positively or negatively regulated by holoenzyme formation and the presence or absence of CSNK2B [45]. In this particular case, the analysis of protein–protein interaction data for CK2 subunits alone is insufficient for assuming holoenzyme-dependent regulation. A recent in silico study relied on text mining for retrieving known holoenzyme-dependent substrates and generated sequence patterns for predicting novel candidates based on structural information of the known substrates [39]. Information on the holoenzyme-dependent substrates can also be obtained from PhosphoSitePlus database [94,95] by querying "substrates of CK2B"; however the list obtained is not comprehensive (accessed February, 2017) when compared to the text mining study [39]. Furthermore, substrates known to be holoenzyme-dependent such as PDX1 [96] and CFTR [97] are cataloged as phosphorylated by the catalytic subunit in this database (query: "substrates of CK2A1"). To avoid such inconsistencies and misleading information, researchers are encouraged to carefully review the evidence provided in databases such as PhosphoSitePlus, which are obtained through automated literature text mining and thus error prone.

A)

B)

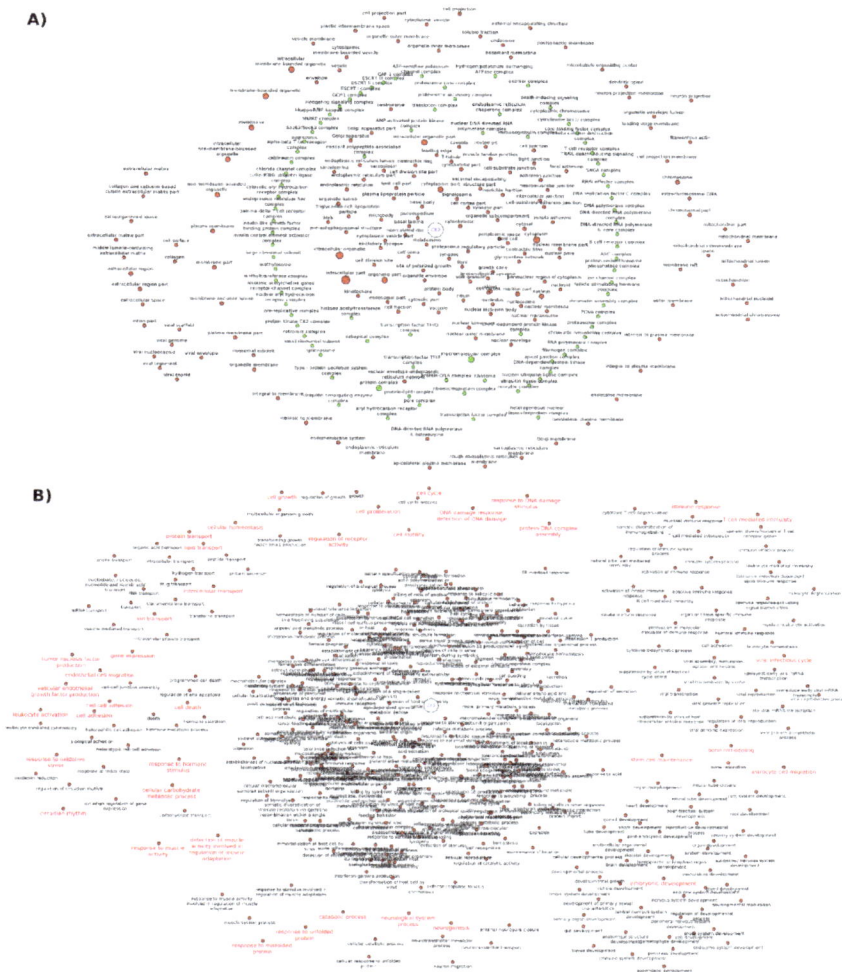

Figure 3. CK2 Functional association networks represented in Cytoscape v3.4.0 for illustrating the: (**A**) Cellular components mentioned together with CK2 in the literature identified by GoPubMed search. The green nodes represent protein complexes and the node size highlights terms frequently co-occurring with CK2; (**B**) Biological processes mentioned together with CK2 in the literature identified by GoPubMed search; the red label-nodes indicate hot topics in CK2 research. Briefly, the term "Casein Kinase II"[Mesh] was queried using the GoPubMed text mining tool and the output was downloaded to generate a network in SIF format [61] for Cytoscape input by specifying CK2 and the GO subcellular components/biological processes as nodes and their co-occurrence in the literature as the interactions (binary type: yes/no). The node size was not set differentially for the biological processes network as this will affect the visualization and readability. A high resolution image of this figure is also available in the Supplementary Materials.

In addition to text mining, systematic proteomic studies represent rich resources for potentially uncovering CK2-regulated biological processes and pathways when datasets from these studies are uploaded to repositories [98] such as PRIDE and MassIVE and/or provided as supplementary information. To explore the availability of proteomics data for CK2, we performed a Pubmed search and, as a result, retrieved two proteome studies [99,100], one interactome study [71], and four phosphoproteome [40,41,101,102] studies. However, a PRIDE search only returned one of these studies, which explores the function of CSNK2A1 from *Ostreococcus tauri* in a minimal circadian system [101] (ID: PXD000975). Consequently, for the remainder of these studies, information available (e.g., protein and/or phosphorylation site identification and/or relative quantification values) is limited to that provided in the original paper or by direct request to the authors. We also searched PhosphoSitePlus and found that only one phosphoproteome study out of the four identified in Pubmed was included (accessed February 2017). This phophoproteomic study explores the short-term response of HEK-293T cells treated with the CK2 inhibitor quinalizarin [102]. However, PhosphoSitePlus only mentions the proteins and phosphosites identified without providing any quantitative results.

The quinalizarin phosphoproteomic study [102] identified 28 downregulated putative CK2 phosphosites with several of the target proteins displaying a role in cell death and/or survival including TPD52 (isoform 2), STX12, BCLAF1, AKAP12, RAD50, and PDCD4 (isoform 2). Overall, the majority of the phosphorylation-modulated substrates were classified as nuclear and were found to be involved in biological processes classified as transcription, mRNA and rRNA processing, gene expression, and DNA replication. Comparable functional annotations were obtained in two of the other CK2 phosphoproteomic studies where the phosphosites identified belong to proteins mostly localized to the nucleus as components of the spliceosome [40,41].

Intriguingly, the quinalizarin phosphoproteomic study also revealed that several "CK2 attributable" phosphosites increased upon treatment with the inhibitor. As this result seems paradoxical, the authors proposed both technical and biological explanations for this observation [102]. Since it is evident that CK2 is connected to a plethora of regulatory hubs through protein–protein interaction and hierarchical phosphorylation, we performed a kinase-motif matching analysis using the PhosphoMotif Finder functionality of the HPRD database [103] to determine if other kinases could in theory be responsible for the upregulation of phosphosites that had been putatively identified as CK2-dependent phosphosites. As a result of this analysis, we identified at least two instances where the modulated phosphosite matched motifs for other kinases besides CK2. For example, the vicinity of the residue S1068 of TP53BP1 matches the minimal CK2 consensus sequence pSXX[E/D] as well as the pSQ and XpSQ substrate motifs of the ATM kinase and the DNA-dependent protein kinase, respectively. Interestingly, TP53BP1 does interact with ATM, which phosphorylates several residues in the protein upon DNA damage to promote its tumor suppressor functions [104]. Another example is AKAP12 where the vicinity of S627 matches substrate recognition motifs pSXX[E/D], RXRXX[pS/pT], [R/K]XRXXpS, RVRRPpSESDK, and RRPpS conforming to CK2, AKT, MAPKAPK1, AMP-activated protein kinase 2, and PKA/PKC motifs, respectively. AKAP12 has been shown to interact at least with PKC and PKA [105], with PKA phosphorylating S627 and three other residues [106] of the protein. Moreover, in proteomic databases, arginine and lysine residues proximal to S627 of AKAP12, are reported to be methylated [98]. Altogether, these observations illustrate the complexity of CK2-signaling networks and the challenges associated with interpreting changes in the phosphoproteome arising from modulation of CK2. Accordingly, all possible sources of information for other kinases and modifying enzymes that may act upon CK2 target sequences (e.g., arginine-methyltransferases and lysine-acetyltransferases) need to be taken into consideration.

2.4. Extension of CK2 Networks to Include Other Constituents of Regulatory Networks

As a logical extension of examining direct interactions with CK2, understanding how CK2 integrates to other signaling networks in the cell requires consideration of how CK2 substrates may be acted upon by other constituents of signaling networks. For example, we have considered phosphorylation information regarding CK2 substrates with other kinases that also modify the CK2 substrates and/or interactors (Figure 4). In this respect, Figure 4 shows that at least 171 other kinases (Table S6) are capable of phosphorylating sites in CK2 interactors, which suggests a likelihood of functional interplay among phosphorylation sites. This is reflected, for example, in the fact that CK2-dependent phosphorylation often participates in hierarchical phosphorylation with other kinases, which generates a CK2 target sequence with a phosphorylated serine that functions as the dominant specificity determinant [36].

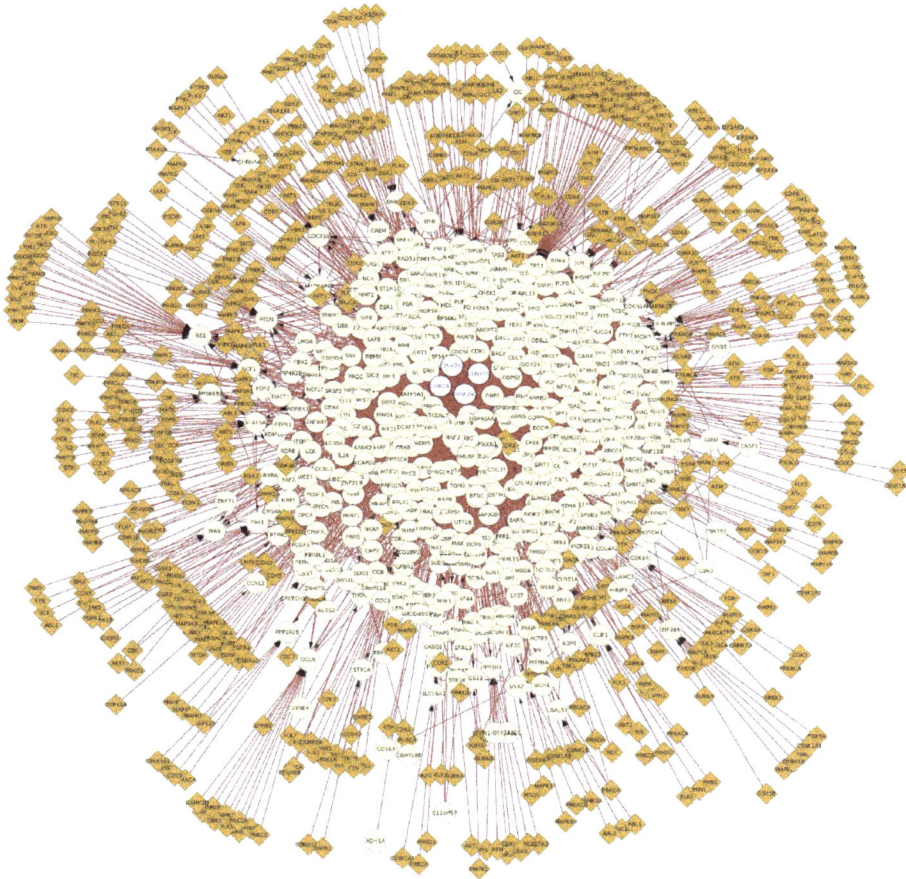

Figure 4. Protein–protein interaction network of CK2 subunits expanded to include kinase information of the interactors retrieved from PhosphositePlus, the network was represented with Cytoscape v3.4.0 using the BisoGenet v3.0.0 plugin and the PhosphositePlus Web Service Client Module. The yellow nodes represent CK2 interactors and the brown nodes represent kinases that phosphorylate (edges with arrow) the interactors. The blue edges represent protein–protein interactions and the red edges represent phosphorylation events. The network was represented as explained in Figure 2. Briefly, all the proteins were selected and the kinase data was added by importing the information from PhosphoSitePlus using the plugin and selecting the gene name as the matching key. A high resolution image of this figure is also available in the Supplementary Materials.

As noted above, there is evidence that many CK2 substrates are also phosphorylated by other kinases. When considering the prospect for hierarchical phosphorylation involving CK2, analysis of the phosphorylation events in the vicinity of the CK2 phosphosites may further contribute to identifying such relationships. Consequently, we searched PhosphoSitePlus database serine, threonine, and tyrosine phosphorylation and CK2 substrate data, mostly reflecting data generated through a proteomics approach [95], for those phosphosites occurring in the primary structure at different distance windows up- or downstream of the CK2 target site (Table 2 and Table S6). This analysis was also extended to other post-translational modifications reported in the PhosphoSitePlus database, such as ubiquitination and acetylation (Table 2 and Table S6). Although this analysis is restricted to CK2 substrate data available in PhosphoSitePlus, it is useful to illustrate the importance of considering the modification status of target sequences when studying CK2-dependent phosphorylation, a concept that also applies to other kinases. For example, the link between AKT-mediated phosphorylation and arginine methylation has been previously reported [107–109]. The post-translational modification analysis indicated that the vicinity of CK2 sites may constitute 'hot spots' for phosphorylation. Consideration of these sites brings together at least 76 different kinases including CDK7, STK1, PRKCA, PLK1, GSK3, CDC7, SRC, CDK2, MAPK3, GRK2, PRKCZ, CDK9, MAPK1, and IKBKE.

Table 2. Post-translational modifications in the vicinity of CK2 [1] target sites retrieved from PhosphoSitePlus (accessed August 2016).

PTM Type	# Sites at −4/+4	# Sites at −7/+7	# Sites at −36/+36
Acetylation	15	25	146
O-N-acetylgalactosamine	2; overlap: 1	5; overlap: 1	19; overlap: 1
O-N-acetylglucosamine	1; overlap: 2	1; overlap: 2	5; overlap: 2
Methylation (m1, m2, m3, me)	4, 3, 1, none	8, 7, 1, none	29, 22, 2, 3
Phosphorylation	262; overlap: 482	395; overlap: 482	1177; overlap: 482
Sumoylation	1	8	50

[1] CK2 sites were retrieved for bovine CSNK2A1 (P68399), human CSNK2A1 (P68400), human CSNK2A2 (P19784), human CSNK2B (P67870), mouse CSNK2A1 (Q60737), rat CSNK2A1 (P19139).

3. Concluding Remarks and Implications

Taken together, systematic analysis of the literature and databases strongly reinforces the view that CK2 is involved in a broad spectrum of biological processes. At the same time, it is important to recognize that there are significant limitations with information that is available both within the peer-reviewed literature and in databases. In this respect, as noted earlier, the literature represents an extensive but 'sparse' body of information generally lacking standard criteria for the identification and characterization of roles for CK2 in biological processes. On the one hand, there are undoubtedly many literature reports with rigorous experimental design and analysis that clearly demonstrate roles for CK2 in specific cellular processes. By comparison, there are also reports where conclusions are drawn exclusively from in vitro studies or experimentally contrived systems that do not reflect what happens under normal physiological conditions in living systems. In a similar vein, databases that are populated primarily from large-scale proteomic studies or high-throughput experimental workflows harbor data of inconsistent integrity. While these databases represent a wealth of information (for example, tens of thousands of phosphorylation sites or protein–protein interactions), the pace at which data is generated dramatically exceeds the pace of validation. Moreover, many of the kinase-substrate relationships that have emerged from large-scale studies have relied on predictions using the CK2 consensus recognition motif rather than experimental validation of these relationships. Consequently, in many instances, these data reflect what 'might happen' rather than rigorous demonstrations of what 'does happen' under normal physiological conditions. Despite this limitation, knowing what 'might happen' can often be a very useful guide for the design of experimental strategies to rigorously define what does happen.

In addition to clearly highlighting the involvement of CK2 in a broad array of biological processes, database mining and network analysis clearly reveals extensive interplay between CK2 and other constituents of signaling networks. This interplay is evident from the identification of 'hot spots' where CK2 phosphorylation sites are localized proximal to other phosphorylation sites or other post-translational modifications within the primary sequence of its substrates. The proximity of post-translational modifications to one another raises the very interesting prospect of one post-translational modification being regulated by others. As noted earlier, we have previously demonstrated that CK2 can modulate cleavage of caspase substrates when CK2 phosphorylates residues adjacent to the cleavage site [48]. This is a clear example of how phosphorylation by CK2 can modulate susceptibility to another post-translational modification. The demonstration that phosphorylated residues can sometimes 'prime' a substrate for hierarchical phosphorylation by CK2 demonstrates that phosphorylation by CK2 can also be regulated by other modifications [36]. Considering the prevalence of post-translational modifications that reside within CK2 substrates within close proximity of the CK2 phosphorylation site (Table 2), it will be important to consider the relationship between CK2 phosphorylation and these other modifications. From the perspective of its participation in regulatory processes, the interplay between CK2 and other pathways could yield very intricate and precise control of processes. Considering the emergence of CK2 as a potential therapeutic target, the intricate relationships of CK2 within the regulatory networks also has important implications for the application of CK2 inhibitors. From this perspective, modulation of CK2 could impact other pathways since phosphorylation by CK2 could have regulatory consequences for other pathways. Similarly, modulation of other pathways could also affect CK2 or its functions as the modification status of the target sequence may ultimately regulate its recognition by CK2.

With the availability of selective new inhibitors for CK2 and elegant strategies for genome engineering based on CRISPR-Cas9, we can expect new opportunities for modulating CK2 under physiological conditions. By combining these strategies with striking advances in analytical technologies such as mass spectrometry to perform proteomic profiling with unrivalled depth, speed, and accuracy, we can anticipate that many gaps in our knowledge of how CK2 is integrated within regulatory and functional networks will be filled to reveal its roles in orchestrating biological processes. Furthermore, given the emergence of CK2 as a potential therapeutic target, we can expect these insights to guide promising applications of CK2 inhibitors in the clinic.

Supplementary Materials: The following are available online at http://www.mdpi.com/1424-8247/10/1/27/s1; Table S1: STRING network, function, and annotations of the top 50 CK2-related genes; Table S2: CK2-interacting proteins in the human interactome; Table S3: CK2-interacting hub proteins; Table S4: CK2-interacting proteins of each subunit; Table S5: CK2-related GO annotations extracted from the literature and protein complex data; Table S6: PTM sites in the vicinity of CK2 phosphorylated sites.

Acknowledgments: Our work on protein kinase CK2 and kinase regulatory networks has been supported by an Operating Grant from the Canadian Institutes of Health Research and a Discovery Grant from the Natural Sciences and Engineering Research Council of Canada. Teresa Nuñez de Villavicencio Diaz has also been supported by a Dean's Doctoral Scholarship from the Schulich School of Medicine & Dentistry. We are also grateful to the members of the Litchfield lab for many helpful discussions related to CK2 and kinase regulatory networks.

Author Contributions: All authors contributed to the ideas for this manuscript as well as editing and writing. TNVD generated all of the figures and tables that are presented.

Conflicts of Interest: The authors declare no conflict of interest.

References

1. Litchfield, D.W. Protein kinase CK2: Structure, regulation and role in cellular decisions of life and death. *Biochem. J.* **2003**, *369*, 1–15. [CrossRef] [PubMed]
2. Cabrejos, M.E.; Allende, C.C.; Maldonado, E. Effects of phosphorylation by protein kinase CK2 on the human basal components of the RNA polymerase II transcription machinery. *J. Cell. Biochem.* **2004**, *93*, 2–10. [CrossRef] [PubMed]
3. Lüscher, B.; Christenson, E.; Litchfield, D.W.; Krebs, E.G.; Eisenman, R.N. Myb DNA binding inhibited by phosphorylation at a site deleted during oncogenic activation. *Nature* **1990**, *344*, 517–522. [CrossRef] [PubMed]

4. Szebeni, A.; Hingorani, K.; Negi, S.; Olson, M.O.J. Role of protein kinase CK2 phosphorylation in the molecular chaperone activity of nucleolar protein b23. *J. Biol. Chem.* **2003**, *278*, 9107–9115. [CrossRef] [PubMed]

5. Borgo, C.; Franchin, C.; Salizzato, V.; Cesaro, L.; Arrigoni, G.; Matricardi, L.; Pinna, L.A.; Donella-Deana, A. Protein kinase CK2 potentiates translation efficiency by phosphorylating eIF3j at Ser127. *Biochim. Biophys. Acta - Mol. Cell Res.* **2015**, *1853*, 1693–1701. [CrossRef] [PubMed]

6. Riera, M.; Roher, N.; Miró, F.; Gil, C.; Trujillo, R.; Aguilera, J.; Plana, M.; Itarte, E. Association of protein kinase CK2 with eukaryotic translation initiation factor eIF-2 and with grp94/endoplasmin. *Mol. Cell. Biochem.* **1999**, *191*, 97–104. [CrossRef] [PubMed]

7. Gandin, V.; Masvidal, L.; Cargnello, M.; Gyenis, L.; McLaughlan, S.; Cai, Y.; Tenkerian, C.; Morita, M.; Balanathan, P.; Jean-Jean, O.; et al. mTORC1 and CK2 coordinate ternary and eIF4F complex assembly. *Nat. Commun.* **2016**, *7*, 11127. [CrossRef] [PubMed]

8. Niechi, I.; Silva, E.; Cabello, P.; Huerta, H.; Carrasco, V.; Villar, P.; Cataldo, L.R.; Marcelain, K.; Armisen, R.; Varas-Godoy, M.; Fernandez, C.; et al. Colon cancer cell invasion is promoted by protein kinase CK2 through increase of endothelin-converting enzyme-1c protein stability. *Oncotarget* **2015**, *6*, 42749–42760. [PubMed]

9. Patsoukis, N.; Li, L.; Sari, D.; Petkova, V.; Boussiotis, V.A. PD-1 Increases PTEN Phosphatase Activity While Decreasing PTEN Protein Stability by Inhibiting Casein Kinase 2. *Mol. Cell. Biol.* **2013**, *33*, 3091–3098. [CrossRef] [PubMed]

10. Zhang, C.; Vilk, G.; Canton, D.A.; Litchfield, D.W. Phosphorylation regulates the stability of the regulatory CK2beta subunit. *Oncogene* **2002**, *21*, 3754–3764. [CrossRef] [PubMed]

11. Shen, J.; Channavajhala, P.; Seldin, D.C.; Sonenshein, G.E. Phosphorylation by the protein kinase CK2 promotes calpain-mediated degradation of IkappaBalpha. *J. Immunol.* **2001**, *167*, 4919–4925. [CrossRef] [PubMed]

12. Scaglioni, P.P.; Yung, T.M.; Choi, S.C.; Baldini, C.; Konstantinidou, G.; Pandolfi, P.P.; Pandolfi, P.P. CK2 mediates phosphorylation and ubiquitin-mediated degradation of the PML tumor suppressor. *Mol. Cell. Biochem.* **2008**, *316*, 149–154. [CrossRef] [PubMed]

13. Homma, M.K.; Homma, Y. Cell cycle and activation of CK2. *Mol. Cell. Biochem.* **2008**, *316*, 49–55. [CrossRef] [PubMed]

14. Ahmed, K.; Gerber, D.A.; Cochet, C. Joining the cell survival squad: An emerging role for protein kinase CK2. *Trends Cell Biol.* **2002**, *12*, 226–230. [CrossRef]

15. Piazza, F.A.; Ruzzene, M.; Gurrieri, C.; Montini, B.; Bonanni, L.; Chioetto, G.; Di Maira, G.; Barbon, F.; Cabrelle, A.; Zambello, R.; et al. Multiple myeloma cell survival relies on high activity of protein kinase CK2. *Blood* **2006**, *108*, 1698–1707. [CrossRef] [PubMed]

16. Duncan, J.S.; Turowec, J.P.; Duncan, K.E.; Vilk, G.; Wu, C.; Luscher, B.; Li, S.S.-C.; Gloor, G.B.; Litchfield, D.W. A Peptide-Based Target Screen Implicates the Protein Kinase CK2 in the Global Regulation of Caspase Signaling. *Sci. Signal.* **2011**, *4*, ra30. [CrossRef] [PubMed]

17. Tsuchiya, Y.; Akashi, M.; Matsuda, M.; Goto, K.; Miyata, Y.; Node, K.; Nishida, E. Involvement of the Protein Kinase CK2 in the Regulation of Mammalian Circadian Rhythms. *Sci. Signal.* **2009**, *2*, ra26. [CrossRef] [PubMed]

18. Trembley, J.H.; Wang, G.; Unger, G.; Slaton, J.; Ahmed, K. Protein Kinase CK2 in Health and Disease: CK2: A key player in cancer biology. *Cell. Mol. Life Sci.* **2009**, *66*, 1858–1867. [CrossRef] [PubMed]

19. Ortega, C.E.; Seidner, Y.; Dominguez, I. Mining CK2 in Cancer. *PLoS ONE* **2014**, *9*, e115609. [CrossRef] [PubMed]

20. Schuck, S.; Ruse, C.; Stenlund, A. CK2 Phosphorylation Inactivates DNA Binding by the Papillomavirus E1 and E2 Proteins. *J. Virol.* **2013**, *87*, 7668–7679. [CrossRef] [PubMed]

21. Marin, O.; Sarno, S.; Boschetti, M.; Pagano, M.A.; Meggio, F.; Ciminale, V.; D'Agostino, D.M.; Pinna, L.A. Unique features of HIV-1 Rev protein phosphorylation by protein kinase CK2 ('casein kinase-2'). *FEBS Lett.* **2000**, *481*, 63–67. [CrossRef]

22. Ohtsuki, K.; Maekawa, T.; Harada, S.; Karino, A.; Morikawa, Y.; Ito, M. Biochemical characterization of HIV-1 Rev as a potent activator of casein kinase II in vitro. *FEBS Lett.* **1998**, *428*, 235–240. [CrossRef]

23. Kim, J.; Kim, S.H. Druggability of the CK2 inhibitor CX-4945 as an anticancer drug and beyond. *Arch. Pharm. Res.* **2012**, *35*, 1293–1296. [CrossRef] [PubMed]

24. Chon, H.J.; Bae, K.J.; Lee, Y.; Kim, J. The casein kinase 2 inhibitor, CX-4945, as an anti-cancer drug in treatment of human hematological malignancies. *Front. Pharmacol.* **2015**, *6*, 70. [CrossRef] [PubMed]
25. Perea, S.E.; Reyes, O.; Baladron, I.; Perera, Y.; Farina, H.; Gil, J.; Rodriguez, A.; Bacardi, D.; Marcelo, J.L.; Cosme, K.; et al. CIGB-300, a novel proapoptotic peptide that impairs the CK2 phosphorylation and exhibits anticancer properties both in vitro and in vivo. *Mol. Cell. Biochem.* **2008**, *316*, 163–167. [CrossRef] [PubMed]
26. Benavent Acero, F.; Capobianco, C.S.; Garona, J.; Cirigliano, S.M.; Perera, Y.; Urtreger, A.J.; Perea, S.E.; Alonso, D.F.; Farina, H.G. CIGB-300, an anti-CK2 peptide, inhibits angiogenesis, tumor cell invasion and metastasis in lung cancer models. *Lung Cancer* **2016**. [CrossRef] [PubMed]
27. Martins, L.R.; Lúcio, P.; Melão, A.; Antunes, I.; Cardoso, B.A.; Stansfield, R.; Bertilaccio, M.T.S.; Ghia, P.; Drygin, D.; Silva, M.G.; et al. Activity of the clinical-stage CK2-specific inhibitor CX-4945 against chronic lymphocytic leukemia. *Leukemia* **2014**, *28*, 179–182. [CrossRef] [PubMed]
28. Martins, L.R.; Perera, Y.; Lúcio, P.; Silva, M.G.; Perea, S.E.; Barata, J.T. Targeting chronic lymphocytic leukemia using CIGB-300, a clinical-stage CK2-specific cell-permeable peptide inhibitor. *Oncotarget* **2014**, *5*, 258–263. [CrossRef] [PubMed]
29. Perea, S.E.; Baladron, I.; Garcia, Y.; Perera, Y.; Lopez, A.; Soriano, J.L.; Batista, N.; Palau, A.; Hernández, I.; Farina, H.; et al. CIGB-300, a synthetic peptide-based drug that targets the CK2 phosphoaceptor domain. Translational and clinical research. *Mol. Cell. Biochem.* **2011**, *356*, 45–50. [CrossRef] [PubMed]
30. Niefind, K.; Raaf, J.; Issinger, O.-G. Protein Kinase CK2 in Health and Disease: Protein Kinase CK2: from structures to insights. *Cell. Mol. Life Sci.* **2009**, *66*, 1800–1816. [CrossRef] [PubMed]
31. Wilson, L.K.; Dhillon, N.; Thorner, J.; Martin, G.S. Casein kinase II catalyzes tyrosine phosphorylation of the yeast nucleolar immunophilin Fpr3. *J. Biol. Chem.* **1997**, *272*, 12961–12967. [CrossRef] [PubMed]
32. Donella-Deana, A.; Cesaro, L.; Sarno, S.; Brunati, A.M.; Ruzzene, M.; Pinna, L.A. Autocatalytic tyrosine-phosphorylation of protein kinase CK2 alpha and alpha' subunits: implication of Tyr182. *Biochem. J.* **2001**, *357*, 563–567. [CrossRef] [PubMed]
33. Basnet, H.; Su, X.B.; Tan, Y.; Meisenhelder, J.; Merkurjev, D.; Ohgi, K.A.; Hunter, T.; Pillus, L.; Rosenfeld, M.G. Tyrosine phosphorylation of histone H2A by CK2 regulates transcriptional elongation. *Nature* **2014**, *516*, 267–271. [CrossRef] [PubMed]
34. Vilk, G.; Weber, J.E.; Turowec, J.P.; Duncan, J.S.; Wu, C.; Derksen, D.R.; Zien, P.; Sarno, S.; Donella-Deana, A.; Lajoie, G.; et al. Protein kinase CK2 catalyzes tyrosine phosphorylation in mammalian cells. *Cell. Signal.* **2008**, *20*, 1942–1951. [CrossRef] [PubMed]
35. Marin, O.; Meggio, F.; Draetta, G.; Pinna, L.A. The consensus sequences for cdc2 kinase and for casein kinase-2 are mutually incompatible. A study with peptides derived from the beta-subunit of casein kinase-2. *FEBS Lett.* **1992**, *301*, 111–114. [CrossRef]
36. St-Denis, N.; Gabriel, M.; Turowec, J.P.; Gloor, G.B.; Li, S.S.-C.; Gingras, A.-C.; Litchfield, D.W. Systematic investigation of hierarchical phosphorylation by protein kinase CK2. *J. Proteomics* **2015**, *118*, 49–62. [CrossRef] [PubMed]
37. Litchfield, D.W.; Arendt, A.; Lozeman, F.J.; Krebs, E.G.; Hargrave, P.A.; Palczewski, K. Synthetic phosphopeptides are substrates for casein kinase II. *FEBS Lett.* **1990**, *261*, 117–120. [CrossRef]
38. Meggio, F.; Pinna, L.A. One-thousand-and-one substrates of protein kinase CK2? *FASEB J.* **2003**, *17*, 349–368. [CrossRef] [PubMed]
39. Nuñez de Villavicencio-Díaz, T.; Mazola, Y.; Yasser, P.; Cruz, Y.; Guirola-Cruz, O.; Perea, S.E. Predicting CK2 beta-dependent substrates using linear patterns. *Rep. Biochem. Biophys.* **2015**, *25*, 20–27. [CrossRef]
40. Wang, C.; Ye, M.; Bian, Y.; Liu, F.; Cheng, K.; Dong, M.; Dong, J.; Zou, H. Determination of CK2 Specificity and Substrates by Proteome-Derived Peptide Libraries. *J. Proteome Res.* **2013**, *12*, 3813–3821. [CrossRef] [PubMed]
41. Bian, Y.; Ye, M.; Wang, C.; Cheng, K.; Song, C.; Dong, M.; Pan, Y.; Qin, H.; Zou, H. Global screening of CK2 kinase substrates by an integrated phosphoproteomics workflow. *Sci. Rep.* **2013**, *3*, 3460. [CrossRef] [PubMed]
42. Salvi, M.; Sarno, S.; Cesaro, L.; Nakamura, H.; Pinna, L.A. Extraordinary pleiotropy of protein kinase CK2 revealed by weblogo phosphoproteome analysis. *Biochim. Biophys. Acta* **2009**, *1793*, 847–859. [CrossRef] [PubMed]

43. Sarno, S.; Ghisellini, P.; Pinna, L.A. Unique activation mechanism of protein kinase CK2. The N-terminal segment is essential for constitutive activity of the catalytic subunit but not of the holoenzyme. *J. Biol. Chem.* **2002**, *277*, 22509–22514. [CrossRef] [PubMed]

44. Olsen, B.B.; Guerra, B.; Niefind, K.; Issinger, O.-G. Structural Basis of the Constitutive Activity of Protein Kinase CK2. *Methods Enzymol.* **2010**, *484*, 515–529.

45. Pinna, L.A. Protein kinase CK2: A challenge to canons. *J. Cell Sci.* **2002**, *115*, 3873–3878. [CrossRef] [PubMed]

46. Olsten, M.E.K.; Weber, J.E.; Litchfield, D.W. CK2 interacting proteins: Emerging paradigms for CK2 regulation? *Mol. Cell. Biochem.* **2005**, *274*, 115–124. [CrossRef] [PubMed]

47. Turowec, J.P.; Duncan, J.S.; French, A.C.; Gyenis, L.; St Denis, N.A.; Vilk, G.; Litchfield, D.W. Protein kinase CK2 is a constitutively active enzyme that promotes cell survival: Strategies to identify CK2 substrates and manipulate its activity in mammalian cells. *Methods Enzymol.* **2010**, *484*, 471–493. [PubMed]

48. Turowec, J.P.; Duncan, J.S.; Gloor, G.B.; Litchfield, D.W. Regulation of caspase pathways by protein kinase CK2: identification of proteins with overlapping CK2 and caspase consensus motifs. *Mol. Cell. Biochem.* **2011**, *356*, 159–167. [CrossRef] [PubMed]

49. Turowec, J.P.; Vilk, G.; Gabriel, M.; Litchfield, D.W. Characterizing the convergence of protein kinase CK2 and caspase-3 reveals isoform-specific phosphorylation of caspase-3 by CK2α': Implications for pathological roles of CK2 in promoting cancer cell survival. *Oncotarget* **2013**, *4*, 560–571. [CrossRef] [PubMed]

50. Duncan, J.S.; Turowec, J.P.; Vilk, G.; Li, S.S.C.; Gloor, G.B.; Litchfield, D.W. Regulation of cell proliferation and survival: Convergence of protein kinases and caspases. *Biochim. Biophys. Acta - Proteins Proteomics* **2010**, *1804*, 505–510. [CrossRef] [PubMed]

51. Lu, Z. PubMed and beyond: A survey of web tools for searching biomedical literature. *Database* **2011**, *2011*, baq036. [CrossRef] [PubMed]

52. Doms, A.; Schroeder, M. GoPubMed: Exploring PubMed with the Gene Ontology. *Nucleic Acids Res.* **2005**, *33*, W783–W786. [CrossRef] [PubMed]

53. Szklarczyk, D.; Morris, J.H.; Cook, H.; Kuhn, M.; Wyder, S.; Simonovic, M.; Santos, A.; Doncheva, N.T.; Roth, A.; Bork, P.; et al. The STRING database in 2017: Quality-controlled protein–protein association networks, made broadly accessible. *Nucleic Acids Res.* **2017**, *45*, D362–D368. [CrossRef] [PubMed]

54. McKendrick, L.; Milne, D.; Meek, D. Protein kinase CK2-dependent regulation of p53 function: Evidence that the phosphorylation status of the serine 386 (CK2) site of p53 is constitutive and stable. *Mol. Cell. Biochem.* **1999**, *191*, 187–199. [CrossRef] [PubMed]

55. Khan, D.H.; He, S.; Yu, J.; Winter, S.; Cao, W.; Seiser, C.; Davie, J.R. Protein Kinase CK2 Regulates the Dimerization of Histone Deacetylase 1 (HDAC1) and HDAC2 during Mitosis. *J. Biol. Chem.* **2013**, *288*, 16518–16528. [CrossRef] [PubMed]

56. Tsai, S.-C.; Seto, E. Regulation of histone deacetylase 2 by protein kinase CK2. *J. Biol. Chem.* **2002**, *277*, 31826–31833. [CrossRef] [PubMed]

57. Dominguez, I.; Sonenshein, G.E.; Seldin, D.C. Protein kinase CK2 in health and disease: CK2 and its role in Wnt and NF-kappaB signaling: Linking development and cancer. *Cell. Mol. Life Sci.* **2009**, *66*, 1850–1857. [CrossRef] [PubMed]

58. Futreal, P.A.; Coin, L.; Marshall, M.; Down, T.; Hubbard, T.; Wooster, R.; Rahman, N.; Stratton, M.R. A census of human cancer genes. *Nat. Rev. Cancer* **2004**, *4*, 177–183. [CrossRef] [PubMed]

59. Chatr-aryamontri, A.; Oughtred, R.; Boucher, L.; Rust, J.; Chang, C.; Kolas, N.K.; O'Donnell, L.; Oster, S.; Theesfeld, C.; Sellam, A.; et al. The BioGRID interaction database: 2017 update. *Nucleic Acids Res.* **2016**, gkw1102. [CrossRef] [PubMed]

60. Killcoyne, S.; Carter, G.W.; Smith, J.; Boyle, J. Cytoscape: A Community-Based Framework for Network Modeling. *Methods Mol. Boil.* **2009**, *563*, 219–239.

61. Cline, M.S.; Smoot, M.; Cerami, E.; Kuchinsky, A.; Landys, N.; Workman, C.; Christmas, R.; Avila-Campilo, I.; Creech, M.; Gross, B.; et al. Integration of biological networks and gene expression data using Cytoscape. *Nat. Protoc.* **2007**, *2*, 2366–2382. [CrossRef] [PubMed]

62. Kuleshov, M.V.; Jones, M.R.; Rouillard, A.D.; Fernandez, N.F.; Duan, Q.; Wang, Z.; Koplev, S.; Jenkins, S.L.; Jagodnik, K.M.; Lachmann, A.; et al. Enrichr: A comprehensive gene set enrichment analysis web server 2016 update. *Nucleic Acids Res.* **2016**, *44*, W90–W97. [CrossRef] [PubMed]

63. Kanehisa, M.; Goto, S. KEGG: kyoto encyclopedia of genes and genomes. *Nucleic Acids Res.* **2000**, *28*, 27–30. [CrossRef] [PubMed]

64. Nersisyan, L.; Samsonyan, R.; Arakelyan, A. CyKEGGParser: Tailoring KEGG pathways to fit into systems biology analysis workflows. *F1000Research* **2014**, *3*, 145. [CrossRef] [PubMed]

65. Martin, A.; Ochagavia, M.E.; Rabasa, L.C.; Miranda, J.; Fernandez-de-Cossio, J.; Bringas, R. BisoGenet: A new tool for gene network building, visualization and analysis. *BMC Bioinform.* **2010**, *11*, 91. [CrossRef] [PubMed]

66. Filhol, O.; Giacosa, S.; Wallez, Y.; Cochet, C. Protein kinase CK2 in breast cancer: The CK2β regulatory subunit takes center stage in epithelial plasticity. *Cell. Mol. Life Sci.* **2015**, *72*, 3305–3322. [CrossRef] [PubMed]

67. Bibby, A.C.; Litchfield, D.W. The multiple personalities of the regulatory subunit of protein kinase CK2: CK2 dependent and CK2 independent roles reveal a secret identity for CK2beta. *Int. J. Biol. Sci.* **2005**, *1*, 67–79. [CrossRef] [PubMed]

68. Vilk, G.; Saulnier, R.B.; St Pierre, R.; Litchfield, D.W. Inducible expression of protein kinase CK2 in mammalian cells. Evidence for functional specialization of CK2 isoforms. *J. Biol. Chem.* **1999**, *274*, 14406–14414. [CrossRef] [PubMed]

69. Messenger, M.M.; Saulnier, R.B.; Gilchrist, A.D.; Diamond, P.; Gorbsky, G.J.; Litchfield, D.W. Interactions between protein kinase CK2 and Pin1. Evidence for phosphorylation-dependent interactions. *J. Biol. Chem.* **2002**, *277*, 23054–23064. [CrossRef] [PubMed]

70. Bosc, D.G.; Graham, K.C.; Saulnier, R.B.; Zhang, C.; Prober, D.; Gietz, R.D.; Litchfield, D.W. Identification and characterization of CKIP-1, a novel pleckstrin homology domain-containing protein that interacts with protein kinase CK2. *J. Biol. Chem.* **2000**, *275*, 14295–14306. [CrossRef] [PubMed]

71. Arrigoni, G.; Pagano, M.A.; Sarno, S.; Cesaro, L.; James, P.; Pinna, L.A. Mass spectrometry analysis of a protein kinase CK2beta subunit interactome isolated from mouse brain by affinity chromatography. *J. Proteome Res.* **2008**, *7*, 990–1000. [CrossRef] [PubMed]

72. Guerra, B.; Siemer, S.; Boldyreff, B.; Issinger, O.G. Protein kinase CK2: Evidence for a protein kinase CK2beta subunit fraction, devoid of the catalytic CK2alpha subunit, in mouse brain and testicles. *FEBS Lett.* **1999**, *462*, 353–357. [CrossRef]

73. Ruepp, A.; Waegele, B.; Lechner, M.; Brauner, B.; Dunger-Kaltenbach, I.; Fobo, G.; Frishman, G.; Montrone, C.; Mewes, H.-W. CORUM: The comprehensive resource of mammalian protein complexes–2009. *Nucleic Acids Res.* **2010**, *38*, D497–D501. [CrossRef] [PubMed]

74. Villavicencio-Diaz, T.N.; Rodriguez-Ulloa, A.; Guirola-Cruz, O.; Perez-Riverol, Y. Bioinformatics tools for the functional interpretation of quantitative proteomics results. *Curr. Top. Med. Chem.* **2014**, *14*, 435–449. [CrossRef] [PubMed]

75. Lou, D.Y.; Dominguez, I.; Toselli, P.; Landesman-Bollag, E.; O'Brien, C.; Seldin, D.C. The alpha catalytic subunit of protein kinase CK2 is required for mouse embryonic development. *Mol. Cell. Biol.* **2008**, *28*, 131–139. [CrossRef] [PubMed]

76. Dominguez, I.; Degano, I.R.; Chea, K.; Cha, J.; Toselli, P.; Seldin, D.C. CK2α is essential for embryonic morphogenesis. *Mol. Cell. Biochem.* **2011**, *356*, 209–216. [CrossRef] [PubMed]

77. Dominguez, I.; Mizuno, J.; Wu, H.; Imbrie, G.A.; Symes, K.; Seldin, D.C. A role for CK2alpha/beta in Xenopus early embryonic development. *Mol. Cell. Biochem.* **2005**, *274*, 125–131. [CrossRef] [PubMed]

78. Bragdon, B.; Thinakaran, S.; Moseychuk, O.; King, D.; Young, K.; Litchfield, D.W.; Petersen, N.O.; Nohe, A. Casein Kinase 2 β-Subunit Is a Regulator of Bone Morphogenetic Protein 2 Signaling. *Biophys. J.* **2010**, *99*, 897–904. [CrossRef] [PubMed]

79. Liu, Y.; Holdbrooks, A.T.; De Sarno, P.; Rowse, A.L.; Yanagisawa, L.L.; McFarland, B.C.; Harrington, L.E.; Raman, C.; Sabbaj, S.; Benveniste, E.N.; et al. Therapeutic efficacy of suppressing the Jak/STAT pathway in multiple models of experimental autoimmune encephalomyelitis. *J. Immunol.* **2014**, *192*, 59–72. [CrossRef] [PubMed]

80. Ulges, A.; Klein, M.; Reuter, S.; Gerlitzki, B.; Hoffmann, M.; Grebe, N.; Staudt, V.; Stergiou, N.; Bohn, T.; Brühl, T.-J.; et al. Protein kinase CK2 enables regulatory T cells to suppress excessive TH2 responses in vivo. *Nat. Immunol.* **2015**, *16*, 267–275. [CrossRef] [PubMed]

81. Ampofo, E.; Rudzitis-Auth, J.; Dahmke, I.N.; Rössler, O.G.; Thiel, G.; Montenarh, M.; Menger, M.D.; Laschke, M.W. Inhibition of protein kinase CK2 suppresses tumor necrosis factor (TNF)-α-induced leukocyte-endothelial cell interaction. *Biochim. Biophys. Acta* **2015**, *1852*, 2123–2136. [CrossRef] [PubMed]

82. Welker, S.; Götz, C.; Servas, C.; Laschke, M.W.; Menger, M.D.; Montenarh, M. Glucose regulates protein kinase CK2 in pancreatic β-cells and its interaction with PDX-1. *Int. J. Biochem. Cell Biol.* **2013**, *45*, 2786–2795. [CrossRef] [PubMed]

83. Al Quobaili, F.; Montenarh, M. CK2 and the regulation of the carbohydrate metabolism. *Metabolism* **2012**, *61*, 1512–1517. [CrossRef] [PubMed]

84. Lupp, S.; Götz, C.; Khadouma, S.; Horbach, T.; Dimova, E.Y.; Bohrer, A.-M.; Kietzmann, T.; Montenarh, M. The upstream stimulatory factor USF1 is regulated by protein kinase CK2 phosphorylation. *Cell. Signal.* **2014**, *26*, 2809–2817. [CrossRef] [PubMed]

85. Spohrer, S.; Dimova, E.Y.; Kietzmann, T.; Montenarh, M.; Götz, C. The nuclear fraction of protein kinase CK2 binds to the upstream stimulatory factors (USFs) in the absence of DNA. *Cell. Signal.* **2016**, *28*, 23–31. [CrossRef] [PubMed]

86. Zaman, M.S.; Johnson, A.J.; Bobek, G.; Kueh, S.; Kersaitis, C.; Bailey, T.D.; Buskila, Y.; Wu, M.J. Protein kinase CK2 regulates metal toxicity in neuronal cells. *Metallomics* **2016**, *8*, 82–90. [CrossRef] [PubMed]

87. Akkiraju, H.; Bonor, J.; Olli, K.; Bowen, C.; Bragdon, B.; Coombs, H.; Donahue, L.R.; Duncan, R.; Nohe, A. Systemic injection of CK2.3, a novel peptide acting downstream of bone morphogenetic protein receptor BMPRIa, leads to increased trabecular bone mass. *J. Orthop. Res.* **2015**, *33*, 208–215. [CrossRef] [PubMed]

88. Kahali, B.; Trott, R.; Paroush, Z.; Allada, R.; Bishop, C.P.; Bidwai, A.P. Drosophila CK2 phosphorylates Hairy and regulates its activity in vivo. *Biochem. Biophys. Res. Commun.* **2008**, *373*, 637–642. [CrossRef] [PubMed]

89. Kuntamalla, P.P.; Kunttas-Tatli, E.; Karandikar, U.; Bishop, C.P.; Bidwai, A.P. Drosophila protein kinase CK2 is rendered temperature-sensitive by mutations of highly conserved residues flanking the activation segment. *Mol. Cell. Biochem.* **2009**, *323*, 49–60. [CrossRef] [PubMed]

90. Ottaviani, D.; Marin, O.; Arrigoni, G.; Franchin, C.; Vilardell, J.; Sandre, M.; Li, W.; Parfitt, D.A.; Pinna, L.A.; Cheetham, M.E.; et al. Protein kinase CK2 modulates HSJ1 function through phosphorylation of the UIM2 domain. *Hum. Mol. Genet.* **2016**. [CrossRef] [PubMed]

91. Schwind, L.; Wilhelm, N.; Kartarius, S.; Montenarh, M.; Gorjup, E.; Götz, C. Protein kinase CK2 is necessary for the adipogenic differentiation of human mesenchymal stem cells. *Biochim. Biophys. Acta* **2015**, *1853*, 2207–2216. [CrossRef] [PubMed]

92. Herrmann, D.; Straubinger, M.; Hashemolhosseini, S. Protein kinase CK2 interacts at the neuromuscular synapse with Rapsyn, Rac1, 14-3-3γ, and Dok-7 proteins and phosphorylates the latter two. *J. Biol. Chem.* **2015**, *290*, 22370–22384. [CrossRef] [PubMed]

93. Cheusova, T.; Khan, M.A.; Schubert, S.W.; Gavin, A.-C.; Buchou, T.; Jacob, G.; Sticht, H.; Allende, J.; Boldyreff, B.; Brenner, H.R.; et al. Casein kinase 2-dependent serine phosphorylation of MuSK regulates acetylcholine receptor aggregation at the neuromuscular junction. *Genes Dev.* **2006**, *20*, 1800–1816. [CrossRef] [PubMed]

94. Hornbeck, P.V.; Kornhauser, J.M.; Tkachev, S.; Zhang, B.; Skrzypek, E.; Murray, B.; Latham, V.; Sullivan, M. PhosphoSitePlus: A comprehensive resource for investigating the structure and function of experimentally determined post-translational modifications in man and mouse. *Nucleic Acids Res.* **2012**, *40*, D261–D270. [PubMed]

95. Hornbeck, P.V.; Zhang, B.; Murray, B.; Kornhauser, J.M.; Latham, V.; Skrzypek, E. PhosphoSitePlus, 2014: Mutations, PTMs and recalibrations. *Nucleic Acids Res.* **2015**, *43*, D512–D520. [CrossRef] [PubMed]

96. Meng, R.; Al-Quobaili, F.; Müller, I.; Götz, C.; Thiel, G.; Montenarh, M. CK2 phosphorylation of Pdx-1 regulates its transcription factor activity. *Cell. Mol. Life Sci.* **2010**, *67*, 2481–2489. [CrossRef] [PubMed]

97. Venerando, A.; Franchin, C.; Cant, N.; Cozza, G.; Pagano, M.A.; Tosoni, K.; Al-Zahrani, A.; Arrigoni, G.; Ford, R.C.; Mehta, A.; et al. Detection of phospho-sites generated by protein kinase CK2 in CFTR: Mechanistic aspects of Thr1471 phosphorylation. *PLoS ONE* **2013**, *8*, e74232. [CrossRef] [PubMed]

98. Deutsch, E.W.; Csordas, A.; Sun, Z.; Jarnuczak, A.; Perez-Riverol, Y.; Ternent, T.; Campbell, D.S.; Bernal-Llinares, M.; Okuda, S.; Kawano, S.; et al. The ProteomeXchange consortium in 2017: Supporting the cultural change in proteomics public data deposition. *Nucleic Acids Res.* **2017**, *45*, D1100–D1106. [CrossRef] [PubMed]

99. Franchin, C.; Salvi, M.; Arrigoni, G.; Pinna, L.A. Proteomics perturbations promoted by the protein kinase CK2 inhibitor quinalizarin. *Biochim. Biophys. Acta* **2015**, *1854*, 1676–1686. [CrossRef] [PubMed]

100. Rodríguez-Ulloa, A.; Ramos, Y.; Gil, J.; Perera, Y.; Castellanos-Serra, L.; García, Y.; Betancourt, L.; Besada, V.; González, L.J.; Fernández-de-Cossio, J.; et al. Proteomic profile regulated by the anticancer peptide CIGB-300 in non-small cell lung cancer (NSCLC) cells. *J. Proteome Res.* **2010**, *9*, 5473–5483. [CrossRef] [PubMed]

101. Le Bihan, T.; Hindle, M.; Martin, S.F.; Barrios-Llerena, M.E.; Krahmer, J.; Kis, K.; Millar, A.J.; van Ooijen, G. Label-free quantitative analysis of the casein kinase 2-responsive phosphoproteome of the marine minimal model species Ostreococcus tauri. *Proteomics* **2015**, *15*, 4135–4144. [CrossRef] [PubMed]

102. Franchin, C.; Cesaro, L.; Salvi, M.; Millioni, R.; Iori, E.; Cifani, P.; James, P.; Arrigoni, G.; Pinna, L. Quantitative analysis of a phosphoproteome readily altered by the protein kinase CK2 inhibitor quinalizarin in HEK-293T cells. *Biochim. Biophys. Acta* **2015**, *1854*, 609–623. [CrossRef] [PubMed]

103. Amanchy, R.; Periaswamy, B.; Mathivanan, S.; Reddy, R.; Tattikota, S.G.; Pandey, A. A curated compendium of phosphorylation motifs. *Nat. Biotechnol.* **2007**, *25*, 285–286. [CrossRef] [PubMed]

104. Jowsey, P.; Morrice, N.A.; Hastie, C.J.; McLauchlan, H.; Toth, R.; Rouse, J. Characterisation of the sites of DNA damage-induced 53BP1 phosphorylation catalysed by ATM and ATR. *DNA Repair. (Amst.)* **2007**, *6*, 1536–1544. [CrossRef] [PubMed]

105. Grove, B.D.; Bruchey, A.K. Intracellular distribution of gravin, a PKA and PKC binding protein, in vascular endothelial cells. *J. Vasc. Res.* **2001**, *38*, 163–175. [CrossRef]

106. Tao, J.; Wang, H.-Y.; Malbon, C.C. Protein kinase A regulates AKAP250 (gravin) scaffold binding to the beta2-adrenergic receptor. *EMBO J.* **2003**, *22*, 6419–6429. [CrossRef] [PubMed]

107. Rust, H.L.; Thompson, P.R. Kinase Consensus Sequences: A Breeding Ground for Crosstalk. *ACS Chem. Biol.* **2011**, *6*, 881–892. [CrossRef] [PubMed]

108. Yamagata, K.; Daitoku, H.; Takahashi, Y.; Namiki, K.; Hisatake, K.; Kako, K.; Mukai, H.; Kasuya, Y.; Fukamizu, A. Arginine Methylation of FOXO Transcription Factors Inhibits Their Phosphorylation by Akt. *Mol. Cell* **2008**, *32*, 221–231. [CrossRef] [PubMed]

109. Sakamaki, J.-i.; Daitoku, H.; Ueno, K.; Hagiwara, A.; Yamagata, K.; Fukamizu, A. Arginine methylation of BCL-2 antagonist of cell death (BAD) counteracts its phosphorylation and inactivation by Akt. *Proc. Natl. Acad. Sci. USA* **2011**, *108*, 6085–6090. [CrossRef] [PubMed]

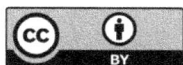

pharmaceuticals

MDPI

Review

The New Role for an Old Kinase: Protein Kinase CK2 Regulates Metal Ion Transport

Adam J. Johnson [1] and Ming J. Wu [1,2,*]

[1] School of Science and Health, Western Sydney University, Locked Bag 1797, Penrith NSW 2751, Australia; a.johnson@westernsydney.edu.au
[2] Molecular Medicine Research Group, School of Medicine, Western Sydney University, Locked Bag 1797, Penrith NSW 2751, Australia
*   Correspondence: m.wu@westernsydney.edu.au; Tel.: +61-2-4620-3089; Fax: +61-2-4620-3025

Academic Editor: Lorenzo Pinna
Received: 18 November 2016; Accepted: 16 December 2016; Published: 21 December 2016

Abstract: The pleiotropic serine/threonine protein kinase CK2 was the first kinase discovered. It is renowned for its role in cell proliferation and anti-apoptosis. The complexity of this kinase is well reflected by the findings of past decades in terms of its heterotetrameric structure, subcellular location, constitutive activity and the extensive catalogue of substrates. With the advent of non-biased high-throughput functional genomics such as genome-wide deletion mutant screening, novel aspects of CK2 functionality have been revealed. Our recent discoveries using the model organism *Saccharomyces cerevisiae* and mammalian cells demonstrate that CK2 regulates metal toxicity. Extensive literature search reveals that there are few but elegant works on the role of CK2 in regulating the sodium and zinc channels. As both CK2 and metal ions are key players in cell biology and oncogenesis, understanding the details of CK2's regulation of metal ion homeostasis has a direct bearing on cancer research. In this review, we aim to garner the recent data and gain insights into the role of CK2 in metal ion transport.

Keywords: protein kinase CK2; metal toxicity; genome-wide screen; metal ion transport; zinc channels; therapeutic targets

1. CK2—A Pleiotropic Kinase

Protein kinase CK2 was first discovered in 1954 [1]. It is one of the earliest kinases in the kinome which currently has about 500 members [1–3]. Over the ensuing decades, its structure, function and substrates have been progressively characterized [4–6]. Despite the enormous progress in characterisation of its roles in cell proliferation, differentiation and anti-apoptosis, several aspects of CK2 are yet to be fully understood such as its regulatory mechanisms in response to extracellular signals. Also scarcely known is its role in metal ion uptake and toxicity, which is the topic of this review.

CK2 is a ubiquitous, pleiotropic, serine/threonine protein kinase with a wide range of substrates, and has been referred to as the most pleiotropic protein kinase existing in eukaryotic organisms [5,6]. Originally the enzyme was termed casein kinase 2 due to its phosphorylation of casein as the first substrate used to assay enzyme activity, and the numerical designation 2 to denotes its elution from DEAE-cellulose after the enzyme CK1 [1,6–8]. However, casein does not appear to be a physiological substrate for CK2 and, therefore, in 1994 it was suggested that the name be changed to protein kinase CK2 to avoid the misnomer confusion [7,8]. CK2 is an unusual protein kinase in several respects. For examples, it is constitutively active and can use both ATP and GTP as the phosphate donor, thus it is different from the other eukaryotic protein kinases [5,7,9–11]. The known substrates of this enzyme are expanding to the thousand [5]. It has been suggested that the proteins phosphorylated by CK2 may make up one quarter of the eukaryotic phosphoproteome [5]. The renowned role of CK2 is its regulation of cell proliferation, including the processes of DNA replication, transcription, tRNA and rRNA synthesis, chromatin remodelling and anti-apoptosis [6,12,13]. With its high pleiotropism, it is not surprising that new aspects of CK2 functionality are continually unravelled, such as we and the others demonstrate that CK2 is involved in metal ion transport [14,15].

2. Structure and Function of CK2

The mammalian CK2 heterotetramer is a protein kinase composed of two catalytic subunits (α and α'), bound to a central homodimer of regulatory β subunits. The fact that the holoenzymes are formed spontaneously in vitro from the mixture of individual subunits tells us that there is probably a built-in code for such action amongst their primary structures. Notably, the affinity of CK2 α' for CK2 β is about 12 times lower than that of CK2 α [16], suggesting that the tetramer $\alpha\alpha\beta\beta$ of CK2 could be the dominant species. The amino acid sequences of human α and α' catalytic subunits are 391 and 350 residues long, respectively. The apparent sizes after purification in vitro are smaller than their theoretical molecular masses (45.144 and 41.213 kDa), due to proteolytic cleavage modifications at the C-terminus [17,18]. The β subunit is much smaller (around 25 kDa) [19,20]. The crystallographic structures of the subunits of CK2 and the holoenzyme demonstrate that the catalytic subunits of CK2 contain the typical architecture found in eukaryotic protein kinases [16,21]. Such architecture consists of two domains: a β-sheet based N-terminal domain, and an α-helical C-terminal domain. The active site is located in a cleft between the two domains [16,17,21]. The main difference between the two catalytic subunits in terms of the three-dimensional structure is found in the CK2 β interface region ($\beta4/\beta5$ loop). Unbound CK2 α typically has a closed $\beta4/\beta5$ loop, while CK2 α' has an open one [16].

A worthwhile notion in the context of this review is that two zinc ions are involved in the holoenzyme. The CK2 β subunit contains a zinc finger that has been shown to be essential for the homodimerisation of the β subunits [22]. The four cysteines (cys^{109}, cys^{114}, cys^{137} and cys^{140}) of CK2 β are in a zinc finger-like arrangement reminiscent of DNA binding proteins [7]. Mutations to cys^{109} and cys^{114} result in disruption of subunit interactions. Each CK2 β monomer consists of an α-helical N-terminal domain and the zinc stabilising area and a C-terminal "tail" [17,23]. The tail crosses the dimer interface and attaches to the other β monomer. This tail segment has been shown to be essential for holoenzyme formation [23]. The holoenzyme complex is shaped like a butterfly, with the catalytic subunits attached to a central dimer of regulatory β subunits [17]. The arrangement is such that both regulatory subunits make contact with each of the catalytic subunits, while neither catalytic subunit contacts the other [17]. The conservation of the active site of unbound CK2 α and the holoenzyme-bound CK2 α supports the idea that CK2 α is catalytically active in isolation and that CK2 β is not an on/off switch as is found in similar kinases such as cyclin-dependent kinase 2 [17,23].

Its extensive list of protein substrates reflects the pleiotropic nature of CK2 functionality, and is structurally due to the acidic consensus sequences (e.g., -SXXE/D-, S for serine which is the most common phosphoacceptor) recognised by the kinase [6,24,25]. The multiple tetrameric forms ($\alpha2\beta2$, $\alpha'2\beta2$, $\alpha\alpha'\beta2$) are present in all animals including mammals, amphibians and insects [17,19,26]. Evidence shows that the formation of human CK2 tetramers occurs via the catalytic subunits attaching independently to a stable dimer of the β subunits [17,23]. The free monomeric α and α' subunits of CK2 are catalytically active as well in the absence of the β subunit and there is evidence that the discrete subunits possess individual functions different to the functions of the tetramer [27–31]. The α and α' subunits are structurally analogous but are encoded by different genes [7]. The β subunits in tetramers may provide stability, protect α-subunits against denaturing agents or conditions, modulate activity of the enzyme or alter substrate specificity and interactions with inhibitors [7,32]. It has been noted that catalytic activity is increased 5–10 fold for certain substrates by the presence of the β subunit [7,33]. Unlike mammalian CK2, yeast cells possess two distinct regulatory subunits (*CKB1* and *CKB2*), while the catalytic subunits are commonly referred to as *CKA1* and *CKA2*. Yeast CK2 tetrameric holoenzymes have been found to require both *CKB1* and *CKB2* subunits [34].

As the yeast *Saccharomyces cerevisiae* contributes to our understanding of mammalian cell biology, such as cell cycle control [35,36], and the signalling serine/threonine kinase TOR (target of rapamycin) [37,38], it proves to be a useful tool again towards understanding CK2. The genes of CK2 were first deleted in *S. cerevisiae* by homologous recombination. The yeast cells with disruption of either *CKA1* or *CKA2* genes are still viable; however, disruption of both *CKA1* and *CKA2* genes at the same time is lethal [39]. It is therefore clear that under normal growth conditions the catalytic subunits are compensatory. However, several studies imply that under certain environmental conditions individual subunits confer different phenotypes [14,40,41], and, therefore, cannot be compensated by one another. In terms of the regulatory subunits, deletion of *CKB1* or *CKB2* or both does not lead to lethality. However, in mammals such as mice, homozygous knockout of CK2 β is fatal at the embryonic development stage [42]. While the CK2 α′ subunit appears to be essential only for normal spermatogenesis [43], the disruption of the CK2 α gene in mice leads to death in mid-gestation [44]. Taken together, these structural and functional data tell us three basic points: (1) the tetrameric holoenzymes are essential since disruption of CK2 β would abolish formation of the CK2 holoenzyme and leads to lethality; (2) between the two catalytic subunits, CK2 α is more critical than CK2 α′; (3) both CK2 α and CK2 α′ have distinctive functions.

Since CK2 is constitutively active, its activity does not need help from any other kinases. The alternative ways to regulate its activity are by level of expression, subcellular location of the enzyme, and extracellular signals. It is evident in cancers where CK2 is highly over-expressed [6,45]. Spatiotemporal dynamics of CK2 in the nucleus and cytoplasm are shown in live cell fluorescence imaging [46]. The remaining question is what triggers up-regulation of CK2 expression or changes its nucleocytoplasmic distribution. Heretofore, there are scant details in terms of what regulates dynamic distribution of CK2. A recent study by Kalathur et al. [47] strongly demonstrates that the transcription factor, STAT3 (Signal Transducer and Activator of Transcription 3), regulates CK2 transcription and the protein level in mammalian cells. STAT3 itself is phosphorylated in response to growth factors or cytokines. The up-regulation of CK2 results in phosphorylation of the tumor suppressor, PML (Promyelocytic Leukemia protein), which in turn leads to PML ubiquitination and degradation. As a result, oncogenesis ensues.

Moreover, its activity can be increased and decreased by certain compounds. Under certain conditions, polyamines are known to increase the activity of CK2 [7]. This activation requires a specific concentration of the polyamine and, therefore, may only occur in certain cells, e.g., the dividing cells due to their increased polyamine concentration [7]. On the other hand, polyanionic compounds such as heparin are inhibitory to CK2. It is therefore possible that CK2 activity in the liver is subject to heparin concentration [7,48]. This suggests that CK2 activity is regulated in specific cells and tissues by activating inhibitory compounds.

In vitro assays have demonstrated that divalent metal ions such as Mg^{2+}, Mn^{2+} and Co^{2+} are required for CK2 activity, but beyond their optimal concentration these metals are actually inhibitory to CK2 [49,50]. These studies were performed using a substrate that precipitates, such as casein, in the presence of metals such as Mg^{2+} and the inhibition of CK2 in the presence of Mg^{2+} concentrations greater than its optimum is due to casein precipitation [51]. The optimal concentration of Mg^{2+} may represent the point at which Mg^{2+}-ATP (required for activity) is highest before precipitation occurs [51]. While this is the case for Mg^{2+}, substrate precipitation in the presence of Co^{2+} and Mn^{2+} does not occur and, therefore, the inhibition of enzyme activity at levels above the optimum of these ions may be a regulatory mechanism [51]. Interestingly, when activity is assayed using Mn^{2+} and Co^{2+} instead of Mg^{2+}, the preferred phosphoryl donor is GTP rather than ATP [49]. Zn^{2+} is inhibitory to CK2 at concentrations above 150 μM [49]. The inhibition of CK2 by zinc, as well as the reported inhibition of activity found when Ni^{2+} is present, is thought to be via direct interaction with the enzyme, perhaps in a manner similar to Mn^{2+} and Co^{2+} [49,51]. Given that the ionic strength of solution greatly impacts enzyme activity [51] and the requirements of CK2 for zinc in order for functional tetramers to form, there might be certain inextricable relationships between CK2 and metal ions.

3. Functional Genomics and Discovery of Novel CK2 Functionality

The yeast *S. cerevisiae* is a pioneering organism in functional genomics and systems biology [52]. Since the publication of its genomic sequence [53], complete collections of yeast gene deletion mutants such as the collection from EUROSCARF have become available for functional annotation of individual genes by genome-wide screening. Such an approach acquires the phenotype of a gene deletion mutant observed under a given condition. Based upon the phenotype, the function of that gene can be revealed. Genome-wide screening of deletion mutants has been applied to nickel [54], cadmium [55], arsenite [56,57], lead [58], aluminium [14,59] and chromium [40]. Significantly, the findings from the yeast system are relevant to human beings due to the genomic homology between the two organisms. They share thousands of orthologous genes, accounting for about one-third of the yeast genome [60,61]. Additionally, there exists a high level of conservation between the cellular processes of yeast and those of mammalian cells [62,63]. By means of *S. cerevisiae* genome-wide deletion mutant screening, we firstly uncovered that deletion of *CKA2* (CKα') leads to resistance to Al^{3+} toxicity [14]. Further, the regulatory subunits (*CKB1* and *CKB2*) were shown to be involved in regulating the toxicity of As^{3+} [56]. Significantly, the role of CK2 in regulating metal toxicity is confirmed in neuronal cells [64]. Intriguingly, CK2 regulates both Zn^{2+} and Ca^{2+} [64]. Considering that CK2 is a key player in carcinogenesis and that dysregulation of Zn^{2+} is observed in cancers such as breast, prostate, pancreatic, ovarian and hepatocellular cancers [65–69], this discovery has significant bearing on cancer research.

4. CK2 and Metal Ion Transport

The ability to transport ions into and out of the cell is essential for life. Herein, we define ion transport as the process of uptake, sequestration into or release from subcellular organelles, and efflux. Approximately 91 of 118 elements in the periodic table are metals or metalloids, many of which are essential to biological functions, whilst some are toxic. Essential metal ions are required for a range of cellular functions, for example, iron is a cofactor for several redox-active metalloenzymes and zinc is required for maintaining protein structures such as in CK2 and the catalytic activity of thousands of enzymes [70,71]. The metal ion uptake, storage and secretion is tightly controlled, and aberrations in this control can lead to cell death and diseases [72,73].

The compendium of recent studies, including the ones of our laboratory aforementioned, demonstrates that CK2 is involved in metal toxicity and transport [64]. We have shown that deletion of *CKA1*, *CKB1* and *CKB2* result in lower accumulation of intracellular chromium, while deletion of *CKA2* leads to higher accumulation than the wild type [40]. We then screened all four deletion mutants of CK2 (*cka1Δ*, *cka2Δ*, *ckb1Δ* and *ckb2Δ*) against Al^{3+}, Zn^{2+}, Co^{2+}, Cr^{6+}, As^{3+} and Cd^{2+}, and found that individual subunits confer distinct profiles for metal resistance (unpublished data). The findings are two-fold. They demonstrate that CK2 is indeed involved in metal uptake and toxicity, and that individual CK2 subunits have specific roles such as *CKA2* against Al^{3+}, and *CKB1* or *CKB2* against As^{3+} and Cr^{6+}. The finding that deletion of CK2 subunits results in metal resistance is supported by the dataset obtained by a different high-throughput profiling approach—transcriptomics. Jin et al. [74] revealed, via transcriptomics of *S. cerevisiae*, that the expression of genes encoding subunits of protein kinase CK2 (*CKB2*, *CKA1*, *CKA2*) was repressed by transitional metal ions, suggesting that CK2 gene expression is undesirable for the cells under metal ion exposure. On the other hand, analysis of the ionomic data generated in a genome-wide yeast screen using overexpression strains indicates that the overexpression of CK2 subunits resulted in an increase of certain metals inside the cell including copper, iron and zinc [75]. Apart from the yeast model organism, a similar finding was demonstrated in mammalian cells [76], in which CK2 transcripts were markedly reduced upon chromium exposure. In a study using mouse epidermal JB6 cells, the phosphorylation of p53 (resulting in p53 DNA binding) by CK2 was found to be reduced in the presence of arsenic [77].

How does CK2 regulate metal ion transport, biochemically? Two studies so far can provide us with some insight. In response to the extracellular stimuli, CK2 was found to phosphorylate the zinc channel, ZIP7 (ZIP is an abbreviation of ZRT, IRT-like Protein), located in the membrane of the endoplasmic reticulum (ER) [15]. Consequently, Zn^{2+} ions in ER stores were released, and cytosolic concentration of Zn^{2+} increased, triggering a cascade of signalling pathways, including the activation of receptor tyrosine kinase and the phosphorylation of AKT and extracellular signal-regulated kinases 1 and 2 (ERK1/2). The end result of such action is enhanced cell proliferation. This finding offers mechanistic explanation, if only partially, to the effect of CK2 on promoting cell proliferation as mentioned previously.

CK2 is also found to regulate epithelial Na^+ channel activity [78]. The Na^+ channel is a trimeric protein, composed of α, β and γ subunits. The phosphorylation sites for CK2 are located in the C terminus of β ($β_{S631}$) and γ subunits ($γ_{T599}$). The channel's activity was inhibited dose-dependently by the selective CK2 inhibitor 4,5,6,7-tetrabromobenzotriazole (TBB). Furthermore, the phosphorylation of the channel by CK2 antagonises the inhibition of Nedd4-2, the E3-ubiquitin ligase, which causes channel ubiquitination and degradation. Intriguingly, CK2 was translocated to the cell membrane upon expression of the wild type Na^+ channel, but not of the mutant channel lacking both of the phosphorylation sites. This notion sheds light on the topic of CK2 distribution as mentioned earlier. There is likely a pulling force or an attraction between CK2 and its substrate, and evidence suggests that this attraction is structurally due to basic residues in key positions of CK2 recognising the acidic determinants in the substrate for phosphorylation. It is expected that more investigations will be carried out on this front.

Another elegant study conducted on CFTR (cystic fibrosis transmembrane conductance regulator) provides more details on the mode of CK2 action [79,80]. Although CFTR is essentially a chloride channel, much can be learned from its interaction with CK2. Inhibition of CK2 closes CFTR wild type but not the cystic fibrosis mutant channel ΔF508-CFTR [81]. The deletion of phenylalanine (F) of the 508th residue in CFTR abolishes the interaction of CK2 with ΔF508-CFTR, suggesting that phenylalanine residue serves as a docking site in the wild type for CK2 action. Furthermore, ΔF508-CFTR mutant is often degraded before reaching the plasma membrane. As for the membrane-bound mutants, they are unstable. Application of the proteostasis regulator cysteamine and the CK2 inhibitor, epigallocatechin gallate (EGCG) or CX-4945, can reduce the degradation of ΔF508-CFTR, resulting in more mutant channels residing in the membrane, hence alleviation of the symptom of cystic fibrosis patients [79]. Such a study serves as an example for future investigations, which could be relevant to the basic understanding of and therapeutic development for many human disorders involving CK2.

Additionally, to understand the cell's regulation of metal ions, we must differentiate the essential ions, such as iron and zinc, from the toxic ones, like arsenic and aluminium. In the evolutionary sense, the cell has become accustomed to the essential ions and has built-in mechanisms to maintain their homeostasis for growth and survival. The cell's response to the toxic metal ions is basically a detoxification process using the cell's defence mechanisms. The data discussed previously clearly show that CK2 is involved in both categories of the metals. The key question is what senses the intracellular level of a particular ion. There is no certain answer to this question thus far. However, it has been shown that in the presence of increased metal ions, the transcription factor MTF-1 (metal transcription factor 1) is phosphorylated by CK2. Upon phosphorylation by CK2, MTF-1 activates metal responsive genes such as metallothioneins [82]. Metallothioneins are a class of cysteine-rich, metal binding proteins that are thought to play a role in essential metal ion homeostasis and detoxification of toxic metal ions [82].

The evidence for CK2's role in metal homeostasis is emerging. As previously mentioned, the work by Taylor et al. [15] demonstrates a role for CK2 in zinc homeostasis through regulation of the ER zinc channel ZIP7. There are 14 ZIP channels responsible for zinc uptake. There also exist 10 ZnT channels responsible for zinc efflux from the cytosol. Given that CK2 is found to directly phosphorylate ZIP7, it is likely that it also phosphorylates other zinc transporters. Table 1 shows the various zinc channels and the possible residues that could be phosphorylated by CK2.

Table 1. Phosphorylated sites predicted in the zinc channels.

Protein	Site	Exemplar Sequence	Score	Location of Phosphorylation Site
ZIP1	None	-	-	-
ZIP2	S87	MVQNRSASERNSSGD	10.179	Extracellular
ZIP2	S91	RSASERNSSGDADSA	15.628	Extracellular
ZIP3	S125	LETFNAGSDVGSDSE	10.216	Cytoplasmic
ZIP3	S129	NAGSDVGSDSEYESP	16.602	Cytoplasmic
ZIP3	S131	GSDVGSDSEYESPFM	12.602	Cytoplasmic
ZIP4	None	-	-	-
ZIP5	None	-	-	-
ZIP6	S100	HHDHDHHSDHEHHSD	11.864	Extracellular
ZIP6	S106	HSDHEHHSDHERHSD	12.672	Extracellular
ZIP6	S112	HSDHERHSDHEHHSE	12.662	Extracellular
ZIP6	S118	HSDHEHHSEHEHHSD	12.807	Extracellular
ZIP6	S124	HSEHEHHSDHDHHSH	12.309	Extracellular
ZIP6	S183	RNVKDSVSASEVTST	10.324	Extracellular
ZIP7	S275	RSTKEKQSSEEEEKE	16.548	Cytoplasmic
ZIP7	S276	RSTKEKQSSEEEEKE	16.548	Cytoplasmic
ZIP8	None	-	-	-
ZIP9	S132	IGNSHVHSTDDPEAA	11.066	Cytoplasmic
ZIP10	None	-	-	-
ZIP11	None	-	-	-
ZIP12	S160	DEDSSFLSQNETEDI	10.412	Extracellular
ZIP12	S197	KKSGIVSSEGANEST	10.888	Extracellular
ZIP12	S293	QDYSNFSSSMEKESE	11.826	Cytoplasmic
ZIP12	S497	LALNSELSDQAGRGK	9.983	Extracellular
ZIP12	S565	AIGAAFSSSSESGVT	10.276	Cytoplasmic
ZIP12	S567	GAAFSSSSESGVTTT	10.409	Cytoplasmic
ZIP13	None	-	-	-
ZIP14	None	-	-	-
ZNT1	None	-	-	-
ZNT2	S322	CQACQGPSD	10.147	Cytoplasmic
ZNT3	S341	SAHLAIDSTADPEAV	9.921	Cytoplasmic
ZNT4	S32	DTSAFDFSDEAGDEG	13.229	Cytoplasmic
ZNT5	None	-	-	-
ZNT6	None	-	-	-
ZNT7	None	-	-	-
ZNT8	S353	SLTIQMESPVDQDPD	10.017	Cytoplasmic
ZNT9	None	-	-	-
ZNT10	S446	TYGSDGLSRRDAREV	11.562	Cytoplasmic

Note: The protein sequence of each zinc channel was analysed for phosphorylation by CK2 using GPS3.0 software [83], using the high threshold option (reported false positive rate of <2%). This threshold correlates with a cut-off value of 9.84. The table shows the predicted residue position, the sequence, the score (higher score means more likely to be phosphorylated) and the location of the predicted phosphorylation sites.

Further from Table 1, a schematic view of the predicted phosphorylation sites in zinc channels is shown in Figure 1. It visualizes that many of the ZIP channels (influx to cytosol) and ZnT channels (efflux from cytosol) can be potentially phosphorylated by CK2. While some of these sites are likely not regulatory in nature (due to their extracellular location), some may indeed regulate the activity of the transporter as is seen in the case of ZIP7 [15].

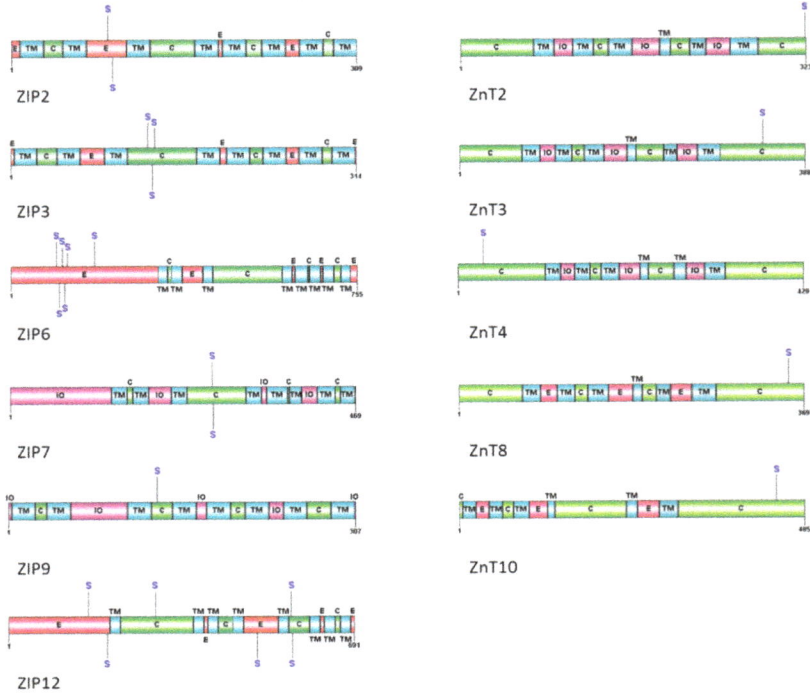

Figure 1. Schematic view of the phosphorylation sites in ZIP and ZnT channels predicted to be phosphorylated by CK2. CK2 phosphorylation sites were predicted using GPS 3.0 software. Transmembrane domains are identified according to Uniprot (http://www.uniprot.org) and the original publications for ZIP2 [84], ZIP3 [84], ZIP6 [84,85], ZIP7 [84,85], ZIP9, ZIP12 [86]. The six TM domains of ZnT2, 3, 4, 8 and 10 are based on an atomic-resolution structure of YiiP [87,88]. TM denotes transmembrane (blue), E for extracellular (red), C for cytoplasmic (green), IO for intra-organellar, S for serine.

5. Metal Transporters Regulated by CK2 Are Potential Therapeutic Targets

In the process of developing therapeutic agents, one of the first steps is to identify a suitable molecular target. For successful precedents, one need look no further than the case of calcium channels. Voltage-gated calcium channels regulate abundant biological functions across various systems and tissues, and numerous drugs have been developed to manipulate calcium channels for treating heart diseases [89–91]. Zinc channels and their regulators are also emerging targets.

Zinc is reported to have proliferative and anti-apoptotic properties [92], whilst some reports show that zinc can also be pro-apoptotic [93]. It is becoming clear that the effects of zinc are concentration and tissue specific. It is for these reasons that the role of zinc in cancer is a somewhat enigmatic one. As previously mentioned, zinc levels vary in different cancers. It has been shown that the zinc level is lower in cancers such as ovarian [67], prostate [94] and hepatocellular cancers [69]. This reduction of zinc has, in the case of prostate and hepatocellular cancers, been linked to altered expression of ZIP channels [95]. Intriguingly, zinc was found to induce apoptosis in these three malignancies [96–98].

In contrast to the above-mentioned cancers, the level of zinc was shown to be markedly increased in cancers such as breast [99,100] and pancreatic cancers [68]. In both cases, the abnormal zinc level was linked to ZIP transporters and this increased zinc level was found to contribute to cancer progression [68,101–104]. In the case of pancreatic cancer, depletion of zinc was found to cause apoptosis [105,106].

While these studies demonstrate contrasting roles for zinc in cancerous tissues, they all point to the fact that zinc channels or the mechanisms that regulate them are potential therapeutic targets for a variety of cancers. We have shown that CK2 is involved in the homeostasis and toxicity of zinc in mouse neuroblastoma cells by a mechanism somewhat similar to *S. cerevisiae* [64], indicating evolutionary conservation. Distribution and availability of zinc is linked to CK2, not only through our studies, but through the work of others [15,82]. Therefore, not just for its roles in cell proliferation but also as a regulator of metal ion homeostasis, CK2 itself should be explored for development of therapeutic agents.

6. Future Perspective

The functional pleiotropism of protein kinase CK2 accentuates the notion that CK2 is at the centre of cellular concatenation, the intricacy of which is still open for delineation. Many questions exist, such as how CK2 regulates metal toxicity. Identification of CK2 substrates, in the context of metal exposure, should be a worthwhile undertaking for future research and drug development. The distinctive effect of CK2 subunits on metal toxicity may serve as a useful tool in understanding the structure and function of the enzyme. We envisage that the current understanding of the role of CK2 in metal transport is merely a prelude to major discoveries in times to come.

Conflicts of Interest: The authors declare no conflict of interest.

References

1. Burnett, G.; Kennedy, E.P. The enzymatic phosphorylation of proteins. *J. Biol. Chem.* **1954**, *211*, 969–980. [PubMed]
2. Fabbro, D.; Cowan-Jacob, S.W.; Moebitz, H. Ten things you should know about protein kinases: IUPHAR Review 14. *Br. J. Pharmacol.* **2015**, *172*, 2675–2700. [CrossRef] [PubMed]
3. Krebs, E.G.; Fischer, E.H. Phosphorylase activity of skeletal muscle extracts. *J. Biol. Chem.* **1955**, *216*, 113–120. [PubMed]
4. Pinna, L. A historical view of protein kinase CK2. *Cell. Mol. Biol. Res.* **1993**, *40*, 383–390.
5. Meggio, F.; Pinna, L.A. One-thousand-and-one substrates of protein kinase CK2? *FASEB J.* **2003**, *17*, 349–368. [CrossRef] [PubMed]
6. Litchfield, D.W. Protein kinase CK2: Structure, regulation and role in cellular decisions of life and death. *Biochem. J.* **2003**, *369 Pt 1*, 1–15. [CrossRef] [PubMed]
7. Allende, J.E.; Allende, C.C. Protein kinases. 4. Protein kinase CK2: An enzyme with multiple substrates and a puzzling regulation. *FASEB J.* **1995**, *9*, 313–323. [PubMed]
8. Venerando, A.; Ruzzene, M.; Pinna, L.A. Casein kinase: The triple meaning of a misnomer. *Biochem. J.* **2014**, *460*, 141–156. [CrossRef] [PubMed]
9. Antonelli, M.; Daniotti, J.L.; Rojo, D.; Allende, C.C.; Allende, J.E. Cloning, expression and properties of the a' subunit of casein kinase 2 from zebrafish (*Danio rerio*). *Eur. J. Biochem.* **1996**, *241*, 272–279. [CrossRef] [PubMed]
10. Niefind, K.; Putter, M.; Guerra, B.; Issinger, O.G.; Schomburg, D. GTP plus water mimic ATP in the active site of protein kinase CK2. *Nat. Struct. Biol.* **1999**, *6*, 1100–1103. [CrossRef] [PubMed]
11. Pinna, L.A. The raison d'etre of constitutively active protein kinases: The Lesson of CK2. *Acc. Chem. Res.* **2003**, *36*, 378–384. [CrossRef] [PubMed]
12. Kappes, F.; Damoc, C.; Knippers, R.; Przybylski, M.; Pinna, L.A.; Gruss, C. Phosphorylation by protein kinase CK2 changes the DNA binding properties of the human chromatin protein DEK. *Mol. Cell. Biol.* **2004**, *24*, 6011–6020. [CrossRef] [PubMed]
13. Guerra, B.; Issinger, O.G. Protein kinase CK2 and its role in cellular proliferation, development and pathology. *Electrophoresis* **1999**, *20*, 391–408. [CrossRef]

14. Tun, N.; O'Doherty, P.; Chen, Z.; Wu, X.; Bailey, T.; Kersaitis, C.; Wu, M. Identification of aluminium transport-related genes via genome-wide phenotypic screening of *Saccharomyces cerevisiae*. *Metallomics* **2014**, *6*, 1558–1564. [CrossRef] [PubMed]

15. Taylor, K.M.; Hiscox, S.; Nicholson, R.I.; Hogstrand, C.; Kille, P. Protein kinase CK2 triggers cytosolic zinc signaling pathways by phosphorylation of zinc channel ZIP7. *Sci. Signal.* **2012**, *5*, ra11. [CrossRef] [PubMed]

16. Bischoff, N.; Olsen, B.; Raaf, J.; Bretner, M.; Issinger, O.-G.; Niefind, K. Structure of the human protein kinase CK2 catalytic subunit CK2α' and interaction thermodynamics with the regulatory subunit CK2β. *J. Mol. Biol.* **2011**, *407*, 1–12. [CrossRef] [PubMed]

17. Niefind, K.; Guerra, B.; Ermakowa, I.; Issinger, O.G. Crystal structure of human protein kinase CK2: Insights into basic properties of the CK2 holoenzyme. *EMBO J.* **2001**, *20*, 5320–5331. [CrossRef] [PubMed]

18. Guerra, B.; Niefind, K.; Ermakowa, I.; Issinger, O.-G. Characterization of CK2 holoenzyme variants with regard to crystallization. *Mol. Cell. Biochem.* **2001**, *227*, 3–11. [CrossRef] [PubMed]

19. Schnitzler, A.; Olsen, B.; Issinger, O.-G.; Niefind, K. The protein kinase CK2 (Andante) holoenzyme structure supports proposed models of autoregulation and trans-autophosphorylation. *J. Mol. Biol.* **2014**, *426*, 1871–1882. [CrossRef] [PubMed]

20. Shi, Y.; Brown, E.D.; Walsh, C.T. Expression of recombinant human casein kinase II and recombinant heat shock protein 90 in *Escherichia coli* and characterization of their interactions. *Proc. Natl. Acad. Sci. USA* **1994**, *91*, 2767–2771. [CrossRef] [PubMed]

21. Pechkova, E.; Zanotti, G.; Nicolini, C. Three-dimensional atomic structure of a catalytic subunit mutant of human protein kinase CK2. *Acta Crystallogr.* **2003**, *59 Pt 12*, 2133–2139. [CrossRef]

22. Chantalat, L.; Leroy, D.; Filhol, O.; Nueda, A.; Benitez, M.J.; Chambaz, E.M.; Cochet, C.; Dideberg, O. Crystal structure of the human protein kinase CK2 regulatory subunit reveals its zinc finger-mediated dimerization. *EMBO J.* **1999**, *18*, 2930–2940. [CrossRef] [PubMed]

23. Raaf, J.; Brunstein, E.; Issinger, O.G.; Niefind, K. The interaction of CK2α and CK2β, the subunits of protein kinase CK2, requires CK2β in a preformed conformation and is enthalpically driven. *Protein Sci.* **2008**, *17*, 2180–2186. [CrossRef] [PubMed]

24. Mazzorana, M.; Pinna, L.; Battistutta, R. A structural insight into CK2 inhibition. *Mol. Cell. Biochem.* **2008**, *316*, 57–62. [CrossRef] [PubMed]

25. Pinna, L.A.; Meggio, F. Protein kinase CK2 ("casein kinase-2") and its implication in cell division and proliferation. *Prog. Cell Cycle Res.* **1997**, *3*, 77–97. [PubMed]

26. Pinna, L.A. Casein kinase 2: An 'eminence grise' in cellular regulation? *Biochim. Biophys. Acta* **1990**, *24*, 267–284. [CrossRef]

27. Blanquet, P.R. Casein kinase 2 as a potentially important enzyme in the nervous system. *Prog. Neurobiol.* **2000**, *60*, 211–246. [CrossRef]

28. Perez, D.I.; Gil, C.; Martinez, A. Protein kinases CK1 and CK2 as new targets for neurodegenerative diseases. *Med. Res. Rev.* **2010**, *31*, 924–954. [CrossRef] [PubMed]

29. Faust, M.; Montenarh, M. Subcellular localization of protein kinase CK2. A key to its function? *Cell Tissue Res.* **2000**, *301*, 329–340. [CrossRef] [PubMed]

30. Bibby, A.C.; Litchfield, D.W. The multiple personalities of the regulatory subunit of protein kinase CK2: CK2 dependent and CK2 independent roles reveal a secret identity for CK2beta. *Int. J. Biol. Sci.* **2005**, *1*, 67–79. [CrossRef] [PubMed]

31. Boldyreff, B.; Issinger, O.G. A-Raf kinase is a new interacting partner of protein kinase CK2 beta subunit. *FEBS Lett.* **1997**, *403*, 197–199. [CrossRef]

32. Guerra, B.; Boldyreff, B.; Sarno, S.; Cesaro, L.; Issinger, O.G.; Pinna, L.A. CK2: A protein kinase in need of control. *Pharmacol. Ther.* **1999**, *82*, 303–313. [CrossRef]

33. Cochet, C.; Chambaz, E.M. Oligomeric structure and catalytic activity of G type casein kinase. Isolation of the two subunits and renaturation experiments. *J. Biol. Chem.* **1983**, *258*, 1403–1406. [PubMed]

34. Kubiński, K.; Domańska, K.; Sajnaga, E.; Mazur, E.; Zieliński, R.; Szyszka, R. Yeast holoenzyme of protein kinase CK2 requires both β and β' regulatory subunits for its activity. *Mol. Cell. Biochem.* **2007**, *295*, 229–236. [CrossRef] [PubMed]

35. Hartwell, L.H.; Mortimer, R.K.; Culotti, J.; Culotti, M. Genetic control of the cell division cycle in yeast: V. genetic analysis of *cdc* mutants. *Genetics* **1973**, *74*, 267–286. [CrossRef]

36. Lee, M.G.; Nurse, P. Complementation used to clone a human homologue of the fission yeast cell cycle control gene *cdc2*. *Nature* **1987**, *327*, 31–35. [CrossRef] [PubMed]
37. Loewith, R. A brief history of TOR. *Biochem. Soc. Trans.* **2011**, *39*, 437–442. [CrossRef] [PubMed]
38. Heitman, J.; Movva, N.; Hall, M. Targets for cell cycle arrest by the immunosuppressant rapamycin in yeast. *Science* **1991**, *253*, 905–909. [CrossRef] [PubMed]
39. Padmanabha, R.; Chen-Wu, J.; Hanna, D.; Glover, C. Isolation, sequencing, and disruption of the yeast CKA2 gene: Casein kinase II is essential for viability in *Saccharomyces cerevisiae*. *Mol. Cell. Biol.* **1990**, *10*, 4089–4099. [CrossRef] [PubMed]
40. Johnson, A.J.; Veljanoski, F.; O'Doherty, P.J.; Zaman, M.S.; Petersingham, G.; Bailey, T.D.; Munch, G.; Kersaitis, C.; Wu, M.J. Revelation of molecular basis for chromium toxicity by phenotypes of *Saccharomyces cerevisiae* gene deletion mutants. *Metallomics* **2016**, *8*, 542–550. [CrossRef] [PubMed]
41. Rethinaswamy, A.; Birnbaum, M.J.; Glover, C.V.C. Temperature-sensitive mutations of the *CKA1* gene reveal a role for casein kinase II in maintenance of cell polarity in *Saccharomyces cerevisiae*. *J. Biol. Chem.* **1998**, *273*, 5869–5877. [CrossRef] [PubMed]
42. Blond, O.; Jensen, H.; Buchou, T.; Cochet, C.; Issinger, O.-G.; Boldyreff, B. Knocking out the regulatory b subunit of protein kinase CK2 in mice: Gene dosage effects in ES cells and embryos. *Mol. Cell. Biochem.* **2005**, *274*, 31–37. [CrossRef] [PubMed]
43. Xu, X.; Toselli, P.A.; Russell, L.D.; Seldin, D.C. Globozoospermia in mice lacking the casein kinase II a' catalytic subunit. *Nat. Genet.* **1999**, *23*, 118–121. [PubMed]
44. Lou, D.Y.; Dominguez, I.; Toselli, P.; Landesman-Bollag, E.; O'Brien, C.; Seldin, D.C. The alpha catalytic subunit of protein kinase CK2 is required for mouse embryonic development. *Mol. Cell. Biol.* **2008**, *28*, 131–139. [CrossRef] [PubMed]
45. Trembley, J.H.; Wang, G.; Unger, G.; Slaton, J.; Ahmed, K. Protein kinase CK2 in health and disease: CK2: A key player in cancer biology. *Cell. Mol. Life Sci.* **2009**, *66*, 1858–1867. [CrossRef] [PubMed]
46. Filhol, O.; Nueda, A.; Martel, V.; Gerber-Scokaert, D.; Benitez, M.J.; Souchie, C.; Saoudi, Y.; Cochet, C. Live-cell fluorescence imaging reveals the dynamics of protein kinase CK2 individual subunits. *Mol. Cell. Biol.* **2003**, *23*, 975–987. [CrossRef] [PubMed]
47. Kalathur, M.; Toso, A.; Chen, J.; Revandkar, A.; Danzer-Baltzer, C.; Guccini, I.; Alajati, A.; Sarti, M.; Pinton, S.; Brambilla, L.; et al. A chemogenomic screening identifies CK2 as a target for pro-senescence therapy in PTEN-deficient tumours. *Nat. Commun.* **2015**, *6*, 7227. [CrossRef] [PubMed]
48. Hathaway, G.M.; Lubben, T.H.; Traugh, J.A. Inhibition of casein kinase II by heparin. *J. Biol. Chem.* **1980**, *255*, 8038–8041. [PubMed]
49. Gatica, M.; Hinrichs, M.V.; Jedlicki, A.; Allende, C.C.; Allende, J.E. Effect of metal ions on the activity of cascein kinase II from *Xenopus laevis*. *FEBS Lett.* **1993**, *315*, 173–177. [CrossRef]
50. Hathaway, G.M.; Traugh, J.A. Interaction of polyamines and magnesium with casein kinase II. *Arch. Biochem. Biophys.* **1984**, *233*, 133–138. [CrossRef]
51. Jiménez, J.; Benítez, M.; Lechuga, C.; Collado, M.; González-Nicólas, J.; Moreno, F. Casein kinase 2 inactivation by Mg^{2+}, Mn^{2+} and Co^{2+} ions. *Mol. Cell. Biochem.* **1995**, *152*, 1–6. [PubMed]
52. Botstein, D.; Fink, G.R. Yeast: An experimental organism for 21st century biology. *Genetics* **2011**, *189*, 695–704. [CrossRef] [PubMed]
53. Goffeau, A.; Barrell, B.; Bussey, H.; Davis, R.; Dujon, B.; Feldmann, H.; Galibert, F.; Hoheisel, J.; Jacq, C.; Johnston, M. Life with 6000 genes. *Science* **1996**, *274*, 546–567. [CrossRef] [PubMed]
54. Arita, A.; Zhou, X.; Ellen, T.P.; Liu, X.; Bai, J.; Rooney, J.P.; Kurtz, A.; Klein, C.B.; Dai, W.; Begley, T.J.; et al. A genome-wide deletion mutant screen identifies pathways affected by nickel sulfate in *Saccharomyces cerevisiae*. *BMC Genom.* **2009**, *10*, 524. [CrossRef] [PubMed]
55. Marmiroli, M.; Pagano, L.; Pasquali, F.; Zappettini, A.; Tosato, V.; Bruschi, C.V.; Marmiroli, N. A genome-wide nanotoxicology screen of *Saccharomyces cerevisiae* mutants reveals the basis for cadmium sulphide quantum dot tolerance and sensitivity. *Nanotoxicology* **2015**, *10*, 84–93. [PubMed]
56. Johnson, A.J.; Veljanoski, F.; O'Doherty, P.J.; Zaman, M.S.; Petersingham, G.; Bailey, T.D.; Munch, G.; Kersaitis, C.; Wu, M.J. Molecular insight into arsenic toxicity via the genome-wide deletion mutant screening of *Saccharomyces cerevisiae*. *Metallomics* **2016**, *8*, 228–235. [CrossRef] [PubMed]

57. Thorsen, M.; Perrone, G.; Kristiansson, E.; Traini, M.; Ye, T.; Dawes, I.; Nerman, O.; Tamas, M. Genetic basis of arsenite and cadmium tolerance in *Saccharomyces cerevisiae*. *BMC Genom.* **2009**, *10*, 105. [CrossRef] [PubMed]

58. Du, J.; Cao, C.; Jiang, L. Genome-scale genetic screen of lead ion-sensitive gene deletion mutations in *Saccharomyces cerevisiae*. *Gene* **2015**, *563*, 155–159. [CrossRef] [PubMed]

59. Tun, N.M.; Lennon, B.R.; O'Doherty, P.J.; Johnson, A.J.; Petersingham, G.; Bailey, T.D.; Kersaitis, C.; Wu, M.J. Effects of metal ions and hydrogen peroxide on the phenotype of yeast *hom6Δ* mutant. *Lett. Appl. Microbiol.* **2015**, *60*, 20–26. [CrossRef] [PubMed]

60. Kachroo, A.H.; Laurent, J.M.; Yellman, C.M.; Meyer, A.G.; Wilke, C.O.; Marcotte, E.M. Systematic humanization of yeast genes reveals conserved functions and genetic modularity. *Science* **2015**, *348*, 921–925. [CrossRef] [PubMed]

61. O'Brien, K.P.; Remm, M.; Sonnhammer, E.L.L. Inparanoid: A comprehensive database of eukaryotic orthologs. *Nucleic Acids Res.* **2005**, *33*, D476–D480. [CrossRef] [PubMed]

62. Simon, J.A.; Bedalov, A. Yeast as a model system for anticancer drug discovery. *Nat. Rev. Cancer* **2004**, *4*, 481–487. [CrossRef] [PubMed]

63. Mager, W.H.; Winderickx, J. Yeast as a model for medical and medicinal research. *Trends Pharmacol. Sci.* **2005**, *26*, 265–273. [CrossRef] [PubMed]

64. Zaman, M.S.; Johnson, A.J.; Bobek, G.; Kueh, S.; Kersaitis, C.; Bailey, T.D.; Buskila, Y.; Wu, M.J. Protein kinase CK2 regulates metal toxicity in neuronal cells. *Metallomics* **2016**, *8*, 82–90. [CrossRef] [PubMed]

65. Alam, S.; Kelleher, S.L. Cellular mechanisms of zinc dysregulation: A perspective on zinc homeostasis as an etiological factor in the development and progression of breast cancer. *Nutrients* **2012**, *4*, 875–903. [CrossRef] [PubMed]

66. Song, Y.; Ho, E. Zinc and prostatic cancer. *Curr. Opin. Clin. Nutr. Metab. Care* **2009**, *12*, 640–645.

67. Lightman, A.; Brandes, J.M.; Binur, N.; Drugan, A.; Zinder, O. Use of the serum copper/zinc ratio in the differential diagnosis of ovarian malignancy. *Clin. Chem.* **1986**, *32*, 101–103. [PubMed]

68. Li, M.; Zhang, Y.; Liu, Z.; Bharadwaj, U.; Wang, H.; Wang, X.; Zhang, S.; Liuzzi, J.P.; Chang, S.-M.; Cousins, R.J. Aberrant expression of zinc transporter ZIP4 (SLC39A4) significantly contributes to human pancreatic cancer pathogenesis and progression. *Proc. Natl. Acad. Sci. USA* **2007**, *104*, 18636–18641. [CrossRef] [PubMed]

69. Ebara, M.; Fukuda, H.; Hatano, R.; Saisho, H.; Nagato, Y.; Suzuki, K.; Nakajima, K.; Yukawa, M.; Kondo, F.; Nakayama, A. Relationship between copper, zinc and metallothionein in hepatocellular carcinoma and its surrounding liver parenchyma. *J. Hepatol.* **2000**, *33*, 415–422. [CrossRef]

70. Eide, D.J. The molecular biology of metal ion transport in *Saccharomyces cerevisiae*. *Annu. Rev. Nutr.* **1998**, *18*, 441–469. [CrossRef] [PubMed]

71. Maret, W. Zinc biochemistry: From a single zinc enzyme to a key element of life. *Adv. Nutr.* **2013**, *4*, 82–91. [CrossRef] [PubMed]

72. Nelson, N. Metal ion transporters and homeostasis. *EMBO J.* **1999**, *18*, 4361–4371. [CrossRef] [PubMed]

73. Zatta, P.; Drago, D.; Bolognin, S.; Sensi, S.L. Alzheimer's disease, metal ions and metal homeostatic therapy. *Trends Pharmacol. Sci.* **2009**, *30*, 346–355. [CrossRef] [PubMed]

74. Jin, Y.H.; Dunlap, P.E.; McBride, S.J.; Al-Refai, H.; Bushel, P.R.; Freedman, J.H. Global transcriptome and deletome profiles of yeast exposed to transition metals. *PLoS Genet.* **2008**, *4*, e1000053. [CrossRef] [PubMed]

75. Yu, D.; Danku, J.M.; Baxter, I.; Kim, S.; Vatamaniuk, O.; Vitek, O.; Ouzzani, M.; Salt, D. High-resolution genome-wide scan of genes, gene-networks and cellular systems impacting the yeast ionome. *BMC Genom.* **2012**, *13*, 623. [CrossRef] [PubMed]

76. Ye, J.; Shi, X. Gene expression profile in response to chromium-induced cell stress in A549 cells. *Mol. Cell. Biochem.* **2001**, *222*, 189–197. [CrossRef] [PubMed]

77. Tang, F.; Liu, G.; He, Z.; Ma, W.Y.; Bode, A.M.; Dong, Z. Arsenite inhibits p53 phosphorylation, DNA binding activity, and p53 target gene p21 expression in mouse epidermal JB6 cells. *Mol. Carcinog.* **2006**, *45*, 861–870. [CrossRef] [PubMed]

78. Bachhuber, T.; Almaça, J.; Aldehni, F.; Mehta, A.; Amaral, M.D.; Schreiber, R.; Kunzelmann, K. Regulation of the epithelial Na$^+$ channel by the protein kinase CK2. *J. Biol. Chem.* **2008**, *283*, 13225–13232. [CrossRef] [PubMed]

79. De Stefano, D.; Villella, V.; Esposito, S.; Tosco, A.; Sepe, A.; de Gregorio, F.; Salvadori, L.; Grassia, R.; Leone, C.; de Rosa, G.; et al. Restoration of CFTR function in patients with cystic fibrosis carrying the F508del-CFTR mutation. *Autophagy* **2014**, *10*, 2053–2074. [CrossRef] [PubMed]

80. Venerando, A.; Pagano, M.A.; Tosoni, K.; Meggio, F.; Cassidy, D.; Stobbart, M.; Pinna, L.A.; Mehta, A. Understanding protein kinase CK2 mis-regulation upon F508del CFTR expression. *Naunyn Schmiedebergs Arch. Pharmacol.* **2011**, *384*, 473–488. [CrossRef] [PubMed]

81. Treharne, K.J.; Xu, Z.; Chen, J.-H.; Best, O.G.; Cassidy, D.M.; Gruenert, D.C.; Hegyi, P.; Gray, M.A.; Sheppard, D.N.; Kunzelmann, K.; et al. Inhibition of protein kinase CK2 closes the CFTR Cl⁻ channel, but has no effect on the cystic fibrosis mutant ΔF508-CFTR. *Cell. Physiol. Biochem.* **2009**, *24*, 347–360. [CrossRef] [PubMed]

82. Adams, T.K.; Saydam, N.; Steiner, F.; Schaffner, W.; Freedman, J.H. Activation of gene expression by metal-responsive signal transduction pathways. *Environ. Health Perspect.* **2002**, *110* (Suppl. 5), S813–S817. [CrossRef]

83. Xue, Y.; Ren, J.; Gao, X.; Jin, C.; Wen, L.; Yao, X. GPS 2.0, a tool to predict kinase-specific phosphorylation sites in hierarchy. *Mol. Cell. Proteom.* **2008**, *7*, 1598–1608. [CrossRef] [PubMed]

84. Wang, K.; Zhou, B.; Kuo, Y.-M.; Zemansky, J.; Gitschier, J. A novel member of a zinc transporter family is defective in acrodermatitis enteropathica. *Am. J. Hum. Genet.* **2002**, *71*, 66–73. [CrossRef] [PubMed]

85. Taylor, K.M.; Muraina, I.A.; Brethour, D.; Schmitt-Ulms, G.; Nimmanon, T.; Ziliotto, S.; Kille, P.; Hogstrand, C. Zinc transporter ZIP10 forms a heteromer with ZIP6 which regulates embryonic development and cell migration. *Biochem. J.* **2016**, *473*, 2531–2544. [CrossRef] [PubMed]

86. Schmitt-Ulms, G.; Ehsani, S.; Watts, J.C.; Westaway, D.; Wille, H. Evolutionary descent of prion genes from the ZIP family of metal ion transporters. *PLoS ONE* **2009**, *4*, e7208. [CrossRef] [PubMed]

87. Huang, L.; Tepaamorndech, S. The SLC30 family of zinc transporters—A review of current understanding of their biological and pathophysiological roles. *Mol. Asp. Med.* **2013**, *34*, 548–560. [CrossRef] [PubMed]

88. Lu, M.; Fu, D. Structure of the zinc transporter YiiP. *Science* **2007**, *317*, 1746–1748. [CrossRef] [PubMed]

89. Monteith, G.R.; Davis, F.M.; Roberts-Thomson, S.J. Calcium channels and pumps in cancer: Changes and consequences. *J. Biol. Chem.* **2012**, *287*, 31666–31673. [CrossRef] [PubMed]

90. Mahe, I.; Chassany, O.; Grenard, A.S.; Caulin, C.; Bergmann, J.F. Defining the role of calcium channel antagonists in heart failure due to systolic dysfunction. *Am. J. Cardiovasc. Drugs* **2003**, *3*, 33–41. [PubMed]

91. Inzitari, M.; Di Bari, M.; Marchionni, N. Calcium channel blockers and coronary heart disease. *Aging Clin. Exp. Res.* **2005**, *17*, S6–S15.

92. Chai, F.; Truong-Tran, A.Q.; Ho, L.H.; Zalewski, P.D. Regulation of caspase activation and apoptosis by cellular zinc fluxes and zinc deprivation: A review. *Immunol. Cell Biol.* **1999**, *77*, 272–278. [CrossRef] [PubMed]

93. Chang, K.-L.; Hung, T.-C.; Hsieh, B.-S.; Chen, Y.-H.; Chen, T.-F.; Cheng, H.-L. Zinc at pharmacologic concentrations affects cytokine expression and induces apoptosis of human peripheral blood mononuclear cells. *Nutrition* **2006**, *22*, 465–474. [CrossRef] [PubMed]

94. Costello, L.C.; Franklin, R.B. The clinical relevance of the metabolism of prostate cancer; zinc and tumor suppression: Connecting the dots. *Mol. Cancer* **2006**, *5*, 17. [CrossRef] [PubMed]

95. Liu, Y.; Zhu, X.; Zhu, J.; Liao, S.; Tang, Q.; Liu, K.; Guan, X.; Zhang, J.; Feng, Z. Identification of differential expression of genes in hepatocellular carcinoma by suppression subtractive hybridization combined cDNA microarray. *Oncol. Rep.* **2007**, *18*, 943–952. [CrossRef] [PubMed]

96. Bae, S.N.; Lee, Y.S.; Kim, M.Y.; Kim, J.D.; Park, L.O. Antiproliferative and apoptotic effects of zinc–citrate compound (CIZAR®) on human epithelial ovarian cancer cell line, OVCAR-3. *Gynecol. Oncol.* **2006**, *103*, 127–136. [CrossRef] [PubMed]

97. Liang, J.-Y.; Liu, Y.-Y.; Zou, J.; Franklin, R.B.; Costello, L.C.; Feng, P. Inhibitory effect of zinc on human prostatic carcinoma cell growth. *Prostate* **1999**, *40*, 200–207. [CrossRef]

98. Xu, J.; Xu, Y.; Nguyen, Q.; Novikoff, P.M.; Czaja, M.J. Induction of hepatoma cell apoptosis by c-myc requires zinc and occurs in the absence of DNA fragmentation. *Am. J. Physiol. Gastrointest. Liver Physiol.* **1996**, *270*, G60–G70.

99. Margalioth, E.J.; Schenker, J.G.; Chevion, M. Copper and zinc levels in normal and malignant tissues. *Cancer* **1983**, *52*, 868–872. [CrossRef]

100. Rizk, S.L.; Sky-Peck, H.H. Comparison between concentrations of trace elements in normal and neoplastic human breast tissue. *Cancer Res.* **1984**, *44*, 5390–5394. [PubMed]
101. Kagara, N.; Tanaka, N.; Noguchi, S.; Hirano, T. Zinc and its transporter ZIP10 are involved in invasive behavior of breast cancer cells. *Cancer Sci.* **2007**, *98*, 692–697. [CrossRef] [PubMed]
102. Manning, D.; Robertson, J.; Ellis, I.; Elston, C.; McClelland, R.A.; Gee, J.M.W.; Jones, R.; Green, C.; Cannon, P.; Blamey, R. Oestrogen-regulated genes in breast cancer: Association of pLIV1 with lymph node involvement. *Eur. J. Cancer* **1994**, *30*, 675–678. [CrossRef]
103. Manning, D.L.; McClelland, R.A.; Knowlden, J.M.; Bryant, S.; Gee, J.M.; Green, C.D.; Robertson, J.F.; Blamey, R.W.; Sutherland, R.L.; Ormandy, C.J. Differential expression of oestrogen regulated genes in breast cancer. *Acta Oncol.* **1995**, *34*, 641–646. [CrossRef] [PubMed]
104. Taylor, K.M.; Morgan, H.E.; Smart, K.; Zahari, N.M.; Pumford, S.; Ellis, I.O.; Robertson, J.F.; Nicholson, R.I. The emerging role of the LIV-1 subfamily of zinc transporters in breast cancer. *Mol. Med.* **2007**, *13*, 396–406. [CrossRef] [PubMed]
105. Donadelli, M.; Dalla Pozza, E.; Costanzo, C.; Scupoli, M.; Scarpa, A.; Palmieri, M. Zinc depletion efficiently inhibits pancreatic cancer cell growth by increasing the ratio of antiproliferative/proliferative genes. *J. Cell. Biochem.* **2008**, *104*, 202–212. [CrossRef] [PubMed]
106. Franklin, R.B.; Costello, L.C. The important role of the apoptotic effects of zinc in the development of cancers. *J. Cell. Biochem.* **2009**, *106*, 750–757. [CrossRef] [PubMed]

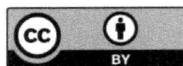

Chapter 2:
CK2 as a therapeutic target

pharmaceuticals

MDPI

Review

CK2—An Emerging Target for Neurological and Psychiatric Disorders

Julia Castello [1,2], Andre Ragnauth [1,3], Eitan Friedman [1,2] and Heike Rebholz [1,*]

1 Department of Physiology, Pharmacology and Neuroscience,
   City University of New York School of Medicine, New York, NY 10031, USA;
   julia.csaval@gmail.com (J.C.); Andre.Ragnauth@gmail.com (A.R.); Friedman@med.cuny.edu (E.F.)
2 Ph.D. Programs in Biochemistry and Biology, The Graduate Center, City University of New York,
   New York, NY 10031, USA
3 Ph.D. Programs at Queens College, City University of New York, New York, NY 11367, USA
* Correspondence: hrebholz@med.cuny.edu; Tel.: +1-212-650-8283

Academic Editor: Lorenzo A. Pinna
Received: 30 November 2016; Accepted: 30 December 2016; Published: 5 January 2017

Abstract: Protein kinase CK2 has received a surge of attention in recent years due to the evidence of its overexpression in a variety of solid tumors and multiple myelomas as well as its participation in cell survival pathways. CK2 is also upregulated in the most prevalent and aggressive cancer of brain tissue, glioblastoma multiforme, and in preclinical models, pharmacological inhibition of the kinase has proven successful in reducing tumor size and animal mortality. CK2 is highly expressed in the mammalian brain and has many bona fide substrates that are crucial in neuronal or glial homeostasis and signaling processes across synapses. Full and conditional CK2 knockout mice have further elucidated the importance of CK2 in brain development, neuronal activity, and behavior. This review will discuss recent advances in the field that point to CK2 as a regulator of neuronal functions and as a potential novel target to treat neurological and psychiatric disorders.

Keywords: CK2; neurodegeneration; synapse; signaling; CK2 inhibitors; GPCRs; CK2 substrates; CK2 knockout

1. Introduction

CK2 (formerly Casein Kinase 2) is a heterotetrameric kinase consisting of two catalytic (α or α') and two regulatory β subunits. It is constitutively active and ubiquitously expressed.

While in some instances several growth factors and neurotrophins have been shown to boost CK2 activity [1–3], the general consensus to date is that CK2 activity is dependent on its microenvironment within multimolecular complexes which can confer substrate specificity [4] or binding and recruitment to activity-regulated proteins such as, for example, Calmodulin [5,6].

CK2 partakes in signal transduction pathways that are crucial for cell survival such as the AKT pathway. It was shown to directly phosphorylate AKT1 (Ser129) to render AKT more active [7]. CK2 also phosphorylates and inactivates the lipid phosphatase PTEN which, by dephosphorylating phosphatidylinositol-3,4,5-trisphosphate (PIP3), reverses the activation of the AKT pathway [8]. Several other modulators of the AKT pathway are also substrates of CK2, making this kinase, clearly, an influential activator of the survival pathway. Studies have demonstrated that overexpression of CK2 potentiates tumor growth through suppression of apoptosis, promotion of angiogenesis, and signaling through PI3K-AKT, Wnt, and NF-kB [9]. Cancer cells and tissue were also shown to undergo necrosis in the presence of CK2 inhibitor [10].

Based on the minimal substrate consensus sequence that requires an acidic residue at position n + 3 [11,12], it is not too surprising that, to date, 356 proteins have been identified that are phosphorylated in vitro and in vivo by CK2 [13] and, thus, represent a large pool of bona fide substrates, attesting to the important role of CK2 as a multifunctional kinase.

In this review, we focus on recent advances in the characterization of brain-derived CK2 substrates that have been studied in an in vivo context and may have an impact in neurodegenerative disorders. We will discuss these substrates first in their roles in the healthy brain, followed by a section on CK2 in the context of brain disorders, and we point out several instances in which CK2 might prove a valid novel target for the treatment of neurological and neuropsychiatric disorders.

2. CK2 Expression in the Adult Mouse Brain

CK2 is ubiquitously expressed in the periphery, and this is true for the brain as well. However, differences in expression in subregions of the brain, both on the transcript level, as can be derived from the Allen Brain Atlas, as well as on the level of protein have been observed [14,15]. Discerning the expression pattern of the individual subunits, CK2β mRNA levels do not appear balanced to the amounts of the combined CK2α and CK2α′ expression, but reflects CKα′ expression more closely. On the protein level, throughout the brain, there is a predominance of α over α′ subunits [14]. For example, in mouse striatum, a region of particular interest due to its role in movement control and reward processing, the molar ratio of CK2α:CK2α′ is 8:1. Even in the region with the highest CK2α′ protein level (hippocampus), the ratio of CK2α:CK2α′ (4:1) favors CK2α. Now, we are adding to the in situ hybridization and western blotting data immunohistochemical analyses of CK2α, α′ and β in adult mouse sagittal slices. These images depict protein expression at a much more detailed level than western blotting analysis, which is limited by the manual dissection technique. Overall, mRNA levels correspond to protein levels of the different subunits across brain regions (Figure 1A), however, some interesting patterns could be detected.

In the hippocampus, CK2α and CK2α′ proteins are present, and protein expression corresponds to mRNA levels. For CK2β, mRNA levels are the highest in the hippocampus when compared to other brain regions, but at the protein level, CK2β appears absent in dentate gyrus or the CA1, CA2, CA3 regions (Figure 1A, CA2 in higher resolution in Figure 1B). In most other regions, CK2β overlaps fully with CK2α, and we show here the prefrontal cortex as a representative example (Figure 1B′).

We found high expression of the three CK2 subunits in the pontine gray nucleus (PG), a part of the brain stem regulating motor function (Figure 1A). This area, however, is also characterized by high cell density (as visualized with a neuron-specific marker NeuN which is present in all neurons with the exception of cerebellar Purkinje cells, olfactory mitral cells, Cajal-Retzius cells, neurons of the inferior olive, and a few others) that causes the elevated immunosignal [16].

In the olfactory bulb, CK2α is very highly expressed, and, thus, the ratio of CK2α:CK2α′ is elevated to 24:1 [14]. Immunohistochemistry confirms this result. On cellular resolution, CK2β and CK2α co-localize, while CK2α′ is not detected despite significant mRNA levels in that region (Figure 1C). CK2β was counterstained with NeuN; the neuronal marker is absent from the CK2β expressing cells, and by deduction also from CK2α expressing cells. These cells supposedly are olfactory mitral cells which cannot be stained with NeuN [16] (Figure 1C).

When examining the cerebellum, we found CK2α and CK2β to be homogenously present in the large GABAergic Purkinje cells, while CK2α′ is expressed in a scattered manner. All isoforms are sporadically present in the molecular and granular layers of the cerebellar folium (Figure 1D).

The fact that no brain region was found where the CK2α′ level dominates does not imply that CK2α′ does not have a specialized vital function in the brain such as the binding to specific partners or localization to specific microdomains or subcellular structures. In fact, for example, the clustered pattern seen in the Purkinje cells of the cerebellum may be of physiological importance.

It will be interesting to take a closer look at the expression profile on a cellular level, including the use of glial markers and assess the differences in subunit expression in different cell types.

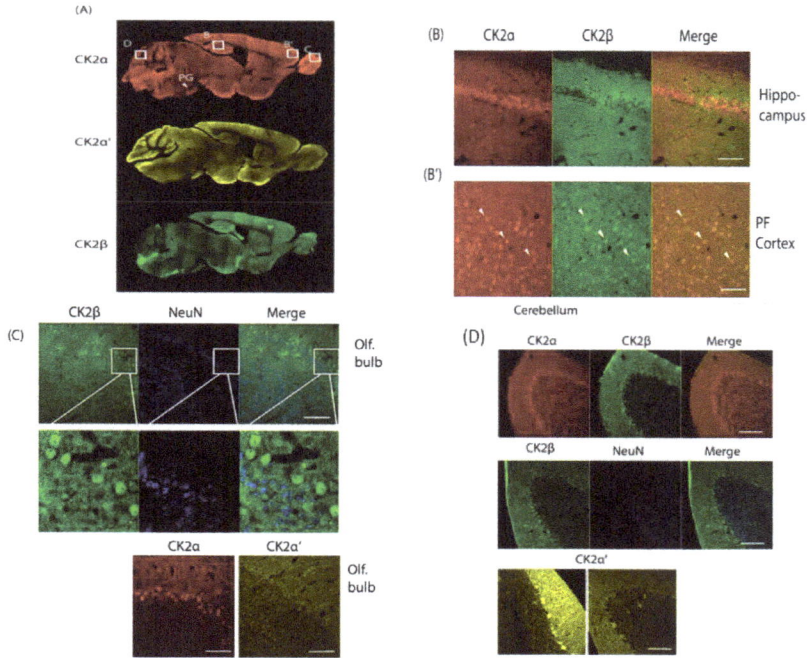

Figure 1. A–D: Immunohistochemical analysis of sagittal brain slices of adult C57BL/6 mice. PFA perfused brains were sliced (40 μm) and incubated with α-CK2α, α-CK2α' (both Abcam), α-CK2β (gift from Dr. O. Filhol Grenoble) and α-NeuN (Cell Signaling) followed by incubation with secondary antibodies, Alexa 546/488 α-rabbit/α-mouse (Fisher Scientific). Imaging was performed using a Zeiss LSM710 laser-scanning confocal microscope. Slices were stained for CK2α, CK2α' and CK2β (**A**), the hippocampal CA1region and PFC were stained for CK2α and CK2β (**B**). Olfactory bulb was stained for CK2β and NeuN, CK2α and CK2α'. (**C**) Cerebellum was stained for CK2α, CK2 β and NeuN (**D**) and for CK2α'. PG: Pontine gray nucleus; white bars = 100 μM.

3. Inhibitors

A multitude of CK2 inhibitors are available, with varying specificities and efficacies [17,18]. Determining the various roles of CK2 in the brain has been difficult in part because of the poor permeability of chemical CK2 inhibitors into the brain due to the blood brain barrier (BBB). This interface separates the brain from the circulatory system, protects it from the influx of potentially harmful chemicals or organisms, and at the same time enables the transport of essential molecules bi-directionally. It is comprised of endothelial cells as well as astrocytes and pericytes adjacent to small capillaries. The high level of expression of efflux transporters (such as P-glycoprotein) in the BBB further prevents many molecules from reaching the brain. Drugs that can diffuse through the BBB must be of small molecular size (less than 500 Da), highly lipophilic, and not ionized at physiological pH [19]. This is not the case for the more specific CK2 inhibitors such as DMAT, TBB, and CX4945 which are relatively hydrophilic.

Thus far, however, one CK2 inhibitor has proven successful in reducing the growth of glioblastoma implanted intracranially in mice [20]. Mice were administered orally with CX4945, the sole CK2 inhibitor to date that has been proven to be safe and efficient in a clinical phase I/II trial in humans (ClinicalTrials.gov Identifier: NCT02128282). It has been shown that glioblastoma hamper the integrity of the BBB and this may have enabled the systemically administered CX4945 to reach the brain tumor in sufficient quantities [21].

In our laboratory, we have performed dose and time course experiments using intraperitoneal (i.p.) injections of CX4945 in adult mice, followed by Western blotting assessment of several CK2 phosphorylation sites or of sites within the AKT pathway. At doses lower or equal 60 mg/kg, no significant reduction of these sites in striatal and prefrontocortical tissue could be detected, however, at a relatively high dose of 75 mg/kg, 2 h post-injection, the direct pS129 Akt site as well as the pS473 AKT and pS235/236 S6 ribosomal protein sites were reliably reduced, indicating that at this dose in healthy adult mice, with an intact BBB, the compound reached the brain (unpublished data). However, i.p. injection of this dose is not advisable when one aims to study CK2-dependency of certain behaviors since the mice become somewhat rigid, which indicates peripheral or central side effects that need to be further studied. The more preferable means of administration is to infuse the drug via implanted cannulae, allowing for intracranial infusion without the need of concurrent anesthesia.

Bi-substrate CK2 inhibitors, interacting with both the adenosine triphosphate (ATP) and the phospho-acceptor substrate-binding sites have been the latest addition to the collection of CK2 inhibitors. While highly effective [22], thus far, these types of compounds are unable to penetrate cells or the BBB.

New strategies are being developed to overcome the restraints of the BBB, such as the use of liposomal, magnetic, or polymeric nanoparticles that are either coated or conjugated with targeting moieties that enable carrier-, receptor-, and absorption-mediated passage through the BBB (for a review see [19]).

One such example for CK2 is the successful delivery of tenfibgen nanocapsules with a siRNA CK2 cargo via intravenous administration, which resulted in significant xenograft tumor reduction in a mouse model of prostate cancer [23]. Recently, a dual approach was tested: CK2 and epidermal growth factor receptor (EGFR), both of which are overexpressed in glioblastoma [24], were targeted by morpholino oligomeres attached to nanobioconjugates [25], in a mouse model of intracranial human glioblastoma. This lead to increased animal survival and concomitantly reduced pro-survival (AKT, STAT, Wnt) signaling. The nanoconjugates were linked to anti-tranferrin antibody that enabled BBB passage and an anti-EGFR antibody to attach to cancer cells [25]. One could envisage the packaging of CK2 inhibitors into nanocapsules as well.

4. CK2 Knockout Mice

Knockout (KO) mice are in many ways superior to inhibitors when one wants to detect physiological functions of a specific gene product since they allow for deletion or insertion of a specific gene through homologous recombination, thus, not affecting other genes. However, one has to be aware that developmental adaptations may occur, especially in full knockout or conditional models with early embryonic Cre recombinase expression. KO mice have clearly shaped our understanding of the crucial role of CK2 in development: full CK2β knockout mice are embryonic lethal. The embryos are absorbed on embryonic day E7.5 [26]. Conditional CK2β KO mice were generated and crossed with a Nestin-Cre driver to generate mice deficient in CK2β in the central nervous system, but mutant pups died shortly after birth [27]. Interestingly, the CK2β protein was detected in KO mice six days after onset of Cre expression, which could be rationalized by the long stability of the CK2β protein once integrated in the CK2 holoenzyme. It is interesting to note that CK2α expression was not altered in the KO mice [27].

A full CK2α KO mouse line was also generated: while the heterozygous offspring are born at the Mendelian ratio, the homozygous embryos die mid-gestation (E11.5) [28]. The strongest defects were seen in the heart and neural tube, pointing towards an important role of CK2 in brain and heart development. Interestingly, expression of CK2β is reduced while CK2α' expression is unaffected in the CK2α KO [28,29].

CK2α' KO mice are viable and do not exhibit an obvious phenotype. Only homozygous males are infertile because spermatocytes frequently undergo apoptosis or have abnormal heads (as in the human condition globozoospermia) [30]. It is of interest to note that due to the lack of apoptosis-positive cells (TUNEL assay) in the CK2α and CK2β KO embryos, it was suggested that, during embryonic development, CK2α and CK2β are mainly controlling cell proliferation and not apoptotic events [29].

To study the role of CK2 in the brain, we generated CK2α$^{fl/fl}$ and CK2α'$^{fl/fl}$ lines. Mice lacking CK2α' in the forebrain (CK2α'$^{fl/fl}$; CaMKII-Cre) were viable and did not display an obvious behavioral or pathological phenotype. In contrast, neither the CK2α$^{fl/fl}$; CaMKII-Cre or CK2α$^{fl/fl}$; CK2α'$^{fl/fl}$; CaMKII-Cre were viable, the mice died perinatally [14]. CaMKII-Cre has been described as readily detectable at postnatal day three [31], however, due to the perinatal death of our offspring, we suspect that sub-threshold expression already occurs days earlier. The non-viability of the Cre-positive offspring indicates that a short depletion of CK2 activity at the developmental stages around birth is crucial for viability.

We also generated cell-specific neuronal KO mice by crossing the CK2α floxed animals with the Drd1a-Cre or the Drd2-Cre driver lines which leads to ablation of CK2α in the dopamine D1 receptor expressing cells of the striatum and cortex, and in the D2 receptor expressing cells of the striatum and midbrain, respectively. Notably, the double KOs, homozygous for CK2α and α' deletion, were not viable with any of the Cre-driver lines tested. However, the single KOs homozygous for CK2α or α' isoforms were viable with both the Drd1a-Cre and the Drd2-Cre driver mouse lines [32]. Cre expression starts at E16 for the Drd1a-Cre and at E14 for Drd2-Cre [33,34]. Interestingly, expression of the β subunit was not affected in the Drd1a-Cre-CK2α KO while it was significantly reduced in Drd2-Cre CK2 KO.

The Drd1a-Cre CK2 KO mice exhibited distinct behavioral phenotypes including novelty-induced hyperlocomotion and exploratory behavior, defective motor control, and motor learning. These traits are indicative of dysregulated dopamine signaling and were rescued by dopamine D1 receptor antagonist [32]. The underlying mechanisms involved in the phenotype are probably manifold: in addition to altered D1 receptor homeostasis, altered synaptic activity may be involved, since, as will be discussed in the next paragraph, CK2 was shown to regulate several glutamate receptors [5,6,35].

The importance of CK2 in the dopaminergic system is further highlighted by preliminary findings indicating that in a mouse model of Parkinson's disease, a response to the antiparkinsonian drug, L-DOPA, namely uncontrollable dyskinesia, is affected in KO mice (unpublished data).

The floxed CK2α, CK2α' and CK2β mouse lines are amenable to focal knockdown of CK2 since Adeno-associated virus (AAV) or Lentivirus can be used to induce Cre recombinase in small to more widespread areas around an injection site, depending on the viral serotype. This approach will certainly be valuable to address whether a specific brain region mediates certain phenotypes.

5. Brain Specific Substrates

CK2 is a pleiotropic kinase with several hundred potential substrates [36]. Many substrates are not only important in the periphery but have similar roles in the brain. An extensive review of such substrates can be found in [37]. In this section, we aim to discuss in vivo substrates of CK2 that are either specific to the brain or are crucial for healthy brain function. Many of these candidates are also involved in brain disorders and suggest that CK2 could be a valid novel target for pharmacotherapy for such disorders, as will be discussed in Section 6 of this review.

5.1. G Protein Coupled Receptors (GPCRs)

G protein coupled receptors (GPCRs) make up the largest protein family in the human genome and consist of over 800 members [38]. These receptors mediate the biological actions of neurotransmitters, hormones, pheromones, light, and calcium through the activation of one or more of the four G protein families: $G\alpha_{i/o}$, $G\alpha_{q/11}$, $G\alpha_s$, and $G\alpha_{12/13}$. GPCR cell surface expression and coupling to G-proteins are regulated by phosphorylation of their third intracellular loop and/or their C-terminal region by various

Ser-Thr kinases, such as G protein-coupled receptor kinases (GRKs1–7) [39]. Binding of arrestins to phosphorylated receptors results in uncoupling of the receptor, desensitization of the response, and endocytosis of the receptor [39,40]. Second messenger-dependent protein kinases, such as protein kinase A and protein kinase C, or CK1α, are also involved in GPCR desensitization [41]. More recently, CK2 joined the pool of kinases that are capable of phosphorylating GPCRs. Torrecilla et al. showed that the muscarinic M3 acetylcholine receptor is phosphorylated by CK2 in the third intracellular loop upon agonist occupation [42]. However, in this case, no internalization except a signaling switch to a Jun-kinase dependent pathway is induced. In pancreatic ß-cells, CK2 was shown to phosphorylate the same receptor, M3 [43], with the effect of reduced insulin release. Both, CK2 inhibition and knockdown of CK2α in β-cells resulted in M3 receptor-stimulated insulin release. Again, in this case, phosphorylation did not affect receptor internalization or signaling. These two papers demonstrate that CK2 is capable of affecting the same receptor, in different cell types, resulting in different outcomes. The determination as to which outcome phosphorylation has most probably depends on the expression of tissue-specific proteins and/or on the specific phosphorylation site.

A different involvement of CK2 in the regulation of GPCRs in the brain was identified following a yeast-two-hybrid screen which yielded the G protein subunit $G\alpha_s$ as a CK2β interacting partner in cultured cells and in brain tissue. The complex also contained CK2α, indicating that the CK2 holoenzyme is bound to $G\alpha_s$ [44]. The interaction was specific to $G\alpha_s$ since no other Gα subunit precipitated with CK2β. Functionally, this interaction suggests negative regulation by CK2 of $G\alpha_s$ signaling since CK2 inhibition or siRNA targeting CK2α reduced agonist-induced receptor endocytosis in cultured cells and concomitantly enhanced receptor signaling. The regulatory effect of CK2 was also observed for the $G\alpha_s$-coupled adenosine A2a receptor [44]. The identity of the substrate for CK2 that is involved in the regulation of $G\alpha_s$-coupled receptor signaling is currently unknown.

The implication of the above studies is that CK2 has the potential to modulate a whole set of GPCRs. It is estimated that roughly 15% of 170 well-studied non-olfactory GPCRs signal via $G\alpha_s$ [45]. Many of these GPCRs are expressed in the brain and are important pharmacological targets involved in a variety of neurological disorders. For example, major depressive disorder, affecting up to 1 in 5 adults in the USA [46] is related to dysfunction in brain serotonergic system. Three of the 14 serotonin receptor subtypes are $G\alpha_s$-linked and are, therefore, candidates for regulation by CK2. We have preliminary evidence showing that one of these serotonin receptors, the 5-HT4 receptor, is regulated by CK2 (unpublished data).

Other neurological diseases in which $G\alpha_s$ coupled receptors play major roles are Parkinson's disease (PD) which is characterized by a hypersensitization of the $G\alpha_s$-coupled dopamine D1 receptor. In PD, adenosine A2a receptors control the activity of neurons that oppose the action of the D1 receptor. A2a antagonists have been shown to exert potent anti-akinetic effects in animal models of PD and are currently being evaluated in clinical trials [47]. One could, therefore, hypothesize that modulation of CK2 could have beneficial effects via regulation of both D1 and A2a receptors in Parkinson's disease.

5.2. CK2 Substrates Involved in Synaptic Transmission

CK2 is present in the nucleus and cytoplasm of neurons, but it is also clearly localized at the plasma membrane [44], and it is accumulated at the post-synaptic density in rat hippocampal and cortical preparations [48]. In vitro, PSD-95 was shown to be a CK2 substrate [48]. CK2 was further shown to co-localize with the N-methyl-D-aspartate receptors (NMDAR) subunit NR1 at the synapse [5]. Finally, CK2 activity was found to be enriched in synaptosomes [15].

Work of several groups has highlighted the importance of CK2 in the regulation of the ionotropic glutamate receptors α-Amino-3-hydroxy-5-methyl-4-isoxazolepropionic acid (AMPA) and NMDAR. With glutamate being the major excitatory neurotransmitter, it is logical that modulation of these receptors impacts neuronal excitability and synaptic transmission. Both glutamate receptor types are CK2 substrates, and their activity is modulated by CK2. For example, pharmacological inhibition of CK2 reduced NMDAR activity [49]. The NR2B subunit of NMDAR is phosphorylated in vitro and in vivo by CK2, which leads to a disruption of receptor interaction with PSD-95 and a reduced cell surface expression of the receptor [5]. This internalization process was a response to receptor activation, suggesting that CK2 is involved in receptor desensitization. Since CK2 is known as a constitutively active kinase, the question was how this subunit internalization may be regulated in an activity-dependent manner. It was shown that the Ca^{2+}/calmodulin-dependent protein kinase II (CaMKII), activated through activity-induced calcium influx, recruits CK2 into a trimeric complex together with NR2B. A NR2B mutant that cannot bind to CaMKII is less phosphorylated at the CK2 site (S1480) and has increased surface expression [6].

While the NR2A subunit of the NMDA receptor is not a CK2 substrate, is it still indirectly regulated by CK2 since phosphorylation-dependent NR2B-endocytosis results in an increase in synaptic NR2A expression. It was shown that this switch from NR2B to NR2A is crucial and corresponds to a surge in CK2 expression during embryonic development and, as was later also shown in hippocampal neurons, was dependent on NMDA receptor activity [35,50]. This switch from a NR2B to NR2A subunit in a CK2 dependent manner, was also detected in adult brain hypothalamic neurons, resulting in increased neuronal excitability [51]. The NMDA activity-dependent action of CK2 should be seen separately from the action of CK2 on activating the receptor, which was proposed to be either mediated through a different phosphorylation site or an indirect mechanism [49].

Recently, a role for CK2 in the regulation of cell surface expression of the AMPA receptor subunit GluA1 was proposed in cultured hippocampal cells; in such a scenario, phosphorylation by CK2 leads cell surface accumulation of GluA1 as opposed to internalization of the NR2B subunit of the NMDAR [52].

Glutamate receptors are not the only molecules involved in synaptic function that are CK2 substrates; others are, for example, synaptotagmin, a transmembrane protein involved in the synaptic vesicle fusion with the presynaptic membrane [53], syntaxin, a synaptotagmin interacting protein [54], and dynamin 1, a microtubule stimulated GTPase involved in endocytosis [53,55,56]. However, these phosphorylation events have not, as yet, been detected in vivo.

Another family of membrane proteins that modulate synaptic activity are the voltage gated sodium channels (NAvs). Recently, the CK2 inhibitor TBB was shown to reduce excitability of neurons by abolishing CK2-mediated phosphorylation of the fibroblast growth factor receptor FGF14 and reduced interaction of FGF14 with voltage gated sodium channels (NAv1.2 and 1.6) [57]. CK2 was further found to directly phosphorylate the voltage gated sodium channel NAv1, thereby enhancing its binding to ankyrin and accumulation at the axon initial element, an event which is necessary for fast propagation of action potentials [58]. Small conductance Calcium-activated K+ (SK) channels are gated by the Ca^{2+} sensor calmodulin. Phosphorylation of calmodulin by CK2 reduces its Ca^{2+} sensitivity and leads to channel deactivation in xenopus oocytes [59].

Molecules involved in slow synaptic transmission are also phosphorylated in vitro by CK2. These include the phosphatases PP2a and PP2c and the kinases PKA and PKC, to mention just a few. For an extensive review on signaling proteins that are CK2 substrates, please refer to [3,36]. One example of an in vivo CK2 substrate that links cyclic AMP (cAMP) signaling to nuclear responses, changes histone phosphorylation and transcription is the dopamine- and cAMP-regulated neuronal phosphoprotein (DARPP-32), a regulator of the phosphatase PP1 that is highly expressed in striatum [60]. CK2 phosphorylation of DARPP-32 enhances its potency to inhibit PP1 [61,62]. DARPP-32's translocation to the nucleus, where it controls histone H3 phosphorylation and transcriptional activation, depends on the phosphorylation state at the CK2 site. Mutation of the CK2 phosphorylation site alters the behavioral effects of drugs of abuse and decreases motivation for food [63].

5.3. Substrates Involved in Proteostasis

Many neurodegenerative disorders originate from protein misfolding processes. Examples are Huntington's disease, spinocerebellar ataxia, Parkinson's and Alzheimer's diseases. The presence of cellular defense mechanisms like molecular chaperones and proteasome degradation systems prevent protein misfolding and aggregation, but these systems may not respond sufficiently under conditions of permanently elevated levels of proteins with high aggregation propensities. Mis- or unfolded proteins first aggregate to soluble oligomers, then to insoluble amyloid fibrils, which are structurally defined by β strands. The capacity of protein quality control and degradation (proteostasis) declines with aging, facilitating neurodegeneration as exemplified by the late onset of excessive accumulation of amyloid-beta peptide (Aβ) and tau in Alzheimer's disease, and α-synuclein in Parkinson's disease [64]. Chaperones have been shown to interfere at various steps of the aggregation cascade including nucleation and fibril elongation and are members of diverse signaling pathways, including the heat shock response activated after acute stress, the ubiquitin-proteasome system, and the autophagosome-lysosome pathway [65,66]. While the aggregated protein itself, often inherited in a mutated version, differs for each disease, the pathways controlling proteostasis are overarching mechanisms of which CK2 has been shown to regulate several major players.

CK2 phosphorylates and modulates several chaperones such as Hsp90 as well as its co-chaperones FKBP51, 52 and Cdc37. CK2-dependent phosphorylation of Cdc37 is essential for the chaperone function of Hsp90-Cdc37 [67]. FKBP51 and 52 regulate, among others, steroid hormone receptor activity: FKBP52 activates while FKBP51 inactivates these types of receptors. Phosphorylation by CK2 completely abrogates FKBP52 regulation of receptor function, thus, leading to a reduction in receptor activation. FKBP51 and FKBP52 are also discussed, together with Hsp90, for their impact on tau phosphorylation and stability. Again, there seems to be an indication that both co-chaperones act in opposing ways, with FKBP51 stabilizing tau and FKBP52 reducing tau stability [68]. To date, these questions are not entirely resolved.

CK2 was shown to phosphorylate Hsf1, leading to nuclear accumulation of Hsf1 in vitro [69], while mutation of phosphosites to alanine inhibited the transcriptional activity of Hsf1. This finding could be of great interest since Hsf1 is the regulator of various chaperones, including Hsp70.

Enhancing the activity of the ubiquitin-proteasome pathway is a promising strategy to ameliorate protein aggregation diseases. In this context, CK2 was found to modulate the expression of proteasome genes via Nrf1 phosphorylation. Knockdown of CK2 enhances the Nrf1-dependent expression of proteasome subunit genes and reduces the accumulation of ubiquitylated proteins in vitro in several cell lines [70]. Like several other kinases, CK2 has been shown to target proteins for degradation through ubiquitin-mediated proteolysis [71].

Taken together, like in other instances, CK2 has a bidirectional effect on the proteasome: phosphorylation of certain substrates enhances their proteasomal degradation, while phosphorylation of transcription factor Nrf1 reduces its activity to mediate expression of members of the proteasome family. It is conceivable that the effect of Nrf1 on the synthesis of proteasome components and, thus, on overall proteasome output, may outweigh the role of CK2 on targeting a handful of substrates to the proteasome. However, one would need to integrate these data, as well as the effects on the proteasome and on heat shock response, to estimate the net effect of CK2 on protein aggregation in several systems, in cell culture, and, ideally, in preclinical models.

6. Diseases of the Human Brain

6.1. Glioblastoma

Glioblastoma multiforme (GBM) comprise 15% of all brain tumors and are the most aggressive human glial tumors with a median survival of 14–15 months [72]. Unfortunately, tumors often become drug-resistant and regrow despite chemotherapy. CK2α is overexpressed in human GBM; this is caused by a gain in gene dosage of approximately 34% [20], while a 4-fold increase in CK2α protein is measured [73].

Inhibition of CK2 activity through small molecule inhibitors or siRNA induced apoptosis, reduced growth in GBM cells in mouse xenograft models of human GBMs [20] as well as in mice that had been injected intracranially with human GBM tumors. Concomitantly, CK2 inhibition lowered JAK/STAT (Janus kinase/signal transducers and activators of transcription pathway) and NFkB activation as well as the activation of survival markers of the AKT pathway and promoted survival of mice [20,25,74]. These data are very promising and clearly warrant clinical trials.

For the remainder of this section, we would like to focus on diseases where not proliferation but rather cellular degeneration occurs, namely neurodegenerative diseases such as Parkinson's and Huntington's diseases, Amyotrophic lateral sclerosis, and Alzheimer's disease.

6.2. Parkinson's Disease

Parkinson's disease (PD) is the second most prevalent neurodegenerative disorder, affecting as many as 2% of people 65 years or older [75]. It is characterized by symptoms such as tremor, rigidity, bradykinesia, and gait disturbances. The major cytopathological markers of the disease are the loss of dopaminergic neurons in the midbrain and the formation of Lewy bodies, mainly composed of aggregated α-synuclein fibrils, in the remaining dopaminergic neurons [76]. Phosphorylation of α-synuclein at Ser-129, close to its C-terminus is held as a hallmark of Parkinson's disease mainly because α-synuclein within Lewy bodies is extensively phosphorylated at this site. It was shown that CK2 as well as polo-like kinase (PLK) phosphorylate soluble α-synuclein at S129, while PLKs are most probably responsible for phosphorylation of aggregated α-synuclein [77]. Overexpression of PLK but not CK2 in cultured cells increased phosphorylation of aggregated α-synuclein at S129 [78]. By employing a series of mutated substrates, in vitro experiments by Salvi et al. demonstrate that the polo-like kinases PLK2 and PLK3 are more efficient at phosphorylating α-synuclein at this site than CK2 [79]. Indeed, using striatal tissue from conditional CK2 KO mice (Drd1-Cre or Drd2-Cre) we could not detect a reduction in pS129 α-synuclein (unpublished data) despite a 50% loss of CK2α protein (and no compensatory upregulation of CK2α'). Thus, one can conclude that while CK2 is an efficient in vitro kinase for this site, it is not the major kinase that performs this phosphorylation in vivo. The physiological relevance of this phosphorylation is still heavily debated since experiments in rats, mice, and drosophila as well as in tissue culture lead to opposing results and do not allow the conclusion that pS129 a-synuclein is causal to the aggregation or to toxic effects [80].

Another protein that is localized to Lewy bodies and binds to α-synuclein is synphilin. It has been reported that, in vitro, CK2 phosphorylates synphilin and thereby alters the interaction to α-synuclein [81].

Based on our work with CK2 KO mice, we hypothesize that in addition to the potential CK2 substrates described above, CK2 may have a central role in modulating the brain's responses to dopamine depletion as well as to anti-parkinsonian treatment. We have shown that the activity of two major dopamine responsive neuronal cell types in the striatum, namely the direct and indirect pathway spiny projection neurons, is modulated by changes in expression and plasma membrane availability of the dopamine D1 and the adenosine A2a receptors, respectively [32,44] Both these receptors are primarily responsible for behavioral responses to dopamine and L-DOPA, therefore, we presume CK2 must have a role in Parkinson's disease; this investigation is currently under way.

6.3. Huntington's Disease

Huntington's disease (HD) is a progressive neurodegenerative disorder mainly affecting medium spiny neurons of the striatum. It is the consequence of an expansion of the CAG sequence in the huntingtin gene that causes the translation of an expanded polyQ tail in the protein. The symptoms are categorized into motor and cognitive in nature, such as frontal lobe dementia, and psychiatric symptoms, including depression, anxiety, and psychosis [82]. Fan et al. have published in vitro evidence that cells overexpressing polyQ-huntingtin, exhibit enhanced CK2 expression [83]. This observation was validated in a mouse model of HD where upregulation of CK2 takes place in the striatum but not in the cortex. When mice were treated with a pharmacological CK2 inhibitor, there was a significant increase in NDMAR mediated toxicity which could be explained by the phosphorylation-induced endocytosis of NMDAR [5]. Taken together, the possible role of CK2 is to counteract the toxic effects of the mutant huntingtin gene on NMDAR activity.

One example of a second polyQ disease with pathophysiological involvement of CK2 is spinocerebellar ataxia type 3. CK2-mediated phosphorylation leads to nuclear accumulation and aggregation of ataxin 3, indicating that, in the context of this disease, inhibition of CK2 could have the desirable effect of reducing its nuclear aggregations [84].

6.4. Amyotrophic Lateral Sclerosis

Amyotrophic lateral sclerosis (ALS) is a neurodegenerative disorder that involves the loss of motor neurons of the cortex, brainstem, and spinal cord leading to paralysis and, ultimately, death by respiratory failure [85]. As in other neurodegenerative diseases, protein aggregates are detected in the affected areas of the brains of patients, although the aggregated protein may vary in different forms of the disease. The nuclear RNA-binding protein TDP-43 is, however, found in cytoplasmic inclusions of all forms of ALS (except in cases of familial ALS with mutations in SOD1).

TDP-43, trapped in the aggregates, undergoes ubiquitination and hyperphosphorylation, and CK2 was found to drive phosphorylation at various sites in cultured cells. Overexpression of CK2 increases phosphorylation, facilitating the solubility of TDP-43 truncated mutants, and this effect is reversed when cells are treated with a CK2 inhibitor. A Drosophila mutant line expressing a non-phosphorylatable point mutant developed aggregates in neurons, while a phosphomimicking mutant failed to do so. These studies suggest that CK2 upregulation and enhanced phosphorylation of TDP-43 may prevent TDP-43 aggregation and be beneficial for disease outcome [86].

6.5. Alzheimer's Disease

Late-onset Alzheimer's disease (AD) is the most common neurodegenerative disorder in the USA and Europe and is characterized by progressive worsening in cognitive functions along with functional and behavioral impairments. The pathophysiological hallmarks of the disease are extracellular insoluble beta amyloid (Aβ) plaques and intracellular neurofibrillary tangles (NFTs) composed of hyperphosphorylated tau aggregates. CK2 activity and protein expression were found to be reduced in Alzheimer's disease [87]. CK2 was detected in association with neurofibrillary tangles whose main component is accumulated and hyperphosphorylated tau [88]. Tau purified from human brain and tau in neuroblastoma cells are CK2 substrates [89,90].

CK2 was found to phosphorylate Apolipoprotein-E at an atypical site involving proline and an acidic residue at +1, and interaction of these two partners rendered CK2 more active towards tau in in vitro kinase assays. However, this data still needs to be confirmed in an in vivo setting [91].

A strong body of evidence suggests that soluble amyloid-β peptide (Aβ) oligomers induce synaptic loss in AD. Aβ-induced synaptic dysfunction is dependent on overstimulation of N-methyl-D-aspartate receptors (NMDARs) resulting in aberrant activation of redox events as well as elevation of cytoplasmic Ca^{2+}, which in turn triggers phosphorylation of tau and the activation of caspases Cdk5/dynamin-related protein 1 (Drp1) and CaMKII [92]. Dysfunction in these pathways leads to mitochondrial dysfunction, synaptic malfunction, impaired long-term potentiation, and cognitive decline. Aβ synaptic toxicity can be partially ameliorated by NMDAR antagonists (such as memantine). As described in the above section on synaptic transmission (Section 5.2), since Aβ was shown to activate CK2 in vitro [93], one could hypothesize that CK2 activation leading to enhanced prolonged NMDA channel opening [49] may be partially responsible for the excessive NMDAR toxicity.

Several laboratories also demonstrated that CK2 is linked to the processing of the amyloid precursor protein (APP). Walter et al. showed that APP is a substrate for the ectokinase CK2 [94], after it had been demonstrated by several groups that CK2 can be shed and can phosphorylate extracellular substrates [95,96]. In neuroblastoma cells, CK2 inhibitor reduced the processing of APP to soluble sAPPα in response to cholinergic stimulation [97]. sAPPα is generated by α-secretase and precludes processing of APP by β and γ-secretases. Thus, this effect caused by CK2 may be desirable, however, further experiments in this direction need to be undertaken.

As mentioned above, CK2 is activated by Aβ in vitro [93]. Such an activation was proposed to result in an inhibition of fast axonal transport (FAT), which is a mechanism by which synaptic proteins and mitochondria are transported from the cell body into axons for proper neuronal function and survival. Inhibition of CK2 rescued axonal transport and overexpression of active CK2 mimicked the inhibitory effects of Aβ on FAT. The effect of CK2 on FAT is believed to be mediated by phosphorylation of kinesin-1 light chains and subsequent release of kinesin from its cargoes, effectively disabling the transport [98].

However, this finding must be evaluated in the light of data showing that in cultured mammalian cells, reduction of CK2 expression decreases the number of active kinesin motors [99]. Thus, CK2 up-regulates kinesin-based transport by enhancing the kinesin number but also releasing kinesin from its cargoes, yielding two functions that counteract each other. Further investigation will help to resolve the question of which of the effects is predominant in vivo.

Recent human and preclinical studies have provided evidence that impaired insulin signaling and glucose utilization are contributing to the pathophysiology in AD [100]. It was shown that insulin and the insulin-sensitizing drug rosiglitazone improve cognitive performance in mouse models of AD and in patients with early AD [101,102] by reducing binding of Aβ oligomers to synapses. In contrast, patients with insulin-resistant type 2 diabetes show an increased risk of developing AD [100]. In this context, it is worthwhile to note that in response to Aβ oligomer binding to hippocampal neurons, CK2 and CaMKII were found to mediate internalization of the insulin receptor. These findings are in several ways reminiscent of CK2's role in NDMAR endocytosis (as discussed in Section 5.2) since both require CaMKII and are dependent on receptor activity.

Other groups have already identified a role for CK2 in the non-neuronal insulin pathway as described in Section 5.1, CK2 negatively modulates insulin release from pancreatic beta cells, in a manner that depends on the M3 receptor [43]. While this work is discussed in the realm of glucose intolerance and diabetes type 2, one could extend a hypothesis here to question if pharmacological CK2 inhibition might benefit Alzheimer's patients.

Neuroinflammation, as detected by the presence of activated complement proteins interleukins and chemokines in microglia, and astrocytes are is increased in AD [103]. Although neuroinflammation in the brain of AD patients is considered primarily beneficial (eliminating injurious stimuli and restoring tissue integrity), a chronic neuroinflammatory response may be harmful due to the constant excess of pro-inflammatory cytokines, prostaglandins, and reactive oxygen species. A recent immunohistochemical study detected increased amounts of CK2α or α' in the hippocampus and temporal cortex of AD patients in astrocytes surrounding amyloid deposits [104]. It remains to be determined whether this increase is of functional consequence.

In summary, CK2 plays a role in several mechanisms that are involved in tau phosphorylation, APP processing, Aβ signaling, and protective responses to Aβ insults such as neuroinflammatory responses and insulin signaling.

7. Conclusions

In summary, it comes as no surprise that CK2 plays a major role in a variety of processes in the brain, as it has been shown to target a vast number of brain proteins. In the context of brain disorders, one would like to assess whether CK2 may be a good target for modifying disease outcome and or progression.

The case for glioblastoma is clear, and several preclinical studies have demonstrated the beneficial effect of CK2 inhibitors on tumor size reduction as well as patient survival.

For Huntington's disease and ALS, there is currently no rationale to argue for CK2 as a target to interfere with disease progression, while in the case of type 3 spinocerebellar ataxia, CK2 inhibition may be desirable and result in a reduction in ataxin aggregation.

In the context of Alzheimer's disease, most known factors would argue that, even though CK2 expression was shown to be reduced, a further inhibition of CK2 through pharmacological means may be beneficial in reducing the burden of hyperphosphorylated tau and neurofibrillary tangles. It may also be beneficial to prevent or reduce insulin receptor internalization and to rescue fast axonal transport that is disabled by Aβ. However, CK2 activity may be desirable due to its endocytotic effect on NMDAR.

In order to ascertain how the various mechanisms of CK2 involvement in neurological disease pathology are integrated in vivo, it is preferable to use a conditional CK2 KO, possibly even in an inducible version, and cross the KO mice into appropriate preclinical models of neurodegenerative diseases. The genetic approach is, in our opinion, preferable for proof of concept experiments because the available inhibitors are not readily blood-brain barrier permeable and, thus, require relatively high-dose administration which will also affect peripheral sites and a variety of centrally mediated behaviors that are unrelated to disease pathologies.

Acknowledgments: This work has been supported by grants PSC-CUNY45, PSC-CUNY46 and PSC-CUNY47 (to HR).

Conflicts of Interest: The authors declare no conflict of interest.

References

1. Ackerman, P.; Glover, C.V.; Osheroff, N. Stimulation of casein kinase II by epidermal growth factor: Relationship between the physiological activity of the kinase and the phosphorylation state of its β subunit. *Proc. Natl. Acad. Sci. USA* **1990**, *87*, 821–825. [CrossRef] [PubMed]
2. Klarlund, J.K.; Czech, M.P. Insulin-like growth factor I and insulin rapidly increase casein kinase II activity in BALB/c 3T3 fibroblasts. *J. Biol. Chem.* **1988**, *263*, 15872–15875. [PubMed]
3. Blanquet, P.R. Neurotrophin-induced activation of casein kinase 2 in rat hippocampal slices. *Neuroscience* **1998**, *86*, 739–749. [CrossRef]
4. Filhol, O.; Cochet, C. Protein kinase CK2 in health and disease: Cellular functions of protein kinase CK2: A dynamic affair. *Cell. Mol. Life Sci.* **2009**, *66*, 1830–1839. [CrossRef] [PubMed]
5. Chung, H.J.; Huang, Y.H.; Lau, L.F.; Huganir, R.L. Regulation of the NMDA receptor complex and trafficking by activity-dependent phosphorylation of the NR2B subunit PDZ ligand. *J. Neurosci.* **2004**, *24*, 10248–10259. [CrossRef] [PubMed]
6. Sanz-Clemente, A.; Gray, J.A.; Ogilvie, K.A.; Nicoll, R.A.; Roche, K.W. Activated CaMKII couples GluN2B and casein kinase 2 to control synaptic NMDA receptors. *Cell Rep.* **2013**, *3*, 607–614. [CrossRef] [PubMed]
7. Di Maira, G.; Salvi, M.; Arrigoni, G.; Marin, O.; Sarno, S.; Brustolon, F.; Pinna, L.A.; Ruzzene, M. Protein kinase CK2 phosphorylates and upregulates Akt/PKB. *Cell Death Differ.* **2005**, *12*, 668–677. [CrossRef] [PubMed]
8. Torres, J.; Pulido, R. The tumor suppressor PTEN is phosphorylated by the protein kinase CK2 at its C terminus. Implications for PTEN stability to proteasome-mediated degradation. *J. Biol. Chem.* **2001**, *276*, 993–998. [CrossRef] [PubMed]
9. Dominguez, I.; Sonenshein, G.E.; Seldin, D.C. Protein kinase CK2 in health and disease: CK2 and its role in Wnt and NF-kappaB signaling: Linking development and cancer. *Cell. Mol. Life Sci.* **2009**, *66*, 1850–1857. [CrossRef] [PubMed]
10. Guerra, B.; Rasmussen, T.D.; Schnitzler, A.; Jensen, H.H.; Boldyreff, B.S.; Miyata, Y.; Marcussen, N.; Niefind, K.; Issinger, O.G. Protein kinase CK2 inhibition is associated with the destabilization of HIF-1alpha in human cancer cells. *Cancer Lett.* **2015**, *356*, 751–761. [CrossRef] [PubMed]
11. Meggio, F.; Marin, O.; Pinna, L.A. Substrate specificity of protein kinase CK2. *Cell. Mol. Biol. Res.* **1994**, *40*, 401–409. [PubMed]
12. Songyang, Z.; Lu, K.P.; Kwon, Y.T.; Tsai, L.H.; Filhol, O.; Cochet, C.; Brickey, D.A.; Soderling, T.R.; Bartleson, C.; Graves, D.J.; et al. A structural basis for substrate specificities of protein Ser/Thr kinases: Primary sequence preference of casein kinases I and II, NIMA, phosphorylase kinase, calmodulin-dependent kinase II, CDK5, and Erk1. *Mol. Cell. Biol.* **1996**, *16*, 6486–6493. [CrossRef] [PubMed]

13. Bian, Y.; Ye, M.; Wang, C.; Cheng, K.; Song, C.; Dong, M.; Pan, Y.; Qin, H.; Zou, H. Global screening of CK2 kinase substrates by an integrated phosphoproteomics workflow. *Sci. Rep.* **2013**, *3*, 3460. [CrossRef] [PubMed]

14. Ceglia, I.; Flajolet, M.; Rebholz, H. Predominance of CK2α over CK2α′ in the mammalian brain. *Mol. Cell. Biochem.* **2011**, *356*, 169–175. [CrossRef] [PubMed]

15. Girault, J.A.; Hemmings, H.C., Jr.; Zorn, S.H.; Gustafson, E.L.; Greengard, P. Characterization in mammalian brain of a DARPP-32 serine kinase identical to casein kinase II. *J. Neurochem.* **1990**, *55*, 1772–1783. [CrossRef] [PubMed]

16. Sarnat, H.B.; Nochlin, D.; Born, D.E. Neuronal nuclear antigen (NeuN): A marker of neuronal maturation in early human fetal nervous system. *Brain Dev.* **1998**, *20*, 88–94. [CrossRef]

17. Cozza, G.; Pinna, L.A.; Moro, S. Kinase CK2 inhibition: An update. *Curr. Med. Chem.* **2013**, *20*, 671–693. [CrossRef] [PubMed]

18. Perez, D.I.; Gil, C.; Martinez, A. Protein Kinases CK1 and CK2 as New Targets for Neurodegenerative Diseases. *Med. Res. Rev.* **2010**, *6*, 924–954. [CrossRef] [PubMed]

19. Tam, V.H.; Sosa, C.; Liu, R.; Yao, N.; Priestley, R.D. Nanomedicine as a non-invasive strategy for drug delivery across the blood brain barrier. *Int. J. Pharm.* **2016**, *515*, 331–342. [CrossRef] [PubMed]

20. Zheng, Y.; McFarland, B.C.; Drygin, D.; Yu, H.; Bellis, S.L.; Kim, H.; Bredel, M.; Benveniste, E.N. Targeting protein kinase CK2 suppresses prosurvival signaling pathways and growth of glioblastoma. *Clin. Cancer Res.* **2013**, *19*, 6484–6494. [CrossRef] [PubMed]

21. Wolburg, H.; Noell, S.; Fallier-Becker, P.; Mack, A.F.; Wolburg-Buchholz, K. The disturbed blood-brain barrier in human glioblastoma. *Mol. Asp. Med.* **2012**, *33*, 579–589. [CrossRef] [PubMed]

22. Cozza, G.; Zanin, S.; Sarno, S.; Costa, E.; Girardi, C.; Ribaudo, G.; Salvi, M.; Zagotto, G.; Ruzzene, M.; Pinna, L.A. Design, validation and efficacy of bisubstrate inhibitors specifically affecting ecto-CK2 kinase activity. *Biochem. J.* **2015**, *471*, 415–430. [CrossRef] [PubMed]

23. Ahmed, K.; Kren, B.T.; Abedin, M.J.; Vogel, R.I.; Shaughnessy, D.P.; Nacusi, L.; Korman, V.L.; Li, Y.; Dehm, S.M.; Zimmerman, C.L.; et al. CK2 targeted RNAi therapeutic delivered via malignant cell-directed tenfibgen nanocapsule: Dose and molecular mechanisms of response in xenograft prostate tumors. *Oncotarget* **2016**. [CrossRef] [PubMed]

24. Ji, H.; Wang, J.; Nika, H.; Hawke, D.; Keezer, S.; Ge, Q.; Fang, B.; Fang, X.; Fang, D.; Litchfield, D.W.; et al. EGF-induced ERK activation promotes CK2-mediated disassociation of α-Catenin from β-Catenin and transactivation of beta-Catenin. *Mol. Cell* **2009**, *36*, 547–559. [CrossRef] [PubMed]

25. Chou, S.T.; Patil, R.; Galstyan, A.; Gangalum, P.R.; Cavenee, W.K.; Furnari, F.B.; Ljubimov, V.A.; Chesnokova, A.; Kramerov, A.A.; Ding, H.; et al. Simultaneous blockade of interacting CK2 and EGFR pathways by tumor-targeting nanobioconjugates increases therapeutic efficacy against glioblastoma multiforme. *J. Control. Release* **2016**, *244 Pt A*, 14–23. [CrossRef] [PubMed]

26. Buchou, T.; Vernet, M.; Blond, O.; Jensen, H.H.; Pointu, H.; Olsen, B.B.; Cochet, C.; Issinger, O.G.; Boldyreff, B. Disruption of the regulatory beta subunit of protein kinase CK2 in mice leads to a cell-autonomous defect and early embryonic lethality. *Mol. Cell. Biol.* **2003**, *23*, 908–915. [CrossRef] [PubMed]

27. Huillard, E.; Ziercher, L.; Blond, O.; Wong, M.; Deloulme, J.C.; Souchelnytskyi, S.; Baudier, J.; Cochet, C.; Buchou, T. Disruption of CK2beta in embryonic neural stem cells compromises proliferation and oligodendrogenesis in the mouse telencephalon. *Mol. Cell. Biol.* **2010**, *30*, 2737–2749. [CrossRef] [PubMed]

28. Lou, D.Y.; Dominguez, I.; Toselli, P.; Landesman-Bollag, E.; O'Brien, C.; Seldin, D.C. The alpha catalytic subunit of protein kinase CK2 is required for mouse embryonic development. *Mol. Cell. Biol.* **2008**, *28*, 131–139. [CrossRef] [PubMed]

29. Dominguez, I.; Degano, I.R.; Chea, K.; Cha, J.; Toselli, P.; Seldin, D.C. CK2alpha is essential for embryonic morphogenesis. *Mol. Cell. Biochem.* **2011**, *356*, 209–216. [CrossRef] [PubMed]

30. Xu, X.; Toselli, P.A.; Russell, L.D.; Seldin, D.C. Globozoospermia in mice lacking the casein kinase II α′ catalytic subunit. *Nat. Genet.* **1999**, *23*, 118–121. [PubMed]

31. Casanova, E.; Fehsenfeld, S.; Mantamadiotis, T.; Lemberger, T.; Greiner, E.; Stewart, A.F.; Schutz, G. A CamKIIalpha iCre BAC allows brain-specific gene inactivation. *Genesis* **2001**, *31*, 37–42. [CrossRef] [PubMed]

32. Rebholz, H.; Zhou, M.; Nairn, A.C.; Greengard, P.; Flajolet, M. Selective knockout of the casein kinase 2 in d1 medium spiny neurons controls dopaminergic function. *Biol. Psychiatry* **2013**, *74*, 113–121. [CrossRef] [PubMed]

33. Araki, K.Y.; Sims, J.R.; Bhide, P.G. Dopamine receptor mRNA and protein expression in the mouse corpus striatum and cerebral cortex during pre- and postnatal development. *Brain Res.* **2007**, *1156*, 31–45. [CrossRef] [PubMed]

34. Mack, K.J.; O'Malley, K.L.; Todd, R.D. Differential expression of dopaminergic D2 receptor messenger RNAs during development. *Brain Res. Dev. Brain Res.* **1991**, *59*, 249–251. [CrossRef]

35. Sanz-Clemente, A.; Matta, J.A.; Isaac, J.T.; Roche, K.W. Casein kinase 2 regulates the NR2 subunit composition of synaptic NMDA receptors. *Neuron* **2010**, *67*, 984–996. [CrossRef] [PubMed]

36. Meggio, F.; Pinna, L.A. One-thousand-and-one substrates of protein kinase CK2? *FASEB J.* **2003**, *17*, 349–368. [CrossRef] [PubMed]

37. Blanquet, P.R. Casein kinase 2 as a potentially important enzyme in the nervous system. *Prog. Neurobiol.* **2000**, *60*, 211–246. [CrossRef]

38. Katritch, V.; Cherezov, V.; Stevens, R.C. Structure-function of the G protein-coupled receptor superfamily. *Annu. Rev. Pharmacol. Toxicol.* **2013**, *53*, 531–556. [CrossRef] [PubMed]

39. Premont, R.T.; Gainetdinov, R.R. Physiological roles of G protein-coupled receptor kinases and arrestins. *Annu. Rev. Physiol.* **2007**, *69*, 511–534. [CrossRef] [PubMed]

40. Ferguson, S.S. Evolving concepts in G protein-coupled receptor endocytosis: The role in receptor desensitization and signaling. *Pharmacol. Rev.* **2001**, *53*, 1–24. [PubMed]

41. Budd, D.C.; Willars, G.B.; McDonald, J.E.; Tobin, A.B. Phosphorylation of the Gq/11-coupled m3-muscarinic receptor is involved in receptor activation of the ERK-1/2 mitogen-activated protein kinase pathway. *J. Biol. Chem.* **2001**, *276*, 4581–4587. [CrossRef] [PubMed]

42. Torrecilla, I.; Spragg, E.J.; Poulin, B.; McWilliams, P.J.; Mistry, S.C.; Blaukat, A.; Tobin, A.B. Phosphorylation and regulation of a G protein-coupled receptor by protein kinase CK2. *J. Cell Biol.* **2007**, *177*, 127–137. [CrossRef] [PubMed]

43. Rossi, M.; Ruiz de Azua, I.; Barella, L.F.; Sakamoto, W.; Zhu, L.; Cui, Y.; Lu, H.; Rebholz, H.; Matschinsky, F.M.; Doliba, N.M.; et al. CK2 acts as a potent negative regulator of receptor-mediated insulin release in vitro and in vivo. *Proc. Natl. Acad. Sci. USA* **2015**, *112*, E6818–E6824. [CrossRef] [PubMed]

44. Rebholz, H.; Nishi, A.; Liebscher, S.; Nairn, A.C.; Flajolet, M.; Greengard, P. CK2 negatively regulates Galphas signaling. *Proc. Natl. Acad. Sci. USA* **2009**, *106*, 14096–140101. [CrossRef] [PubMed]

45. Alexander, S.P.; Mathie, A.; Peters, J.A. Guide to Receptors and Channels (GRAC), 5th edition. *Br. J. Pharmacol.* **2011**, *164* (Suppl. 1), S1–S324. [CrossRef] [PubMed]

46. Kessler, R.C.; Demler, O.; Frank, R.G.; Olfson, M.; Pincus, H.A.; Walters, E.E.; Wang, P.; Wells, K.B.; Zaslavsky, A.M. Prevalence and treatment of mental disorders, 1990 to 2003. *N. Engl. J. Med.* **2005**, *352*, 2515–2523. [CrossRef] [PubMed]

47. Kondo, T.; Mizuno, Y.; Japanese Istradefylline Study Group. A long-term study of istradefylline safety and efficacy in patients with Parkinson disease. *Clin. Neuropharmacol.* **2015**, *38*, 41–46. [CrossRef] [PubMed]

48. Soto, D.; Pancetti, F.; Marengo, J.J.; Sandoval, M.; Sandoval, R.; Orrego, F.; Wyneken, U. Protein kinase CK2 in postsynaptic densities: Phosphorylation of PSD-95/SAP90 and NMDA receptor regulation. *Biochem. Biophys. Res. Commun.* **2004**, *322*, 542–550. [CrossRef] [PubMed]

49. Lieberman, D.N.; Mody, I. Casein kinase-II regulates NMDA channel function in hippocampal neurons. *Nat. Neurosci.* **1999**, *2*, 125–132. [CrossRef] [PubMed]

50. Kimura, R.; Matsuki, N. Protein kinase CK2 modulates synaptic plasticity by modification of synaptic NMDA receptors in the hippocampus. *J. Physiol.* **2008**, *586*, 3195–3206. [CrossRef] [PubMed]

51. Ye, Z.Y.; Li, L.; Li, D.P.; Pan, H.L. Casein kinase 2-mediated synaptic GluN2A up-regulation increases N-methyl-D-aspartate receptor activity and excitability of hypothalamic neurons in hypertension. *J. Biol. Chem.* **2012**, *287*, 17438–17446. [CrossRef] [PubMed]

52. Lussier, M.P.; Gu, X.; Lu, W.; Roche, K.W. Casein kinase 2 phosphorylates GluA1 and regulates its surface expression. *Eur. J. Neurosci.* **2014**, *39*, 1148–1158. [CrossRef] [PubMed]

53. Bennett, M.K.; Miller, K.G.; Scheller, R.H. Casein kinase II phosphorylates the synaptic vesicle protein p65. *J. Neurosci.* **1993**, *13*, 1701–1707. [PubMed]

54. Littleton, J.T.; Bellen, H.J. Synaptotagmin controls and modulates synaptic-vesicle fusion in a Ca^{2+}-dependent manner. *Trends Neurosci.* **1995**, *18*, 177–183. [CrossRef]

55. Robinson, P.J.; Sontag, J.M.; Liu, J.P.; Fykse, E.M.; Slaughter, C.; McMahon, H.; Sudhof, T.C. Dynamin GTPase regulated by protein kinase C phosphorylation in nerve terminals. *Nature* **1993**, *365*, 163–166. [CrossRef] [PubMed]

56. Graham, M.E.; Anggono, V.; Bache, N.; Larsen, M.R.; Craft, G.E.; Robinson, P.J. The in vivo phosphorylation sites of rat brain dynamin I. *J. Biol. Chem.* **2007**, *282*, 14695–14707. [CrossRef] [PubMed]

57. Hsu, W.C.; Scala, F.; Nenov, M.N.; Wildburger, N.C.; Elferink, H.; Singh, A.K.; Chesson, C.B.; Buzhdygan, T.; Sohail, M.; Shavkunov, A.S.; et al. CK2 activity is required for the interaction of FGF14 with voltage-gated sodium channels and neuronal excitability. *FASEB J.* **2016**, *30*, 2171–2186. [CrossRef] [PubMed]

58. Hien, Y.E.; Montersino, A.; Castets, F.; Leterrier, C.; Filhol, O.; Vacher, H.; Dargent, B. CK2 accumulation at the axon initial segment depends on sodium channel Nav1. *FEBS Lett.* **2014**, *588*, 3403–3408. [CrossRef] [PubMed]

59. Bildl, W.; Strassmaier, T.; Thurm, H.; Andersen, J.; Eble, S.; Oliver, D.; Knipper, M.; Mann, M.; Schulte, U.; Adelman, J.P.; et al. Protein kinase CK2 is coassembled with small conductance Ca^{2+}-activated K+ channels and regulates channel gating. *Neuron* **2004**, *43*, 847–858. [CrossRef] [PubMed]

60. Nishi, A.; Snyder, G.L.; Greengard, P. Bidirectional regulation of DARPP-32 phosphorylation by dopamine. *J. Neurosci.* **1997**, *17*, 8147–8155. [PubMed]

61. Girault, J.A.; Hemmings, H.C., Jr.; Williams, K.R.; Nairn, A.C.; Greengard, P. Phosphorylation of DARPP-32, a dopamine- and cAMP-regulated phosphoprotein, by casein kinase II. *J. Biol. Chem.* **1989**, *264*, 21748–21759. [PubMed]

62. Desdouits, F.; Cheetham, J.J.; Huang, H.B.; Kwon, Y.G.; da Cruz e Silva, E.F.; Denefle, P.; Ehrlich, M.E.; Nairn, A.C.; Greengard, P.; Girault, J.A. Mechanism of inhibition of protein phosphatase 1 by DARPP-32: Studies with recombinant DARPP-32 and synthetic peptides. *Biochem. Biophys. Res. Commun.* **1995**, *206*, 652–658. [CrossRef] [PubMed]

63. Stipanovich, A.; Valjent, E.; Matamales, M.; Nishi, A.; Ahn, J.H.; Maroteaux, M.; Bertran-Gonzalez, J.; Brami-Cherrier, K.; Enslen, H.; Corbille, A.G.; et al. A phosphatase cascade by which rewarding stimuli control nucleosomal response. *Nature* **2008**, *453*, 879–884. [CrossRef] [PubMed]

64. Balchin, D.; Hayer-Hartl, M.; Hartl, F.U. In vivo aspects of protein folding and quality control. *Science* **2016**, *353*, aac4354. [CrossRef] [PubMed]

65. Kundu, M.; Thompson, C.B. Autophagy: Basic principles and relevance to disease. *Annu. Rev. Pathol.* **2008**, *3*, 427–455. [CrossRef] [PubMed]

66. Takalo, M.; Salminen, A.; Soininen, H.; Hiltunen, M.; Haapasalo, A. Protein aggregation and degradation mechanisms in neurodegenerative diseases. *Am. J. Neurodegener. Dis.* **2013**, *2*, 1–14. [PubMed]

67. Miyata, Y. Protein kinase CK2 in health and disease: CK2: The kinase controlling the Hsp90 chaperone machinery. *Cell. Mol. Life Sci.* **2009**, *66*, 1840–1849. [CrossRef] [PubMed]

68. Storer, C.L.; Dickey, C.A.; Galigniana, M.D.; Rein, T.; Cox, M.B. FKBP51 and FKBP52 in signaling and disease. *Trends Endocrinol. Metab.* **2011**, *22*, 481–490. [CrossRef] [PubMed]

69. Soncin, F.; Zhang, X.; Chu, B.; Wang, X.; Asea, A.; Ann Stevenson, M.; Sacks, D.B.; Calderwood, S.K. Transcriptional activity and DNA binding of heat shock factor-1 involve phosphorylation on threonine 142 by CK2. *Biochem. Biophys. Res. Commun.* **2003**, *303*, 700–706. [CrossRef]

70. Tsuchiya, Y.; Taniguchi, H.; Ito, Y.; Morita, T.; Karim, M.R.; Ohtake, N.; Fukagai, K.; Ito, T.; Okamuro, S.; Iemura, S.; et al. The casein kinase 2-nrf1 axis controls the clearance of ubiquitinated proteins by regulating proteasome gene expression. *Mol. Cell. Biol.* **2013**, *33*, 3461–3472. [CrossRef] [PubMed]

71. Hunter, T. The age of crosstalk: Phosphorylation, ubiquitination, and beyond. *Mol. Cell* **2007**, *28*, 730–738. [CrossRef] [PubMed]

72. Johnson, D.R.; Ma, D.J.; Buckner, J.C.; Hammack, J.E. Conditional probability of long-term survival in glioblastoma: A population-based analysis. *Cancer* **2012**, *118*, 5608–5613. [CrossRef] [PubMed]

73. Ferrer-Font, L.; Alcaraz, E.; Plana, M.; Candiota, A.P.; Itarte, E.; Arus, C. Protein Kinase CK2 Content in GL261 Mouse Glioblastoma. *Pathol. Oncol. Res.* **2016**, *22*, 633–637. [CrossRef] [PubMed]

74. Dixit, D.; Ahmad, F.; Ghildiyal, R.; Joshi, S.D.; Sen, E. CK2 inhibition induced PDK4-AMPK axis regulates metabolic adaptation and survival responses in glioma. *Exp. Cell Res.* **2016**, *344*, 132–142. [CrossRef] [PubMed]

75. Massano, J.; Bhatia, K.P. Clinical approach to Parkinson's disease: Features, diagnosis, and principles of management. *Cold Spring Harb. Perspect. Med.* **2012**, *2*, a008870. [CrossRef] [PubMed]
76. Dauer, W.; Przedborski, S. Parkinson's disease: Mechanisms and models. *Neuron* **2003**, *39*, 889–909. [CrossRef]
77. Waxman, E.A.; Giasson, B.I. Specificity and regulation of casein kinase-mediated phosphorylation of alpha-synuclein. *J. Neuropathol. Exp. Neurol.* **2008**, *67*, 402–416. [CrossRef] [PubMed]
78. Waxman, E.A.; Giasson, B.I. Characterization of kinases involved in the phosphorylation of aggregated alpha-synuclein. *J. Neurosci. Res.* **2011**, *89*, 231–247. [CrossRef] [PubMed]
79. Salvi, M.; Trashi, E.; Marin, O.; Negro, A.; Sarno, S.; Pinna, L.A. Superiority of PLK-2 as α-synuclein phosphorylating agent relies on unique specificity determinants. *Biochem. Biophys. Res. Commun.* **2012**, *418*, 156–160. [CrossRef] [PubMed]
80. Tenreiro, S.; Eckermann, K.; Outeiro, T.F. Protein phosphorylation in neurodegeneration: Friend or foe? *Front. Mol. Neurosci.* **2014**, *7*, 42. [CrossRef] [PubMed]
81. Lee, G.; Tanaka, M.; Park, K.; Lee, S.S.; Kim, Y.M.; Junn, E.; Lee, S.H.; Mouradian, M.M. Casein kinase II-mediated phosphorylation regulates alpha-synuclein/synphilin-1 interaction and inclusion body formation. *J. Biol. Chem.* **2004**, *279*, 6834–6839. [CrossRef] [PubMed]
82. Ross, C.A.; Aylward, E.H.; Wild, E.J.; Langbehn, D.R.; Long, J.D.; Warner, J.H.; Scahill, R.I.; Leavitt, B.R.; Stout, J.C.; Paulsen, J.S.; et al. Huntington disease: Natural history, biomarkers and prospects for therapeutics. *Nat. Rev. Neurol.* **2014**, *10*, 204–216. [CrossRef] [PubMed]
83. Fan, M.M.; Zhang, H.; Hayden, M.R.; Pelech, S.L.; Raymond, L.A. Protective up-regulation of CK2 by mutant huntingtin in cells co-expressing NMDA receptors. *J. Neurochem.* **2008**, *104*, 790–805. [CrossRef] [PubMed]
84. Mueller, T.; Breuer, P.; Schmitt, I.; Walter, J.; Evert, B.O.; Wullner, U. CK2-dependent phosphorylation determines cellular localization and stability of ataxin-3. *Hum. Mol. Genet.* **2009**, *18*, 3334–3343. [CrossRef] [PubMed]
85. Peters, O.M.; Ghasemi, M.; Brown, R.H., Jr. Emerging mechanisms of molecular pathology in ALS. *J. Clin. Investig.* **2015**, *125*, 2548. [CrossRef] [PubMed]
86. Li, H.Y.; Yeh, P.A.; Chiu, H.C.; Tang, C.Y.; Tu, B.P. Hyperphosphorylation as a defense mechanism to reduce TDP-43 aggregation. *PLoS ONE* **2011**, *6*, e23075. [CrossRef] [PubMed]
87. Iimoto, D.S.; Masliah, E.; DeTeresa, R.; Terry, R.D.; Saitoh, T. Aberrant casein kinase II in Alzheimer's disease. *Brain Res.* **1990**, *507*, 273–280. [CrossRef]
88. Baum, L.; Masliah, E.; Iimoto, D.S.; Hansen, L.A.; Halliday, W.C.; Saitoh, T. Casein kinase II is associated with neurofibrillary tangles but is not an intrinsic component of paired helical filaments. *Brain Res.* **1992**, *573*, 126–132. [CrossRef]
89. Avila, J.; Ulloa, L.; Gonzalez, J.; Moreno, F.; Diaz-Nido, J. Phosphorylation of microtubule-associated proteins by protein kinase CK2 in neuritogenesis. *Cell. Mol. Biol. Res.* **1994**, *40*, 573–579. [PubMed]
90. Greenwood, J.A.; Scott, C.W.; Spreen, R.C.; Caputo, C.B.; Johnson, G.V. Casein kinase II preferentially phosphorylates human tau isoforms containing an amino-terminal insert. Identification of threonine 39 as the primary phosphate acceptor. *J. Biol. Chem.* **1994**, *269*, 4373–4380. [PubMed]
91. Raftery, M.; Campbell, R.; Glaros, E.N.; Rye, K.A.; Halliday, G.M.; Jessup, W.; Garner, B. Phosphorylation of apolipoprotein-E at an atypical protein kinase CK2 PSD/E site in vitro. *Biochemistry* **2005**, *44*, 7346–7353. [CrossRef] [PubMed]
92. Tu, S.; Okamoto, S.; Lipton, S.A.; Xu, H. Oligomeric Aβ-induced synaptic dysfunction in Alzheimer's disease. *Mol. Neurodegener.* **2014**, *9*, 48. [CrossRef] [PubMed]
93. Chauhan, A.; Chauhan, V.P.; Murakami, N.; Brockerhoff, H.; Wisniewski, H.M. Amyloid beta-protein stimulates casein kinase I and casein kinase II activities. *Brain Res.* **1993**, *629*, 47–52. [CrossRef]
94. Walter, J.; Schindzielorz, A.; Hartung, B.; Haass, C. Phosphorylation of the beta-amyloid precursor protein at the cell surface by ectocasein kinases 1 and 2. *J. Biol. Chem.* **2000**, *275*, 23523–23529. [CrossRef] [PubMed]
95. Rodriguez, F.; Allende, C.C.; Allende, J.E. Protein kinase casein kinase 2 holoenzyme produced ectopically in human cells can be exported to the external side of the cellular membrane. *Proc. Natl. Acad. Sci. USA* **2005**, *102*, 4718–4723. [CrossRef] [PubMed]
96. Stepanova, V.; Jerke, U.; Sagach, V.; Lindschau, C.; Dietz, R.; Haller, H.; Dumler, I. Urokinase-dependent human vascular smooth muscle cell adhesion requires selective vitronectin phosphorylation by ectoprotein kinase CK2. *J. Biol. Chem.* **2002**, *277*, 10265–10272. [CrossRef] [PubMed]

97. Lenzken, S.C.; Stanga, S.; Lanni, C.; de Leonardis, F.; Govoni, S.; Racchi, M. Recruitment of casein kinase 2 is involved in AbetaPP processing following cholinergic stimulation. *J. Alzheimers Dis.* **2010**, *20*, 1133–1141. [PubMed]

98. Pigino, G.; Morfini, G.; Atagi, Y.; Deshpande, A.; Yu, C.; Jungbauer, L.; LaDu, M.; Busciglio, J.; Brady, S. Disruption of fast axonal transport is a pathogenic mechanism for intraneuronal amyloid beta. *Proc. Natl. Acad. Sci. USA* **2009**, *106*, 5907–5912. [CrossRef] [PubMed]

99. Xu, J.; Reddy, B.J.; Anand, P.; Shu, Z.; Cermelli, S.; Mattson, M.K.; Tripathy, S.K.; Hoss, M.T.; James, N.S.; King, S.J.; et al. Casein kinase 2 reverses tail-independent inactivation of kinesin-1. *Nat. Commun.* **2012**, *3*, 754. [CrossRef] [PubMed]

100. Craft, S. Insulin resistance and Alzheimer's disease pathogenesis: Potential mechanisms and implications for treatment. *Curr. Alzheimer Res.* **2007**, *4*, 147–152. [CrossRef] [PubMed]

101. Pedersen, W.A.; McMillan, P.J.; Kulstad, J.J.; Leverenz, J.B.; Craft, S.; Haynatzki, G.R. Rosiglitazone attenuates learning and memory deficits in Tg2576 Alzheimer mice. *Exp. Neurol.* **2006**, *199*, 265–273. [CrossRef] [PubMed]

102. Reger, M.A.; Watson, G.S.; Green, P.S.; Wilkinson, C.W.; Baker, L.D.; Cholerton, B.; Fishel, M.A.; Plymate, S.R.; Breitner, J.C.; DeGroodt, W.; et al. Intranasal insulin improves cognition and modulates beta-amyloid in early AD. *Neurology* **2008**, *70*, 440–448. [CrossRef] [PubMed]

103. Wyss-Coray, T.; Rogers, J. Inflammation in Alzheimer disease-a brief review of the basic science and clinical literature. *Cold Spring Harb. Perspect. Med.* **2012**, *2*, a006346. [CrossRef] [PubMed]

104. Rosenberger, A.F.; Morrema, T.H.; Gerritsen, W.H.; van Haastert, E.S.; Snkhchyan, H.; Hilhorst, R.; Rozemuller, A.J.; Scheltens, P.; van der Vies, S.M.; et al. Increased occurrence of protein kinase CK2 in astrocytes in Alzheimer's disease pathology. *J. Neuroinflamm.* **2016**, *13*, 4. [CrossRef] [PubMed]

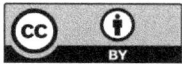

pharmaceuticals

MDPI

Review

CK2 in Cancer: Cellular and Biochemical Mechanisms and Potential Therapeutic Target

Melissa M.J. Chua [†], Charina E. Ortega [†], Ayesha Sheikh, Migi Lee, Hussein Abdul-Rassoul, Kevan L. Hartshorn and Isabel Dominguez *

Department of Medicine, School of Medicine, Boston University, Boston, MA 02118, USA; mel98791@bu.edu (M.M.J.C.); ceortega@bu.edu (C.E.O.); Ayesha.Sheikh@bmc.org (A.S.); migi0430@bu.edu (M.L.); habdulra@bu.edu (H.A.-R.); khartsho@bu.edu (K.L.H.)
* Correspondence: isdoming@bu.edu; Tel.: +1-617-414-1829
† These authors contributed equally to this work.

Academic Editor: Marc Le Borgne
Received: 2 December 2016; Accepted: 23 January 2017; Published: 28 January 2017

Abstract: CK2 genes are overexpressed in many human cancers, and most often overexpression is associated with worse prognosis. Site-specific expression in mice leads to cancer development (e.g., breast, lymphoma) indicating the oncogenic nature of CK2. CK2 is involved in many key aspects of cancer including inhibition of apoptosis, modulation of signaling pathways, DNA damage response, and cell cycle regulation. A number of CK2 inhibitors are now available and have been shown to have activity against various cancers in vitro and in pre-clinical models. Some of these inhibitors are now undergoing exploration in clinical trials as well. In this review, we will examine some of the major cancers in which CK2 inhibition has promise based on in vitro and pre-clinical studies, the proposed cellular and signaling mechanisms of anti-cancer activity by CK2 inhibitors, and the current or recent clinical trials using CK2 inhibitors.

Keywords: CK2; cancer; proliferation; apoptosis; migration; invasion; signaling pathways; signaling cascades; preclinical models; clinical trials; therapy

1. Introduction

There is strong evidence that CK2 plays a role in the pathogenesis of cancer [1–5]. Thus, CK2 functions as an oncogene when overexpressed in mice [2,4–6]. CK2 can regulate essential cellular processes, many of which are deregulated in cancer cells. In particular, CK2 increases cell proliferation [7,8], cell growth [9], and cell survival [10,11], changes cell morphology [12,13], enhances cellular transformation [4,5] and promotes angiogenesis [14,15].

CK2 kinases are a highly conserved serine/threonine kinase family, and in mammals, is composed of 2 genes: *CK2α* (*CSNK2A1*) and *CK2α'* (*CSNK2A2*). CK2α protein has higher levels and more extensive expression in mouse tissues than CK2α' has [16]. CK2 kinases can function as monomeric kinases, and also within a tetrameric complex (Figure 1). This tetrameric complex is composed of two CK2 units (CK2α and/or CK2α') and two regulatory units (CK2β). The regulatory protein CK2β is coded by a different gene, *CSNK2B*, and within the CK2 tetrameric complex, it alters CK2 kinase substrate specificity [17]. In addition, an intronlesss *CK2α* pseudogene (*CK2αP*) can be expressed in mammalian cells and somehow it is relevant in cancer [18,19]. Importantly, CK2 proteins regulate each other's levels. For example, knockdown of *CK2α* decreases CK2β protein levels, and knockdown of *CK2β* decreases CK2α' levels [4,20–22].

As we will discuss in this review, *CK2* transcripts and proteins are upregulated in many forms of cancer. In some cases CK2 protein is increased without corresponding transcript level changes [23]. However, a recent study in five cancer types (lung and bronchus, prostate, breast, colon and rectum, ovarian and pancreatic cancers) found *CK2* transcript expression upregulated in some tumors, suggesting that transcriptional mechanisms may also play a role in the increase in CK2 proteins found in human tumors [19]. In general, CK2 transcript and/or protein upregulation correlates with worse prognosis. However, it should be noted that not all published data supports the general hypothesis that *CK2* gene over-expression is a driver of cancer progression and is associated with poor prognosis. One study found that some tumors show under-expression of *CK2* genes (e.g., CK2α' in breast, ovarian, and pancreatic cancer), and that over-expression of the *CK2* gene correlated with higher patient survival in some tumors (e.g., lung adenocarcinoma) [19].

CK2's ability to promote tumors in animal models may be largely due to its ability to regulate signal transduction pathways, which may vary in different cancers [24]. CK2 can regulate signal transduction cascades such as Wnt signaling [5,25,26], Hedgehog signaling (Hh) [27], JAK/STAT [28], NF-κB [5], and PTEN/PI3K/Akt-PKB [29–32]. Modulation of these signaling transduction pathways and cascades leads to tumorigenesis, indicating avenues that CK2 can induce cancer. For example, CK2 can activate Wnt signaling by phosphorylating and upregulating the transcriptional co-factor, β-catenin [25,26]. Indeed, β-catenin is upregulated in mice overexpressing *CK2α* in mammary glands [4]. CK2 may also promote tumorigenesis through stabilization of the proto-oncogene myc [33], activation of NF-κB, an anti-apoptotic factor in breast cancer [34], and inactivation of PTEN, a tumor suppressor phosphatase [31,32]. CK2 can inhibit Notch signaling in lung cancer cells and T cell acute lymphoblastic leukemia cells in vitro. This is particularly important since Notch1 regulates myc expression [35]. CK2 itself is also regulated by other tumor-promoting oncogenes, including Bcr-Abl [36]. Additionally, CK2 can downregulate the activity of tumor suppressors [37,38]. Moreover, CK2 inhibits DNA repair in some models, providing a rationale for combining CK2 inhibitors with chemotherapy agents that cause DNA damage (see cholangiocarcinoma trial). It is plausible that there are still unidentified additional biological effects of CK2 in cancer cells.

An ample variety of cell-permeable chemical CK2 inhibitors have been developed. The most frequently used are TBB, Quinalizarin, hematein, TBCA, CIGB-300, CX-4945, DRB, apigenin, DMAT, emodin, and TF [39–49]. We will discuss the use of these inhibitors in different cancers in vitro and in vivo, and the cellular processes and signaling pathways that they affect in each type of cancer. We will also discuss the two CK2 inhibitors, CX-4945 and CIGB-300, that have made into clinical trials.

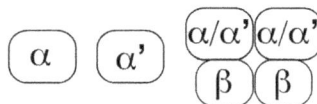

Figure 1. CK2 kinases can function as monomeric kinases and in a tetrameric complex.

2. Discussion

2.1. Solid Tumors in Which Over-Expression of CK2 Appears to Contribute to the Cancer Phenotype

Evidence is increasing that CK2 expression is linked to adverse prognosis in many common solid tumor types. These include tumors associated with chronic carcinogen exposure like non-small cell lung cancer, head and neck cancer, bladder cancer, or mesothelioma. CK2 is also involved in the pathogenesis of gastrointestinal cancers including biliary, liver, esophageal and gastric cancer, some of which may arise due to longstanding inflammation (e.g., hepatitis viruses for liver cancer or *H. pylori* for gastric cancer). CK2 is also linked to kidney cancer, HPV-related cancer (i.e., cervical cancer) and glioblastoma multiforme. As we review below, it is possible that CK2 contributes to these cancers in different ways. It is likely that initial trials of CK2 inhibitors will focus on patients with cancers that lack other effective treatments or are in advanced stages with recurrence after standard therapies.

2.1.1. Environmentally Induced Cancers

Lung Cancer

Lung cancer is a leading cause of death in the United States. It can be divided into two broad categories—small cell (SCLC) and non-small cell (NSCLC) lung cancers. Numerous studies have shown the connection of lung cancer to smoking. Survival can be extended to some extent by chemotherapy in advanced or metastatic disease. The major clinical breakthrough is the emergence of FDA approval of immunotherapy agents like Nivolumab. However, more novel therapeutic approaches are strongly needed.

Rationale for CK2 inhibitors in lung cancers: *CK2α*, *CK2α'*, *CK2β* and *CK2αP* transcripts are significantly overexpressed in lung cancer [19,50–53]. Importantly, *CK2* gene expression is proposed as a prognostic marker [19,50]. For example, in lung squamous cell carcinoma, high *CK2α* transcript expression correlates with unfavorable prognosis for relapsed free survival, disease specific survival, and overall survival [50].

CK2 may play diverse cellular roles in lung cancer progression, including the control of cell proliferation, survival, migration and invasion. In vitro studies suggest differential cellular responses depending of the subtype of cancer. For example, CK2 inhibitors decrease cell migration and invasion in human adenocarcinoma and NSCLC cell lines, seemingly through downregulation of MMP-2 transcript expression and activity via the ERK pathway [54]. In SCLC and LCLC (large cell lung cancer), cell proliferation, but not cell invasion, is highly sensitive to Quinalizarin [55]. In contrast, in one adenocarcinoma cell line, invasion and apoptosis, but not proliferation, were sensitive to Quinalizarin [55]. In other adenocarcinoma cell lines, Quinalizarin only leads to increased apoptosis [55]. Hematein, a new inhibitor of CK2, also increases apoptosis in a human lung adenocarcinoma, corroborating the results obtained with Quinalizarin [41].

CK2 may play a role in metastatic lung cancer. For example, in adenocarcinoma cell lines, CK2 activity is necessary for TGFβ-1-induced invasion [56]. This effect correlated with changes in expression of EMT (epithelial to mesenchymal transition) markers such as E-cadherin, N-cadherin, vimentin, phospho-FAK (focal adhesion kinase), phospho-Src, Twist, and Snail, and MMP-2 and MMP9 [56]. In addition, CX-4945 inhibits TGFβ-1 induced-Smad2/3 activation and β-catenin activation, suggesting that CK2 is working downstream of TGFβ receptor activation [56]. Interestingly, TGFβ-1 significantly increases CK2α, but not CK2β, protein levels in the cytosol and the nucleus, and this effect is inhibited by CX-4945. This suggests that CK2 activity is required for the increase of CK2α protein levels promoted by TGFβ-1 [56].

CK2 may also be linked to stem cell maintenance through Notch signaling, which is found activated in lung cancer [35]. Thus, CK2 activity is sufficient and necessary for Notch reporter and gene target transactivation in adenocarcinoma cell lines, at least in part due to effects in Notch1 protein levels [35].

Integration of CK2 inhibition into treatment of lung cancers: The different cellular effects of CK2 inhibitors in different lung cancer cell lines indicate that CK2 inhibitors could be specifically used in particular cancer subtypes or genotypes for lung cancer treatment. For example, CK2 inhibitors (TBB, TBCA, and hematein) alone and in combination with irradiation have variable effects on cell numbers in four different LCLC and adenocarcinoma cell lines [57]. Quinalizarin also had variable effects in a panel of cell adenocarcinoma lines with or without EGFR mutations. However, an adenocarcinoma cell line with an EGFR L858R + T790M mutation is unaffected by Quinalizarin [55].

CK2 inhibitors alone or in combination with anticancer agents have been successful in decreasing tumor burden in mouse models. Hematein prevents tumor growth in lung adenocarcinoma xenograft models as compared to controls [58]. In vitro, hematein decreases colony formation, phospho-AKT and surviving levels, and increases cleaved PARP [58].

Benavent et al. show that intravenous administration of CIGB-300 (10 mg/kg) in mouse models, markedly decreased lung colonization and metastasis development of murine 3LL cells [59].

Interestingly, after five days of systemic treatment with CIGB-300, tumor cell-driven neovascularization was significantly reduced in comparison to control group. The mechanism could be due to decrease cell adhesion, migration and invasion, MMP-2 and uPA (urokinase plasminogen activator) activity. Altogether their data suggest an important role of CK2 in lung tumor development, suggesting a potential use of CIGB-300 as a novel therapeutic agent against lung cancer. In 2014, Perera et al. studied the synergistic interactions of the anti-casein kinase 2 CIGB-300 peptide and chemotherapeutic agents in lung and cervical preclinical cancer models [60]. They studied agents such as cisplatin (alkylating), paclitaxel (antimitotic), doxorubicin (anti-topoisomerase II) or 5-fluorouracil (DNA/RNA antimetabolite) in cell lines derived from lung and cervical cancer. They observed that paclitaxel and cisplatin exhibited the best synergistic/additive profile when combined with CIGB-300, according to the combination and dose reduction indices. Such therapeutically favorable profiles may be explained by a direct cytotoxic effect and also by the observed cell cycle impairment (arrest in S and G2/M phases) following incubation of tumor cells with selected drug combinations. Paclitaxel displayed the strongest synergism with CIGB-300 in NCI-H125 and SiHa cell lines, with 5 fold less peptide required to show similar anti-proliferative effects. These findings provide a rationale for combining the anti-CK2 CIGB-300 peptide with currently available anticancer agents in the clinical setting and indicate platins and taxanes as compounds with major prospects.

Similarly, there have been studies combining CX-4945 with Erlotinib, an EGFR tyrosine kinase inhibitor used to treat advanced or metastatic non-small cell lung cancer. Bliesath et al. studied combining CX-4945 and Erlotinib, in vitro and in vivo in models of non-small cell lung carcinoma and squamous cell carcinoma, and demonstrated that it inhibited tumor growth via enhanced inhibition of the PI3K-Akt-mTOR pathway [61]. They also observed a decrease in proliferation, an increase in apoptosis, a synergistic killing of cancer cells in vitro, and an improved antitumor efficacy in vivo. Taken together, these data position CK2 as a valid pharmacologic target for drug combinations and support further evaluation of CX-4945 in combination with EGFR targeting agents [61].

There is currently an open clinical trial using CX-4945 in advanced cancers including lung cancer, Castleman's disease and multiple myeloma (trial designation: NCT00891280).

Urothelial Cancer

Urothelial carcinoma is the most common type of bladder cancer and occurs in the urinary tract system (bladder and related organs). The National Cancer Institute (NCI) estimates 76,960 new cases of bladder cancer and 16,390 deaths from the disease in 2016. It is linked to smoking and some chemical exposures. It can be well managed in early stages with surgery and other approaches (e.g., intravesicle BCG (Bacillus Calmette-Guérin immunotherapy). Advanced disease is responsive to chemotherapy but this does not extend survival markedly. The latest in the treatment is FDA approval of Atezolizumab (anti PD-L1 antibody). Atezolizumab showed partial response in at least 14.8 percent of participants and the effect lasted from more than 2.1 to more than 13.8 months at the time of the response analysis. However, we still need more options for those who are not eligible, do not respond to that or develop intolerable toxicity.

Rationale of CK2 inhibition: CK2α could play a role in invasive bladder cancer. First, immunohistochemical analysis shows that CK2α protein is overexpressed in high-grade invasive urothelial carcinomas as well as carcinoma in situ (pT2-4, CIS), but not in low-grade and noninvasive phenotypes (pTa, pT1) [62]. Second, cyclooxygenase 2 (COX2) and phospho-AKT (phospho-AKT), two proteins that may play a role in the transition to an invasive phenotype as they start to be overexpressed in noninvasive phenotypes (pT1), could be upstream of CK2α expression [62]. Indeed, *COX2* knockdown with *COX2*-siRNA decreased expression of CK2α protein and lead to cell cycle arrest at the G1 phase in urothelial carcinoma cell line, UMUC2. In addition, COX2 inhibitor, Meloxicam, suppresses the growth of invasive orthotropic bladder cancer (established by inoculating KU-7 low-grade papillary bladder cancer cells into the urinary bladder of nude mice) correlating with dowregulation of CK2α protein and phospho-AKT level [62]. Third, *CK2α* knockdown with

CK2α-siRNA fully eliminates uPA activity in UMUC2 cells and reduces uPA activity by half in a human urothelial carcinoma cell line, UMUC6, generated by long-term culture in doxorubicin [62]. uPA has several functions, including the remodeling of extracellular matrix and decreasing cellular adhesion. Fourth, CK2α protein was also increased in the lumen of exosomes secreted from human metastatic transitional cell carcinoma cells in contrast with non-metastatic cells [63]. This is significant because exosomes are proposed to facilitate invasion and metastasis [64]. These data indicate a possible role for CK2α in bladder cancer metastasis.

CK2α' and CK2β transcript levels are deregulated in bladder cancer tissues [65], suggesting the possibility that CK2α' and CK2β proteins are also deregulated in bladder cancer. Determining the levels of these two other proteins during bladder cancer progression will help determine the extent of use of CK2 inhibitors in bladder cancer.

Integration into treatment of bladder cancer: To our knowledge there are no studies on CK2 inhibition in preclinical models of bladder cancer or open clinical trials specifically focused on urothelial cancer. Promising areas for study could include combination of CK2 inhibitors with COX2 inhibitors (see above), immunotherapy or chemotherapy.

Head and Neck

Head and neck squamous cell cancers are linked to smoking and human papilloma virus (HPV) (see below). Early stage cancers are well managed with surgery, radiation and chemotherapy. However, advanced or recurrent head and neck cancer is a major problem since chemotherapy provides little survival benefit. A recent study showed benefit of immunotherapy with pembrolizumab (a PD-1 antibody) in advanced head and neck squamous cell cancer. Nonetheless there is a strong need for new therapies in advanced or recurrent head and neck cancer when surgery or radiation are no longer possible.

Rationale of CK2 inhibition: CK2 transcripts, proteins and activity are elevated in head and neck squamous cell carcinoma (HNSCC) tumors and cell lines [37,38,65–68], and are proposed to be a prognostic marker for HNSCC [65–68]. The increase in CK2α, CK2α' and CK2β transcript in HNSCC could be due, at least in part, to DNA amplification [38]. As for CK2 proteins, normal oral mucosa and HNSCC tumor samples show staining of CK2α, CK2α' and CK2β in cytoplasm and, prominently, in the nucleus [37].

CK2 is essential for HNSCC cell viability, proliferation and cell cycle regulation. Thus, antisense CK2α reduce cell numbers [37,69] and induces apoptosis [37,70] and antisense CK2β induced apoptosis in HNSCC [37,69]. Individual knockdown of *CK2α, CK2α'* and *CK2β* arrests HNSCC cells at G0/G1. Similarly, CX-4945 decreases cell numbers, induces cell cycle arrest at S or G2/M, and increases apoptosis in HNSCC cell lines [38].

The differential effects of knockdown of CK2α, CK2α' and CK2β suggest that these proteins play independent roles in HNSSC. For example, CK2α and CK2β knockdown, but not CK2α', leads to decreased cell migration of HNSCC cell lines [37]. Individual knockdown of CK2α, CK2α' and CK2β differentially affect gene expression of key cell proliferation, survival and tumor suppressor genes in HNSCC that are WT for P53, further suggesting that the three genes play independent roles in HNSSC [37]. Similar effects on cell proliferation, survival and tumor suppressor genes are shown using CX-4945 in HNSCC cells WT for P53. However, gene expression changes in mutant P53 cells exposed to CX-4945 were qualitatively different [38].

Several mechanisms for CK2's action in head and neck cancer are proposed including activation of signaling pathways, EMT processes and cancer stem cell regulation. Thus, HNSCC show elevated levels of NFκB, a factor required for HNSCC cell survival [71]. In HNSCC, NFκB increases could be due to CK2α activity through activation IκB kinase (IKK), a known activator of NF-κB [72]. Indeed, knockdown with siRNA of *CK2α, CK2α'* and *CK2β* independently decreased NF-κB activity [37]. This suggests the importance of CK2 in HNSCC, and, moreover, the importance of CK2α' and *CK2β*, both understudied CK2 genes in cancer.

CK2 activity is required for post-translational stabilization of Twist, a transcription factor involved in EMT processes [73]. CK2 also regulates other EMT-linked proteins. For example, CK2 knockdown also decreases protein levels of slug, snail and vimentin, and increases E-cadherin levels in laryngeal carcinoma cells [74]. CK2 is also required for IL-6 dependent cell migration of HNSCC cells [73]. This is significant because IL-6, a cytokine, is upregulated in HNSCC correlating with recurrence and low patient survival [75–77]. These data indicate a role for CK2 in the metastatic potential of head and neck cancers.

CK2 activity is required for cancer stem cell-like cell maintenance, tumor sphere formation and proliferation, and for the expression of cancer stem cell genes and proteins (e.g., Nanog, Oct4, and Sox2) in HNSCC [78]. Cancer stem cell genes are important in tumor initiation and therapeutic resistance, positing a role for CK2 in tumorigenesis and therapy resistance in HNSCC.

Integration into clinical care of head and neck cancer: Preclinical models show that CK2 inhibitors reduce tumor burden in head and neck cancer. HNSCC xenograft tumor models (tongue, hypopharyngeal and laryngeal carcinomas) show that treatment with CK2 inhibitors (RNAi-CK2α/α′containing nanocapsules) can significantly reduce tumor volume, reduce number of metastasis and increase the survival of mice [79]. In addition, tumors from CK2α/α′-RNAi-treated mice show reduced staining of pro-proliferative proteins (e.g., Cyclin D1) and increased levels of tumor suppressors (e.g., P53) compared to tumors from control mice [37]. Nanoencapsulated CK2α/α′ RNAi did not affect mouse body weight [79]. In contrast, CX-4945 had no effect on the survival of mice and minimal effect on tumor volume in a HNSCC xenograft tumor model, and did not synergize in a combination with a MEK inhibitor (PD-901). This lack of effect of CX-4945 in vivo could be due to an ineffective drug dose scheme, lack of intake in tumor cells, or the particular cell line genotype.

The likely first use in clinical trials will be in advanced head and neck cancer given the limited treatment options for this type of tumors. To our knowledge there are no active trials of CK2 inhibitors directed against head and neck specifically. CK2 inhibitors could be tested out as single agents in refractory disease or combined with chemotherapy or immunotherapy. In cases where the cancer is linked to HPV, there may be an additional rationale for use of CK2 inhibitors (see discussion below of HPV related cancers).

Mesothelioma

Malignant mesothelioma is a rare neoplasm linked to asbestos exposure. It has an extremely poor prognosis with median survival of 4 to 13 months for untreated patients and 6 to 18 months for treated patients, regardless of therapeutic approach. Combination chemotherapy using cisplatin and pemetrexed is the standard regimen for patients with unresectable disease. For selected minority of patients, a monoclonal antibody, bevacizumab has shown some promise but still awaiting regulatory approval.

Rationale of CK2 inhibition: CK2α transcript is deregulated in mesothelioma tissues and cell lines [65,80]. CK2α staining is elevated in mesothelioma tissue sections and cell lines [80]. Moreover, the *CK2α pseudogene (CK2αP)* could be a prognostic factor in mesothelioma [65].

CK2 plays a role in the control of Hedgehog (Hh)/Gli1 signaling, a pathway that is aberrantly upregulated in mesothelioma [81,82]. Thus, CK2α upregulation in mesothelioma correlates with upregulation of the transcript and protein for Gli1, the transcription factor of Hh signaling. CK2α activity is sufficient and necessary (CK2α-siRNA, CX-4945) to activate a Gli1 reporter in mesothelioma cell lines [80]. Furthermore, CX-4945 treatment led to a decrease in mesothelioma cell proliferation [80]. These indicate that CK2 inhibition is a potential treatment for mesothelioma potentially through the regulation of Hh signaling.

Integration into clinical care of mesothelioma—To our knowledge there are no active trials of CK2 inhibitors in mesothelioma. However, this is certainly a disease in need of new therapies, especially in the advanced stages. Potential approaches would include use of CX-4945 or CIGB 300 in combination with cisplatin or pemetrexed.

2.1.2. Gastrointestinal Cancers (Often Related to Chronic Inflammation)

Hepatocellular Cancer

The major etiological factors for hepatocellular cancer include chronic infection with hepatitis B or C, alcohol cirrhosis, or steatohepatitis. There are limited options for treatment for hepatocellular cancer when not amenable to transplant or surgery. Local ablative therapies or tyrosine kinase inhibitors are used often and these measures improve survival by several months in general. Immunotherapy is also being studied for advanced hepatocellular cancer. Clearly there is need for additional therapies.

Rationale of CK2 inhibition: Hepatocellular cancer (HCC) samples show high expression of CK2 gene transcripts, proteins and activity [6,65,83–85]. Levels of CK2 transcripts and proteins are proposed as prognostic markers for HCC [6,65,83]. Interestingly, a variant of CK2α, CK2α", is highly expressed in the liver and is required for membrane protein trafficking and has limited nuclear localization [86]. The role of CK2α" in HCC has not been studied.

In mouse xenograft models, injection of hepatoma cells overexpressing CK2α leads to higher tumor volume than injection of the corresponding untransfected hepatoma cells, further indicating the oncogenic nature of CK2α [6]. In vitro, CK2α overexpression increases proliferation, colony formation, migration and invasion, and inhibits apoptosis in HCC cell lines [6]. This suggests that CK2 may be involved in the control of diverse cellular processes during HCC progression.

Conversely, *CK2α* knockdown decreases proliferation and colony formation, causes G2/M arrest, and increases apoptosis in HCC cell lines [6,83,85]. *CK2α* knockdown also inhibits migration and invasion in HCC cell lines [6,84]. Several mechanisms have been proposed for these effects of *CK2α* knockdown in HCC cell lines. Among the mechanisms proposed are downregulation of MMP and EMT-linked proteins (snail, slug, vimentin) and increasing E-cadherin expression [84]; inhibition of Hedgehog signaling [84]; and downregulation of phospho-Akt, apoptotic-marker genes and p53 [6]. Additionally, CK2 inhibition can increase Natural Killer (NK) cell-mediated apoptosis of liver cancer cells suggesting that CK2 could increase tumor immunity [87]. Similarly, chemical inhibition of CK2 in HCC cells leads to decreased proliferation (e.g., DMAT [85]) and increased apoptosis (e.g., emodin, [87]).

Integration into clinical care of HCC: Preclinical studies show that CK2 inhibitors reduce tumor burden alone and in combination with other agents. Thus, in mouse xenograft models of HCC, DMAT and shCK2α inhibit tumor growth [6,85]. DMAT acts by decreasing proliferation but not cell survival or angiogenesis and, importantly, did not induce liver damage [85]. DMAT's effects may be mediated by reducing NFκB and Wnt/β-catenin signaling activation [85]. Moreover, CK2 inhibitors increase the effectiveness of chemotherapeutics on HCC proliferation (5-fluorouracil (5-FU), doxorubicin or sorafenib) [85,87]. These suggest that CK2 inhibitors could be used as potential therapeutics for liver cancers, alone or in combination in other drugs.

Gastric Cancer

Gastric adenocarcinoma is a major cause of cancer death worldwide, and its development is linked to *Helicobacter pylori* infection and chronic atrophic gastritis. There are several lines of chemotherapy available to extend survival in advanced disease. Anti-HER 2 antibodies are also useful in subset of patients, and anti VEGF receptor antibodies are a part of second line therapy. Additional therapies are clearly needed since survival in advanced gastric cancer is limited to approximately 1 year even when using all available treatments.

Rationale of CK2 inhibition: CK2 transcripts and proteins are elevated in gastric cancer [88], and CK2 is proposed as a prognostic marker for gastric cancer [65,88,89]. Interestingly, CK2 activity is upregulated after *H. pylori* infection of gastric epithelial cells [90]. The upregulation of CK2 activity is not due to increased CK2α protein levels, however, CK2α' and CK2β expression are still to be studied in these tumors [90].

CK2 inhibition leads to decreased cell proliferation and migration of gastric cancer cells by decreasing MMP expression [88]. CK2 inhibition also leads to apoptosis in human gastric carcinoma cells [91].

Importantly, CK2 is associated with *H. pylori*-infection in gastric cells. In gastric epithelial cells, CK2 is necessary for *H. pylori*-induced cell migration and invasion [90]. The underlying mechanism is the phosphorylation of α-catenin by CK2 that results in the depletion of α-catenin at the membrane and subsequently, the disruption of the α-catenin/β-catenin complexes at the membrane. Indeed in *H. pylori*-infected patient tissue sections, membrane α-catenin, β-catenin and E-cadherin levels are decreased compared with non-infected tissue samples [90]. The disruption of these membrane complexes leads to β-catenin accumulation in the nucleus of *H. pylori*–infected tissue sections. This is important because, nuclear accumulation of β-catenin is a requisite for activation of Wnt/β-catenin signaling. Indeed, in gastric epithelial cells, *H. pylori*-infection leads to increased Wnt/β-catenin reporter activity and Wnt target gene MMP7, a secreted protein that breaks down the extracellular matrix, in gastric cells [90]. Additionally, CK2 could be associated to gastric carcinoma also through phosphorylation of DBC1 (deleted in breast cancer 1) [88].

Integration into clinical care of gastric cancer: CK2 may play a role in resistance to chemotherapy. Thus, CK2α protein levels are elevated in cisplatin resistant gastric cancer cells. Moreover, CK2 has been proposed to help mediate cisplatin resistance in gastric cancer cells [92].

There are no active trials of CK2 inhibitors focused specifically on gastric cancer. However, there is a strong need for novel therapies for this common cancer. The likely area for initial trials of CK2 inhibitors will be in advanced disease after progression on the first two approved lines of therapy.

Esophageal Cancer

There are two major types of esophageal cancer: adenocarcinoma and squamous cell carcinoma. The main epidemiological link for adenocarcinoma is chronic reflux esophagitis, and the incidence of this cancer is increasing. Squamous cell carcinoma is mainly linked to alcohol and tobacco use, and its incidence is declining. Localized disease is curable in some cases with combinations of chemotherapy, radiation and surgery but there are limited options for treatment of advanced or recurrent disease.

Rationale of CK2 inhibition: To our knowledge there is no data on expression of CK2 proteins in esophageal cancer. However, CK2 gene transcripts are deregulated in esophageal cancer [65]. Importantly, esophageal cancer cell lines show differences in CK2 activity levels despite similar levels of CK2α expression [93]. This suggests that expression of the other CK2 proteins may be deregulated, although other mechanisms are possible. CK2 activity is also found elevated in TRAIL (TNF-related apoptosis-inducing ligand)-resistant esophageal cancer cell lines compared to non-resistant cell lines [94]. This suggests that CK2 may play a role in resistance to therapy in esophageal cancer.

CK2 has been linked to invasive phenotypes in esophageal cancer cells. Thus, *CK2α* overexpression increases invasiveness in esophageal cancer cells through the nuclear receptor corepressor (NCoR) [93]. NCoR represses transcription of the chemokine IFNγ-inducible protein-10 (IP-10), an antitumoral gene that inhibits tumor proliferation and metastasis [93]. The ability of CK2α to promote invasion is also linked to EMT-linked genes. Thus, CK2α overexpression results in decreased E-cadherin expression and increased N-cadherin and vimentin expression [93,95]. These changes in EMT-linked proteins lead to resistance to anoikis, a type of induced programmed cell death when anchorage-dependent cells detach from the surrounding extracellular matrix [95]. This suggests that CK2 could act to promote metastasis in esophageal cancer.

CK2 may be mediating inhibition of 5-fluorouracil (5-Fu)-induced apoptosis by IGF-1 in esophageal carcinoma cells [96]. Since 5-FU is a key ingredient in treatment of esophageal cancers (and other gastrointestinal tract cancers), this suggests that combining CK2 inhibition with 5-FU may be an effective strategy.

Integration into clinical care of esophageal cancer: There are no active trials of CK2 inhibitors focused specifically on esophageal cancers. The most likely initial use is in advanced or recurrent cancer, where survival is poor and chemotherapy is of limited effectiveness.

Cholangiocarcinoma

Cholangiocarcinomas are rare malignancies arising from the epithelial cells of the intrahepatic and extrahepatic bile ducts. The etiology is not clear, but there is a linkage to chronic liver fluke infection, chronic hepatitis C infection and possibly to Hepatitis B and HIV. The first line chemotherapy regimen in advanced disease includes gemcitabine plus cisplatin, which yields an approximate 4-month survival benefit compared to gemcitabine alone. Overall cures are rare when the cancer is not resectable and there is a strong need for new agents, especially in advanced or recurrent disease.

Rationale of CK2 inhibition: CK2 has been linked to cholangiocarcinoma (CCA) tumorigenesis. CK2β staining is higher in CCA tumor sections compared to normal tissue liver sections [97]. CK2β staining is found in the cytoplasm and more prominently in the nucleus. In addition, high CK2β staining is associated with higher tumor stage, higher histological grade and high serum CEA (carcinoembryonic antigen) level. These suggest a role for CK2 in CCA progression and invasion. High CK2β staining correlates with lower patient survival, and it is an independent prognostic factor in CCA [97]. In addition, CK2α was specifically detected in plasma of CCA patients suggesting that CK2α is a potential biomarker for CCA diagnosis [98].

It has been proposed that XIAP (X-Linked inhibitor of apoptosis protein) could be downstream of CK2β upregulation in CCA, as CK2 activity is required for XIAP levels [99]. This is important because XIAP is upregulated in CAA, and high levels of XIAP correlate with low patient survival [97].

Integration into clinical care of cholangiocarcinoma: Currently, CX-4945 is being tested in phase I/II study in combination with gemcitabine and cisplatin in patients with cholangiocarcinoma. In this context, CX-4945 may inhibit DNA repair, and be particularly effective when combined with agents such as cisplatin that cause DNA damage. The objective of this trial is to determine the maximum tolerated dose (MTD), followed by a randomized study that compares antitumor activity in cholangiocarcinoma patients receiving the standard of care gemcitabine plus cisplatin versus CX-4945 at the combination MTD with gemcitabine plus cisplatin. This is a multicenter study in the United States, South Korea and Taiwan with estimated study completion date of December 2017(NCT02108282).

Colorectal Cancer

The most common type of colorectal cancer is adenocarcinoma (95%). The precursor to adenocarcinoma is adenomatous polyps (adenomas), which are a precancerous condition. Treatment includes surgery, chemotherapy, biological therapy, and radiation therapy.

Rationale of CK2 inhibition: CK2 gene transcripts are elevated in colorectal cancer [19,89]. Notably, CK2α protein is overexpressed in the nucleus of cells in tumor tissue sections, compared to normal colorectal and adenoma tissue sections [100]. Elevated levels of nuclear CK2α correlate with poor prognosis in patients with colorectal cancer, with increased invasion depth, node involvement, American Joint Committee on Cancer (AJCC) stage, poorer differentiation and overall decreased survival rate [101].

Inhibition of CK2α, by siRNA or CK2α inhibitor emodin, led to inhibition of colorectal carcinoma cell proliferation, G0/G1 cell cycle phase arrest, inhibition of cell division, increase in p53/p21 expression, downregulation of c-myc, and decreased cell motility and invasion [100].

CK2 has been shown to regulate Wnt/β-catenin signaling [5]. Importantly, Wnt/β-catenin signaling is major player in colorectal cancer, as it is proposed to be the first hit to be deregulated in colon cancer progression [102]. CK2 also promotes colon cancer cell invasion by increasing stability of a membrane metalloprotease, endothelin-converting enzyme-1c (ECE-1c) [103]. ECE-1c is involved in endothelin-1 synthesis, which also participates in invasion in vivo in breast, ovary, and prostate cancer cells [104–107]. CK2 phosphorylates ECE-1c at the N-terminal end, stabilizing it. Expression of full-length ECE-1c mutants mimicking CK2 phosphorylation led to increased invasion of colon cancer cells. Conversely, expression of full-length ECE-1c mutants that cannot be phosphorylated by CK2 led to decreased invasion of colon cancer cells. Together these demonstrated the relation of CK2 and ECE-1c protein stabilization by phosphorylation in increasing invasion of colon cancer cells, demonstrating a mechanism by which CK2 can promote invasion of colon cancer.

Integration of CK2 inhibition into therapy of colorectal cancer: There are no active trials of CK2 inhibitors focused specifically on colon cancer. In vitro data suggest that CK2 may play a role in resistance to chemotherapy. Thus, CK2 protects against colon carcinoma cell apoptosis induced by TRAIL (TNF-related apoptosis-inducing ligand) [108]. Indeed, CK2 inhibition with DRB leads to increased TRAIL-induced apoptosis in colon carcinoma cells, correlating with increased TRAIL-induced death-inducing signaling complex (DISC) formation, caspase-8 cleavage, and Bid cleavage, leading to proapoptotic factor release from the mitochondria. *CK2α* knockdown with *CK2α* shRNA also increased TRAIL sensitivity in human colorectal adenocarcinoma cells. These suggest a potential for CK2 inhibition in overcoming tumor resistance to therapy.

Pancreatic Cancer

Pancreatic adenocarcinoma remains a common and still highly lethal malignancy. Most cases are not amenable to curative surgery and there is no screening modality to detect this cancer in the general population at risk. Treatments for advanced disease have limited survival impact, so new therapies are desperately needed.

Rationale for CK2 inhibition: *CK2α* and *CK2α'* knockdown, DRB, and apigenin induce apoptosis of pancreatic cancer cells [109–111]. Some of these effects can be mediated by a reduction of NF-κB-dependent transcriptional activity [109]. In addition, D11, a potential inhibitor of CK2, reduced phosphorylation of two biomarkers for CK2 activity, CDC37 and PTEN [110].

There may be an important role for CK2α' in pancreatic cancer. Thus, knockdown of *CK2α'* was more efficient in inducing apoptosis than *CK2α* knockdown in PANC-1 cells, a gemcitabine resistant cell line. *CK2α* or *CK2α'* knockdown sensitizes cells to gemcitabine, correlating with increased Jun-amino-terminal kinase (JNK) phosphorylation and phospho-p70S6K (T389), respectively. Authors speculate that CK2α may be sequester in an inactive from in oligomers of the tetrameric CK2α2β2 while, CK2α'2β2 tetramers, that cannot oligomerize, will be active in these cells [112].

Integration of CK2 inhibition into therapy of pancreatic cancer: Preclinical studies show that CK2 inhibitors reduce tumor burden, alone or in combination with other inhibitors. Thus, in a mouse xenograft model of pancreatic cancer, CX-4945 inhibits tumor growth and decreases p21 staining [44]. Moreover, in an orthotopic mouse xenograft model of pancreatic cancer, intraperitoneal injection of *O*-methyl modified CK2α siRNA together with a transfection reagent results in a trend towards decreased tumor volume, and a significant increase in apoptosis [111]. A larger and significant decrease in tumor volume is found when CK2α siRNA is used in combination with PAK7 and/or MAP3K7 siRNAs [111]. None of these treatments affect mouse weight. These suggest that CK2 inhibitors could be used as potential therapeutics for pancreatic cancers.

2.1.3. HPV-Related Cancers: Cervical, Head and Neck, Anal and Penile

Cancers related to HPV infection are highly prevalent worldwide and do not respond well to treatment in advanced stages. Cervical cancer and anal cancer are particularly prevalent and problematic in patients with HIV infection and AIDS. There is evidence that CK2 plays a specific role in the mechanisms through which HPV induces cancer, and hence CK2 inhibition has received special attention in these cancers.

Rationale for use of CK2 inhibition in cervical cancer: CK2 gene transcripts are deregulated in cervical cancer, and the *CK2α* pseudogene, *CK2αP*, could be a prognostic marker in cervical cancer [65]. To our knowledge there are no studies showing expression of CK2 proteins in cervical cancer, nonetheless, CK2 activity is higher in HPV-immortalized cell lines compared to normal keratinocytes [113]. Conversely, CK2 regulates HPV through the HPV-16 E7 viral oncoprotein [113,114].

CK2 inhibitors affect cervical cancer cells. Thus, CIGB-300 inhibits cervical cancer cell line proliferation [60]. Moreover, CIGB-300 synergized with paclitaxel and doxorubicin, and was additive in combination with cisplatin (CDDP) [60]. CK2 could also play a role in cervical stem cancer cell maintenance, as apigenin inhibits HeLa tumorsphere formation and self-renewal capacity while, conversely, CK2α overexpression increases self-renewal capacity [115]. The tumorsphere assay is an analysis of the self-renewal capability of cancer stem cells, which is a population with tumor initiation, drug resistance, and metastasis properties.

Integration into clinical care of cervical cancer and by extension other HPV related cancers: CK2 could be a potential therapeutic target in cervical cancer. The efficacy of CK2 inhibitor in cervical tumor remission was first tested on mouse xenograft models. CIGB-300 diminished tumor growth, even after cessation of treatment [43,60]. In addition, CIGB-300 plus cisplatin significantly reduced tumor growth and increased mouse survival in a cervical mouse xenograft model [60].

Moreover, the first human clinical trial of the CK2 inhibitor CIGB-300 demonstrated potential clinical benefit for cervical cancer [116]. In this study, thirty-one women with cervical cancer were administered CIGB-300 intralesionally at four increasing doses over five consecutive days. Side effects were minimal even with the highest dose, and 75% of patients had significant lesion reduction. Strikingly, 19% of patients had full histological regression and 48% of patients who were previously HPV DNA-positive were negative at the end of the trial [116]. At the one-year follow up, there were no recurrences or adverse events. Interestingly, four patients conceived, of which two were infertile prior to the intervention. Pharmacokinetic studies with CIGB-300 have established a treatment plan for phase II trials [117]. Therefore CK2 inhibition is tolerable in humans, and is a promising treatment for cervical cancers, alone or in combination with chemotherapeutic agents [60].

There is currently an open clinical trial in Argentina, where investigators are using CIGB-300 in patients with squamous cell carcinoma or adenocarcinoma of the cervix stage IIA and IIB FIGO classification in a concurrent fashion with external radiotherapy, endocavitary brachytherapy and weekly systemic cisplatin (trial designation: NCT01639625)

2.1.4. Other Solid Tumors: Glioblastoma, Melanoma, Ovarian Cancer, Prostate Cancer, Breast Cancer and Renal Cell Carcinoma

Glioblastoma

Glioblastoma (GBM) is a highly lethal cancer and there are limited treatment options once it recurs after surgery and radiation (combined with chemotherapy). Cure rates for this cancer are low and there is a strong need for new therapies.

Rationale of CK2 inhibition: Numerous reports have recently shown a role for CK2 in GBM tumorigenesis. First, CK2 transcripts and proteins are overexpressed in GBM samples. Thus, CK2α transcript and protein levels and staining are elevated in GBM tumor samples [21,65,118–120]. The increase in CK2α transcripts may be due to changes in gene dosage. *CK2α* had gene dosage gains in more than fifty percent of human GBM cases [21]. CK2α' gene dosage gains have also been reported in GBM [21]. Expression of CK2α transcripts correlates with lower survival [119], although this may be controversial [65]. In addition, CK2α but not CK2β is overexpressed in tumors from a preclinical model of GBM (GL261 cells) compared to normal tissue. The authors suggest that the unbalance in the ratio CK2α/CK2β in GL261 tumors should be considered in preclinical studies [121].

Second, CK2α or CK2β overexpression is sufficient to increase GBM cell proliferation and colony formation in GBM cell lines [119].

Third, CK2 is necessary in GBM for cellular processes and signaling pathway activation. Thus, CK2 inhibition (CX-4945, siRNA, RNAi, TBB, DMAT, DRB, apigenin, etc.) in GBM cell lines leads to increased apoptosis, S or G2/M cell cycle phase arrest, and decreased adhesion, migration and colony formation [20,21,118,119,122–124]. The downstream mechanism by which CK2 inhibition causes these effects in GBMs is still being studied. Among the proposed mechanisms are the downregulation of the Wnt/β-catenin, JAK/STAT-3, NF-κB and PI3K/Akt pathways, and enhanced DNA-PK activity and autophagy [20,21,119,120,125].

CK2 inhibition sensitized GBM cells to TNFα-induced apoptosis, through mechanisms involving NFκB, p53 and SIRT1 [118]. This is relevant because GBM cells are often resistant to TNFα-induced apoptosis mediated through NF-κB activation [118]. Recently a phospho-proteomic study indicated that a constitutively active epidermal growth factor receptor (EGFRvIII) overexpressed in GBM may regulate the activity of CK2α in GBM [126].

In addition, CK2α is necessary for expression of Oct4 and Nanog, two genes involved in glioblastoma-initiating cell proliferation, in cells and tumor spheres from GBM patient cell lines [119]. These data suggests that CK2 activity is required to maintain stem cell phenotypes and self-renewal in GBM [119]. Therefore, CK2 could be a potential target for the treatment of GBM.

Integration of CK2 inhibition into treatment of glioblastoma: Preclinical GBM xenograft models show that several CK2 inhibitors are effective in inhibiting glioblastoma tumor growth and increasing the survival of mice [21,119,123,124,127]. In addition, *CK2* knockdown alone or in combination with *EGFR* knockdown increased mouse survival and necrosis in the tumor tissue of GBM xenograft mouse models [127]. CK2 inhibition in xenograft GBM tumors lead to decreased activation of STAT-3, NF-κB, c-myc and AKT, and decreased EGFR expression, suggesting that CK2 controls several pro-survival and pro-proliferative signals in vivo [21,127]. Hence, CK2 inhibitors may have a role in preventing recurrence after surgical resection along with radiotherapy with concurrent and adjuvant Temozolomide.

Melanoma

Therapy for advanced melanoma has been improving with use of signal transduction inhibitors for tumors expressing BRAF mutations. The other recent major advance in therapy of advanced melanoma or melanoma at high risk of recurrence after surgery is the use of immune checkpoint inhibitor antibodies. However, melanoma is still an aggressive and often lethal disease and its incidence is increasing.

Rationale of CK2 inhibition: *CK2α* transcript is upregulated in 15% of melanoma tumor samples [128]. To our knowledge there is no data on expression of CK2 proteins in melanoma. However, CK2 activity is elevated in metastatic melanoma samples compared to dermal nevus [129], suggesting that there is aberrant expression of CK2 transcripts and/or proteins in melanoma. Strengthening this notion, protein levels of CK2α are increased in melanoma cell lines [128].

CK2 inhibition with 7,7'-Diazaindirubin diminishes proliferation in melanoma cell lines [130]. Importantly, CK2 has been linked to sensitivity to BRAF inhibitors. First, CK2α overexpression in BRAF-mutant melanoma cells decreased sensitivity to BRAF inhibitors (vemurafenib, dabrafenib) and MEK inhibitor (trametinib) [128]. Conversely, *CK2α* knockdown sensitized BRAF-mutant melanoma cells to vemurafenib. Interestingly, combination of CK2 inhibitor CX-4945 and BRAF inhibitor vemurafenib additively inhibited proliferation in BRAF mutant patient-derived melanoma cell lines [131]. This is significant because patients with BRAF mutations become resistant to vemurafenib, and the novel therapies being explored aim to target several signaling pathways. One interesting finding is that the effect of CK2α overexpression in melanoma is not dependent on its catalytic activity [128].

Integration of CK2 inhibition into clinical care of melanoma: It is still true that most patients with metastatic melanoma succumb to their disease, therefore trials in advanced melanoma either as single agents or in combination with signal transduction inhibitors or immunotherapy will be of great interest.

Ovarian Cancer

Ovarian cancer is hard to detect in early stages and difficult to cure with current modalities in advanced stages.

Rationale for CK2 inhibition in ovarian cancer: CK2α transcript expression is elevated in 518 serous cystadenocarcinomas samples as compared to 8 fallopian tube sample controls [132]. In a culture model of epithelial ovarian tumorigenesis, CK2α protein expression is highest in a metastatic cell line compared to a neoplastic and tumorigenic cell line, and to the control (normal and pre-neoplastic, non-tumorigenic) cell lines [133], suggesting a role for CK2 in ovarian cancer progression.

CK2 may play a role in the maintenance of cancer stem cells, as CK2α protein levels are higher in the tumorspheres from SKOV3 cells that are contain only cancer-stem cells, compared with the parental cells that are a mix of cancer stem and non-stem cells. In addition, CK2α overexpression increases the sphere formation of SKOV3 cells over two fold, and inhibition of CK2 (apigenin and CK2α siRNA) decrease sphere forming efficiency. These two effects correlate with increased and decreased expression of *Gli1*, which is amplified in ovarian cancer stem-like cells respectively [134].

Integration of CK2 inhibitors into treatment of ovarian cancer: Combination therapies with CK2 inhibitors have studied in cell cultures and xenograft models. In cell cultures, CX-4945 synergizes with cisplatin and gemcitabine to increase apoptosis in p53 WT (A2780) but not in p53 null (SKOV-3) cells, and to increase mitotic catastrophe in SKOV-3 cells [135].

CX-4945 in combination with dasatinib, a tyrosine kinase inhibitor of the Src-family kinases, promote apoptosis in a panel of human epithelial ovarian carcinoma cell lines. Cell lines with low *CSNK2A1* transcript expression had lower viability in the presence of dasatinib, therefore *CSNK2A1* transcript levels are proposed to be a predictor for dasatinib sensitivity. Indeed, a 3:1 ratio of CX-4945:Dasatinib were better in cell lines with low *CSNK2A1* transcript expression, while a 8:1 or 20:1 ratio was synergistic for cell lines with high transcript levels of *CSNK2A1*. Authors suggest that CSNK2A1 levels should be analyzed before treatment with dasatinib [132].

In a mouse xenograft model of non-high grade ovarian cancer (IGROV-1 cells), CX-4945 treatment prevented tumor growth, decreased vascular area and proliferative index, and prevented mRNA expression of TNF, IL-6, and VEGF. CK2 inhibition reduces the release of these factors in IGROV-1 and SKOV3ip1 cells, and in primary ovarian cancer cells from ascites [136].

In a xenograft model of high-grade ovarian cancer (A2780 cells), a combination of CX-4945 with three drugs (cisplatin, Carboplatin, and gemcitabine) extended the time-to-endpoint two fold as compared to the untreated mice. Specifically, carboplatin synergizes with CX-4945 while cisplatin and gemcitabine had an additive effect on tumor growth inhibition However, the combination of cisplatin and CX-4945 resulted in mouse weight loss [135]. Hence, CK2 inhibitors could be used for the treatment of advanced ovarian cancer.

Prostate Cancer

Prostate cancer is the second most common cancer in men (after lung cancer) and remains lethal in advanced stages despite recent advances in therapy.

Rationale for CK2 inhibition in prostate cancer: CK2 protein levels and activity are deregulated in prostate cancer and prostate cancer-derived cells. Human benign prostatic hyperplasia (BPH; $n = 31$) and prostate cancer ($n = 30$) tissue sections had higher staining for CK2α and NF-κB compared to normal prostate tissue specimens [137]. Furthermore, CK2α staining in sections is higher in malignant compared to normal human prostate glandular cells. Total CK2α immunostaining correlated with poorly differentiated tumors (high Gleason scores) and locally aggressive tumors (high cT). In both normal and tumoral glands, there is higher staining in the nucleus than in the cytoplasm. However, nuclear, but not cytoplasmic, staining of CK2α in prostate cancers correlates with high cT stages, higher Gleason scores, and more potential capsular involvement (lymphatic or perineural invasion). All these are established prognostic factors for prostate cancer, therefore CK2α nuclear staining can be a prognostic marker [138].

In contrast, decreased CK2α and CK2α' protein levels are observed in xenograft tumors relative to cultured cells from cell lines including C4-2 cells, a metastatic subline of LNCaP (androgen-sensitive human prostate adenocarcinoma cells) and PC3-LN4 cells, a lymph node derived cell line from repeated orthotopic injections of PC-3 cells (bone-metastatic derived prostate adenocarcinoma cells). Intriguingly, the transcript levels in the xenograft tumors doubled compared to their respective cultured cell lines. Authors speculate that this decrease in CK2α/α' protein levels in xenograft tumors is due to the presence of mouse stromal cells within the lysate. Intriguingly, CK2α' protein levels were greater in BPH-1 cells compared to prostate cancer cell lines [139]. It is possible that CK2α' overexpression explains the intense staining in human BPH tissue sections compared to controls found by other authors [140]. As it is found in other tumor types, despite having the same amount of CK2α protein and mRNA levels, some prostate cell lines show different CK2 activity. For example, PC-3 (bone-metastatic derived prostate adenocarcinoma) cells have 8 times more CK2 activity than RWPEI (normal prostate) cells and 3 times more activity than LNCaP cells (androgen-sensitive human prostate adenocarcinoma cells) [141]. Importantly, CK2 activity levels correlate with increased of invasion potential (matrigel invasion assay) in these cell lines [141].

CK2 inhibition (DMAT, TF, TBB, TBCA, siRNA, apigenin, and KI-CK2α) reduces cell proliferation in prostate cancer cell lines [49,142–146], and TF, CX-4945, DMAT, TBB, TBCA, and apigenin increase apoptosis [49,142,146–150]. CX-4945, apigenin, and TBCA induced cell cycle arrest in G2/M phase [146,148]. Interestingly, only when DMAT and CK2α/α' siRNA are nanoencapsulated, they specifically decreases proliferation in prostate cancer cell lines (PC3-LN4), but not benign cell lines (BPH-1) [144]. In addition to PC3-LN4, nanoencapsulated CK2α/α' siRNA also affects prostate cancer cell line C4-2, but not normal prostate epithelial cell lines (PrEC) [144].

A number of mechanisms are proposed to underlie the role of CK2 in prostate cancer. For example, apigenin, TBCA, and CK2α or CK2α' siRNA decrease nuclear translocation of AR (androgen-receptor) and AR-mediated gene expression in response to an AR agonist, R1881, treatment [146]. TBB sensitizes cells to TRAIL (tumor-necrosis factor-related ligand)/induced apoptosis and glycolysis inhibitors (2-DG) in PC-3 and ALVA-41 cells in a synergistic manner [150,151]. Conversely, overexpression of CK2α partially blocks TRAIL-induced apoptosis, caspase activity and caspase protein levels in ALVA-41 and PC-3 cells [152]. In addition, reactive oxygen species were detected after 6 h of DMAT but not with TBB treatment. After 24 h of TBB or DMAT treatment, γH2AX levels increase in LNCaP cells [142].

Integration of CK2 inhibition into clinical care of prostate cancer: Xenograft models show that CK2 inhibition can decrease tumor burden in mice. Nanoencapsulated-CK2α/α' siRNA and RNAi [139], and CX-4945 [148] decreased tumor volumes in metastatic PC-3 derived-xenograft tumors. Nanoencapsulated-DMAT, decrease proliferation and CK2α and CK2α' proteins levels in PC3-LN 4 cells derived-xenograft tumors [143].

To date there are no reported human trials of CK2 inhibitors in prostate cancer, but such trials would be reasonable in patients with advanced disease that have progressed on other approved lines of therapy (which include various anti-androgen therapies and chemotherapy). In addition, CK2α nuclear staining may be tried as a prognostic factor in patients with early disease to tailor how closely they should be monitored.

Breast Cancer

Breast cancer treatment is now very complex and in many ways highly successful, especially in early stage disease. There are many agents available for treatment of advanced, metastatic breast cancer and molecular typing is key in deciding on the appropriate therapy. Estrogen receptor positive (ER+) breast cancer is largely approached with anti-estrogen therapies which can result in years of disease control even in metastatic disease. Many patients with metastatic, ER+ breast cancer eventually develop resistance to anti-estrogenic approaches, representing a challenge for treatment. HER2 positive (HER2+) breast cancers can be targeted with a range of agents directed against this receptor. Finally, patients lacking receptors for estrogen, progesterone and also lacking over-expression of HER2 (triple negative breast cancer) have currently fever options for therapy apart from chemotherapy and, more recently, PARP inhibitors for some patients. Hence, there are several areas of need for new therapy in advanced or metastatic breast cancer as nearly all such patients eventually succumb to their disease.

Rationale for CK2 inhibition: There is strong evidence for a role for CK2 in the pathophysiology of breast cancer as CK2 is overexpressed or mutated in breast cancer. In general, human breast tumors show high levels of *CK2α* and *CK2β* and low levels of *CK2α'* transcripts [19,153–155]. *CK2α* and *CK2β* transcripts were higher in basal tumors while *CK2α'* was lower in luminal A and B and *HER2* tumors [155]. These aberrations in *CK2* gene transcript expression correlate with changes in copy number variation [153]. In particular, basal tumors had higher gain on *CK2β* and Luminal A tumors show higher loss on *CK2α'* [153,155]. High levels of *CK2α* and *CK2β* transcripts predict lower survival rates [19]. In addition, high *CK2α* transcript expression correlates with increased risk of relapse among breast cancer patients with ERα+ grade 1 or 2 tumors and those receiving hormonal therapy [156]. Moreover, *CK2α* is part of an "invasiveness" gene signature associated with overall survival and metastasis-free survival in breast cancer patients [157].

CK2α activity and protein are elevated in human breast tumors [158,159]. CK2α staining is increased prominently in the nucleus and also in the cytoplasm in breast tumor sections [154,159–161]. Importantly, high CK2α staining is an independent prognostic indicator of patient survival and relapse-free survival [154]. High CK2α staining is also associated with distant metastatic relapse and *HER2* expression, and negatively correlated with progesterone receptor (*PR*) expression [154].

Similar alterations in expression can be found in breast cancer cell lines. CK2α, CK2α' and CK2β proteins are expressed in variable levels in breast cancer cell lines [44,153,155]. CK2 transcript and protein expression levels do not correlate in a number of cell lines suggesting that post-transcriptional mechanisms regulate CK2 expression [155]. Similar to tumors samples, breast cancer cell lines (MDA-MB-231 and MCF7) show loss of heterozygosity on *CK2α'*, however, CK2α' protein was still expressed at high levels [153]. Immunostaining show CK2α and CK2α' located in the nuclei and cytoplasm in the non-transformed immortalized triple-negative breast cell line MCF10A [155].

Elevated levels on CK2α could play an important role in breast cancer, since elevated levels of CK2α have been show to be oncogenic in mouse models. Thus, transgenic overexpression of CK2α in mammary glands causes mammary gland tumors with upregulated β-catenin and c-myc protein levels and NF-κB reporter activity [158]. In addition, CK2α activity and protein are elevated in carcinogen-induced mammary tumors in rats and mice [158,162].

CK2 inhibition alters cellular processes and blocks important signaling cascades. Thus, CK2 inhibition and knockdown of *CK2* lead to decreased cell numbers due to G2/M or G0/G1 arrest, apoptosis or senescence [44,153,154,163–165]. CK2 inhibition and knockdown of *CK2* also lead to changes in cell morphology, migration and invasion [153,154]. In addition, unbalanced expression of *CK2* genes promotes epithelial to mesenchymal transition in cell lines [13]. Importantly, *CK2α/α'* downregulation in triple negative (SUM-149) and *HER2* negative (MCF-7L) breast cancer cell lines resulted in increased apoptosis [155]. In addition, *CK2α/α'* downregulation lead to decreased clonal survival in triple negative SUM-149 and MDA-MB-231 [155]. These suggest that CK2 could be a therapeutic target even in triple negative breast tumors.

CK2 could act through several signaling pathways and mechanisms in breast cancer such as NF-κB, JAK/STAT, MAPK, Akt/MTOR, SIRT6, and miRNA expression [5,44,153,154,166,167]. Intriguingly, *CK2α* is among the targets of miR-125b, a miRNA that is decreased in breast tumor tissue. miR-125b inhibition promotes proliferation and reduced anchorage-independent proliferation [159].

CK2 also has links to breast cancer relevant proteins. For example, levels of CK2α and ERα proteins show a positive correlation in human breast cancer samples, human breast cancer cell lines and tumors from DMBA-treated rats [161]. Intriguingly, estrogen increases CK2α transcript and protein levels in an ERα-dependent manner through ERE sites in the *CK2α* promoter [161]. In turn, CK2α upregulation leads to increase proliferation, migration and anchorage-independent proliferation, and to PML degradation and AKT activation [161]. Additionally, CK2 phosphorylates PR, and this phosphorylation is necessary for anchorage-independent proliferation and expression of specific PR target genes [168].

Integration of CK2 inhibitors into treatment of breast cancer: The most likely clinical usage of CK2 inhibitors in the near future will be in the setting of hormone refractory or triple negative metastatic breast cancer. Thus far, there have not been dedicated breast cancer studies in humans but the pre-clinical data suggests strong potential for this approach. Thus, preclinical studies show that CK2 inhibitors reduce tumor burden. CX-4945 reduces tumor growth in orthotopic xenograft mouse models of breast cancer but did not affect mouse body weight or lead to overt toxicity [44]. Interestingly, CK2 activity decreased in tumors from a breast cancer xenograft model (MCF-7 cells) treated with dexamethasone, a chemosensitizer for breast cancer [169].

Importantly, CK2 inhibition has an effect in triple negative breast cancer xenograft models. Thus, nanocapsulated CK2α/α' siRNA treatment reduces tumor growth in a mouse xenograft model correlating with reduced proliferation rates, but did not affect mouse body weight [155]. In addition, CX-4945 reduced IL-6 expression in a triple negative inflammatory breast cancer patient, in a xenograft model and triple negative breast cancer cell lines [170].

CK2 inhibition could help prevent resistance to anti-tumor drugs in breast cancer. Thus, overexpression of CK2α inhibits tamoxifen induced-senescence [165]. DMAT reduced cell numbers, increased apoptosis and changed morphology of tamoxifen-resistant breast cancer cells more efficiently than anti-estrogen sensitive MCF-7 parental line [171]. However, there were no differences in the protein levels of CK2α, CK2α and CK2β in tamoxifen-resistant versus nonresistant cells [171]. In contrast, breast cancer cell lines resistant to high levels of the antineoplastic agent VP-16 had CK2α transcript and protein elevated correlating with increase levels of phospho-topoisomerase IIα [172]. All together these data indicate that CK2 inhibitors could be used as potential therapeutics for triple negative and anti-estrogen resistant breast cancer.

Renal Cell Carcinoma

Renal cell carcinoma is a highly vascular cancer, which is responsible for approximately 14,000 deaths per year in the USA (out of approximately 61,000 cases). Clear cell carcinoma is the most common subtype of renal cell carcinoma and it is frequently accompanied by loss of expression of the Von Hippel-Lindau (VHL) gene which is a tumor suppressor gene that suppresses hypoxia-inducible factor (HIF) resulting in down-regulation of vascular growth factor (VEGF) production. When VHL expression is lost either through inherited or sporadic mutations, marked rise in VEGF and PDGF occurs which is major factor promoting growth and survival of renal cell carcinoma. Chemotherapy and radiation therapy have minimal benefit in advanced renal cell carcinoma; however, survival is extended by treatment with tyrosine kinase inhibitors targeting VEGF, MTOR inhibitors, and immunotherapy. There is unmet need for patients who progress on these therapies.

Rationale for CK2 inhibition in renal cell carcinoma: There is strong rationale for exploring CK2 inhibition in renal cell carcinoma. Renal cell carcinoma (RCC) samples show high expression of CK2α, *CK2α'* and *CK2β* transcripts [65,173,174]. Higher *CK2α* transcript expression correlated with higher grade and stage and with rate of metastasis [173,174]. Higher *CK2α'* transcript expression correlated with higher grade [173]. High *CK2α* transcript levels were a strong indicator of a poor overall survival, disease specific survival and progression free survival ($n = 96$) [173].

RCC samples show high CK2α, *CK2α'* and *CK2β* protein levels [173,175] and high levels of CK2 activity [173,176]. Importantly, in half of the samples there is unbalanced CK2α-α'/CK2β ratio that is due to increased CK2α-α' expression and/or decreased CK2β expression. High nuclear CK2α staining was a strong indicator of a poor overall survival, disease specific survival and progression free survival ($n = 40$) [173]. In one study, the increase in CK2 proteins in RCC samples did not correlate with increased transcript levels; indeed, transcript levels decreased 1.5–16 times [175]. This is in contrast with the microarray data presented above.

CK2 can regulate VHL directly. CK2 inhibition stabilizes VHL, and therefore decreases HIF levels, although the mechanism is not yet defined [177,178]. CK2 phosphorylates VHL specifically at 3 N-terminal serine residues and stabilizes it [177,179]. Mutation of these 3 serine residues prevents the N-terminal protease cleavage that seems required for further proteasomal degradation of VHL [178]. However, mutation of the 3 serine residues only increased VHL half-life by 30% [177,178]. This suggests that additional mechanisms could be contributing to the increased VHL stability by CK2 inhibition. Importantly, expression of this mutation of these 3 serine residues delayed tumor onset by 6 weeks in a xenograft model [179].

Importantly, in VHL-deficient cells, CK2 inhibition results in decreased cell numbers and cell survival, correlating with decreased phosho-Akt and phosho-p21 and with increase phosho-p38 MAPK [173,175]. Together, these demonstrate a potential role for CK2 as a therapeutic target in renal cell carcinoma.

Integration in clinical care of renal cell carcinoma: The most active areas of clinical investigation in renal cell carcinoma of late include targeted drugs and immunotherapy. However, there remains an unmet need for patients who progress after use of these therapies. CK2 inhibition would be worth exploring in these patients and perhaps as well as a combination therapy with currently approved agents.

2.2. Hematological Malignancies

There has been a dramatic increase in new therapies for lymphomas and myeloma, and it may be harder for CK2 inhibitors to find niche in this setting. However there is rationale for use in these cancers (see below). In particular, acute leukemia has a greater need for new options since progress has been slower in this area.

2.2.1. Leukemia

There is good evidence for a role for CK2 in acute myeloid leukemia (AML), acute lymphoid leukemia (ALL), and in chronic lymphocytic leukemia (CLL).

Rationale for CK2 inhibition: CK2 protein levels and activity are also deregulated in leukemias. B-ALL cell lines and primary B-ALL cells show upregulation of CK2 activity and CK2α and CK2α' protein levels [180,181]. Primary T-ALL cells, show increased CK2 activity and CK2α and CK2β protein levels [182]. Primary AML cells and leukemia cell lines show increased levels of CK2 activity and CK2α protein [183,184]. Importantly, in patients with AML, high CK2α protein levels were a predictor of decreased overall and disease-free survival [183]. Primary CLL cells show increased CK2 activity and CK2α and CK2β proteins [185]. In summary, oncomine transcript expression and CK2 protein expression do not always correlate.

CK2 inhibition with CX-4945 resulted in increased apoptosis in B-ALL cell lines and primary B-ALL cells but, importantly, not primary normal bone marrow cells [180]. CK2 inhibition with CX-4945 resulted in decreased proliferation [186]. Two potential mechanisms have been proposed for the effect of CK2 inhibition in B-ALL: decreased PTEN and phospho-PTEN levels [180] and decreased expression of target genes of the tumor suppressor gene ikaros [186]. Importantly, xenograft models of primary B-ALL cells and cell lines, show that CX-4945 inhibits leukemia cell growth and increased mouse survival [186].

CK2 inhibitors TBB and DRB decreased cell viability in primary T-ALL cells while normal T-cells were unaffected [182]; CX-4945 also decreased cell viability [187]. CK2 overexpressed in T ALL cell lines and this correlates with increased Notch1 and myc activity in these cells. CX-4945 inhibits CK2 activity and has pro-apoptotic effect on these cells. CX-4549 promotes proteosomal degradation of Notch1 and decreases myc transcripts in the cells. Myc is downstream of Notch, hence CK2 inhibition could be an mechanism to inhibit myc. The target of CK2 action may be PTEN as CK2 can phosphorylate PTEN [32], CK2α overexpression correlates with PTEN phosphorylation in T-ALL primary cells, inhibition of CK2 led to increased PTEN activity, and subsequently decreased Akt phosphorylation [182,187]. CX-4945 decreased tumor growth in a xenograft model [187].

In AML cell lines, overexpression of CK2α leads to decreased proportion of cells in G0/G1 while inhibition of CK2 with apigenin, K27 and CX-4945 or with CK2α siRNA resulted in increased apoptosis [183,184]. Importantly, normal bone marrow cells were almost unaffected by apigenin [183]. In addition, CK2 inhibitors or CK2α/β siRNA sensitized AML cells to daunorubicin, an AML chemoterapeutic agent [184].

In CLL, CK2 inhibition with TBB and DRB led to decreased cell viability while leaving normal T and B cells unaffected [185]; CX-4945 also decreased cell viability [188]. Similar to ALL, primary CLL cells show phospho-PTEN upregulation, and *CK2* knockdown or inhibition decreased phospho-PTEN and PTEN expression [185].

Integration of CK2 inhibitors in treatment of leukemias: CIGB-300 promotes activation of the tumor suppressor PTEN and abrogates PI3K-mediated downstream signaling in CLL cells. In accordance, CIGB-300 decreases the viability and proliferation of CLL cell lines, promotes apoptosis of primary leukemia cells and displays antitumor efficacy in a xenograft mouse model of human CLL [187].

These experiments indicate a potential role for CK2 as a target for therapy in leukemia. Researchers have determined that two Phase 1 drugs (CX-4945 and JQ1) can work together to efficiently kill T-cell acute lymphoblastic leukemia cells while having minimal impact on normal blood cells. Despite treatment improvement, T-cell leukemia remains fatal in 20 percent of pediatric and 50 percent of adult patients. Both CX-4945 and JQ1 are currently in clinical trials as single agents to treat solid and hematological cancers. Based on a recent in vitro study it has been suggested that the combination treatment of CX-4945 and JQ1 could be an effective strategy to refractory/relapsed T-cell leukemia.

2.2.2. Non-Hodgkin Lymphoma (NHL)

Many new agents are emerging for treatment of NHL, but there remains a strong need for new therapies. There are many variants of NHL so our discussion can only highlight specific findings relevant to CK2. T cell lymphomas are particularly difficult to treat.

Rationale of CK2 inhibition: Interestingly, overexpression of CK2α in lymphocytes of transgenic mice leads to T cell lymphoma [33,189,190]. A recently published study demonstrated increased CK2α and CK2β protein levels by immunoblot in follicular lymphoma, Burkitt's lymphoma, and DLBCL, and in lymphoma cell lines [191].

Integration of CK2 inhibitors in treatment of lymphomas: Pharmacological inhibition of CK2 activity with CX-4945 led to dose-dependent increase in apoptosis in both Burkitt's lymphoma and DLBCL cell lines [191]. In contrast, normal peripheral blood mononuclear cells were not affected by CX-4945. These data indicate a role of CK2 in NHL, and suggest that CK2 inhibitors could be used to diminish the survival of NHL tumor cells.

2.2.3. Myeloma

The therapeutic options for multiple myeloma have expanded dramatically in recent years. However, this remains a very important malignancy, which is ultimately fatal in most cases. Hence, new options for therapy are still needed.

Rationale for CK2 inhibition: CK2α protein levels and CK2 kinase activity are increased in plasma cells from patients with multiple myeloma and in cell lines [192,193], and higher CK2α and CK2β staining in multiple myeloma tissues [192]. Furthermore, CK2 inhibition with TBB, IQA, a TBB-derivative K27 (2-amino-4,5,6,7-tetrabromo–1H-benzimidazole) and apigenin [194] led to decreased viability and increased apoptosis of myeloma cells. This indicates a role for CK2α in cell survival in myeloma [193–195]. CK2 inhibitors could be acting through decreasing NF-κB activation and transactivation activity [193]. CK2 inhibitors also decrease the endoplasmic reticulum (ER)-stress response leading to increased apoptosis [196]. The ER-stress/unfolded protein response is need for myeloma cells survival, due to the fact that myeloma cells produce abnormally large amounts of protein antibodies.

Integration of CK2 inhibitors into treatment of myeloma: CK2 inhibitors synergize with melphalan, the conventional chemotherapeutic agent used in myeloma treatment, to increase cytotoxicity [193]. CK2 inhibitors have an additive effect to geldanamycin, an antitumoral drug, to increase apoptosis [196]. Therefore, CK2 inhibitors may increase sensitivity (i.e., decrease dosage) to chemotherapy for myeloma [193].

3. Conclusions

CK2 is overexpressed in many cancers and often overexpression is associated with worse prognosis, although the opposite may be true in some cancer types as reviewed above [19]. CK2 can be used as a diagnostic and prognostic marker in certain malignancies, such as prostate cancer [19,137]. However, we the potential for CK2 expression as a prognostic and diagnostic marker could be greater as only a few studies analyze all three CK2 proteins, CK2 activity and localization. In addition, only a few studies analyze levels of CK2αP transcript that, as it was reviewed above, in some cancers are proposed as a prognostic marker. Analysis of all these parameters in future studies in cancer will realize the potential for CK2 as a diagnostic and prognostic marker. The mechanisms underlying the increases in CK2 transcript and protein levels are still unknown in many cancer types, although gene dosage alterations, epigenetic mechanisms and post-translational regulation have been proposed. In addition, in some cancers there are differences in CK2 activity without changes in levels of CK2α expression [93,144], suggesting additional post-translational mechanisms. Importantly, CK2 protein localization in the nucleus is found in a number of tumors, in some cases correlating with clinical parameters. This suggests that phosphorylation of nuclear target proteins is important for CK2's role in cancer. However, we know less about the nuclear targets of CK2 during tumorigenesis compared to the cytoplasmic targets.

Individual knockdown of the *CK2* genes result effects on cellular processes, signaling pathway activation and gene expression that are qualitatively different in diverse tumors [37,38]. Therefore it will be important to develop CK2 inhibitors that could target specifically the monomeric or tetrameric complexes [197]. The development of specific inhibitors of the different CK2 forms for clinical use is being paralleled by targeted drug delivery methods, such as nanocapsules that are targeted to cancer cells [79].

CK2 has emerged as a potential anticancer target. As discussed above, an ample variety of cell-permeable CK2 inhibitors have been developed, and two of these CX-4945 and CIGB-300 have made into preclinical and clinical trials. This review shows how these inhibitors are already being employed in phase I/II trials in certain malignancies like lung, head and neck cancer, cholangiocarcinoma, cervical cancer and multiple myeloma with promising results for the future. With respect to the toxicity observed so far in clinical trials, CIGB-300 was fairly well tolerated in clinical trial of cervical cancer. The most frequent local events were pain, bleeding, hematoma and erythema at the injection site. The systemic adverse events were rash, facial edema, itching, hot flashes and localized cramps. CX-4945 was also fairly well tolerated in a phase 1 trial at MD Anderson cancer center involving patients with various advanced solid tumors and multiple myeloma. Diarrhea and hypokalemia were the dose limiting toxicities, and these toxicities were reversible with drug discontinuation, antidiarrheal use, and potassium supplementation.

These data also gives future perspective on how these two inhibitors can potentially be deployed for further clinical studies. They can be used as a single agent approach, like other signal transduction protein inhibitors in some cancers. They can also be combined with other signal transduction inhibitors, as CK2 regulates several signaling pathways that are key for tumorigenesis. They can be combined with chemotherapy or radiation therapy to prevent repair of DNA damage and increase cancer cell death. They can potentially be used either independently or in combination with other treatment modalities like immunotherapy and even with other Phase 1 drugs like JQ1. These two inhibitors have shown to enhance anti-proliferative effects as well as overcome resistance to the established chemotherapeutic agents, requiring much lower dosage, thus also possibly decreasing the toxic side effects, though not yet studied. CK2 inhibitors are also highly promising for specific use in HPV-related cancers and perhaps incorporation with other therapies for hematological malignancies.

Acknowledgments: This work was supported with funding from the National Institutes of General Medical Sciences (NIGMS) (1R01GM098367). This project was supported by a Boston University School of Medicine Medical Student Summer Research Program (MSSRP) and Barbur Kalique Scholarship (to M.M.J.C.), and a Boston University Undergraduate Research Opportunities Program (UROP) fellowship (to M.L.).

Author Contributions: I.D. and K.L.H. conceived the manuscript; all the authors reviewed the literature, and contributed to the writing of the manuscript.

Conflicts of Interest: The authors declare no conflict of interest.

References

1. Trembley, J.H.; Wu, J.; Unger, G.M.; Kren, B.T.; Ahmed, K. *Ck2 Suppression of Apoptosis and Its Implication in Cancer Biology and Therapy*; Wiley-Blackwell: Ames, IA, USA, 2013; pp. 219–343.
2. Seldin, D.C.; Landesman-Bollag, E. *The Oncogenic Potential of CK2*; Wiley-Blackwell: Ames, IA, USA, 2013.
3. Ruzzene, M.; Pinna, L.A. Addiction to protein kinase ck2: A common denominator of diverse cancer cells? *Biochim. Biophys. Acta* **2010**, *1804*, 499–504. [CrossRef] [PubMed]
4. Seldin, D.C.; Landesman-Bollag, E.; Farago, M.; Currier, N.; Lou, D.; Dominguez, I. Ck2 as a positive regulator of wnt signalling and tumourigenesis. *Mol. Cell. Biochem.* **2005**, *274*, 63–67. [CrossRef] [PubMed]
5. Dominguez, I.; Sonenshein, G.E.; Seldin, D.C. Protein kinase ck2 in health and disease: Ck2 and its role in wnt and nf-kappab signaling: Linking development and cancer. *Cell. Mol. Life Sci.* **2009**, *66*, 1850–1857. [CrossRef] [PubMed]
6. Zhang, H.X.; Jiang, S.S.; Zhang, X.F.; Zhou, Z.Q.; Pan, Q.Z.; Chen, C.L.; Zhao, J.J.; Tang, Y.; Xia, J.C.; Weng, D.S. Protein kinase ck2α catalytic subunit is overexpressed and serves as an unfavorable prognostic marker in primary hepatocellular carcinoma. *Oncotarget* **2015**, *6*, 34800–34817. [PubMed]
7. Pinna, L.A.; Meggio, F. Protein kinase ck2 ("casein kinase-2") and its implication in cell division and proliferation. *Prog. Cell. Cycle Res.* **1997**, *3*, 77–97. [PubMed]
8. Ahmed, K.; Davis, A.T.; Wang, H.; Faust, R.A.; Yu, S.; Tawfic, S. Significance of protein kinase ck2 nuclear signaling in neoplasia. *J. Cell. Biochem.* **2000**, *79* (Suppl. 35), 130–135. [CrossRef]
9. Litchfield, D.W. Protein kinase ck2: Structure, regulation and role in cellular decisions of life and death. *Biochem. J.* **2003**, *369*, 1–15. [CrossRef] [PubMed]
10. Ahmad, K.A.; Wang, G.; Unger, G.; Slaton, J.; Ahmed, K. Protein kinase ck2—A key suppressor of apoptosis. *Adv. Enzyme Regul.* **2008**, *48*, 179–187. [CrossRef] [PubMed]
11. Ahmed, K.; Gerber, D.A.; Cochet, C. Joining the cell survival squad: An emerging role for protein kinase ck2. *Trends Cell. Biol.* **2002**, *12*, 226–230. [CrossRef]
12. Canton, D.A.; Litchfield, D.W. The shape of things to come: An emerging role for protein kinase ck2 in the regulation of cell morphology and the cytoskeleton. *Cell. Signal.* **2006**, *18*, 267–275. [CrossRef] [PubMed]
13. Filhol, O.; Deshiere, A.; Cochet, C. *Role of CK2 in the Control of Cell Plasticity in Breast Carcinoma Progression*; Wiley-Blackwell: Ames, IA, USA, 2013.
14. Kramerov, A.A.; Saghizadeh, M.; Caballero, S.; Shaw, L.C.; Li Calzi, S.; Bretner, M.; Montenarh, M.; Pinna, L.A.; Grant, M.B.; Ljubimov, A.V. Inhibition of protein kinase ck2 suppresses angiogenesis and hematopoietic stem cell recruitment to retinal neovascularization sites. *Mol. Cell. Biochem.* **2008**, *316*, 177–186. [CrossRef] [PubMed]
15. Montenarh, M. Protein kinase ck2 and angiogenesis. *Adv. Clin. Exp. Med.* **2014**, *23*, 153–158. [CrossRef] [PubMed]
16. Xu, X.; Toselli, P.A.; Russell, L.D.; Seldin, D.C. Globozoospermia in mice lacking the casein kinase ii α' catalytic subunit. *Nat. Genet.* **1999**, *23*, 118–121. [PubMed]
17. Bibby, A.C.; Litchfield, D.W. The multiple personalities of the regulatory subunit of protein kinase ck2: Ck2 dependent and ck2 independent roles reveal a secret identity for ck2β. *Int. J. Biol. Sci.* **2005**, *1*, 67–79. [CrossRef] [PubMed]

18. Wirkner, U.; Voss, H.; Lichter, P.; Weitz, S.; Ansorge, W.; Pyerin, W. Human casein kinase ii subunit α: Sequence of a processed (pseudo)gene and its localization on chromosome 11. *Biochim. Biophys. Acta* **1992**, *1131*, 220–222. [CrossRef]

19. Ortega, C.E.; Seidner, Y.; Dominguez, I. Mining ck2 in cancer. *PLoS ONE* **2014**, *9*, e115609. [CrossRef] [PubMed]

20. Olsen, B.B.; Issinger, O.G.; Guerra, B. Regulation of DNA-dependent protein kinase by protein kinase ck2 in human glioblastoma cells. *Oncogene* **2010**, *29*, 6016–6026. [CrossRef] [PubMed]

21. Zheng, Y.; McFarland, B.C.; Drygin, D.; Yu, H.; Bellis, S.L.; Kim, H.; Bredel, M.; Benveniste, E.N. Targeting protein kinase CK2 suppresses prosurvival signaling pathways and growth of glioblastoma. *Clin. Cancer Res.* **2013**, *19*, 6484–6494. [CrossRef] [PubMed]

22. Zhang, C.; Vilk, G.; Canton, D.A.; Litchfield, D.W. Phosphorylation regulates the stability of the regulatory ck2β subunit. *Oncogene* **2002**, *21*, 3754–3764. [CrossRef] [PubMed]

23. Tawfic, S.; Yu, S.; Wang, H.; Faust, R.; Davis, A.; Ahmed, K. Protein kinase CK2 signal in neoplasia. *Histol. Histopathol.* **2001**, *16*, 573–582. [PubMed]

24. Macias Alvarez, L.; Revuelta-Cervantes, J.; Dominguez, I. CK2 in embryonic development. In *The Wiley-IUBMB Series on Biochemistry and Molecular Biology: Protein Kinase CK2*; Wiley: New York, NY, USA, 2013.

25. Dominguez, I.; Mizuno, J.; Wu, H.; Song, D.H.; Symes, K.; Seldin, D.C. Protein kinase CK2 is required for dorsal axis formation in xenopus embryos. *Dev. Biol.* **2004**, *274*, 110–124. [CrossRef] [PubMed]

26. Dominguez, I.; Mizuno, J.; Wu, H.; Imbrie, G.A.; Symes, K.; Seldin, D.C. A role for CK2α/β in Xenopus early embryonic development. *Mol. Cell. Biochem.* **2005**, *274*, 125–131. [CrossRef] [PubMed]

27. Jia, H.; Liu, Y.; Xia, R.; Tong, C.; Yue, T.; Jiang, J.; Jia, J. Casein kinase 2 promotes hedgehog signaling by regulating both smoothened and cubitus interruptus. *J. Biol. Chem.* **2010**, *285*, 37218–37226. [CrossRef] [PubMed]

28. Zheng, Y.; Qin, H.; Frank, S.J.; Deng, L.; Litchfield, D.W.; Tefferi, A.; Pardanani, A.; Lin, F.T.; Li, J.; Sha, B.; et al. A ck2-dependent mechanism for activation of the jak-stat signaling pathway. *Blood* **2011**, *118*, 156–166. [CrossRef] [PubMed]

29. Di Maira, G.; Salvi, M.; Arrigoni, G.; Marin, O.; Sarno, S.; Brustolon, F.; Pinna, L.A.; Ruzzene, M. Protein kinase CK2 phosphorylates and upregulates akt/pkb. *Cell Death Differ.* **2005**, *12*, 668–677. [CrossRef] [PubMed]

30. Park, J.H.; Kim, J.J.; Bae, Y.S. Involvement of pi3k-akt-mtor pathway in protein kinase ckii inhibition-mediated senescence in human colon cancer cells. *Biochem. Biophys. Res. Commun.* **2013**, *433*, 420–425. [CrossRef] [PubMed]

31. Torres, J.; Pulido, R. The tumor suppressor pten is phosphorylated by the protein kinase CK2 at its C terminus. Implications for pten stability to proteasome-mediated degradation. *J. Biol. Chem.* **2001**, *276*, 993–998. [CrossRef] [PubMed]

32. Miller, S.J.; Lou, D.Y.; Seldin, D.C.; Lane, W.S.; Neel, B.G. Direct identification of pten phosphorylation sites. *FEBS Lett.* **2002**, *528*, 145–153. [CrossRef]

33. Channavajhala, P.; Seldin, D.C. Functional interaction of protein kinase CK2 and c-myc in lymphomagenesis. *Oncogene* **2002**, *21*, 5280–5288. [CrossRef] [PubMed]

34. Romieu-Mourez, R.; Landesman-Bollag, E.; Seldin, D.C.; Sonenshein, G.E. Protein kinase CK2 promotes aberrant activation of nuclear factor-kappab, transformed phenotype, and survival of breast cancer cells. *Cancer Res.* **2002**, *62*, 6770–6778. [PubMed]

35. Zhang, S.; Long, H.; Yang, Y.L.; Wang, Y.; Hsieh, D.; Li, W.; Au, A.; Stoppler, H.J.; Xu, Z.; Jablons, D.M.; et al. Inhibition of ck2α down-regulates notch1 signalling in lung cancer cells. *J. Cell. Mol. Med.* **2013**, *17*, 854–862. [CrossRef] [PubMed]

36. Heriche, J.K.; Chambaz, E.M. Protein kinase CK2α is a target for the Abl and Bcr-Abl tyrosine kinases. *Oncogene* **1998**, *17*, 13–18. [CrossRef] [PubMed]

37. Brown, M.S.; Diallo, O.T.; Hu, M.; Ehsanian, R.; Yang, X.; Arun, P.; Lu, H.; Korman, V.; Unger, G.; Ahmed, K.; et al. CK2 modulation of Nf-kappaB, TP53, and the malignant phenotype in head and neck cancer by anti-CK2 oligonucleotides in vitro or in vivo via sub-50-nm nanocapsules. *Clin. Cancer Res.* **2010**, *16*, 2295–2307. [CrossRef] [PubMed]

38. Bian, Y.; Han, J.; Kannabiran, V.; Mohan, S.; Cheng, H.; Friedman, J.; Zhang, L.; VanWaes, C.; Chen, Z. Mek inhibitor PD-0325901 overcomes resistance to CK2 inhibitor CX-4945 and exhibits anti-tumor activity in head and neck cancer. *Int. J. Biol. Sci.* **2015**, *11*, 411–422. [CrossRef] [PubMed]

39. Sarno, S.; Reddy, H.; Meggio, F.; Ruzzene, M.; Davies, S.P.; Donella-Deana, A.; Shugar, D.; Pinna, L.A. Selectivity of 4,5,6,7-tetrabromobenzotriazole, an ATP site-directed inhibitor of protein kinase CK2 ('casein kinase-2'). *FEBS Lett.* **2001**, *496*, 44–48. [CrossRef]

40. Cozza, G.; Mazzorana, M.; Papinutto, E.; Bain, J.; Elliott, M.; di Maira, G.; Gianoncelli, A.; Pagano, M.A.; Sarno, S.; Ruzzene, M.; et al. Quinalizarin as a potent, selective and cell-permeable inhibitor of protein kinase ck2. *Biochem. J.* **2009**, *421*, 387–395. [CrossRef] [PubMed]

41. Hung, M.S.; Xu, Z.; Lin, Y.C.; Mao, J.H.; Yang, C.T.; Chang, P.J.; Jablons, D.M.; You, L. Identification of hematein as a novel inhibitor of protein kinase CK2 from a natural product library. *BMC Cancer* **2009**, *9*, 135. [CrossRef] [PubMed]

42. Pagano, M.A.; Poletto, G.; Di Maira, G.; Cozza, G.; Ruzzene, M.; Sarno, S.; Bain, J.; Elliott, M.; Moro, S.; Zagotto, G.; et al. Tetrabromocinnamic acid (TBCA) and related compounds represent a new class of specific protein kinase CK2 inhibitors. *Chembiochem* **2007**, *8*, 129–139. [CrossRef] [PubMed]

43. Perea, S.E.; Reyes, O.; Baladron, I.; Perera, Y.; Farina, H.; Gil, J.; Rodriguez, A.; Bacardi, D.; Marcelo, J.L.; Cosme, K.; et al. Cigb-300, a novel proapoptotic peptide that impairs the CK2 phosphorylation and exhibits anticancer properties both in vitro and in vivo. *Mol. Cell. Biochem.* **2008**, *316*, 163–167. [CrossRef] [PubMed]

44. Siddiqui-Jain, A.; Drygin, D.; Streiner, N.; Chua, P.; Pierre, F.; O'Brien, S.E.; Bliesath, J.; Omori, M.; Huser, N.; Ho, C.; et al. CX-4945, an orally bioavailable selective inhibitor of protein kinase CK2, inhibits prosurvival and angiogenic signaling and exhibits antitumor efficacy. *Cancer Res.* **2010**, *70*, 10288–10298. [CrossRef] [PubMed]

45. Zandomeni, R.; Zandomeni, M.C.; Shugar, D.; Weinmann, R. Casein kinase type II is involved in the inhibition by 5,6-dichloro-1-β-D-ribofuranosylbenzimidazole of specific RNA polymerase II transcription. *J. Biol. Chem.* **1986**, *261*, 3414–3419. [PubMed]

46. Hagiwara, M.; Inoue, S.; Tanaka, T.; Nunoki, K.; Ito, M.; Hidaka, H. Differential effects of flavonoids as inhibitors of tyrosine protein kinases and serine/threonine protein kinases. *Biochem. Pharmacol.* **1988**, *37*, 2987–2992. [PubMed]

47. Pagano, M.A.; Meggio, F.; Ruzzene, M.; Andrzejewska, M.; Kazimierczuk, Z.; Pinna, L.A. 2-Dimethylamino-4,5,6,7-tetrabromo-1H-benzimidazole: A novel powerful and selective inhibitor of protein kinase CK2. *Biochem. Biophys. Res. Commun.* **2004**, *321*, 1040–1044. [CrossRef] [PubMed]

48. Yim, H.; Lee, Y.H.; Lee, C.H.; Lee, S.K. Emodin, an anthraquinone derivative isolated from the rhizomes of rheum palmatum, selectively inhibits the activity of casein kinase ii as a competitive inhibitor. *Planta Med.* **1999**, *65*, 9–13. [CrossRef] [PubMed]

49. Gotz, C.; Gratz, A.; Kucklaender, U.; Jose, J. Tf—A novel cell-permeable and selective inhibitor of human protein kinase CK2 induces apoptosis in the prostate cancer cell line LNCaP. *Biochim. Biophys. Acta* **2012**, *1820*, 970–977. [CrossRef] [PubMed]

50. O-charoenrat, P.; Rusch, V.; Talbot, S.G.; Sarkaria, I.; Viale, A.; Socci, N.; Ngai, I.; Rao, P.; Singh, B. Casein kinase ii α subunit and c1-inhibitor are independent predictors of outcome in patients with squamous cell carcinoma of the lung. *Clin. Cancer Res.* **2004**, *10*, 5792–5803. [CrossRef] [PubMed]

51. Hung, M.S.; Lin, Y.C.; Mao, J.H.; Kim, I.J.; Xu, Z.; Yang, C.T.; Jablons, D.M.; You, L. Functional polymorphism of the CK2α intronless gene plays oncogenic roles in lung cancer. *PLoS ONE* **2010**, *5*, e11418. [CrossRef] [PubMed]

52. Daya-Makin, M.; Sanghera, J.S.; Mogentale, T.L.; Lipp, M.; Parchomchuk, J.; Hogg, J.C.; Pelech, S.L. Activation of a tumor-associated protein kinase (p40TAK) and casein kinase 2 in human squamous cell carcinomas and adenocarcinomas of the lung. *Cancer Res.* **1994**, *54*, 2262–2268. [PubMed]

53. Yaylim, I.; Isbir, T. Enhanced casein kinase II (CK II) activity in human lung tumours. *Anticancer Res.* **2002**, *22*, 215–218. [PubMed]

54. Ku, M.J.; Park, J.W.; Ryu, B.J.; Son, Y.J.; Kim, S.H.; Lee, S.Y. CK2 inhibitor CX4945 induces sequential inactivation of proteins in the signaling pathways related with cell migration and suppresses metastasis of a549 human lung cancer cells. *Bioorg. Med. Chem. Lett.* **2013**, *23*, 5609–5613. [CrossRef] [PubMed]

55. Zhou, Y.; Li, K.; Zhang, S.; Li, Q.; Li, Z.; Zhou, F.; Dong, X.; Liu, L.; Wu, G.; Meng, R. Quinalizarin, a specific CK2 inhibitor, reduces cell viability and suppresses migration and accelerates apoptosis in different human lung cancer cell lines. *Indian J. Cancer* **2015**, *52* (Suppl. 2), 119–124.

56. Kim, J.; Hwan Kim, S. CK2 inhibitor CX-4945 blocks TGF-β1-induced epithelial-to-mesenchymal transition in A549 human lung adenocarcinoma cells. *PLoS ONE* **2013**, *8*, e74342.

57. Lin, Y.C.; Hung, M.S.; Lin, C.K.; Li, J.M.; Lee, K.D.; Li, Y.C.; Chen, M.F.; Chen, J.K.; Yang, C.T. CK2 inhibitors enhance the radiosensitivity of human non-small cell lung cancer cells through inhibition of stat3 activation. *Cancer Biother. Radiopharm.* **2011**, *26*, 381–388. [CrossRef] [PubMed]

58. Hung, M.S.; Xu, Z.; Chen, Y.; Smith, E.; Mao, J.H.; Hsieh, D.; Lin, Y.C.; Yang, C.T.; Jablons, D.M.; You, L. Hematein, a casein kinase II inhibitor, inhibits lung cancer tumor growth in a murine xenograft model. *Int. J. Oncol.* **2013**, *43*, 1517–1522. [PubMed]

59. Benavent, F.; Capobianco, C.S.; Garona, J.; Cirigliano, S.M.; Perera, Y.; Urtreger, A.J.; Perea, S.E.; Alonso, D.F.; Farina, H.G. CIGB-300, an anti-CK2 peptide, inhibits angiogenesis, tumor cell invasion and metastasis in lung cancer models. *Lung Cancer* **2016**. [CrossRef] [PubMed]

60. Perera, Y.; Toro, N.D.; Gorovaya, L.; Fernandez, D.E.C.J.; Farina, H.G.; Perea, S.E. Synergistic interactions of the anti-casein kinase 2 CIGB-300 peptide and chemotherapeutic agents in lung and cervical preclinical cancer models. *Mol. Clin. Oncol.* **2014**, *2*, 935–944. [CrossRef] [PubMed]

61. Bliesath, J.; Huser, N.; Omori, M.; Bunag, D.; Proffitt, C.; Streiner, N.; Ho, C.; Siddiqui-Jain, A.; O'Brien, S.E.; Lim, J.K.; et al. Combined inhibition of EGFR and CK2 augments the attenuation of pi3k-akt-mtor signaling and the killing of cancer cells. *Cancer Lett.* **2012**, *322*, 113–118. [CrossRef] [PubMed]

62. Shimada, K.; Anai, S.; Marco, D.A.; Fujimoto, K.; Konishi, N. Cyclooxygenase 2-dependent and independent activation of Akt through casein kinase 2α contributes to human bladder cancer cell survival. *BMC Urol.* **2011**, *11*, 8. [CrossRef] [PubMed]

63. Jeppesen, D.K.; Nawrocki, A.; Jensen, S.G.; Thorsen, K.; Whitehead, B.; Howard, K.A.; Dyrskjot, L.; Orntoft, T.F.; Larsen, M.R.; Ostenfeld, M.S. Quantitative proteomics of fractionated membrane and lumen exosome proteins from isogenic metastatic and nonmetastatic bladder cancer cells reveal differential expression of EMT factors. *Proteomics* **2014**, *14*, 699–712. [CrossRef] [PubMed]

64. Weidle, U.H.; Birzele, F.; Kollmorgen, G.; Ruger, R. The multiple roles of exosomes in metastasis. *Cancer Genom. Proteom.* **2017**, *14*, 1–15. [CrossRef] [PubMed]

65. Chua, M.M.J.; Dominguez, I. Cancer-type dependent miss-expression of CK2 genes. **2017**, in preparation.

66. Gapany, M.; Faust, R.A.; Tawfic, S.; Davis, A.; Adams, G.L.; Ahmed, K. Association of elevated protein kinase CK2 activity with aggressive behavior of squamous cell carcinoma of the head and neck. *Mol. Med.* **1995**, *1*, 659–666. [PubMed]

67. Faust, R.A.; Gapany, M.; Tristani, P.; Davis, A.; Adams, G.L.; Ahmed, K. Elevated protein kinase CK2 activity in chromatin of head and neck tumors: Association with malignant transformation. *Cancer Lett.* **1996**, *101*, 31–35. [CrossRef]

68. Faust, R.A.; Niehans, G.; Gapany, M.; Hoistad, D.; Knapp, D.; Cherwitz, D.; Davis, A.; Adams, G.L.; Ahmed, K. Subcellular immunolocalization of protein kinase CK2 in normal and carcinoma cells. *Int. J. Biochem. Cell. Biol.* **1999**, *31*, 941–949. [CrossRef]

69. Faust, R.A.; Tawfic, S.; Davis, A.T.; Bubash, L.A.; Ahmed, K. Antisense oligonucleotides against protein kinase CK2-α inhibit growth of squamous cell carcinoma of the head and neck in vitro. *Head Neck* **2000**, *22*, 341–346. [CrossRef]

70. Wang, H.; Davis, A.; Yu, S.; Ahmed, K. Response of cancer cells to molecular interruption of the CK2 signal. *Mol. Cell. Biochem.* **2001**, *227*, 167–174. [CrossRef] [PubMed]

71. Allen, C.; Duffy, S.; Teknos, T.; Islam, M.; Chen, Z.; Albert, P.S.; Wolf, G.; Van Waes, C. Nuclear factor-kappaB-related serum factors as longitudinal biomarkers of response and survival in advanced oropharyngeal carcinoma. *Clin. Cancer Res.* **2007**, *13*, 3182–3190. [CrossRef] [PubMed]

72. Yu, M.; Yeh, J.; Van Waes, C. Protein kinase casein kinase 2 mediates inhibitor-kappaB kinase and aberrant nuclear factor-kappaB activation by serum factor(s) in head and neck squamous carcinoma cells. *Cancer Res.* **2006**, *66*, 6722–6731. [CrossRef] [PubMed]

73. Su, Y.W.; Xie, T.X.; Sano, D.; Myers, J.N. IL-6 stabilizes twist and enhances tumor cell motility in head and neck cancer cells through activation of casein kinase 2. *PLoS ONE* **2011**, *6*, e19412. [CrossRef] [PubMed]

74. Zhang, F.; Yang, B.; Shi, S.; Jiang, X. RNA interference (RNAi) mediated stable knockdown of protein casein kinase 2-α (CK2α) inhibits migration and invasion and enhances cisplatin-induced apoptosis in HEp-2 laryngeal carcinoma cells. *Acta Histochem.* **2014**, *116*, 1000–1006. [CrossRef] [PubMed]

75. Chen, Z.; Malhotra, P.S.; Thomas, G.R.; Ondrey, F.G.; Duffey, D.C.; Smith, C.W.; Enamorado, I.; Yeh, N.T.; Kroog, G.S.; Rudy, S.; et al. Expression of proinflammatory and proangiogenic cytokines in patients with head and neck cancer. *Clin. Cancer Res.* **1999**, *5*, 1369–1379. [PubMed]

76. Hosono, S.; Kajiyama, H.; Terauchi, M.; Shibata, K.; Ino, K.; Nawa, A.; Kikkawa, F. Expression of Twist increases the risk for recurrence and for poor survival in epithelial ovarian carcinoma patients. *Br. J. Cancer* **2007**, *96*, 314–320. [CrossRef] [PubMed]

77. Duffy, S.A.; Taylor, J.M.; Terrell, J.E.; Islam, M.; Li, Y.; Fowler, K.E.; Wolf, G.T.; Teknos, T.N. Interleukin-6 predicts recurrence and survival among head and neck cancer patients. *Cancer* **2008**, *113*, 750–757. [CrossRef] [PubMed]

78. Lu, H.; Yan, C.; Quan, X.X.; Yang, X.; Zhang, J.; Bian, Y.; Chen, Z.; Van Waes, C. CK2 phosphorylates and inhibits TAp73 tumor suppressor function to promote expression of cancer stem cell genes and phenotype in head and neck cancer. *Neoplasia* **2014**, *16*, 789–800. [CrossRef] [PubMed]

79. Unger, G.M.; Kren, B.T.; Korman, V.L.; Kimbrough, T.G.; Vogel, R.I.; Ondrey, F.G.; Trembley, J.H.; Ahmed, K. Mechanism and efficacy of sub-50-nm tenfibgen nanocapsules for cancer cell-directed delivery of anti-CK2 RNAi to primary and metastatic squamous cell carcinoma. *Mol. Cancer Ther.* **2014**, *13*, 2018–2029. [CrossRef] [PubMed]

80. Zhang, S.; Yang, Y.L.; Wang, Y.; You, B.; Dai, Y.; Chan, G.; Hsieh, D.; Kim, I.J.; Fang, L.T.; Au, A.; et al. CK2α, over-expressed in human malignant pleural mesothelioma, regulates the Hedgehog signaling pathway in mesothelioma cells. *J. Exp. Clin. Cancer Res.* **2014**, *33*, 93. [PubMed]

81. Shi, Y.; Moura, U.; Opitz, I.; Soltermann, A.; Rehrauer, H.; Thies, S.; Weder, W.; Stahel, R.A.; Felley-Bosco, E. Role of hedgehog signaling in malignant pleural mesothelioma. *Clin. Cancer Res.* **2012**, *18*, 4646–4656. [CrossRef] [PubMed]

82. Zhang, Y.; He, J.; Zhang, F.; Li, H.; Yue, D.; Wang, C.; Jablons, D.M.; He, B.; Lui, N. SMO expression level correlates with overall survival in patients with malignant pleural mesothelioma. *J. Exp. Clin. Cancer Res.* **2013**, *32*, 7. [CrossRef] [PubMed]

83. Kim, H.S.; Chang, Y.G.; Bae, H.J.; Eun, J.W.; Shen, Q.; Park, S.J.; Shin, W.C.; Lee, E.K.; Park, S.; Ahn, Y.M.; et al. Oncogenic potential of CK2α and its regulatory role in EGF-induced HDAC2 expression in human liver cancer. *FEBS J.* **2014**, *281*, 851–861. [CrossRef] [PubMed]

84. Wu, D.; Sui, C.; Meng, F.; Tian, X.; Fu, L.; Li, Y.; Qi, X.; Cui, H.; Liu, Y.; Jiang, Y. Stable knockdown of protein kinase CK2-α (CK2α) inhibits migration and invasion and induces inactivation of hedgehog signaling pathway in hepatocellular carcinoma Hep G2 cells. *Acta Histochem.* **2014**, *116*, 1501–1508. [CrossRef] [PubMed]

85. Sass, G.; Klinger, N.; Sirma, H.; Hashemolhosseini, S.; Hellerbrand, C.; Neureiter, D.; Wege, H.; Ocker, M.; Tiegs, G. Inhibition of experimental HCC growth in mice by use of the kinase inhibitor DMAT. *Int. J. Oncol.* **2011**, *39*, 433–442. [CrossRef] [PubMed]

86. Shi, X.; Potvin, B.; Huang, T.; Hilgard, P.; Spray, D.C.; Suadicani, S.O.; Wolkoff, A.W.; Stanley, P.; Stockert, R.J. A novel casein kinase 2 α-subunit regulates membrane protein traffic in the human hepatoma cell line HuH-7. *J. Biol. Chem.* **2001**, *276*, 2075–2082. [CrossRef] [PubMed]

87. Kim, H.R.; Kim, K.; Lee, K.H.; Kim, S.J.; Kim, J. Inhibition of casein kinase 2 enhances the death ligand- and natural kiler cell-induced hepatocellular carcinoma cell death. *Clin. Exp. Immunol.* **2008**, *152*, 336–344. [CrossRef] [PubMed]

88. Bae, J.S.; Park, S.H.; Kim, K.M.; Kwon, K.S.; Kim, C.Y.; Lee, H.K.; Park, B.H.; Park, H.S.; Lee, H.; Moon, W.S.; et al. CK2α phosphorylates DBC1 and is involved in the progression of gastric carcinoma and predicts poor survival of gastric carcinoma patients. *J. Int. Cancer* **2015**, *136*, 797–809. [CrossRef] [PubMed]

89. Lin, K.Y.; Fang, C.L.; Chen, Y.; Li, C.F.; Chen, S.H.; Kuo, C.Y.; Tai, C.; Uen, Y.H. Overexpression of nuclear protein kinase CK2 Beta subunit and prognosis in human gastric carcinoma. *Ann. Surg. Oncol.* **2010**, *17*, 1695–1702. [CrossRef] [PubMed]

90. Lee, Y.S.; Lee do, Y.; Yu da, Y.; Kim, S.; Lee, Y.C. Helicobacter pylori induces cell migration and invasion through casein kinase 2 in gastric epithelial cells. *Helicobacter* **2014**, *19*, 465–475. [CrossRef] [PubMed]

91. Chen, S.H.; Lin, K.Y.; Chang, C.C.; Fang, C.L.; Lin, C.P. Aloe-emodin-induced apoptosis in human gastric carcinoma cells. *Food Chem. Toxicol.* **2007**, *45*, 2296–2303. [CrossRef] [PubMed]

92. Xu, W.; Chen, Q.; Wang, Q.; Sun, Y.; Wang, S.; Li, A.; Xu, S.; Roe, O.D.; Wang, M.; Zhang, R.; et al. JWA reverses cisplatin resistance via the CK2-XRCC1 pathway in human gastric cancer cells. *Cell Death Dis.* **2014**, *5*, e1551. [CrossRef] [PubMed]

93. Yoo, J.Y.; Choi, H.K.; Choi, K.C.; Park, S.Y.; Ota, I.; Yook, J.I.; Lee, Y.H.; Kim, K.; Yoon, H.G. Nuclear hormone receptor corepressor promotes esophageal cancer cell invasion by transcriptional repression of interferon-gamma-inducible protein 10 in a casein kinase 2-dependent manner. *Mol. Biol. Cell.* **2012**, *23*, 2943–2954. [CrossRef] [PubMed]

94. Shin, S.; Lee, Y.; Kim, W.; Ko, H.; Choi, H.; Kim, K. Caspase-2 primes cancer cells for TRAIL-mediated apoptosis by processing procaspase-8. *EMBO J.* **2005**, *24*, 3532–3542. [CrossRef] [PubMed]

95. Ko, H.; Kim, S.; Jin, C.H.; Lee, E.; Ham, S.; Yook, J.I.; Kim, K. Protein kinase casein kinase 2-mediated upregulation of N-cadherin confers anoikis resistance on esophageal carcinoma cells. *Mol. Cancer Res.* **2012**, *10*, 1032–1038. [CrossRef] [PubMed]

96. Juan, H.C.; Tsai, H.T.; Chang, P.H.; Huang, C.Y.; Hu, C.P.; Wong, F.H. Insulin-like growth factor 1 mediates 5-fluorouracil chemoresistance in esophageal carcinoma cells through increasing survivin stability. *Apoptosis* **2011**, *16*, 174–183. [CrossRef] [PubMed]

97. Zhou, F.; Xu, J.; Ding, G.; Cao, L. Overexpressions of CK2β and XIAP are associated with poor prognosis of patients with cholangiocarcinoma. *Pathol. Oncol. Res.* **2014**, *20*, 73–79. [CrossRef] [PubMed]

98. Kotawong, K.; Thitapakorn, V.; Roytrakul, S.; Phaonakrop, N.; Viyanant, V.; Na-Bangchang, K. Plasma peptidome as a source of biomarkers for diagnosis of cholangiocarcinoma. *Asian Pac. J. Cancer Prev.* **2016**, *17*, 1163–1168. [CrossRef] [PubMed]

99. Izeradjene, K.; Douglas, L.; Delaney, A.; Houghton, J.A. Influence of casein kinase II in tumor necrosis factor-related apoptosis-inducing ligand-induced apoptosis in human rhabdomyosarcoma cells. *Clin. Cancer Res.* **2004**, *10*, 6650–6660. [CrossRef] [PubMed]

100. Zou, J.; Luo, H.; Zeng, Q.; Dong, Z.; Wu, D.; Liu, L. Protein kinase CK2α is overexpressed in colorectal cancer and modulates cell proliferation and invasion via regulating EMT-related genes. *J. Transl. Med.* **2011**, *9*, 97. [CrossRef] [PubMed]

101. Lin, K.Y.; Tai, C.; Hsu, J.C.; Li, C.F.; Fang, C.L.; Lai, H.C.; Hseu, Y.C.; Lin, Y.F.; Uen, Y.H. Overexpression of nuclear protein kinase CK2 α catalytic subunit (CK2α) as a poor prognosticator in human colorectal cancer. *PLoS ONE* **2011**, *6*, e17193.

102. Duncan, J.S.; Litchfield, D.W. Too much of a good thing: The role of protein kinase CK2 in tumorigenesis and prospects for therapeutic inhibition of CK2. *Biochim. Biophys. Acta* **2008**, *1784*, 33–47. [CrossRef] [PubMed]

103. Niechi, I.; Silva, E.; Cabello, P.; Huerta, H.; Carrasco, V.; Villar, P.; Cataldo, L.R.; Marcelain, K.; Armisen, R.; Varas-Godoy, M.; et al. Colon cancer cell invasion is promoted by protein kinase CK2 through increase of endothelin-converting enzyme-1c protein stability. *Oncotarget* **2015**, *6*, 42749–42760. [PubMed]

104. Lambert, L.A.; Whyteside, A.R.; Turner, A.J.; Usmani, B.A. Isoforms of endothelin-converting enzyme-1 (ECE-1) have opposing effects on prostate cancer cell invasion. *Br. J. Cancer* **2008**, *99*, 1114–1120. [CrossRef] [PubMed]

105. Smollich, M.; Gotte, M.; Kersting, C.; Fischgrabe, J.; Kiesel, L.; Wulfing, P. Selective ETAR antagonist atrasentan inhibits hypoxia-induced breast cancer cell invasion. *Breast Cancer Res. Treat.* **2008**, *108*, 175–182. [CrossRef] [PubMed]

106. Smollich, M.; Gotte, M.; Yip, G.W.; Yong, E.S.; Kersting, C.; Fischgrabe, J.; Radke, I.; Kiesel, L.; Wulfing, P. On the role of endothelin-converting enzyme-1 (ECE-1) and neprilysin in human breast cancer. *Breast Cancer Res. Treat.* **2007**, *106*, 361–369. [CrossRef] [PubMed]

107. Rayhman, O.; Klipper, E.; Muller, L.; Davidson, B.; Reich, R.; Meidan, R. Small interfering RNA molecules targeting endothelin-converting enzyme-1 inhibit endothelin-1 synthesis and the invasive phenotype of ovarian carcinoma cells. *Cancer Res.* **2008**, *68*, 9265–9273. [CrossRef] [PubMed]

108. Izeradjene, K.; Douglas, L.; Delaney, A.; Houghton, J.A. Casein kinase II (CK2) enhances death-inducing signaling complex (DISC) activity in TRAIL-induced apoptosis in human colon carcinoma cell lines. *Oncogene* **2005**, *24*, 2050–2058. [CrossRef] [PubMed]

109. Hamacher, R.; Saur, D.; Fritsch, R.; Reichert, M.; Schmid, R.M.; Schneider, G. Casein kinase II inhibition induces apoptosis in pancreatic cancer cells. *Oncol. Rep.* **2007**, *18*, 695–701. [CrossRef] [PubMed]

110. Guerra, B.; Hochscherf, J.; Jensen, N.B.; Issinger, O.G. Identification of a novel potent, selective and cell permeable inhibitor of protein kinase CK2 from the NIH/NCI diversity set library. *Mol. Cell. Biochem.* **2015**, *406*, 151–161. [CrossRef] [PubMed]

111. Giroux, V.; Iovanna, J.L.; Garcia, S.; Dagorn, J.C. Combined inhibition of PAK7, MAP3K7 and CK2α kinases inhibits the growth of MiaPaCa2 pancreatic cancer cell xenografts. *Cancer Gene Ther.* **2009**, *16*, 731–740. [CrossRef] [PubMed]

112. Kreutzer, J.N.; Ruzzene, M.; Guerra, B. Enhancing chemosensitivity to gemcitabine via RNA interference targeting the catalytic subunits of protein kinase CK2 in human pancreatic cancer cells. *BMC Cancer* **2010**, *10*, 440. [CrossRef] [PubMed]

113. Tugizov, S.; Berline, J.; Herrera, R.; Penaranda, M.E.; Nakagawa, M.; Palefsky, J. Inhibition of human papillomavirus type 16 E7 phosphorylation by the s100 MRP-8/14 protein complex. *J. Virol.* **2005**, *79*, 1099–1112. [CrossRef] [PubMed]

114. Massimi, P.; Banks, L. Differential phosphorylation of the HPV-16 E7 oncoprotein during the cell cycle. *Virology* **2000**, *276*, 388–394. [CrossRef] [PubMed]

115. Liu, J.; Cao, X.C.; Xiao, Q.; Quan, M.F. Apigenin inhibits HeLa sphere-forming cells through inactivation of casein kinase 2α. *Mol. Med. Rep.* **2015**, *11*, 665–669. [PubMed]

116. Solares, A.M.; Santana, A.; Baladron, I.; Valenzuela, C.; Gonzalez, C.A.; Diaz, A.; Castillo, D.; Ramos, T.; Gomez, R.; Alonso, D.F.; et al. Safety and preliminary efficacy data of a novel casein kinase 2 (CK2) peptide inhibitor administered intralesionally at four dose levels in patients with cervical malignancies. *BMC Cancer* **2009**, *9*, 146. [CrossRef] [PubMed]

117. Sarduy, M.R.; Garcia, I.; Coca, M.A.; Perera, A.; Torres, L.A.; Valenzuela, C.M.; Baladron, I.; Solares, M.; Reyes, V.; Hernandez, I.; et al. Optimizing CIGB-300 intralesional delivery in locally advanced cervical cancer. *Br. J. Cancer* **2015**, *112*, 1636–1643. [CrossRef] [PubMed]

118. Dixit, D.; Sharma, V.; Ghosh, S.; Mehta, V.S.; Sen, E. Inhibition of Casein kinase-2 induces p53-dependent cell cycle arrest and sensitizes glioblastoma cells to tumor necrosis factor (TNFα)-induced apoptosis through SIRT1 inhibition. *Cell. Death Dis.* **2012**, *3*, e271. [CrossRef] [PubMed]

119. Nitta, R.T.; Gholamin, S.; Feroze, A.H.; Agarwal, M.; Cheshier, S.H.; Mitra, S.S.; Li, G. Casein kinase 2α regulates glioblastoma brain tumor-initiating cell growth through the β-catenin pathway. *Oncogene* **2015**, *34*, 3688–3699. [CrossRef] [PubMed]

120. Mandal, T.; Bhowmik, A.; Chatterjee, A.; Chatterjee, U.; Chatterjee, S.; Ghosh, M.K. Reduced phosphorylation of Stat3 at Ser-727 mediated by casein kinase 2 - Protein phosphatase 2A enhances Stat3 Tyr-705 induced tumorigenic potential of glioma cells. *Cell. Signal.* **2014**, *26*, 1725–1734. [CrossRef] [PubMed]

121. Ferrer-Font, L.; Alcaraz, E.; Plana, M.; Candiota, A.P.; Itarte, E.; Arus, C. Protein kinase CK2 content in GL261 mouse glioblastoma. *Pathol. Oncol. Res.* **2016**, *22*, 633–637. [CrossRef] [PubMed]

122. Kaminska, B.; Ellert-Miklaszewska, A.; Oberbek, A.; Wisniewski, P.; Kaza, B.; Makowska, M.; Bretner, M.; Kazimierczuk, Z. Efficacy and mechanism of anti-tumor action of new potential CK2 inhibitors toward glioblastoma cells. *Int. J. Oncol.* **2009**, *35*, 1091–1100. [CrossRef] [PubMed]

123. Prudent, R.; Moucadel, V.; Nguyen, C.H.; Barette, C.; Schmidt, F.; Florent, J.C.; Lafanechere, L.; Sautel, C.F.; Duchemin-Pelletier, E.; Spreux, E.; et al. Antitumor activity of pyridocarbazole and benzopyridoindole derivatives that inhibit protein kinase CK2. *Cancer Res.* **2010**, *70*, 9865–9874. [CrossRef] [PubMed]

124. Moucadel, V.; Prudent, R.; Sautel, C.F.; Teillet, F.; Barette, C.; Lafanechere, L.; Receveur-Brechot, V.; Cochet, C. Antitumoral activity of allosteric inhibitors of protein kinase CK2. *Oncotarget* **2011**, *2*, 997–1010. [CrossRef] [PubMed]

125. Olsen, B.B.; Svenstrup, T.H.; Guerra, B. Downregulation of protein kinase CK2 induces autophagic cell death through modulation of the mTOR and MAPK signaling pathways in human glioblastoma cells. *Int. J. Oncol.* **2012**, *41*, 1967–1976. [PubMed]

126. Joughin, B.A.; Naegle, K.M.; Huang, P.H.; Yaffe, M.B.; Lauffenburger, D.A.; White, F.M. An integrated comparative phosphoproteomic and bioinformatic approach reveals a novel class of MPM-2 motifs upregulated in EGFRvIII-expressing glioblastoma cells. *Mol. Biosyst.* **2009**, *5*, 59–67. [CrossRef] [PubMed]

127. Chou, S.T.; Patil, R.; Galstyan, A.; Gangalum, P.R.; Cavenee, W.K.; Furnari, F.B.; Ljubimov, V.A.; Chesnokova, A.; Kramerov, A.A.; Ding, H.; et al. Simultaneous blockade of interacting CK2 and EGFR pathways by tumor-targeting nanobioconjugates increases therapeutic efficacy against glioblastoma multiforme. *J. Control. Release* **2016**, *244*, 14–23. [CrossRef] [PubMed]

128. Zhou, B.; Ritt, D.A.; Morrison, D.K.; Der, C.J.; Cox, A.D. Protein kinase CK2α maintains extracellular signal-regulated kinase (ERK) activity in a CK2α kinase-independent manner to promote resistance to inhibitors of RAF and MEK but not ERK in BRAF mutant melanoma. *J. Biol. Chem.* **2016**, *291*, 17804–17815. [CrossRef] [PubMed]

129. Mitev, V.; Miteva, L.; Botev, I.; Houdebine, L.M. Enhanced Casein kinase II activity in metastatic melanoma. *J. Dermatol. Sci.* **1994**, *8*, 45–49. [CrossRef]

130. Cheng, X.; Merz, K.H.; Vatter, S.; Christ, J.; Wolfl, S.; Eisenbrand, G. 7,7'-diazaindirubin—A small molecule inhibitor of Casein kinase 2 in vitro and in cells. *Bioorg. Med. Chem.* **2014**, *22*, 247–255. [CrossRef] [PubMed]

131. Parker, R.; Clifton-Bligh, R.; Molloy, M.P. Phosphoproteomics of mapk inhibition in braf-mutated cells and a role for the lethal synergism of dual braf and ck2 inhibition. *Mol Cancer Ther* **2014**, *13*, 1894–1906. [CrossRef] [PubMed]

132. Pathak, H.B.; Zhou, Y.; Sethi, G.; Hirst, J.; Schilder, R.J.; Golemis, E.A.; Godwin, A.K. A synthetic lethality screen using a focused siRNA library to identify sensitizers to dasatinib therapy for the treatment of epithelial ovarian cancer. *PLoS ONE* **2015**, *10*, e0144126. [CrossRef] [PubMed]

133. Wong, A.S.; Kim, S.O.; Leung, P.C.; Auersperg, N.; Pelech, S.L. Profiling of protein kinases in the neoplastic transformation of human ovarian surface epithelium. *Gynecol. Oncol.* **2001**, *82*, 305–311. [CrossRef] [PubMed]

134. Tang, A.Q.; Cao, X.C.; Tian, L.; He, L.; Liu, F. Apigenin inhibits the self-renewal capacity of human ovarian cancer SKOV3derived sphere-forming cells. *Mol. Med. Rep.* **2015**, *11*, 2221–2226. [PubMed]

135. Siddiqui-Jain, A.; Bliesath, J.; Macalino, D.; Omori, M.; Huser, N.; Streiner, N.; Ho, C.B.; Anderes, K.; Proffitt, C.; O'Brien, S.E.; et al. CK2 inhibitor CX-4945 suppresses DNA repair response triggered by DNA-targeted anticancer drugs and augments efficacy: Mechanistic rationale for drug combination therapy. *Mol. Cancer Ther.* **2012**, *11*, 994–1005. [CrossRef] [PubMed]

136. Kulbe, H.; Iorio, F.; Chakravarty, P.; Milagre, C.S.; Moore, R.; Thompson, R.G.; Everitt, G.; Canosa, M.; Montoya, A.; Drygin, D.; et al. Integrated transcriptomic and proteomic analysis identifies protein kinase CK2 as a key signaling node in an inflammatory cytokine network in ovarian cancer cells. *Oncotarget* **2016**, *7*, 15648–15661. [CrossRef] [PubMed]

137. Qaiser, F.; Trembley, J.H.; Sadiq, S.; Muhammad, I.; Younis, R.; Hashmi, S.N.; Murtaza, B.; Rector, T.S.; Naveed, A.K.; Ahmed, K. Examination of CK2α and NF-kappaB p65 expression in human benign prostatic hyperplasia and prostate cancer tissues. *Mol. Cell. Biochem.* **2016**, *420*, 43–51. [CrossRef] [PubMed]

138. Laramas, M.; Pasquier, D.; Filhol, O.; Ringeisen, F.; Descotes, J.L.; Cochet, C. Nuclear localization of protein kinase CK2 catalytic subunit (CK2α) is associated with poor prognostic factors in human prostate cancer. *Eur. J. Cancer* **2007**, *43*, 928–934. [CrossRef] [PubMed]

139. Ahmed, K.; Kren, B.T.; Abedin, M.J.; Vogel, R.I.; Shaughnessy, D.P.; Nacusi, L.; Korman, V.L.; Li, Y.; Dehm, S.M.; Zimmerman, C.L.; et al. CK2 targeted RNAi therapeutic delivered via malignant cell-directed tenfibgen nanocapsule: Dose and molecular mechanisms of response in xenograft prostate tumors. *Oncotarget* **2016**, *7*, 61789–61805. [CrossRef] [PubMed]

140. Yenice, S.; Davis, A.T.; Goueli, S.A.; Akdas, A.; Limas, C.; Ahmed, K. Nuclear casein kinase 2 (CK-2) activity in human normal, benign hyperplastic, and cancerous prostate. *Prostate* **1994**, *24*, 11–16. [CrossRef] [PubMed]

141. Yoo, J.Y.; Lim, B.J.; Choi, H.K.; Hong, S.W.; Jang, H.S.; Kim, C.; Chun, K.H.; Choi, K.C.; Yoon, H.G. CK2-NcoR signaling cascade promotes prostate tumorigenesis. *Oncotarget* **2013**, *4*, 972–983. [CrossRef] [PubMed]

142. Schneider, C.C.; Hessenauer, A.; Gotz, C.; Montenarh, M. DMAT, an inhibitor of protein kinase CK2 induces reactive oxygen species and DNA double strand breaks. *Oncol. Rep.* **2009**, *21*, 1593–1597. [PubMed]

143. Trembley, J.H.; Unger, G.M.; Gomez, O.C.; Abedin, J.; Korman, V.L.; Vogel, R.I.; Niehans, G.; Kren, B.T.; Ahmed, K. Tenfibgen-DMAT nanocapsule delivers CK2 inhibitor DMAT to prostate cancer xenograft tumors causing inhibition of cell proliferation. *Mol. Cell. Pharmacol.* **2014**, *6*, 15–25. [PubMed]

144. Trembley, J.H.; Unger, G.M.; Korman, V.L.; Tobolt, D.K.; Kazimierczuk, Z.; Pinna, L.A.; Kren, B.T.; Ahmed, K. Nanoencapsulated anti-CK2 small molecule drug or siRNA specifically targets malignant cancer but not benign cells. *Cancer Lett.* **2012**, *315*, 48–58. [CrossRef] [PubMed]

145. Wang, G.; Unger, G.; Ahmad, K.A.; Slaton, J.W.; Ahmed, K. Downregulation of CK2 induces apoptosis in cancer cells—A potential approach to cancer therapy. *Mol. Cell. Biochem.* **2005**, *274*, 77–84. [CrossRef] [PubMed]

146. Yao, K.; Youn, H.; Gao, X.; Huang, B.; Zhou, F.; Li, B.; Han, H. Casein kinase 2 inhibition attenuates androgen receptor function and cell proliferation in prostate cancer cells. *Prostate* **2012**, *72*, 1423–1430. [CrossRef] [PubMed]

147. Hessenauer, A.; Schneider, C.C.; Gotz, C.; Montenarh, M. CK2 inhibition induces apoptosis via the ER stress response. *Cell. Signal.* **2011**, *23*, 145–151. [CrossRef] [PubMed]

148. Pierre, F.; Chua, P.C.; O'Brien, S.E.; Siddiqui-Jain, A.; Bourbon, P.; Haddach, M.; Michaux, J.; Nagasawa, J.; Schwaebe, M.K.; Stefan, E.; et al. Pre-clinical characterization of CX-4945, a potent and selective small molecule inhibitor of CK2 for the treatment of cancer. *Mol. Cell. Biochem.* **2011**, *356*, 37–43. [CrossRef] [PubMed]

149. Qaiser, F.; Trembley, J.H.; Kren, B.T.; Wu, J.J.; Naveed, A.K.; Ahmed, K. Protein kinase CK2 inhibition induces cell death via early impact on mitochondrial function. *J. Cell. Biochem.* **2014**, *115*, 2103–2115. [CrossRef] [PubMed]

150. Wang, G.; Ahmad, K.A.; Harris, N.H.; Ahmed, K. Impact of protein kinase CK2 on inhibitor of apoptosis proteins in prostate cancer cells. *Mol. Cell. Biochem.* **2008**, *316*, 91–97. [CrossRef] [PubMed]

151. Orzechowska, E.; Kozlowska, E.; Staron, K.; Trzcinska-Danielewicz, J. Time schedule-dependent effect of the CK2 inhibitor TBB on PC-3 human prostate cancer cell viability. *Oncol. Rep.* **2012**, *27*, 281–285. [PubMed]

152. Wang, G.; Ahmad, K.A.; Ahmed, K. Role of protein kinase CK2 in the regulation of tumor necrosis factor-related apoptosis inducing ligand-induced apoptosis in prostate cancer cells. *Cancer Res.* **2006**, *66*, 2242–2249. [CrossRef] [PubMed]

153. Gray, G.K.; McFarland, B.C.; Rowse, A.L.; Gibson, S.A.; Benveniste, E.N. Therapeutic CK2 inhibition attenuates diverse prosurvival signaling cascades and decreases cell viability in human breast cancer cells. *Oncotarget* **2014**, *5*, 6484–6496. [CrossRef] [PubMed]

154. Bae, J.S.; Park, S.H.; Jamiyandorj, U.; Kim, K.M.; Noh, S.J.; Kim, J.R.; Park, H.J.; Kwon, K.S.; Jung, S.H.; Park, H.S.; et al. CK2α/CSNK2A1 phosphorylates SIRT6 and is involved in the progression of breast carcinoma and predicts shorter survival of diagnosed patients. *Am. J. Pathol.* **2016**, *186*, 3297–3315. [CrossRef] [PubMed]

155. Kren, B.T.; Unger, G.M.; Abedin, M.J.; Vogel, R.I.; Henzler, C.M.; Ahmed, K.; Trembley, J.H. Preclinical evaluation of cyclin dependent kinase 11 and casein kinase 2 survival kinases as RNA interference targets for triple negative breast cancer therapy. *Breast Cancer Res.* **2015**, *17*, 19. [CrossRef] [PubMed]

156. Williams, M.D.; Nguyen, T.; Carriere, P.P.; Tilghman, S.L.; Williams, C. Protein kinase CK2 expression predicts relapse survival in ERα dependent breast cancer, and modulates erα expression in vitro. *Int. J. Environ. Res. Public Health* **2015**, *13*. [CrossRef] [PubMed]

157. Liu, R.; Wang, X.; Chen, G.Y.; Dalerba, P.; Gurney, A.; Hoey, T.; Sherlock, G.; Lewicki, J.; Shedden, K.; Clarke, M.F. The prognostic role of a gene signature from tumorigenic breast-cancer cells. *N. Engl. J. Med.* **2007**, *356*, 217–226. [CrossRef] [PubMed]

158. Landesman-Bollag, E.; Romieu-Mourez, R.; Song, D.H.; Sonenshein, G.E.; Cardiff, R.D.; Seldin, D.C. Protein kinase CK2 in mammary gland tumorigenesis. *Oncogene* **2001**, *20*, 3247–3257. [CrossRef] [PubMed]

159. Feliciano, A.; Castellvi, J.; Artero-Castro, A.; Leal, J.A.; Romagosa, C.; Hernandez-Losa, J.; Peg, V.; Fabra, A.; Vidal, F.; Kondoh, H.; et al. miR-125b acts as a tumor suppressor in breast tumorigenesis via its novel direct targets ENPEP, CK2-α, CCNJ, and MEGF9. *PLoS ONE* **2013**, *8*, e76247. [CrossRef] [PubMed]

160. Munstermann, U.; Fritz, G.; Seitz, G.; Lu, Y.P.; Schneider, H.R.; Issinger, O.G. Casein kinase II is elevated in solid human tumours and rapidly proliferating non-neoplastic tissue. *Eur. J. Biochem.* **1990**, *189*, 251–257. [CrossRef] [PubMed]

161. Das, N.; Datta, N.; Chatterjee, U.; Ghosh, M.K. Estrogen receptor α transcriptionally activates casein kinase 2 α: A pivotal regulator of promyelocytic leukaemia protein (PML) and AKT in oncogenesis. *Cell Signal.* **2016**, *28*, 675–687. [CrossRef] [PubMed]

162. Currier, N.; Solomon, S.E.; Demicco, E.G.; Chang, D.L.; Farago, M.; Ying, H.; Dominguez, I.; Sonenshein, G.E.; Cardiff, R.D.; Xiao, Z.X.; et al. Oncogenic signaling pathways activated in DMBA-induced mouse mammary tumors. *Toxicol. Pathol.* **2005**, *33*, 726–737. [CrossRef] [PubMed]

163. Ford, H.L.; Landesman-Bollag, E.; Dacwag, C.S.; Stukenberg, P.T.; Pardee, A.B.; Seldin, D.C. Cell cycle-regulated phosphorylation of the human SIX1 homeodomain protein. *J. Biol. Chem.* **2000**, *275*, 22245–22254. [CrossRef] [PubMed]

164. Tapia, J.C.; Torres, V.A.; Rodriguez, D.A.; Leyton, L.; Quest, A.F. Casein kinase 2 (CK2) increases survivin expression via enhanced β-catenin-T cell factor/lymphoid enhancer binding factor-dependent transcription. *Proc. Natl. Acad. Sci. USA* **2006**, *103*, 15079–15084. [CrossRef] [PubMed]

165. Lee, Y.H.; Kang, B.S.; Bae, Y.S. Premature senescence in human breast cancer and colon cancer cells by tamoxifen-mediated reactive oxygen species generation. *Life Sci.* **2014**, *97*, 116–122. [CrossRef] [PubMed]

166. Eddy, S.F.; Guo, S.; Demicco, E.G.; Romieu-Mourez, R.; Landesman-Bollag, E.; Seldin, D.C.; Sonenshein, G.E. Inducible IkappaB kinase/IkappaB kinase epsilon expression is induced by CK2 and promotes aberrant nuclear factor-kappaB activation in breast cancer cells. *Cancer Res.* **2005**, *65*, 11375–11383. [CrossRef] [PubMed]

167. Li, D.; Chen, L.; Hu, Z.; Li, H.; Li, J.; Wei, C.; Huang, Y.; Song, H.; Fang, L. Alterations of microRNAs are associated with impaired growth of MCF-7 breast cancer cells induced by inhibition of casein kinase 2. *Int. J. Clin. Exp. Pathol.* **2014**, *7*, 4008–4015. [PubMed]

168. Hagan, C.R.; Regan, T.M.; Dressing, G.E.; Lange, C.A. CK2-dependent phosphorylation of progesterone receptors (PR) on Ser81 regulates PR-B isoform-specific target gene expression in breast cancer cells. *Mol. Cell. Biol.* **2011**, *31*, 2439–2452. [CrossRef] [PubMed]

169. McManaway, M.E.; Eckberg, W.R.; Anderson, W.A. Characterization and hormonal regulation of casein kinase II activity in heterotransplanted human breast tumors in nude mice. *Exp. Clin. Endocrinol.* **1987**, *90*, 313–323. [CrossRef] [PubMed]

170. Drygin, D.; Ho, C.B.; Omori, M.; Bliesath, J.; Proffitt, C.; Rice, R.; Siddiqui-Jain, A.; O'Brien, S.; Padgett, C.; Lim, J.K.; et al. Protein kinase CK2 modulates IL-6 expression in inflammatory breast cancer. *Biochem. Biophys. Res. Commun.* **2011**, *415*, 163–167. [CrossRef] [PubMed]

171. Yde, C.W.; Frogne, T.; Lykkesfeldt, A.E.; Fichtner, I.; Issinger, O.G.; Stenvang, J. Induction of cell death in antiestrogen resistant human breast cancer cells by the protein kinase CK2 inhibitor DMAT. *Cancer Lett.* **2007**, *256*, 229–237. [CrossRef] [PubMed]

172. Matsumoto, Y.; Takano, H.; Fojo, T. Cellular adaptation to drug exposure: Evolution of the drug-resistant phenotype. *Cancer Res.* **1997**, *57*, 5086–5092. [PubMed]

173. Rabjerg, M.; Guerra, B.; Olivan-Viguera, A.; Nedergaard Mikkelsen, M.L.; Kohler, R.; Issinger, O.G.; Marcussen, N. Nuclear localization of the CK2α-subunit correlates with poor prognosis in clear cell renal cell carcinoma. *Oncotarget* **2016**, *8*, 1613–1627.

174. Rabjerg, M.; Bjerregaard, H.; Halekoh, U.; Jensen, B.L.; Walter, S.; Marcussen, N. Molecular characterization of clear cell renal cell carcinoma identifies CSNK2A1, SPP1 and DEFB1 as promising novel prognostic markers. *APMIS* **2016**, *124*, 372–383. [CrossRef] [PubMed]

175. Caroline Roelants, S.G.; Duchemin-Pelletier, E.; McLeer-Florin, A.; Tisseyre, C.; Aubert, C.; Champelovier, P.; Boutonnat, J.; Descotes, J.L.; Rambeaud, J.-J.; Arnoux, V.; et al. Dysregulated expression of protein kinase ck2 in renal cancer. In *Protein Kinase CK2 Cellular Function in Normal and Disease States*; Khalil, O.-G.I., Ryszard Szyszka, A., Eds.; Springer: Cham, Switzerland, 2015; Volume 12, pp. 241–257.

176. Stalter, G.; Siemer, S.; Becht, E.; Ziegler, M.; Remberger, K.; Issinger, O.G. Asymmetric expression of protein kinase CK2 subunits in human kidney tumors. *Biochem. Biophys. Res. Commun.* **1994**, *202*, 141–147. [CrossRef] [PubMed]

177. Ampofo, E.; Kietzmann, T.; Zimmer, A.; Jakupovic, M.; Montenarh, M.; Gotz, C. Phosphorylation of the von Hippel-Lindau protein (VHL) by protein kinase CK2 reduces its protein stability and affects p53 and HIF-1α mediated transcription. *Int. J. Biochem. Cell. Biol.* **2010**, *42*, 1729–1735. [CrossRef] [PubMed]

178. German, P.; Bai, S.; Liu, X.D.; Sun, M.; Zhou, L.; Kalra, S.; Zhang, X.; Minelli, R.; Scott, K.L.; Mills, G.B.; et al. Phosphorylation-dependent cleavage regulates von Hippel Lindau proteostasis and function. *Oncogene* **2016**, *35*, 4973–4980. [CrossRef] [PubMed]

179. Lolkema, M.P.; Gervais, M.L.; Snijckers, C.M.; Hill, R.P.; Giles, R.H.; Voest, E.E.; Ohh, M. Tumor suppression by the von Hippel-Lindau protein requires phosphorylation of the acidic domain. *J. Biol. Chem.* **2005**, *280*, 22205–22211. [CrossRef] [PubMed]

180. Gomes, A.M.; Soares, M.V.; Ribeiro, P.; Caldas, J.; Povoa, V.; Martins, L.R.; Melao, A.; Serra-Caetano, A.; de Sousa, A.B.; Lacerda, J.F.; et al. Adult B-cell acute lymphoblastic leukemia cells display decreased PTEN activity and constitutive hyperactivation of PI3K/Akt pathway despite high PTEN protein levels. *Haematologica* **2014**, *99*, 1062–1068. [CrossRef] [PubMed]

181. Song, C.; Gowda, C.; Pan, X.; Ding, Y.; Tong, Y.; Tan, B.H.; Wang, H.; Muthusami, S.; Ge, Z.; Sachdev, M.; et al. Targeting casein kinase II restores Ikaros tumor suppressor activity and demonstrates therapeutic efficacy in high-risk leukemia. *Blood* **2015**, *126*, 1813–1822. [CrossRef] [PubMed]

182. Silva, A.; Yunes, J.A.; Cardoso, B.A.; Martins, L.R.; Jotta, P.Y.; Abecasis, M.; Nowill, A.E.; Leslie, N.R.; Cardoso, A.A.; Barata, J.T. PTEN posttranslational inactivation and hyperactivation of the PI3K/Akt pathway sustain primary t cell leukemia viability. *J. Clin. Investig.* **2008**, *118*, 3762–3774. [CrossRef] [PubMed]

183. Kim, J.S.; Eom, J.I.; Cheong, J.-W.; Choi, A.J.; Lee, J.K.; Yang, W.I.; Min, Y.H. Protein kinase CK2α as an unfavorable prognostic marker and novel therapeutic target in acute myeloid leukemia. *Clin. Cancer Res.* **2007**, *13*, 1019–1028. [CrossRef] [PubMed]

184. Quotti Tubi, L.; Gurrieri, C.; Brancalion, A.; Bonaldi, L.; Bertorelle, R.; Manni, S.; Piazza, F. Inhibition of protein kinase CK2 with the clinical-grade small ATP-competitive compound CX-4945 or by RNA interference unveils its role in acute myeloid leukemia cell survival, p53-dependent apoptosis and daunorubicin-induced cytotoxicity. *J. Hematol. Oncol.* **2013**, *6*, 78. [CrossRef] [PubMed]

185. Martins, L.R.; Lucio, P.; Silva, M.C.; Anderes, K.L.; Gameiro, P.; Silva, M.G.; Barata, J.T. Targeting CK2 overexpression and hyperactivation as a novel therapeutic tool in chronic lymphocytic leukemia. *Blood* **2010**, *116*, 2724–2731. [CrossRef] [PubMed]

186. Gowda, C.; Sachdev, M.; Muthisami, S.; Kapadia, M.; Petrovic-Dovat, L.; Hartman, M.; Ding, Y.; Song, C.; Payne, J.L.; Tan, B.H.; et al. Casein kinase II (CK2) as a therapeutic target for hematological malignancies. *Curr. Pharm. Des.* **2016**, in press. [CrossRef]

187. Buontempo, F.; Orsini, E.; Martins, L.R.; Antunes, I.; Lonetti, A.; Chiarini, F.; Tabellini, G.; Evangelisti, C.; Evangelisti, C.; Melchionda, F.; et al. Cytotoxic activity of the casein kinase 2 inhibitor CX-4945 against T-cell acute lymphoblastic leukemia: Targeting the unfolded protein response signaling. *Leukemia* **2014**, *28*, 543–553. [CrossRef] [PubMed]

188. Martins, L.R.; Lucio, P.; Melao, A.; Antunes, I.; Cardoso, B.A.; Stansfield, R.; Bertilaccio, M.T.; Ghia, P.; Drygin, D.; Silva, M.G.; et al. Activity of the clinical-stage CK2-specific inhibitor CX-4945 against chronic lymphocytic leukemia. *Leukemia* **2014**, *28*, 179–182. [CrossRef] [PubMed]

189. Seldin, D.C. New models of lymphoma in transgenic mice. *Curr. Opin. Immunol.* **1995**, *7*, 665–673. [CrossRef]

190. Seldin, D.C.; Leder, P. Casein kinase II α transgene-induced murine lymphoma: Relation to theileriosis in cattle. *Science* **1995**, *267*, 894–897. [CrossRef] [PubMed]

191. Pizzi, M.; Piazza, F.; Agostinelli, C.; Fuligni, F.; Benvenuti, P.; Mandato, E.; Casellato, A.; Rugge, M.; Semenzato, G.; Pileri, S.A. Protein kinase CK2 is widely expressed in follicular, burkitt and diffuse large b-cell lymphomas and propels malignant B-cell growth. *Oncotarget* **2015**, *6*, 6544–6552. [CrossRef] [PubMed]

192. Manni, S.; Brancalion, A.; Mandato, E.; Tubi, L.Q.; Colpo, A.; Pizzi, M.; Cappellesso, R.; Zaffino, F.; Di Maggio, S.A.; Cabrelle, A.; et al. Protein kinase CK2 inhibition down modulates the NF-kappaB and STAT3 survival pathways, enhances the cellular proteotoxic stress and synergistically boosts the cytotoxic effect of bortezomib on multiple myeloma and mantle cell lymphoma cells. *PLoS ONE* **2013**, *8*, e75280. [CrossRef] [PubMed]

193. Piazza, F.A.; Ruzzene, M.; Gurrieri, C.; Montini, B.; Bonanni, L.; Chioetto, G.; Di Maira, G.; Barbon, F.; Cabrelle, A.; Zambello, R.; et al. Multiple myeloma cell survival relies on high activity of protein kinase CK2. *Blood* **2006**, *108*, 1698–1707. [CrossRef] [PubMed]

194. Zhao, M.; Ma, J.; Zhu, H.Y.; Zhang, X.H.; Du, Z.Y.; Xu, Y.J.; Yu, X.D. Apigenin inhibits proliferation and induces apoptosis in human multiple myeloma cells through targeting the trinity of CK2, Cdc37 and Hsp90. *Mol. Cancer* **2011**, *10*, 104. [CrossRef] [PubMed]

195. Piazza, F.; Manni, S.; Semenzato, G. Novel players in multiple myeloma pathogenesis: Role of protein kinases CK2 and GSK3. *Leukemia Res.* **2013**, *37*, 221–227. [CrossRef] [PubMed]

196. Manni, S.; Brancalion, A.; Tubi, L.Q.; Colpo, A.; Pavan, L.; Cabrelle, A.; Ave, E.; Zaffino, F.; Di Maira, G.; Ruzzene, M.; et al. Protein kinase CK2 protects multiple myeloma cells from ER stress-induced apoptosis and from the cytotoxic effect of HSP90 inhibition through regulation of the unfolded protein response. *Clin. Cancer Res.* **2012**, *18*, 1888–1900. [CrossRef] [PubMed]

197. Cozza, G.; Venerando, A.; Sarno, S.; Pinna, L.A. The selectivity of CK2 inhibitor quinalizarin: A reevaluation. *Biomed. Res. Int.* **2015**, *2015*, 734127. [CrossRef] [PubMed]

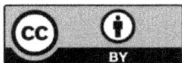

pharmaceuticals

MDPI

Review

CK2 Molecular Targeting—Tumor Cell-Specific Delivery of RNAi in Various Models of Cancer

Janeen H. Trembley [1,2,3,*], Betsy T. Kren [1,2,3], Md. Joynal Abedin [1,2], Rachel I. Vogel [3,4], Claire M. Cannon [5], Gretchen M. Unger [6] and Khalil Ahmed [1,2,3,7]

[1] Research Service, Minneapolis VA Health Care System, Minneapolis, MN 55417, USA; krenx@umn.edu (B.T.K.); mdjoynal@yahoo.com (M.J.A.); ahmedk@umn.edu (K.A.)
[2] Department of Laboratory Medicine and Pathology, University of Minnesota, Minneapolis, MN 55455, USA
[3] Masonic Cancer Center, University of Minnesota, Minneapolis, MN 55455, USA; isak0023@umn.edu
[4] Department of Obstetrics, Gynecology and Women's Health, University of Minnesota, Minneapolis, MN 55455, USA
[5] School of Veterinary Medicine, University of Minnesota, Minneapolis, MN 55455, USA; clairemcannon@gmail.com
[6] GeneSegues Therapeutics, Minnetonka, MN 55343, USA; gmu@genesegues.com
[7] Department of Urology, University of Minnesota, Minneapolis, MN 55455, USA
*   Correspondence: trem0005@umn.edu, Tel.: +1-612-467-2877

Academic Editor: Mathias Montenarh
Received: 7 December 2016; Accepted: 14 February 2017; Published: 21 February 2017

Abstract: Protein kinase CK2 demonstrates increased protein expression relative to non-transformed cells in the majority of cancers that have been examined. The elevated levels of CK2 are involved in promoting not only continued proliferation of cancer cells but also their resistance to cell death; thus, CK2 has emerged as a plausible target for cancer therapy. Our focus has been to target CK2 catalytic subunits at the molecular level using RNA interference (RNAi) strategies to achieve their downregulation. The delivery of oligonucleotide therapeutic agents warrants that they are protected and are delivered specifically to cancer cells. The latter is particularly important since CK2 is a ubiquitous signal that is essential for survival. To achieve these goals, we have developed a nanocapsule that has the properties of delivering an anti-CK2 RNAi therapeutic cargo, in a protected manner, specifically to cancer cells. Tenfibgen (TBG) is used as the ligand to target tenascin-C receptors, which are elevated in cancer cells. This strategy is effective for inhibiting growth and inducing death in several types of xenograft tumors, and the nanocapsule elicits no safety concerns in animals. Further investigation of this therapeutic approach for its translation is warranted.

Keywords: CK2; nanocapsules; nanoparticles; anti-CK2; RNAi; siRNA; tenfibgen; TBG; TBG-RNAi-CK2; therapy; cancer; targeting; cancer-specific; tumor-specific; prostate cancer; breast cancer; HNSCC

1. Introduction

Protein kinase CK2 (acronym for the former casein kinase II or 2) is a ubiquitous protein serine/threonine kinase consisting of two catalytic subunits (42 kDa α and 38 kDa α') linked through two regulatory subunits (28 kDa β). The kinase is present in the nuclear and cytoplasmic fractions of the cell, including numerous cellular organelles. The distribution of the kinase in normal cells is diffuse in both the nuclear and cytoplasmic compartments; however, in cancer cells the overall expression and nuclear localization of CK2 is significantly enhanced [1–4].

Over time, several investigations recognized the association of protein kinase CK2 with cell growth and proliferation in normal and cancer cells (reviewed in, e.g., [1,4–7]). However, its link to cancer biology was firmly established only when it was discovered that CK2 not only promotes cell growth and proliferation but also is an effective suppressor of cell death, originally revealed by this laboratory [8–11]. Likewise, it was recognized that the treatment of cells with antisense to CK2 resulted in potent cell death, thus prompting the notion, for the first time, that CK2 downregulation might serve as cancer therapy strategy [12]. The potential of CK2 as a druggable target for cancer therapy has been documented with several recent studies on its targeting primarily using small molecular inhibitors or by peptide-mediated inhibition of its phosphorylation site(s), (see, e.g., [13–15]).

2. Discussion

2.1. Features of CK2 Pertinent to Cancer

CK2 is present in all cells and its activity appears to be stable at a certain level depending on the organ. CK2 (activity/level) is elevated in cells during proliferation, and in normal cell proliferation the CK2 activity returns to the basal level on cessation of proliferation. The basal CK2 activity is involved in a wide range of cellular activities as has been reviewed in several publications (e.g., [2,3]). The possible involvement of CK2 in cancer is supported by a wide range of observations. First, CK2 has been found to be elevated in the vast majority of cancers that have been examined [5,7,16]. Its elevation, however, is not simply an indicator of cell proliferation but rather indicates a state of dysplasia [17] and contributes to transformation [18–20]. The intracellular distribution of CK2 proteins in cancer cells is also distinct from that in normal cells such that the level of CK2 in the nuclear compartment of cancer cells is much higher than that in normal cells [7,17,21].

Second, CK2 is a potent regulator of cell death such that its elevation serves as a potent suppressor of apoptosis while its downregulation results in the induction of cell death—this characteristic of CK2 may be regarded as the key functional link of this enzyme to the cancer cell phenotype [5,8–10]. A number of hallmarks of cancer have been described [22]. However, two consistent characteristics of cancer cells are a dysregulation of cell growth and proliferation as well as a resistance to cell death. Thus, it is reasonable to surmise that up-regulation of CK2 in cancer cells not only provides the environment for their continued proliferation but also contributes to their suppression of cell death [8–10,23]. Considering the dysregulation of CK2 in all cancers that have been examined, we previously presented discussions of the studies suggesting involvement of CK2 in several of the hallmarks of cancer (besides the two mentioned above) [24,25]. It is also important to note that the level of CK2 dysregulation in a given cancer has been linked to prognosis (e.g., [26–30]). Here we present further discussion on the roles for CK2 in proliferation and malignancy, and the results of molecular targeting of CK2 in cancer, based on our recent research publications.

2.2. CK2 Elevation in Benign Prostate Proliferation versus in Prostate Cancer

The aforementioned observations describe that CK2 elevation has been uniformly observed in various cancers. In general, CK2 level/activity is elevated during normal cell proliferation as well [1,4,31]; however, there are cases of benign pathologic cell proliferation where CK2 is present at an elevated level as observed, e.g., in benign prostatic hyperplasia (BPH) [27,30,32]. This raises a question as to the nature of functionality of CK2 in prostatic cancer (PCa) versus BPH. To address this issue, we examined the combined expression of CK2α and NFκB p65 in PCa and BPH, considering that both are elevated in each of these diseases and that NFκB p65 is a known substrate of CK2α [33,34]. We thus wanted to determine if there was a differential expression of CK2α and NFκB p65 that may provide a means of distinction between the two diseases. An analysis of both of these signals in human PCa and BPH specimens revealed a number of observations. First, the amount of nuclear staining for CK2α and NFκB p65 was much higher in PCa than BPH. Second, expression levels of nuclear NFκB p65 and nuclear CK2α were correlated in both disease states. Correlation between CK2α and NFκB p65 expression observed at the protein level was generally not evident at the mRNA level in PCa based on comparison of mRNA expression for CSNK2A1 and RELA (information for mRNA expression in BPH was not readily available [35–37]). Third, increased nuclear CK2α protein expression in cancer was at least partially responsible for increased nuclear localization of NFκB p65 in PCa. Fourth, we found that PCa specimens demonstrated higher proliferation (Ki-67 immunostaining) than BPH specimens. Interestingly, nuclear NFκB p65 levels correlated with cytoplasmic NFκB p65 as well as Ki-67 signals in BPH, but not in PCa. It is noteworthy that these various correlations were apparent at the protein level and require the ability to determine nuclear and cytoplasmic localization of the signals [33]. Together, these observations suggest that with respect to their combined activity CK2 and NFκB have different modes of functionality in the biology of benign prostate growth and malignancy.

2.3. CK2 as a Target of Cancer Therapy

As mentioned, CK2 expression and activity are altered in most cancers that have been examined, and its molecular downregulation results in potent induction of cell death in cancer cells in culture or in vivo [7,12,38,39]. These observations from our laboratory prompted us to propose the notion that CK2 may serve as a target for cancer therapy, provided means for its effective targeting are developed (discussed subsequently). Since that time, CK2 has gained general acceptance as a target for cancer therapy, and currently diverse methods to achieve this targeting are being investigated [40,41]. Among the various approaches to targeting CK2 are the use of small molecule inhibitors, use of a peptide to block CK2 phosphorylation sites, and molecular downregulation employing RNAi to catalytic subunits of CK2 [13,42–48]. CK2 as a therapy target is particularly appealing because of its potent and rapid effect on activation of the apoptotic machinery [49], while also likely affecting the activity of a large number of downstream intracellular substrates and pathways as a consequence of its downregulation [6,50].

The nature of CK2 as ubiquitous and essential for cell survival has raised concerns regarding its targeting for cancer therapy, as its inhibition or loss might result in considerable toxicity to the host [12]. However, it has been observed that normal cells are significantly more resistant to CK2 inhibition or molecular downregulation [38,44]. These observations would suggest a pharmacological window for using CK2 as a target for cancer therapy. Regardless, we have been focused on the therapeutic targeting of CK2 in a cancer cell-specific manner, as discussed subsequently.

2.4. Desirability of Targeting CK2 Specifically in Cancer Cells and Utility of the TBG Nanocapsule to Accomplish This Goal

The relative resistance of normal cells to downregulation of CK2 has prompted considerable interest in the possible utility of small molecule inhibitors (such as CX-4945) as therapeutic agents. However, since CK2 is a ubiquitous survival signal, it would seem appropriate to employ strategies that are specific for downregulating CK2 in cancer cells, avoiding normal cells in vivo. Secondly, cancer cells may eventually develop drug resistance by various mechanisms, as has been a common observation in cancer chemotherapy (see, e.g., [22,51]). To avoid such a situation for CK2 targeted therapy, we have focused on blocking the production of CK2 by employing anti-CK2 RNAi strategies designed to block the generation of the two catalytic subunits. Such an approach warrants that systemic RNAi delivery is achieved in a protected manner and further that this delivery mechanism is cancer cell-specific. To that end, we have developed a nanocapsule that satisfies these requirements.

Our nanocapsule is based on a protein shell containing tenfibgen (TBG) peptide which is the C-terminal fibrinogen globe domain of the 225 kDa fibronectin-like extracellular matrix protein tenascin-C (TN-C) (Figure 1, with permission of Springer [52]). The preparation of the TBG nanocapsules incorporating various types of anti-CK2 oligonucleotide molecules as well as dysprosium (Dy) has been described previously [47,48,53,54]. These nanocapsules are generally between 14 to 28 nm in size, and display uniform morphology (appearing as uniform single capsules) as determined by atomic force microscopy and transmission electron microscopy. They carry neutral or slightly negatively charge. The targeting of the TBG nanocapsules is based on the knowledge that TN-C receptors are elevated in cancer cells and thus the TBG nanocapsules hone to cancer cells but not to normal/benign cells [55–61]; this malignant cell specificity has been demonstrated in cultured cells as well as in xenograft models of PCa, breast cancer, and head and neck squamous cell carcinoma (HNSCC) [24,47,48,54,62–64]. The uptake of the nanocapsules into the cancer cells is via the lipid raft pathway [47]. Of note, the TBG nanocapsules are also capable of delivering their cargo effectively to tumor cells metastasized to lymph node and spleen [47,64]. A microscopy approach using TBG-encapsulated Dy (TBG-Dy), which takes advantage of the innate fluorescence of this lanthanide element, established that the nanocapsule was detected in xenograft tumor localized to tibia but not in normal counterpart tibia [64]. Further, analysis of several normal tissues in tumor-bearing animals treated with various types of TBG nanocapsules demonstrated the accumulation of the nanocapsule in primary and metastatic tumors, but not in tissue such as liver, brain, and kidney where no tumor was present, consistent with an absence of nonspecific uptake or trapping of the nanocapsule [40,47,63,64].

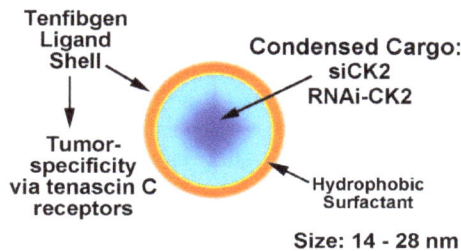

Figure 1. Nanocapsule concept and design and functional aspects are depicted.

2.5. Response of Xenograft Tumors to TBG-RNAi-CK2

We investigated CK2 molecular downregulation for several types of cancer xenograft models by utilizing TBG nanocapsule based delivery of anti-CK2 oligomers (such as double-stranded siRNA or single-stranded RNAi) that target both of the catalytic subunits of CK2. Comparison of oligomer types was carried out because it is possible that single-stranded or double-stranded RNAi oligomers might show differential efficacy in vivo as they might distinctively employ lalternate RNAi processing mechanisms. For controls in these studies, TBG nanocapsules carrying non-targeted siRNA (TBG-siCON1) or carrying oligomers targeting mouse factor VII (TBG-RNAi-F7) were employed [46]. The siCON1 control oligomer is a non-targeting double-stranded siRNA, which was rigorously established [65]. The mouse factor VII sequence was chosen as a negative control for single-stranded oligomer as this sequence was previously shown to engage the RNAi machinery in mouse liver and because factor VII is not expressed in prostate tumor [66]. Studies on acute dose-response in prostate PC3-LN4 xenograft tumors suggested that TBG-RNAi-CK2 was most effective at reducing tumor growth in the dose range of 0.01 to 0.1 mg/kg given three times over a period of 10 days. Under similar experimental conditions, the TBG-siCK2 nanocapsules demonstrated the most effective dose level to be 0.01 mg/kg. In the castration-resistant prostate cancer (CRPC) 22Rv1 model, the most effective dose of TBG-RNAi-CK2 was 0.1 mg/kg. TBG-siCK2 treatment using 0.01 mg/kg also reduced tumor growth in the MDA-MB-231 model of triple negative breast cancer [48]. In all of these studies, the nanocapsule was delivered by intravenous tail vein injection. These data are summarized in Table 1.

Table 1. Comparison of oligomer-based anti-CK2 TBG nanocapsule effects on tumor volumes in multiple cancer models.

Tumor Model	Treatment	Tumor Volume on Final Day [a]	p-Value
PC3-LN4	TBG-RNAi-CK2—0.01 mg/kg TBG-RNAi-F7—0.01 mg/kg	5.2 ± 3.2 12.2 ± 4.2	0.005
PC3-LN4	TBG-siCK2—0.01 mg/kg TBG-siCON1—1.0 mg/kg	4.0 ± 2.5 10.6 ± 5.5	0.007
22Rv1	TBG-RNAi-CK2—0.1 mg/kg TBG-RNAi-F7—1.0 mg/kg	2.5 ± 1.5 4.0 ± 1.5	0.11
MDA-MB-231	TBG-siCK2—0.01 mg/kg TBG-siCON1—0.01 mg/kg	1.4 ± 0.32 2.1 ± 0.55	0.026

[a] Tumor volume at sacrifice (days 10 or 11) relative to start of treatment (mean $\pm$ standard deviation).

In examining the tumor volume changes over time for both TBG-RNAi-CK2 and TBG-siCK2 dose response studies in the PC3-LN3 model, we noted that the time period from days 5 through 7 showed a dramatic separation in tumor growth rates between the anti-CK2 treated and the control treated mice (Figure 2). We set up another therapy study in which mice were treated with TBG-RNAi-CK2 or TBG-RNAi-F7 nanocapsules at 0.01 mg/kg on days 1 and 4, and tumors were collected on days 5, 6 and 7. These tumors were then used to examine the molecular and cellular responses within the treated tumors over the time course.

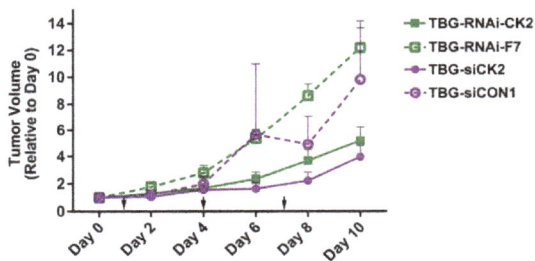

Figure 2. Comparison of xenograft tumor volumes over time in anti-CK2 and control TBG nanocapsule treated mice. The changes in PC3-LN4 tumor volumes relative to day 0 are shown following three nanocapsule drug treatments. Nanocapsule doses were 0.01 mg/kg for anti-CK2 and F7 nanocapsules and 1 mg/kg for TBG-siCON1 nanocapsules. Means + standard error of the mean are presented. Group sizes TBG-RNAi-CK2 $n = 9$; TBG-RNAi-F7 $n = 8$; TBG-siCK2 $n = 9$. TBG-siCON1 $n = 8$. Arrows indicate days that nanocapsule treatment injections occurred. Statistical significance for day 10 is given in Table 1.

After performing immunoblot analyses on nuclear and cytosolic fractions from the time course tumors, we noted a biphasic response (Figure 3). On day 5, 24 h following the TBG-RNAi-CK2 treatment on day 4, CK2α and CK2α' protein levels were notably reduced in both the nuclear and cytosolic compartments. At the same time, there was loss of NFκB p65 phosphorylation on S529, a CK2 phosphorylation site, as well as decreased levels of full length caspase 3 and the survival protein Bcl-xL. These markers indicate that some cell death was occurring, as well as loss of CK2 signaling. On day 6, there were decreased CK2α and CK2α' protein levels in cytosol, although not statistically significant. On day 7, 72 h after TBG-RNAi-CK2 treatment, a second wave of cell death markers was noted. These markers included loss of total NFκB p65 as well as NFκB p65 P-S529, decreased nuclear survivin and cytosolic Bcl-xL. A further marker was loss of pro-caspase 3, suggesting probable activation of caspase 3 through cleavage. In addition to these events, immunohistochemical Ki-67 analysis demonstrated a dramatic decreased in proliferative cells in day 7 TBG-RNAi-CK2-treated tumors relative to day 5 tumors [46].

In the TBG-RNAi-CK2 dose response studies using the prostate models PC3-LN4 and 22Rv1, several interesting observations were made [46]. For example, we observed that the higher dose level (0.1 mg/kg) required for best repression of 22Rv1 tumor growth compared with PC3-LN4 tumor response (0.01 mg/kg) related to the higher levels of caveolin 1 in PC3-LN4 tumors compared with that in 22Rv1 tumors, suggesting more effective uptake of the drug in the PC3-LN4 model. Other factors influencing the tumor response to TBG-RNAi-CK2 in these two prostate models related to the levels of argonaute 1 (Ago 1), Ago 2, and GW182, which were present in higher amounts in the PC3-LN4 xenograft tumors compared with 22Rv1. In these in vivo studies of the TBG-RNAi-CK2 therapy of xenograft tumors, there was no evidence of the uptake of the nanocapsules in non-cancer tissues such as liver and spleen. Likewise, there was no evidence of a change in the blood serum chemistry for urea nitrogen, creatinine, total serum protein, alanine aminotransferase, and aspartate aminotransferase. Finally, no tissue damage to liver, spleen, or kidney has been observed in multiple studies [46,63].

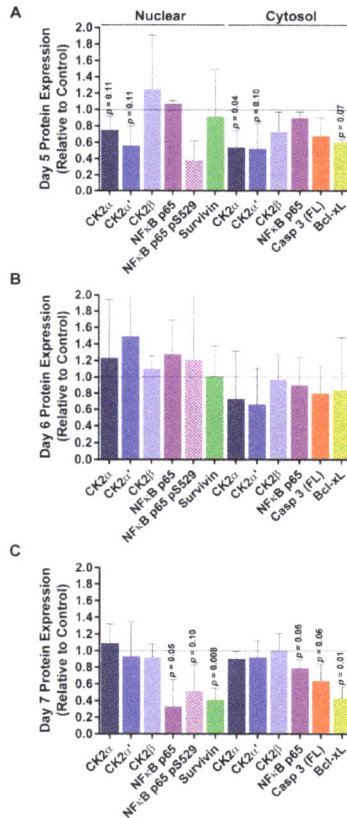

Figure 3. Protein expression response over time to TBG-RNAi-CK2 treatment in PC3-LN4 xenograft tumors. Immunoblot analysis of nuclear and cytosol fractionated PC3-LN4 tumor lysates following intravenous treatments of 0.01 mg/kg TBG-RNAi-CK2 or TBG-RNAi-F7 was performed. Protein signals were quantitated and means and standard deviations are graphed for (**A**) day 5, (**B**) day 6, and (**C**) day 7 following initiation of nanocapsule treatments. Group sizes TBG-RNAi-CK2 $n = 3$; TBG-RNAi-F7 $n = 6$ (days 5 and 6) or 7 (day 7). The grey line at expression level of "1" marks the expression for control treated tumors.

Direct quantitative analysis of the entry of TBG nanocapsules into tumor cells was undertaken by testing the uptake of TBG encapsulated dysprosium (TBG-Dy). The presence of dysprosium cargo (a fluorescent lanthanide element) in dissociated tumor cells was detected by fluorescence activated cell sorting (FACS) analysis. The results revealed that more than 46% of the cells demonstrated the presence of the nanocapsules in LNCaP orthotopic tumor cells examined at 20 h after just one nanocapsule injection via either intravenous or intraperitoneal routes [46]. Uptake of TBG-Dy nanocapsules was also analyzed by FACS in two models of triple negative breast cancer, demonstrating an average of 33.9% positive cells in SUM-149 tumors and 11% positive cells in one MDA-MB-231 tumor [48].

A complimentary analysis was undertaken to quantify the amount of bioavailable oligomer that is released into tumor cells following nanocapsule entry and proteolytic breakdown. In this study, mice carrying PC3-LN4 xenograft flank tumors were injected with TBG-RNAi-CK2 nanocapsules or with a combination of naked RNAi-CK2 oligomer plus TBG-erythritol. The naked oligomer/sugar nanocapsule combination was used to formally test that the RNAi-CK2 oligomers are entering tumor cells due to TBG encapsulation and not due to non-specific association with TBG. Released RNAi-CK2 oligomer was measured in RNA purified from tumor homogenates using quantitative stem-loop reverse transcriptase PCR. The results demonstrated that six of six tumors from mice receiving TBG-RNAi-CK2 contained an average of 152 fmols of released oligomer per gram of tumor. In contrast, none of the six tumors from mice receiving naked RNAi-CK2/TBG-erythritol contained detectable oligomer, indicating the utility and necessity of the TBG encapsulation. Taking the TBG-Dy uptake data together with the oligomer release data, and using the generally accepted value of 10^9 cells per gram of tumor, we calculate that approximately 197 RNAi-CK2 oligomers were contained per tumor cell. The nanocapsule uptake and oligomer release data from prostate cancer xenograft tumors is summarized in Figure 4.

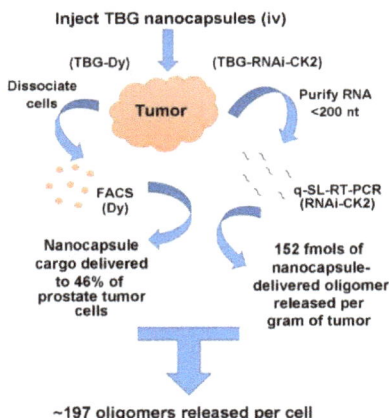

Figure 4. Quantitative analyses for TBG nanocapsule delivery to tumor and for release of RNAi-CK2 oligomer within tumors. Mice carrying LNCaP orthotopic xenograft tumors were injected via tail vein or intraperitoneal routes with TBG-Dy nanocapsules. The tumors were collected 20 h post-injection, the cells were dissociated, and the Dy signal was detected by FACS. For detection of oligomer within tumors, mice carrying PC3-LN4 xenograft flank tumors were treated once by tail vein injection at 1 mg/kg dose. Twenty-four hours after injection, RNAi-CK2 oligomer with a standard 3'-OH chemistry was detected by quantitative stem-loop RT-PCR on RNA purified from tissues. The number of oligomers released per cell was based on the mean percentage of Dy(+) prostate cells per tumor, the mean fmols of oligomer released per gram of tumor, and the mean theoretical number of cells per gram of tumor as 10^9. q-SL-RT-PCR, quantitative stem-loop reverse transcriptase polymerase chain reaction. FACS, fluorescence activated cell sorting.

The above-described studies clearly established the potential of the TBG-based nanocapsule as a means of delivering the anti-CK2 RNAi therapy in a protected and cancer-cell-specific manner. We have also examined the effects of TBG nanoencapsulated anti-CK2 therapy in HNSCC. Similar to the data discussed for prostate and breast cancer, short-term studies in HNSCC demonstrated the efficacy of TBG nanoencapsulated RNAi-CK2 in multiple models of HNSCC [62]. A significant reduction in tumor growth was demonstrated concordant with modulation of CK2 targets including NFκB regulated molecules, TP53 protein, and apoptosis pathway proteins [62]. In follow-up studies, evidence was produced to show that TBG nanocapsule-delivered RNAi-CK2 co-opted the Ago 2/RISC pathway to target the CK2α/α' mRNAs. The TBG-RNAi-CK2 nanocapsules reduced the growth of three different xenograft models of HNSCC affecting not only the primary tumor but also the metastases [47]. In these studies, a 6-month host survival was achieved at relatively low doses of the therapeutic agent without any apparent adverse effect in normal tissues, further supporting the translational potential of the TBG-RNAi-CK2 therapeutic for diverse cancers.

2.6. Phase I Trial of TBG-RNAi-CK2 in Large Animal Patients

Recently, we demonstrated that feline oral squamous cell carcinoma (FOSCC) and feline breast cancer cell lines have high expression of CK2 and that downregulation of CK2 in these cells resulted in induction of apoptosis analogous to observations on various cancer cell lines of human origin [7,67]. For the TBG-RNAi-CK2 nanocapsule to enter human clinical translation, an important step is to test its effects in large animals. FOSCC is commonly observed in domestic cats and has many features in common with human HNSCC; accordingly, FOSCC has been proposed as a large animal model for human HNSCC [68]. We decided to undertake a preclinical phase I trial of TBG-RNAi-CK2 use in FOSCC patients. The primary goal of this trial was to evaluate safety of the nanocapsule use, and a secondary goal was to assess for evidence of anti-CK2 targeting and tumor response. RNAi-CK2 oligomers were designed to specifically target feline CK2α and α' and were formulated into TBG nanocapsules. Our study involved nine FOSCC patients with advanced disease and these patients were given two intravenous treatments per week of the therapeutic agent over a total period of three weeks. Two dose levels of the therapeutic were employed for two groups divided between the nine enrolled cats. Tumor and normal oral mucosal tissue biopsies were collected zero to seven days before treatment was initiated and again three to four days after the last treatment. Tumors were measured at treatment initiation and completion, and blood was collected for analyses at treatment start, once per week during treatment, and after treatment ceased. Tumor response was evaluated by RECIST criteria. Results from this initial large animal study are promising (our unpublished data), and together with the mouse studies provide a strong impetus for the pursuit of the TBG-RNAi-CK2 based nanomedicine approach for further studies to enter human clinical trials.

3. Conclusions

We have provided a brief overview of our work that contributed to the linking of CK2 to the cancer cell phenotype. Overexpression of CK2 in cancer cells at the protein level is a consistent observation, and much evidence now supports the notion that CK2 is a desirable target for cancer therapy. The elevation of CK2 in benign proliferation, as observed in BPH compared with PCa, suggests a complex role and possible involvement of other signals (such as NFκB p65) in the biology of CK2 in benign growth versus cancer cell growth. Since CK2 is essential for cell survival, one would surmise that loss of its physical presence and/or its lack of function would result in an effective mode of cancer therapy. Chemical or molecular downregulation of CK2 results in potent induction of cell death in cancer cells but normal cells tend to be somewhat resistant to downregulation of CK2, suggesting a possible therapeutic window that may be utilized for use of small molecule inhibitors of CK2 as chemotherapeutic agents. However, therapeutic targeting of CK2 through its molecular downregulation (using RNAi methods) warrants that the anti-CK2 therapeutic agent delivery is achieved in a protected and cancer cell-specific manner. Towards that end, we have described the application of a TBG nanocapsule that has the properties of delivering CK2 RNAi oligomers to primary and metastatic sites in several types of xenograft tumor models resulting in inhibition of tumor growth. The TBG-RNAi-CK2 drug has essentially no adverse effects in normal cells, and in a small study of naturally occurring feline oral cancer we found the drug to be well tolerated without any serious adverse events. Our studies on PCa therapy have highlighted the observation that downregulation of CK2 is effective in treatment of the therapy resistant form of prostate cancer, namely, CRPC, thus highlighting the utility of this therapeutic approach to hormonal cancers regardless of the activity of various receptors present therein.

Based on our observations in cultured cells, where precise and/or very short timed effects are more feasible, and in xenograft tumor models, we propose that loss of CK2 holoenzyme proteins and/or enzymatic activity induces cell death in at least two ways. First, acute loss of CK2 function (greater than 30% loss) causes rapid induction of cell death via decreased mitochondrial health, induction of reactive oxygen species (ROS), and loss of survival proteins such as Bcl-xL. Second, sustained but less severe loss of CK2 function over time causes cell cycle arrest, decreased proliferative signaling such as NFκB p65 activation and localization, induction of cell death through loss of survival proteins such as survivin and Bcl-xL, and through caspase 3 activation. This general theory on the function of the TBG-CK2-RNAi nanocapsules as a cancer therapeutic is described in the following flow diagram (Figure 5), and references for this diagram are found here [46–49,62–64,69–76].

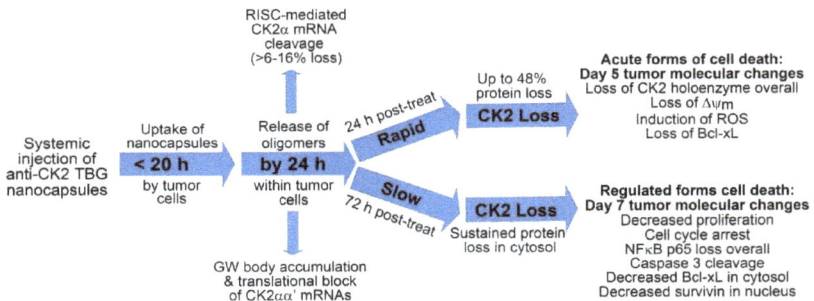

Figure 5. Flow chart illustrating proposed timeline of response and mechanisms of drug action and cell death within tumors. Notes: translational block of CK2αα' mRNAs is inferred; loss of Δψ m (mitochondrial membrane potential) and induction of ROS in tumors on day 5 are based on data in cultured cells, not tumor data; decreased proliferation is based on published Ki-67 data in tumors; cell cycle arrest is based on cultured cell data.

Thus, based on the various observations described in the foregoing we propose that the TBG nanocapsule delivery of RNAi-CK2 specifically to cancer cells merits further consideration as a therapeutic agent for various cancers. Future work will broaden our elucidation of the timing and steps in death pathway mechanisms induced by acute and chronic CK2 signaling loss.

Acknowledgments: This work was supported by Merit Review research funds BX001731 awarded by the Department of Veterans Affairs (K.A.); research grant CA150182 awarded by the National Cancer Institute, NIH, Department of Health and Human Services (K.A.); University of Minnesota Clinical and Translational Sciences Award 1UL1-RR033183-01 (K.A.); research grants CA158730 and DK067436 awarded by NCI and NIDDK, respectively, NIH, Department of Health and Human Services (B.T.K.); and research grants HHS-N261-2008-00027/N42CM-2008-00027C, CA99366, and CA119556 awarded by National Cancer Institute, NIH, Department of Health and Human Services (G.M.U.).

Author Contributions: J.H.T. designed and performed experiments, analyzed data, and wrote the manuscript; B.T.K. designed and performed experiments, analyzed data, and edited the manuscript; M.J.A. designed and performed experiments; R.I.V. performed statistical analyses and edited the manuscript; C.M.C. designed and performed experiments, responsible for all clinical aspects of the cat study; G.M.U. designed and performed experiments and synthesized the nanocapsules; K.A. advised on experimental design, discussed results, and wrote the manuscript.

Conflicts of Interest: G.M. Unger has ownership interest (including patents) in GeneSegues Therapeutics. Other authors declare no conflict of interest. The views expressed in this article are those of the authors and do not necessarily reflect the position or policy of the U.S. Department of Veterans Affairs or the U.S. government.

References

1. Guerra, B.; Issinger, O.-G. Protein kinase CK2 and its role in cellular proliferation, development and pathology. *Electrophoresis* **1999**, *20*, 391–408. [CrossRef]
2. Guerra, B.; Issinger, O.-G. Protein kinase CK2 in human diseases. *Curr. Med. Chem.* **2008**, *15*, 1870–1886. [CrossRef] [PubMed]
3. Pinna, L.A. Protein kinase CK2: A challenge to canons. *J. Cell Sci.* **2002**, *115*, 3873–3878. [CrossRef] [PubMed]
4. Ahmed, K. Significance of the casein kinase system in cell growth and proliferation with emphasis on studies of the androgenic regulation of the prostate. *Cell. Mol. Biol. Res.* **1994**, *40*, 1–11. [PubMed]
5. Ruzzene, M.; Pinna, L.A. Addiction to protein kinase CK2: A common denominator of diverse cancer cells? *Biochim. Biophys. Acta* **2010**, *1804*, 499–504. [CrossRef] [PubMed]
6. Meggio, F.; Pinna, L.A. One-thousand-and-one substrates of protein kinase CK2? *FASEB J.* **2003**, *17*, 349–368. [CrossRef] [PubMed]
7. Tawfic, S.; Yu, S.; Wang, H.; Faust, R.; Davis, A.; Ahmed, K. Protein kinase CK2 signal in neoplasia. *Histol. Histopathol.* **2001**, *16*, 573–582. [PubMed]
8. Guo, C.; Yu, S.; Davis, A.T.; Wang, H.; Green, J.E.; Ahmed, K. A potential role of nuclear matrix-associated protein kinase CK2 in protection against drug-induced apoptosis in cancer cells. *J. Biol. Chem.* **2001**, *276*, 5992–5999. [CrossRef] [PubMed]
9. Ahmed, K.; Gerber, D.A.; Cochet, C. Joining the cell survival squad: An emerging role for protein kinase CK2. *Trends Cell Biol.* **2002**, *12*, 226–230. [CrossRef]
10. Ahmad, K.A.; Wang, G.; Unger, G.; Slaton, J.; Ahmed, K. Protein kinase CK2—A key suppressor of apoptosis. *Adv. Enzyme Regul.* **2008**, *48*, 179–187. [CrossRef] [PubMed]
11. Trembley, J.H.; Qaiser, F.; Kren, B.T.; Ahmed, K. CK2—A global regulator of cell death. In *Protein Kinase CK2 Cellular Function in Normal and Disease States*; Ahmed, K., Issinger, O.-G., Szyszka, R., Eds.; Springer: Cham, Switzerland, 2015; Volume 12, pp. 159–181.
12. Wang, H.; Davis, A.; Yu, S.; Ahmed, K. Response of cancer cells to molecular interruption of the CK2 signal. *Mol. Cell. Biochem.* **2001**, *227*, 167–174. [CrossRef] [PubMed]
13. Perea, S.E.; Baladron, I.; Garcia, Y.; Perera, Y.; Lopez, A.; Soriano, J.L.; Batista, N.; Palau, A.; Hernández, I.; Farina, H.; et al. CIGB-300, a synthetic peptide-based drug that targets the CK2 phosphoaceptor domain. Translational and clinical research. *Mol. Cell. Biochem.* **2011**, *356*, 45–50. [CrossRef] [PubMed]
14. Pinna, L.A.; Allende, J.E. Protein kinase CK2 in health and disease: Protein kinase CK2: An ugly duckling in the kinome pond. *Cell. Mol. Life Sci.* **2009**, *66*, 1795–1799. [CrossRef] [PubMed]
15. Pierre, F.; Chua, P.C.; O'Brien, S.E.; Siddiqui-Jain, A.; Bourbon, P.; Haddach, M.; Michaux, J.; Nagasawa, J.; Schwaebe, M.K.; Stefan, E.; et al. Discovery and SAR of 5-(3-chlorophenylamino)benzo[c][2,6]naphthyridine-8-carboxylic acid (CX-4945), the first clinical stage inhibitor of protein kinase CK2 for the treatment of cancer. *J. Med. Chem.* **2011**, *54*, 635–654. [CrossRef] [PubMed]
16. Ortega, C.E.; Seidner, Y.; Dominguez, I. Mining CK2 in cancer. *PLoS ONE* **2014**, *9*, e115609. [CrossRef] [PubMed]
17. Faust, R.A.; Niehans, G.; Gapany, M.; Hoistad, D.; Knapp, D.; Cherwitz, D.; Davis, A.; Adams, G.L.; Ahmed, K. Subcellular immunolocalization of protein kinase CK2 in normal and carcinoma cells. *Int. J. Biochem. Cell Biol.* **1999**, *31*, 941–949. [CrossRef]
18. Dominguez, I.; Sonenshein, G.E.; Seldin, D.C. Protein kinase CK2 in health and disease: CK2 and its role in Wnt and NF-κB signaling: Linking development and cancer. *Cell. Mol. Life Sci.* **2009**, *66*, 1850–1857. [CrossRef] [PubMed]
19. Seldin, D.C.; Landesman-Bollag, E.; Farago, M.; Currier, N.; Lou, D.; Dominguez, I. CK2 as a positive regulator of Wnt signalling and tumourigenesis. *Mol. Cell. Biochem.* **2005**, *274*, 63–67. [CrossRef] [PubMed]

20. Zhang, H.-X.; Jiang, S.-S.; Zhang, X.-F.; Zhou, Z.-Q.; Pan, Q.-Z.; Chen, C.-L.; Zhao, J.-J.; Tang, Y.; Xia, J.-C.; Weng, D.-S. Protein kinase CK2α catalytic subunit is overexpressed and serves as an unfavorable prognostic marker in primary hepatocellular carcinoma. *Oncotarget* **2015**, *6*, 34800. [PubMed]

21. Ahmed, K.; Davis, A.T.; Wang, H.; Faust, R.A.; Yu, S.; Tawfic, S. Significance of protein kinase CK2 nuclear signaling in neoplasia. *J. Cell. Biochem. Suppl.* **2000**, *35*, 130–135. [CrossRef]

22. Hanahan, D.; Weinberg, R.A. Hallmarks of cancer: The next generation. *Cell* **2011**, *144*, 646–674. [CrossRef] [PubMed]

23. Wang, G.; Ahmad, K.A.; Ahmed, K. Modulation of death receptor-mediated apoptosis by CK2. *Mol. Cell. Biochem.* **2005**, *274*, 201–205. [CrossRef] [PubMed]

24. Trembley, J.H.; Wang, G.; Unger, G.; Slaton, J.; Ahmed, K. Protein kinase CK2 in health and disease: CK2: A key player in cancer biology. *Cell. Mol. Life Sci.* **2009**, *66*, 1858–1867. [CrossRef] [PubMed]

25. Trembley, J.H.; Wu, J.; Unger, G.M.; Kren, B.T.; Ahmed, K. CK2 suppression of apoptosis and its implications in cancer biology and therapy. In *Protein Kinase CK2*; the Wiley-IUBMB Series on Biochemistry and Molecular Biology; Pinna, L.A., Ed.; Wiley: Hoboken, NJ, USA, 2013; pp. 319–333.

26. Gapany, M.; Faust, R.A.; Tawfic, S.; Davis, A.; Adams, G.L.; Ahmed, K. Association of elevated protein kinase CK2 activity with aggressive behavior of squamous cell carcinoma of the head and neck. *Mol. Med.* **1995**, *1*, 659–666. [PubMed]

27. Yenice, S.; Davis, A.T.; Goueli, S.A.; Akdas, A.; Limas, C.; Ahmed, K. Nuclear casein kinase 2 (CK-2) activity in human normal, benign hyperplastic, and cancerous prostate. *Prostate* **1994**, *24*, 11–16. [CrossRef] [PubMed]

28. Faust, R.A.; Gapany, M.; Tristani, P.; Davis, A.; Adams, G.L.; Ahmed, K. Elevated protein kinase CK2 activity in chromatin of head and neck tumors: Association with malignant transformation. *Cancer Lett.* **1996**, *101*, 31–35. [CrossRef]

29. Giusiano, S.; Cochet, C.; Filhol, O.; Duchemin-Pelletier, E.; Secq, V.; Bonnier, P.; Carcopino, X.; Boubli, L.; Birnbaum, D.; Garcia, S.; et al. Protein kinase CK2α subunit over-expression correlates with metastatic risk in breast carcinomas: Quantitative immunohistochemistry in tissue microarrays. *Eur. J. Cancer* **2011**, *47*, 792–801. [CrossRef] [PubMed]

30. Laramas, M.; Pasquier, D.; Filhol, O.; Ringeisen, F.; Descotes, J.L.; Cochet, C. Nuclear localization of protein kinase CK2 catalytic subunit (CK2α) is associated with poor prognostic factors in human prostate cancer. *Eur. J. Cancer* **2007**, *43*, 928–934. [CrossRef] [PubMed]

31. Ahmed, K.; Yenice, S.; Davis, A.; Goueli, S.A. Association of casein kinase 2 with nuclear chromatin in relation to androgenic regulation of rat prostate. *Proc. Natl. Acad. Sci. USA* **1993**, *90*, 4426–4430. [CrossRef] [PubMed]

32. Rayan, A.; Goueli, S.A.; Lange, P.; Ahmed, K. Chromatin-associated protein kinases in human normal and benign hyperplastic prostate. *Cancer Res.* **1985**, *45*, 2277–2282. [PubMed]

33. Qaiser, F.; Trembley, J.H.; Sadiq, S.; Muhammad, I.; Younis, R.; Hashmi, S.N.; Murtaza, B.; Rector, T.S.; Naveed, A.K.; Ahmed, K. Examination of CK2α and NF-κB p65 expression in human benign prostatic hyperplasia and prostate cancer tissues. *Mol. Cell. Biochem.* **2016**, *420*, 43–51. [CrossRef] [PubMed]

34. Wang, D.; Westerheide, S.D.; Hanson, J.L.; Baldwin, A.S. Tumor necrosis factor α-induced phosphorylation of RelA/p65 on Ser529 is controlled by casein kinase II. *J. Biol. Chem.* **2000**, *275*, 32592–32597. [CrossRef] [PubMed]

35. Taylor, B.S.; Schultz, N.; Hieronymus, H.; Gopalan, A.; Xiao, Y.; Carver, B.S. Integrative genomic profiling of human prostate cancer. *Cancer Cell* **2010**, *18*, 11–22. [CrossRef] [PubMed]

36. Robinson, D.; Van Allen, E.M.; Wu, Y.M.; Schultz, N.; Lonigro, R.J.; Mosquera, J.M.; Montgomery, B.; Taplin, M.E.; Pritchard, C.C.; Attard, G.; et al. Integrative clinical genomics of advanced prostate cancer. *Cell* **2015**, *161*, 1215–1228. [CrossRef] [PubMed]

37. Cancer Genome Atlas Research Network. The molecular taxonomy of primary prostate cancer. *Cell* **2015**, *163*, 1011–1025.

38. Slaton, J.W.; Unger, G.M.; Sloper, D.T.; Davis, A.T.; Ahmed, K. Induction of apoptosis by antisense CK2 in human prostate cancer xenograft model. *Mol. Cancer Res.* **2004**, *2*, 712–721. [PubMed]

39. Wang, G.; Unger, G.; Ahmad, K.A.; Slaton, J.W.; Ahmed, K. Downregulation of CK2 induces apoptosis in cancer cells—A potential approach to cancer therapy. *Mol. Cell. Biochem.* **2005**, *274*, 77–84. [CrossRef] [PubMed]

40. Trembley, J.H.; Chen, Z.; Unger, G.; Slaton, J.; Kren, B.T.; Van Waes, C.; Ahmed, K. Emergence of protein kinase CK2 as a key target in cancer therapy. *Biofactors* **2010**, *36*, 187–195. [CrossRef] [PubMed]

41. Sarno, S.; Pinna, L.A. Protein kinase CK2 as a druggable target. *Mol. Biosyst.* **2008**, *4*, 889–894. [CrossRef] [PubMed]

42. Sarno, S.; Ruzzene, M.; Frascella, P.; Pagano, M.A.; Meggio, F.; Zambon, A.; Mazzorana, M.; Di Maira, G.; Lucchini, V.; Pinna, L.A. Development and exploitation of CK2 inhibitors. *Mol. Cell. Biochem.* **2005**, *274*, 69–76. [CrossRef] [PubMed]

43. Cozza, G.; Zanin, S.; Sarno, S.; Costa, E.; Girardi, C.; Ribaudo, G.; Salvi, M.; Zagotto, G.; Ruzzene, M.; Pinna, L.A. Design, validation and efficacy of bisubstrate inhibitors specifically affecting ecto-CK2 kinase activity. *Biochem. J.* **2015**, *471*, 415–430. [CrossRef] [PubMed]

44. Siddiqui-Jain, A.; Drygin, D.; Streiner, N.; Chua, P.; Pierre, F.; O'Brien, S.E.; Bliesath, J.; Omori, M.; Huser, N.; Ho, C.; et al. CX-4945, an orally bioavailable selective inhibitor of protein kinase CK2, inhibits prosurvival and angiogenic signaling and exhibits antitumor efficacy. *Cancer Res.* **2010**, *70*, 10288–10298. [CrossRef] [PubMed]

45. Siddiqui-Jain, A.; Bliesath, J.; Macalino, D.; Omori, M.; Huser, N.; Streiner, N.; Ho, C.B.; Anderes, K.; Proffitt, C.; O'Brien, S.E.; et al. CK2 inhibitor CX-4945 suppresses DNA repair response triggered by DNA-targeted anticancer drugs and augments efficacy: Mechanistic rationale for drug combination therapy. *Mol. Cancer Ther.* **2012**, *11*, 994–1005. [CrossRef] [PubMed]

46. Ahmed, K.; Kren, B.T.; Abedin, M.J.; Vogel, R.I.; Shaughnessy, D.P.; Nacusi, L.; Korman, V.L.; Li, Y.; Dehm, S.M.; Zimmerman, C.L.; et al. CK2 targeted RNAi therapeutic delivered via malignant cell-directed tenfibgen nanocapsule: Dose and molecular mechanisms of response in xenograft prostate tumors. *Oncotarget* **2016**, *7*, 61789–61805. [CrossRef] [PubMed]

47. Unger, G.M.; Kren, B.T.; Korman, V.L.; Kimbrough, T.G.; Vogel, R.I.; Ondrey, F.G.; Trembley, J.H.; Ahmed, K. Mechanism and efficacy of sub-50-nm tenfibgen nanocapsules for cancer cell-directed delivery of anti-CK2 RNAi to primary and metastatic squamous cell carcinoma. *Mol. Cancer Ther.* **2014**, *13*, 2018–2029. [CrossRef] [PubMed]

48. Kren, B.; Unger, G.; Abedin, M.; Vogel, R.; Henzler, C.; Ahmed, K.; Trembley, J. Preclinical evaluation of cyclin dependent kinase 11 and casein kinase 2 survival kinases as RNA interference targets for triple negative breast cancer therapy. *Breast Cancer Res.* **2015**, *17*, 19. [CrossRef] [PubMed]

49. Qaiser, F.; Trembley, J.H.; Kren, B.T.; Wu, J.J.; Naveed, A.K.; Ahmed, K. Protein kinase CK2 inhibition induces cell death via early impact on mitochondrial function. *J. Cell. Biochem.* **2014**, *115*, 2103–2115. [CrossRef] [PubMed]

50. Girardi, C.; Ottaviani, D.; Pinna, L.A.; Ruzzene, M. Different persistence of the cellular effects promoted by protein kinase CK2 inhibitors CX-4945 and TDB. *Biomed. Res. Int.* **2015**, *2015*, 185736. [CrossRef] [PubMed]

51. Cree, I.A.; Charlton, P. Molecular chess? Hallmarks of anti-cancer drug resistance. *BMC Cancer* **2017**, *17*, 10. [CrossRef] [PubMed]

52. Ahmed, K.; Unger, G.M.; Kren, B.T.; Trembley, J.H. Targeting CK2 for Cancer Therapy Using A Nanomedicine Approach. In *Protein Kinase CK2 in Cellular Function in Normal and Disease States*; Ahmed, K., Issinger, O.-G., Szyszka, R., Eds.; Springer International Publishing Switzerland: Gewerbestrasse, Switzerland, 2015; Volume 12, pp. 299–315.

53. Unger, G.; Trembley, J.; Kren, B.; Ahmed, K. Nanoparticles in cancer therapy. In *Encyclopedia of Cancer: SpringerReference*; Schwab, M., Ed.; Springer: Heidelberg, Germany, 2012; pp. 1–4.

54. Trembley, J.H.; Unger, G.M.; Korman, V.L.; Tobolt, D.K.; Kazimierczuk, Z.; Pinna, L.A.; Kren, B.T.; Ahmed, K. Nanoencapsulated anti-CK2 small molecule drug or sirna specifically targets malignant cancer but not benign cells. *Cancer Lett.* **2012**, *315*, 48–58. [CrossRef] [PubMed]

55. Tuxhorn, J.A.; Ayala, G.E.; Rowley, D.R. Reactive stroma in prostate cancer progression. *J. Urol.* **2001**, *166*, 2472–2483. [CrossRef]

56. Erickson, H.P.; Bourdon, M.A. Tenascin: An extracellular matrix protein prominent in specialized embryonic tissues and tumors. *Annu. Rev. Cell Biol.* **1989**, *5*, 71–92. [CrossRef] [PubMed]

57. Chiquet-Ehrismann, R.; Chiquet, M. Tenascins: Regulation and putative functions during pathological stress. *J. Pathol.* **2003**, *200*, 488–499. [CrossRef] [PubMed]

58. Yokoyama, K.; Erickson, H.P.; Ikeda, Y.; Takada, Y. Identification of amino acid sequences in fibrinogen gamma -chain and tenascin C C-terminal domains critical for binding to integrin $\alpha\nu\beta3$. *J. Biol. Chem.* **2000**, *275*, 16891–16898. [CrossRef] [PubMed]

59. Desgrosellier, J.S.; Cheresh, D.A. Integrins in cancer: Biological implications and therapeutic opportunities. *Nat. Rev. Cancer* **2010**, *10*, 9–22. [CrossRef] [PubMed]
60. Guttery, D.; Shaw, J.; Lloyd, K.; Pringle, J.; Walker, R. Expression of tenascin-C and its isoforms in the breast. *Cancer Metastasis Rev.* **2010**, 1–12. [CrossRef] [PubMed]
61. Oskarsson, T.; Acharyya, S.; Zhang, X.H.; Vanharanta, S.; Tavazoie, S.F.; Morris, P.G.; Downey, R.J.; Manova-Todorova, K.; Brogi, E.; Massague, J. Breast cancer cells produce tenascin C as a metastatic niche component to colonize the lungs. *Nat. Med.* **2011**, *17*, 867–874. [CrossRef] [PubMed]
62. Brown, M.S.; Diallo, O.T.; Hu, M.; Ehsanian, R.; Yang, X.; Arun, P.; Lu, H.; Korman, V.; Unger, G.; Ahmed, K.; et al. CK2 modulation of NF-κB, TP53, and the malignant phenotype in head and neck cancer by anti-CK2 oligonucleotides in vitro or in vivo via sub-50-nm nanocapsules. *Clin. Cancer Res.* **2010**, *16*, 2295–2307. [CrossRef] [PubMed]
63. Trembley, J.H.; Unger, G.M.; Gomez, O.C.; Abedin, J.; Korman, V.L.; Vogel, R.I.; Niehans, G.; Kren, B.T.; Ahmed, K. Tenfibgen-DMAT nanocapsule delivers CK2 inhibitor dmat to prostate cancer xenograft tumors causing inhibition of cell proliferation. *Mol. Cell. Pharmacol.* **2014**, *6*, 15–25. [PubMed]
64. Trembley, J.H.; Unger, G.M.; Korman, V.L.; Abedin, M.J.; Nacusi, L.P.; Vogel, R.I.; Slaton, J.W.; Kren, B.T.; Ahmed, K. Tenfibgen ligand nanoencapsulation delivers bi-functional anti-CK2 RNAi oligomer to key sites for prostate cancer targeting using human xenograft tumors in mice. *PLoS ONE* **2014**, *9*, e109970. [CrossRef] [PubMed]
65. Bartlett, D.W.; Davis, M.E. Impact of tumor-specific targeting and dosing schedule on tumor growth inhibition after intravenous administration of sirna-containing nanoparticles. *Biotechnol. Bioeng.* **2008**, *99*, 975–985. [CrossRef] [PubMed]
66. Kren, B.T.; Korman, V.L.; Tobolt, D.K.; Unger, G.M. Subcutaneous delivery of hepatocyte targeted sub-50 nm nanoencapsulated sirna mediates gene silencing. *Mol. Ther.* **2011**, *19*, S319–S320.
67. Cannon, C.M.; Trembley, J.H.; Kren, B.T.; Unger, G.M.; O'Sullivan, M.G.; Cornax, I.; Modiano, J.F.; Ahmed, K. Protein kinase CK2 as a promising new therapeutic target in feline squamous cell carcinoma. *Am. J. Vet. Res.* **2017**, in press.
68. Wypij, J.M. A naturally occurring feline model of head and neck squamous cell carcinoma. *Pathol. Res. Int.* **2013**, *2013*, 7. [CrossRef] [PubMed]
69. Hanif, I.M.; Ahmad, K.A.; Ahmed, K.; Pervaiz, S. Involvement of reactive oxygen species in apoptosis induced by pharmacological inhibition of protein kinase CK2. *Ann. N. Y. Acad. Sci.* **2009**, *1171*, 591–599. [CrossRef] [PubMed]
70. Tapia, J.C.; Torres, V.A.; Rodriguez, D.A.; Leyton, L.; Quest, A.F. Casein kinase 2 (CK2) increases survivin expression via enhanced beta-catenin-T cell factor/lymphoid enhancer binding factor-dependent transcription. *Proc. Natl. Acad. Sci. USA* **2006**, *103*, 15079–15084. [CrossRef] [PubMed]
71. Wang, H.; Yu, S.; Davis, A.T.; Ahmed, K. Cell cycle dependent regulation of protein kinase CK2 signaling to the nuclear matrix. *J. Cell. Biochem.* **2003**, *88*, 812–822. [CrossRef] [PubMed]
72. Ahmad, K.A.; Wang, G.; Ahmed, K. Intracellular hydrogen peroxide production is an upstream event in apoptosis induced by down-regulation of casein kinase 2 in prostate cancer cells. *Mol. Cancer Res.* **2006**, *4*, 331–338. [CrossRef] [PubMed]
73. Ahmad, K.A.; Harris, N.H.; Johnson, A.D.; Lindvall, H.C.; Wang, G.; Ahmed, K. Protein kinase CK2 modulates apoptosis induced by resveratrol and epigallocatechin-3-gallate in prostate cancer cells. *Mol. Cancer Ther.* **2007**, *6*, 1006–1012. [CrossRef] [PubMed]
74. Yu, S.; Wang, H.; Davis, A.; Ahmed, K. Consequences of CK2 signaling to the nuclear matrix. *Mol. Cell. Biochem.* **2001**, *227*, 67–71. [CrossRef] [PubMed]
75. Wang, G.; Ahmad, K.A.; Harris, N.H.; Ahmed, K. Impact of protein kinase CK2 on inhibitor of apoptosis proteins in prostate cancer cells. *Mol. Cell. Biochem.* **2008**, *316*, 91–97. [CrossRef] [PubMed]
76. Trembley, J.H.; Unger, G.M.; Tobolt, D.K.; Korman, V.L.; Wang, G.; Ahmad, K.A.; Slaton, J.W.; Kren, B.T.; Ahmed, K. Systemic administration of antisense oligonucleotides simultaneously targeting CK2α and α' subunits reduces orthotopic xenograft prostate tumors in mice. *Mol. Cell. Biochem.* **2011**, *356*, 21–35. [CrossRef] [PubMed]

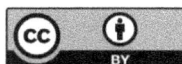

pharmaceuticals

MDPI

Article

Targeting Protein Kinase CK2: Evaluating CX-4945 Potential for GL261 Glioblastoma Therapy in Immunocompetent Mice

Laura Ferrer-Font [1,2,3], Lucia Villamañan [1], Nuria Arias-Ramos [1,2], Jordi Vilardell [4], Maria Plana [1], Maria Ruzzene [4], Lorenzo A. Pinna [4,5], Emilio Itarte [1], Carles Arús [1,2,3] and Ana Paula Candiota [2,1,3,*]

[1] Departament de Bioquímica i Biologia Molecular, Unitat de Bioquímica de Biociències, Edifici C, Universitat Autònoma de Barcelona, Cerdanyola del Vallès 08193, Spain; Laura.Ferrer@uab.cat (L.F.-F.); Lucia.Villamanan@uab.cat (L.V.); Nuria.Arias@uab.cat (N.A.-R.); Maria.Plana@uab.cat (M.P.); Emili.Itarte@uab.cat (E.I.); Carles.Arus@uab.es (C.A.)
[2] Centro de Investigación Biomédica en Red en Bioingeniería, Biomateriales y Nanomedicina (CIBER-BBN), Cerdanyola del Vallès 08193, Spain
[3] Institut de Biotecnologia i de Biomedicina (IBB), Universitat Autònoma de Barcelona, Cerdanyola del Vallès 08193, Spain
[4] Department of Biomedical Sciences, University of Padova, Padova 35131, Italy; jordivilardellvila@gmail.com (J.V.); maria.ruzzene@unipd.it (M.R.); lorenzo.pinna@unipd.it (L.A.P.)
[5] Consiglio Nazionale delle Ricerche (CNR), Neuroscience Institute, Padova 35131, Italy
[*] Correspondence: AnaPaula.Candiota@uab.cat; Tel.: +34-93-581-4126; Fax: +34-93-581-1264

Academic Editor: Marc Le Borgne
Received: 30 November 2016; Accepted: 6 February 2017; Published: 12 February 2017

Abstract: Glioblastoma (GBM) causes poor survival in patients even with aggressive treatment. Temozolomide (TMZ) is the standard chemotherapeutic choice for GBM treatment but resistance always ensues. Protein kinase CK2 (CK2) contributes to tumour development and proliferation in cancer, and it is overexpressed in human GBM. Accordingly, targeting CK2 in GBM may benefit patients. Our goal has been to evaluate whether CK2 inhibitors (iCK2s) could increase survival in an immunocompetent preclinical GBM model. Cultured GL261 cells were treated with different iCK2s including CX-4945, and target effects evaluated in vitro. CX-4945 was found to decrease CK2 activity and Akt(S129) phosphorylation in GL261 cells. Longitudinal in vivo studies with CX-4945 alone or in combination with TMZ were performed in tumour-bearing mice. Increase in survival ($p < 0.05$) was found with combined CX-4945 and TMZ metronomic treatment (54.7 ± 11.9 days, $n = 6$) when compared to individual metronomic treatments (CX-4945: 24.5 ± 2.0 and TMZ: 38.7 ± 2.7, $n = 6$) and controls (22.5 ± 1.2, $n = 6$). Despite this, CX-4945 did not improve mice outcome when administered on every/alternate days, either alone or in combination with 3-cycle TMZ. The highest survival rate was obtained with the metronomic combined TMZ+CX-4945 every 6 days, pointing to the participation of the immune system or other ancillary mechanism in therapy response.

Keywords: glioma; preclinical brain tumour; GBM therapeutic target; CK2 inhibitors; CX-4945; metronomic therapy; immune system

1. Introduction

Glioblastoma (GBM) is the most common aggressive glial primary brain tumour with an average survival of 14–15 months, even after aggressive treatment [1,2]. Temozolomide (TMZ) plus radiotherapy is the standard therapeutic choice for GBM treatment and, at present, produces the best survival rates [3]. TMZ is an alkylating agent with a mechanism of action based in damaging DNA through methylation of guanine residues, finally leading to cell death. Methylation of the O6 of guanine (O6-MeG) accounts for only about 5%–10% of DNA adducts, but is the primary responsible for the cytotoxic effects of TMZ. The O6-MeG lesion leads to DNA double-strand breaks (DSBs) and subsequent cell death via apoptosis and/or autophagy [4]. In our group, GL261 GBM tumour-bearing mice treated with TMZ showed a survival rate of 33.8 ± 8.7 days [5] versus control mice, 20.0 ± 4.1 days. Unfortunately, cancer stem cells (CSCs) are known to mediate chemoresistance, indicating GBM CSCs persistence even after standard treatment [6]. In addition, cellular exposure to DNA damaging agents (such as TMZ) may cause mutations and clastogenic effects, potentially resulting in additional malignant transformation [7]. Due to the poor outcome and resistance to standard therapy, efficient alternative non-mutagenic treatments are urgently needed for these tumours.

Inhibition of protein kinases has become a standard of modern clinical oncology, and it could improve GBM patients' survival. Protein kinase CK2 (CK2), an oncogenic protein kinase, contributes to tumour development, proliferation, and apoptosis suppression in cancer [8]. It is a constitutively active serine-threonine kinase and elevated CK2 expression levels have been demonstrated in several cancer types in comparison with normal tissue [9–11]. Its overexpression has been also proved in human GBM biopsies compared to adjacent normal tissue [12], regulating signalling pathways involved in tumour cell survival, proliferation, migration and invasion [13]. Furthermore, we have demonstrated that CK2 catalytic subunit (CK2α) expression level was higher in preclinical GL261 GBM tumour and in contralateral brain parenchyma than in wild type C57BL/6 brain parenchyma [14]. These characteristics identify CK2 as an active therapeutic target, and targeting CK2 in GBM treatment could benefit patients.

Different CK2 inhibitors (iCK2) have been studied for cancer applications, such as 4,5,6,7-tetrabromobenzotriazole (TBB) [15,16] or apigenin (APG) [17,18]. Additionally, a more specific CK2 inhibitor, 5-(3-chlorophenylamino)benzo[c][2,6] naphthyridine-8-carboxylic acid (CX-4945) [19–23] has been reported as the first CK2 inhibitor in clinical stage [24,25]. In vitro studies of breast cancer [21] and studies with an intracranial xenograft murine glioma model [23] have also presented successful results for CX-4945. In addition, it has been reported that CX-4945 decreases GBM initiating cell growth and stemness through β-catenin [26]. Moreover, other promising CK2 inhibitors are in development, such as tetrabromo-deoxyribofuranosyl-benzimidazole (TDB), a dual inhibitor of CK2 and proviral integration of Moloney virus (PIM-1) [27]. These results highlight the relevance of CK2 and its interwoven signalling targets in tumour growth and progression.

Moreover, new therapeutic schedules are being investigated using chemotherapeutic drugs in a metronomic-like approach, referring to administrations of low and equally spaced doses of chemotherapeutics without long rest periods in between [28,29], to try to activate immune responses to potentiate tumour regression and avoid regrowth [29]. For instance, cyclophosphamide (CPA) metronomic therapy has been shown to activate antitumour CD8+ T-cell response, and also induce specific long-term T-cell tumour memory in GL261 GBM tumours growing subcutaneously in immunocompetent mice [30].

The use of animal models in tumour research is mandatory in the search for new therapeutic targets due to obvious ethical restrictions related to human patients. One of the most investigated immunocompetent murine brain tumour models is GL261 growing into C57BL/6 mice, used for more than 20 years in different therapy evaluation approaches [5,31,32].

In this work, we have evaluated iCK2 effects over cultured GL261 cells viability to select the best candidates for in vivo preclinical studies. Also, preliminary in vivo work with preclinical GBM was performed, regarding maximum tolerated doses (MTD), tumour targeting effects assessment and survival rate evaluation in longitudinal studies with C57BL/6 mice bearing GL261 tumours treated with iCK2.

2. Results

2.1. GL261 Cell Viability under CK2 Inhibition Treatment

Cultured GL261 cells sensitivity to different treatments was assessed. Figure 1A,B showed a low half maximal effective concentration (EC_{50}) (12.9 ± 2.3 μM) for APG, similar to CX-4945 (16.5 ± 5.5 μM), but the final viability reached with APG was only up to 40% of the initial value. Instead, TBB and CX-4945 both decreased viability to about 20% of the initial value. Regarding to TBB, a concentration of 91.4 ± 8.3 μM produced a 50% viability decrease, whereas for CX-4945, a concentration of 16.5 ± 5.5 μM produced the same results. In the case of TDB, it showed the lowest EC_{50} (8.1 ± 1.5 μM), and the final viability obtained was similar to CX-4945. TMZ EC_{50} was 747.6 ± 63.3 μM.

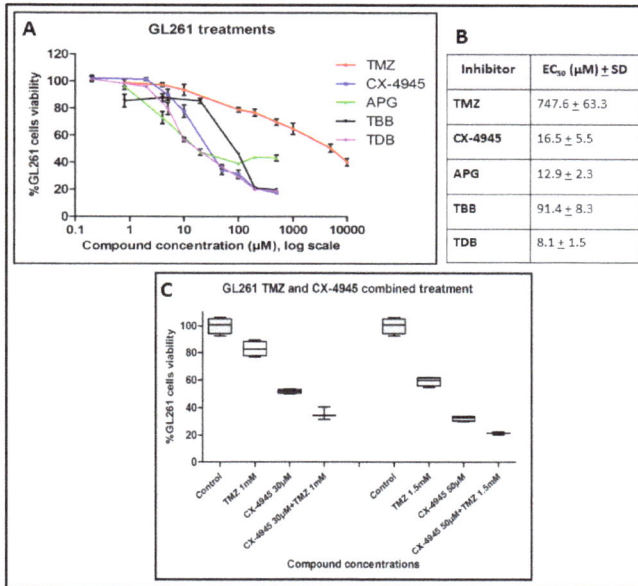

Figure 1. GL261 cells viability after treatment; (**A**) GL261 cells viability (%) "XTT assay" after 72 h of treatment with temozolomide (TMZ): 0 μM, 0.8 μM, 4 μM, 20 μM, 100 μM, 200 μM, 500 μM, 1000 μM, 5000 μM and 10,000 μM, apigenin (APG) and tetrabromobenzotriazole (TBB): 0 μM, 0.8 μM, 4 μM, 20 μM, 100 μM, 200 μM and 500 μM, CX-4945 and tetrabromo-deoxyribofuranosyl-benzimidazole (TDB): 0 μM, 0.2 μM, 2 μM, 5 μM, 20 μM, 50 μM, 100 μM, 200 μM and 500 μM); 100% cell viability was assigned to control cells treated with 0.8% dimethyl sulfoxide (DMSO) (*v/v*). Experiments were performed with $n = 3$–9, and mean ± SD values are shown; (**B**) EC_{50} (Half maximal, 50% viability decrease, effective concentration) mean ± SD values obtained with the different treatments to GL261 cells after 72 h of incubation with the drug; (**C**) Boxplot of GL261 cells viability after TMZ and CX-4945 treatment. GL261 cells viability (%) "MTT assay" after 72 h of treatment. On the left side, control ($n = 4$), CX-4945 30 μM ($n = 4$), TMZ 1 mM ($n = 4$) and CX-4945 30 μM plus TMZ 1 mM ($n = 3$); on the right side, control ($n = 4$), CX-4945 50 μM ($n = 4$), TMZ 1.5 mM ($n = 4$) and CX-4945 50 μM and TMZ 1.5 mM ($n = 3$); 100% cell viability was assigned to control cells treated with 0.8% DMSO (*v/v*). As both experiments were performed at the same time, controls were acquired only once and, accordingly, the same control cells results are shown for both experimental conditions. Experiments were performed with $n = 3$–4, and mean ± SD values are shown. Boxplot (the limits of the box represent quartiles 1 (Q1) and 3 (Q3) of the distribution, the central line corresponds to the median (quartile 2). The whiskers symbolize the maximum and minimum values in each distribution.

Additionally, an in vitro experiment with combined treatment of GL261 cells was outlined, and as it can be seen in Figure 1C, we could demonstrate that the combined administration of CX-4945 and TMZ to GL261 cultured cells presented an increased efficacy in comparison with treatments of single substances alone. TMZ alone reduced cell viability to 82.8% ± 5.6% (at 1 mM) and 59.2% ± 3.2% (at 1.5 mM) in comparison to controls, whereas CX-4945 alone reduced cell viability to 52.0% ± 1.4% (at 30 µM) and 31.9% ± 2.1% (at 50 µM). The combined administration of both therapeutic agents resulted in a cell viability reduction to 35.6% ± 4.7% (TMZ 1 mM + CX-4945 30 µM), and to 21.5% ± 1.0% (TMZ 1.5 mM + CX-4945 50 µM) in comparison to controls, being clearly superior to the efficacy of each substance separately. Concentrations chosen were above the EC50 (Figure 1A,B), to ensure enough cell viability reduction. In the remainder of this study, we decided to focus first on CX-4945, one of the two most effective CK2 inhibitors tested on GL261 cell viability (Figure 1) because unlike the other one, TDB, it has been already used in clinical trials [24,25].

2.2. CK2 Activity in GL261 Cells Treated with CX-4945

CK2 activity was analysed in GL261 cells treated with CX-4945 and in control, non-treated cells. As a reporter of endocellular CK2 activity, the phosphorylation state of the well-known CK2 target Akt (S129) [33] was analysed. In Figure 2A, p-Akt (S129) normalized to total Akt1 expression was obtained (at 8 h and 24 h post-treatment) and CX-4945 presented a dose-scale response, being p-Akt (S129) lower when higher concentrations of the inhibitor were applied. In addition, Figure 2B,C shows that p-Akt (S129), normalized to total Akt1, is significantly ($p < 0.05$) less phosphorylated in GL261 cells treated with 67.2 µM CX-4945 compared to control cells. No differences were found for CK2α and CK2β expression ($p > 0.05$) between treated and non-treated cells. CK2 activity was also measured in cell lysates, exploiting a highly specific peptide substrate [34] and significant differences ($p < 0.05$) were found between CX-4945 treated cells (Figure 2D) and control cells (pre-treatment). These results indicate that CX-4945 reduces endogenous CK2 activity when used to treat cultured GL261 cells, but not the total amount of CK2 subunits present in those cells.

2.3. CX-4945 Mice Tolerability

Before starting longitudinal in vivo treatment experiments, tolerability evaluation was performed for CX-4945 and TMZ. As it can be observed in Figure S1A, in the first phase, an MTD of 920 mg/kg was estimated for TMZ and of 1200 mg/kg for CX-4945. These MTD values were chosen because the doses of 1840 mg/kg (TMZ) and 2400 mg/kg (CX-4945) produced toxicity/adverse effects to the treated mice. In phase 2, when $n = 3$ mice where administered with a dosage of 920 mg/kg of TMZ, 9 days after this single TMZ administration, noticeable body weight decrease was detected in all mice. For this reason, the experiment was repeated with an $n = 3$ at the next lower dose, 480 mg/kg (Figure S1B). A similar situation was observed for CX-4945 when 1200 mg/kg of CX-4945 were administered per $n = 3$, one mouse was found dead, the day after administration so the experiment was repeated at 600 mg/kg (Figure S1C). These results indicate that the MTD (acute dose) is 480 mg/kg for TMZ and 600 mg/Kg for CX-4945, under our experimental conditions.

2.4. CK2 Activity in CX-4945 Treated Mice

In preliminary in vivo target validation studies, CK2 activity was found significantly ($p < 0.05$) reduced in all samples analysed, in comparison to controls (Figure 2E). Values obtained at the different time points (2 h, 6 h and 24 h) did not present significant differences when compared ($p > 0.05$), and results were grouped in $n = 6$ treated and $n = 6$ control mice. These results indicate that CX-4945 successfully reached tumours and exerted the expected effect on its target.

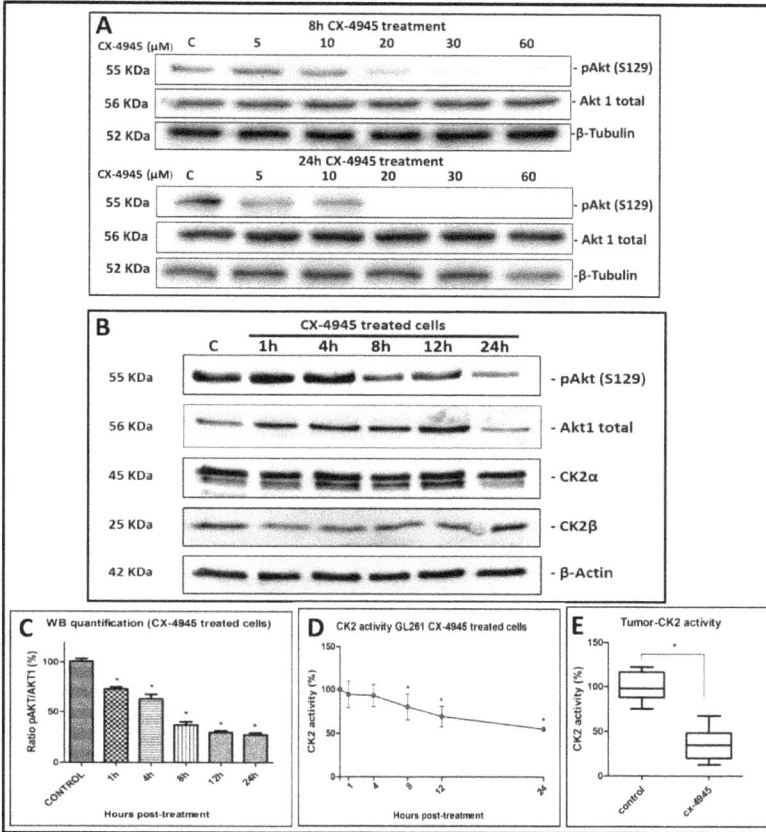

Figure 2. CK2 activity in GL261 cells and tumour samples. (**A**) Western blot for GL261 cell protein extracts (25 μg) treated with increasing doses of CX-4945 (from left to right: control (C) and CX-4945 treated cells 5 μM, 10 μM, 20 μM, 30 μM and 60 μM). This experiment was performed with $n = 1$ for each condition and for 8 h (upper part) or 24 h (lower part). p-Akt(S129), Akt1 total and β-Tubulin proteins were analysed; (**B**) Western blot for GL261 cell protein extracts (25 μg) treated with 67.2 μM CX-4945 (from left to right: control (C) and CX-4945 treated cells for 1 h, 4 h, 8 h, 12 h and 24 h). The experiment was performed with $n = 3$ for each condition. p-Akt(S129), Akt1 total, CK2α, CK2β and β-Actin proteins were analysed; (**C**) Quantification of western blot (WB) for GL261 cell protein extracts (25 μg) treated with CX-4945 ($n = 3$ per each condition). Ratio (%) of p-Akt(S129) content divided by Akt1 total content, while the control values (C) for this ratio are taken as the 100% start value. * = $p < 0.05$ for Student's *t*-test for the comparison of control and treated groups; (**D**) CK2 activity measured on a CK2-specific synthetic peptide in lysates from GL261 cells treated with 67.2 μM CX-4945 ($n = 3$ for each condition). Treatment during 1 h, 4 h, 8 h, 12 h and 24 h. * = $p < 0.05$ for Student's *t*-test for the comparison of control (100% initial value) and treated groups; (**E**) Boxplot of CK2 activity in CX-4945 treated mice compared to control mice. CX-4945 was administered to treated mice during 3 days (a total of 150 mg/Kg/day split into two administrations per day) and mice were euthanized 2 h, 6 h and 24 h after the last CX-4945 administration. As no CK2 activity differences ($p > 0.05$) were detected between euthanization time points (2 h, 6 h and 24 h), they were grouped in a single CX-4945 treated group. (* = $p > 0.05$ for Student's *t*-test for the comparison of control and treated groups). CK2 activity was measured on tissue homogenates by means of radioactive assays towards a CK2-specific peptide. Boxplot features as in Figure 1 legend.

2.5. Metronomic Longitudinal Treatments with CX-4945 and/or TMZ in Tumour-Bearing Mice

Three metronomic (every 6 days) administration treatments were performed: CX-4945 ($n = 6$), TMZ ($n = 6$) and a combination of CX-4945 and TMZ ($n = 6$), Figure 3. For the CX-4945 metronomic treatment, a survival rate of 24.5 ± 2.0 days was found, whereas for TMZ treatment, the survival rate was 38.7 ± 2.7. For the combined TMZ and CX-metronomic treatment, a provisional survival rate (right censored data) of 54.7 ± 11.9 days was found (three mice were still alive at day 65 p.i.). All groups offered significantly higher survival rate ($p < 0.05$) compared to control mice group (22.5 ± 1.2 days), Figure 3A. Besides, TMZ alone produced better survival than CX-4945 alone, while combined TMZ and CX-4945 was better than any of the two alone. Moreover, tumour volume evolution (Figure 3B–E) was significantly different ($p < 0.05$) when comparing treated groups with control group. Body weight was also inspected every day (Figure S3D). At the time of comparing the different treated groups, significant differences were found regarding weight, tumour volume evolution and survival rate, being the best results always obtained with the metronomic treatment combining TMZ with CX-4945.

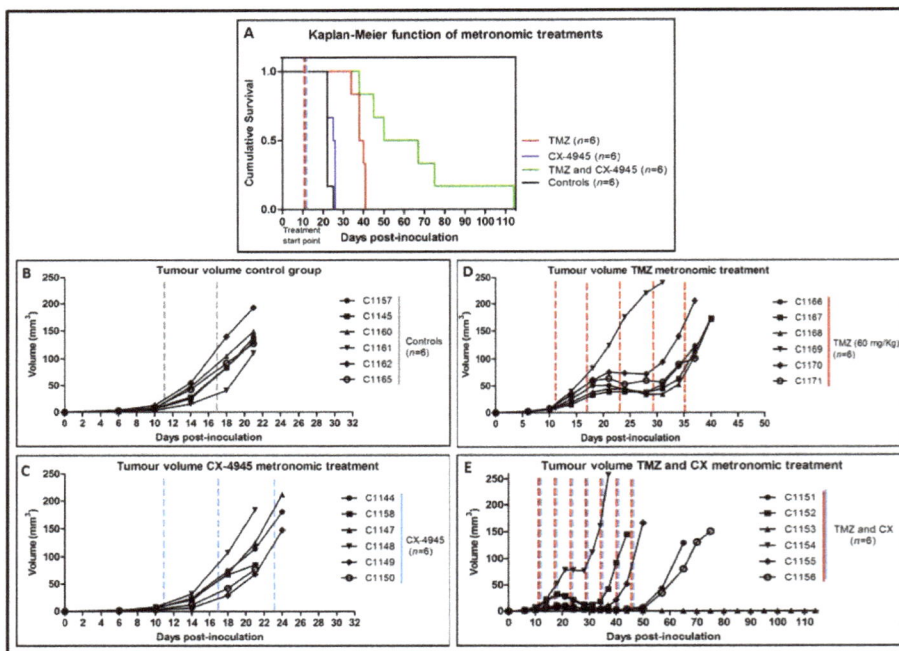

Figure 3. Tumour volumes and survival rates for 6-day metronomic treatment. (**A**) Survival Kaplan-Meier curve for metronomic CX-4945 treated mice ($n = 6$), blue line, metronomic TMZ treated mice ($n = 6$), red line, CX-4945 and TMZ metronomic treated mice ($n = 6$), green line, and control mice ($n = 6$), black line. Significant differences ($p < 0.05$) were observed between all treatment groups analysed in comparison with control mice; (**B**) Tumour volumes of control mice ($n = 6$); (**C**) Tumour volumes of metronomic CX-treated mice ($n = 6$); (**D**) Tumour volumes of metronomic TMZ-treated mice ($n = 6$); (**E**) Tumour volumes of metronomic CX and TMZ- treated mice ($n = 6$). Significant differences were found between groups ($p < 0.05$) when comparing control mice with treated mice, and when comparing different treatments between them (TMZ, CX-4945 and combined TMZ and CX-4945). The dashed lines indicate therapy administration points. Cxxxx corresponds to a unique alpha-numeric animal identifier code in the GABRMN group.

2.6. Non-Metronomic Longitudinal Treatments with CX-4945 and/or TMZ in Tumour-Bearing Mice

Despite having demonstrated that CX-4945 produces a better effect in GL261 implanted mice when administered in combination with TMZ and administered every 6 days, additional results of longitudinal mice experiments must be taken into account to better understand its causes, as in some cases, antagonistic effects can be observed.

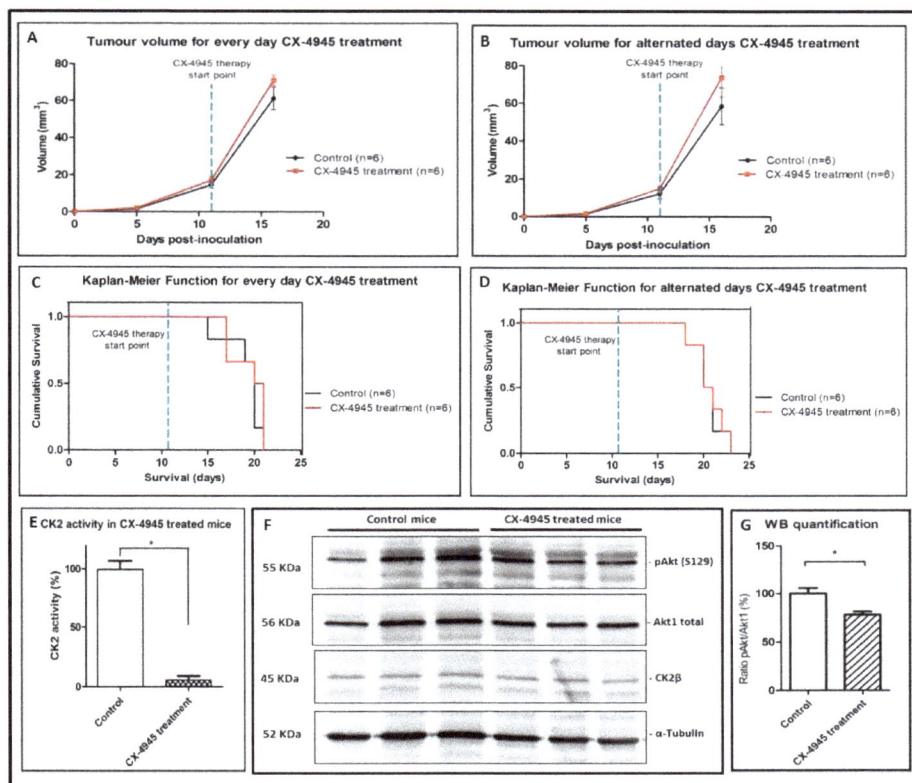

Figure 4. Tumour volumes, survival rates and CK2 activity and expression in CX-4945 treated mice. Tumour volumes (recorded at days 5, 11 and 16 p.i.) of treated ($n = 6$, black line) and control non-treated bearing tumour mice ($n = 6$, red line) for (**A**) CX-4945 treated every day GL261 implanted mice and (**B**) CX-4945 treated alternated days GL261 implanted mice. No significant differences were observed between groups ($p > 0.05$). The dashed blue line indicates the CX-4945 therapy start point; (**C**) Survival Kaplan-Meier curve for CX-4945 treated every day mice ($n = 6$) and control mice ($n = 6$); (**D**) Survival Kaplan-Meier curve for CX-4945 treated alternated days mice ($n = 6$) and control mice ($n = 6$). No significant differences were found between groups ($p > 0.05$). The dashed blue line indicates the CX-4945 therapy start point; (**E**) Tumour CK2 activity (%) in mice treated with CX-4945, $n = 3$, compared with control mice, $n = 3$. (* = $p < 0.05$ for Student's *t*-test for the comparison of control and treated groups); (**F**) Western blot for tumour total protein homogenate (40 µg) from different mice treated with CX-4945, $n = 3$, compared with control mice, $n = 3$. p-Akt(S129), Akt1 total, CK2α, and α-tubulin proteins were analyzed; (**G**) Quantification of Western blot for tumour total protein homogenate (40 µg) from mice treated with CX-4945, $n = 3$, compared with control mice, $n = 3$. Ratio (%) of p-Akt (S129) content divided by Akt1 total content. * = $p < 0.05$ for Student's *t*-test for the comparison of control and treated groups.

In this respect, CX-4945 treatment (either every day or alternated days administration at the classical dose/schedule described by others [21–23]) was performed in GL261 tumour-bearing mice, and no improvement was detected regarding tumour evolution (Figure 4A,B) or survival rate ($p > 0.05$, Figure 4C,D) in comparison with control mice. Figure 4C,D show the survival rate for every day CX-4945 treatment (20.5 ± 2.0 vs. 20.0 ± 2.1 days for control mice) and for alternated days CX-4945 treatment (20.5 ± 1.8 days vs. 20.5 ± 1.6 days for control mice). Body weight was inspected every day and no significant differences ($p > 0.05$) were observed between groups (Figure S3A). Examples of T_{2w} images for CX-4945 treated mice are shown in Figure S4. To ensure that CX-4945 reached the tumour, even when no effect on survival could be detected, 6 arbitrarily chosen tumour samples from the CX-4945 treatment every day ($n = 3$ treated, $n = 3$ controls) were analysed for CK2 activity and p-Akt (S129) WB. The CK2 activity was more than seventeen-fold reduced in CX-4945 treated tumour compared to control tumour after 10.0 ± 2.0 days of treatment (Figure 4E) and p-Akt (S129)/Akt1 ratio (Figure 4F,G) was found around 20% reduced in CX-4945 treated mice, indicating that CX-4945 had reached the desired target and inhibited CK2 activity, despite no increase of the survival rate was observed.

An additional experiment with three cycles TMZ and CX-4945 combined administered every day, produced significantly worse results than TMZ treatment alone (see [5] and Figure S5). In other words, CX-4945 treatment in vivo, in these conditions, seems to inhibit the beneficial effect produced by TMZ. Tumour volume curves are shown in Figure 5A. As stated in Figure S3B, three out of the six treated mice died around day 16 p.i., without noticeable weight reduction. Control mice weight evolution can be observed in Figure S3C. To compare survival rates between groups, Kaplan-Meier survival curves were elaborated, and no significant differences were found between TMZ 3 cycles + CX-4945 every day treated group and control group ($p > 0.05$, Figure 5B). The average survival rate was 21.3 ± 9.0 days for treated mice (TMZ 3 cycles + CX-4945 every day) vs. 19.8 ± 1.5 days for control mice, while for TMZ three cycles only treated mice from previous work (Figure S5) average survival time found was 33.9 ± 11.7 days. In addition, no significant differences were found when comparing TMZ 3 cycles+CX-4945 every day and CX-4945 everyday alone (survival rates of 19.8 ± 1.5 vs. 20.5 ± 2.0 days, respectively). C984 mouse was proven to be an outlier both in Grubbs' and Dixon's tests for single outliers (survival rate of 39 days, $p < 0.05$), but still it was maintained for survival analysis calculations. Overall average survival for control (untreated) GL261 harbouring mice was 20.8 ± 1.8 days, $n = 18$, while previous work from our group had obtained 21.5 ± 3.7 days, $n = 61$ (Figure S5), without significant difference ($p > 0.05$) with the present cohort of mice.

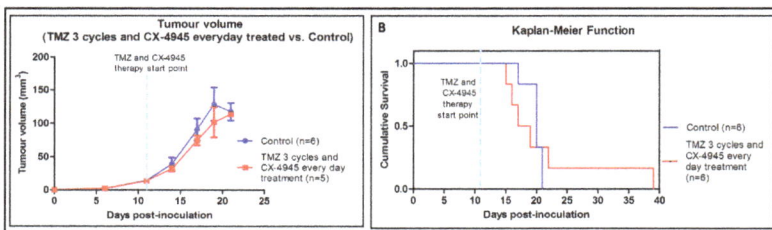

Figure 5. Tumour volume and Kaplan-Meier survival curve of mice treated with TMZ combined with CX-4945; (**A**) Tumour volumes (recorded at days 6, 11, 14, 17, 19 and 21 p.i.) of control GL261 implanted mice ($n = 6$, blue line) and combined TMZ-CX-4945 cycles in GL261 implanted mice ($n = 5$, red line). The dashed blue line indicates TMZ and CX-4945 therapy start point. No significant differences were observed between groups for comparisons of control and treated mice tumour volumes at each time point ($p > 0.05$). C984 has been excluded from tumour volume comparisons because it has been proven an outlier with Grubb's and Dixon's tests; (**B**) Survival Kaplan-Meier curves for TMZ and CX-4945 treated mice ($n = 6$) and control mice ($n = 6$). No significant differences were found between groups ($p > 0.05$). The dashed blue line indicates TMZ and CX-4945 therapy start point.

3. Discussion

3.1. Effect of iCK2 on GL261 Cultured Cells

GL261 cultured cells sensitivity was variable for the different iCK2 evaluated. CX-4945 decreased cell viability to about 20% of the control value. The EC_{50} found for CX-4945 (16.5 ± 5.5 µM) is similar to the EC_{50} found in breast cancer cell lines by others [21], who reported values between 1.7 and 20 µM. The lowest EC_{50} (8.1 ± 1.5) was found for TDB, concurring with a previous study [27], where a half maximal cell death concentration (DC_{50}) of 2.45 ± 0.84 µM was observed for the human HeLa cell line and of 3.45 ± 0.2 µM for human T lymphoblastoid cells. The standard GBM chemotherapeutic agent, TMZ, reached the EC_{50} at 747.6 ± 63.3 µM, which agrees with high values of half maximal inhibitory concentration (IC_{50}) found by others [35].

In addition, the combined TMZ and CX-4945 treatment carried out with GL261 cells in vitro presented increased efficacy regarding cell viability reduction, in comparison with both therapeutic agents administered separately (Figure 1C). The low EC_{50} of CX-4945 and TDB, combined with a significant decrease in cell viability, indicated that they should be suitable for future preclinical evaluation with GL261 tumours in vivo. CX-4945 was eventually chosen because it has been already described in clinical and preclinical studies [24,25].

As expected, we observed a significant reduction of CK2 activity in CX-4945 treated GL261 cells (Figure 2D). This was accompanied by the decrease of the phosphorylation of the CK2 target Akt (S129) (Figure 2B,C), similarly to [22] in prostate PC3 cancer cells. In addition, the Akt phosphorylation was found reduced as the CX-4945 concentration was increased, in a dose-dependent manner (Figure 2A). It has been described that the antiapoptotic effect of CK2 can be partially mediated by upregulation of the Akt/PKB pathway [33], thus the reduced viability found in GL261 cultured cells treated with CX-4945 can be also related to the down-regulation of this pathway, although the involvement of other pathways could also have an effect in the overall results observed [36]. These results reinforced the idea that CX-4945 could be a promising candidate for non-mutagenic brain tumour therapy in our preclinical GBM model.

3.2. Effects of CX-4945 in In Vivo Studies

In in vivo studies, CX-4945 was described to inhibit the activation of STAT-3, NF-κB p65 and Akt, in nude mice with intracranial human GBM X1046 xenografts [23]. In our work, we could demonstrate that 3 days of CX-4945 administration to GL261 tumour-bearing mice caused a decrease in CK2 activity of tumour samples analysed to 35% of control values (Figure 2E). This confirms that CX-4945 reached the target organ and caused the expected effect, as also reported in [23], although no further detailed study of the affected pathway was performed in our case. Regarding CX-4945 pharmacokinetics, described extensively elsewhere [37], it has a long half-life (more than 5 h) and high oral bioavailability (20%) in mice, without detectable mutagenicity, genotoxicity or cardiac toxicity. The results described in our work agree with this, showing that CX-4945 was well tolerated in mice as assessed by minimal changes in body weight during the course of treatment compared to control vehicle (Figure S3A).

3.3. Non-Metronomic CX-4945 Longitudinal In Vivo Studies

Although in vitro results indicated that CX-4945 should be a promising candidate for preclinical GBM therapy, unexpectedly, the non-metronomic in vivo treatment of GL261 tumour-bearing mice did not produce a better outcome. No tumour growth arrest and no survival improvement were detected (Figure 4A–D). This is in contrast to a previous in vivo study [23] with intracranial human xenografts treated with CX-4945 which showed significant effects in mice survival (50.2–67.8 days for treated mice, versus 35.6–40.4 days for control mice). However, there are relevant differences between work reported in [23] and our work, which could explain, at least partially, the differences observed. In [23], athymic nude mice were used, while in our experiment, immunocompetent C57BL/6 mice have been used, because we consider that they mimic better the clinical patient situation. Moreover, despite authors in [23] inoculated more cells for tumour generation (5×10^5 cells vs. 10^5 cells, in our study), their tumour growth pattern was much slower (survival rate for their control mice, 35.6–40.4 days, whereas our control mice survived 17–21 days). In this sense, it is widely accepted that small, slow-growing tumours are easier to treat than established, fast-growing tumour [38,39].

It is also worth mentioning that longitudinal in vivo studies reported by other authors did not present satisfactory results with CX-4945 alone in the same doses used in this work, although they studied other tumour types [36]. In this sense, using a drug combination for therapy involving CX-4945 was already suggested by authors in [36,40], with an additive effect recorded, which is also in line with our decision to study a drug combination (CX-4945 and TMZ) in order to perhaps improve the therapy response results produced by CX-4945 alone.

3.4. Non-Metronomic Combined CX-4945 and TMZ Longitudinal In Vivo Studies

Thus, the unexpected result obtained with the in vivo longitudinal study using CX-4945 alone in GL261 tumour-bearing mice lead us to hypothesize that a combined therapy with CX-4945 superimposed with TMZ could produce better results. The TMZ treatment in preclinical GBM mice has been proved useful in our group [5] with an average survival of 33.9 ± 11.7 days for treated animals (see also Figure S5), significantly higher than control mice (21.5 ± 3.7 days). TMZ cytotoxicity is predominantly mediated by O6-methylguanine (O6-MG) DNA lesions, which are repaired by the DNA repair protein O(6)-methylguanine-DNA methyltransferase (MGMT) [41]. Consequently, GBM patients whose tumours express low MGMT level, due to promoter hypermethylation, are more responsive to TMZ based therapy [42,43]. Protein Kinase CK2 is a novel interaction partner of JAK1/2, potentiating janus kinase (JAK) and signal transducer and activator of transcription (STAT-3) activation [44]. A CK2 inhibitor could reduce STAT-3, which has been implicated in the resistance of GBM to TMZ, downregulating MGMT and diminishing TMZ resistance [45], highlighting the potential of use of iCK2 combined with standards of care like TMZ. Nevertheless, the combined treatment (standard 3-cycle TMZ described by our group [5] superimposed with non-metronomic schedule for CX-4945) did not produce the expected improvement, except by case C984, classified as an outlier (Figure S3C), which followed an evolution pattern similar to TMZ-treated cases described in [5]. Except for this case, the combined TMZ+CX-4945 therapy showed similar results than control mice (survival of 17.8 ± 2.8 days for treated mice vs. 19.8 ± 1.5 days for control mice), reversing the beneficial effect of TMZ 3 cycles treatment. However, the combined TMZ and CX-4945 treatment carried out with GL261 cells in vitro presented increased efficacy regarding cell viability reduction, in comparison with both therapeutic agents administered separately (Figure 1C). This reinforced the idea that an increased efficacy, instead of an antagonistic effect, should have been observed in vivo with the combined therapy.

One of the possible explanations for those results could be due to dramatic CX-4945 'off target' effects, e.g., leading to strong splicing inhibition [46]. We cannot discard that these effects, rather than CK2 inhibition, are responsible for reversing TMZ efficacy. Another explanation could be related to the role of the immune system in therapy response [47] (see below), which would help to explain why a synergistic effect was observed with GL261 treated in vivo cells but it was not seen in our early non-metronomic in vivo approach.

3.5. Metronomic CX-4945 and/or TMZ Longitudinal In Vivo Studies and Possible Implication of the Immune System

The disappointing results obtained with non-metronomic administration schedules of CX-4945 both alone or in combination with TMZ lead us to raise the hypothesis that a possible interference with the host immune system was taking place, and it was the cause of the unfavourable outcome. Thus, we decided to move to a metronomic approach to discard or confirm this hypothesis. The so-called "metronomic therapy" [28], referring to equally spaced, low doses of chemotherapeutic drugs without extended rest periods, has been studied by several groups in the preceding years. Also, new therapeutic regimens with conventional drugs have been evaluated in order to activate immune responses that enhance tumour regression and prevent tumour regrowth. Recent studies with cyclophosphamide (CPA) metronomic therapy proved that this type of administration not only activates antitumour CD8+ T-cell response, but also induces long-term, specific T-cell tumour memory in GL261 tumours growing subcutaneously in immunocompetent mice [30,48]. These authors have also proven that a 6-day intermittent was the optimum timing for this therapy and this could agree with the 7-day cycle for immune cell recruitment described in [49], and accordingly this was the schedule chosen for our metronomic treatments. Indeed, the metronomic (every 6 days) therapy carried out in our study offered a better mice outcome, being the best results produced by CX-4945 and TMZ combined (54.7 ± 11.9 days) metronomic therapy, which was better than CX-4945 or TMZ metronomic therapies alone. These results reinforce the idea of the role of the immune system in therapy response [47] in GBM, and could explain the variation in our results depending on the therapy administration protocol used. Regarding the immune system cycle involved in tumour response, we should consider that the cytotoxic T-lymphocytes (CTLs) have a relevant role in the defence against cancer recognizing antigens presented on the surface of transformed cells, following a complex cycle described in [50]. Also, the whole cycle for immune cell response could take around 7 days in mouse brain [49], which is in agreement with the 6-day interleave that we have used in our work. It was also described the need of a functional CD5-dependent CK2 signalling for efficient differentiation of naive CD4+ T cells into Th2 and Th17 cells [50,51], involved in monocytes differentiation into dendritic cell subsets [52]. Moreover, authors in [53] have recently described impairment of Th17 cells development by CK2 inhibition with CX-4945 in a C57BL/6 mouse model of experimental autoimmune encephalomyelitis. Accordingly, CK2 inhibition (which could take place in every day or alternated days CX-4945 administration) could impair proper attraction of immune response triggered by immunogenic cell death signals. In this respect, several authors have described immunogenic death caused by TMZ therapy in GBM [54,55] and it could explain the reversal of beneficial effects observed in the non-metronomic combined therapy. Additionally, CK2 inhibition in vitro has been shown to compromise normal T-cell viability of cultured peripheral blood T-lymphocytes harvested from chronic lymphocytic leukemia patients [56], while other authors [36] demonstrated cytotoxic effects of CX-4945 administration, alone, in head and neck cancer cultured cell lines and xenograft models. Further work will be needed to clarify, in vitro and in vivo, the extent of immunogenic cell death produced by TMZ and CX-4945, alone or in combination, in the GL261 GBM model.

In summary, it is tempting to speculate that when CX-4945 is administered every day or in alternated days, it could cause an impairment of immune system elements needed for tumour response. Furthermore, when it is administered combined with TMZ (three cycles of therapy), CX-4945 reversed the beneficial effect of TMZ. When TMZ and CX-4945 are administered in a metronomic scheme every 6 days, the activation of the immune cell recruitment and response, which can take around 7 days [49], would not be significantly compromised. Accordingly, a word of caution should be said when treating immunocompetent preclinical tumours with CX-4945: the continued administration of a drug could impair the proper attraction of immune response contributing to therapeutic effects being evaluated.

4. Materials and Methods

4.1. GL261 Cells

GL261 mouse glioma cells were obtained from the Tumour Bank Repository at the National Cancer Institute (Frederick, MD, USA) and were grown as previously described in [57].

4.2. Cell Viability Assay

GL261 cells were plated in 96-well multiwell plates (Sigma Aldrich, Madrid, Spain) and allowed to adhere for 24 h before adding drugs to the medium (TMZ, APG, TBB, CX-4945 and TDB). Controls included cell culture medium and 0.4%–0.8% range of dimethyl sulfoxide (DMSO). After 72 h of drug exposure, cell viability was measured using XTT or MTT Assay (Sigma Aldrich). Half maximal effective concentration (EC_{50}) was calculated using GraphPad Prism software [58] See Supplementary Material file for further details.

4.3. Antibodies

CK2α-subunit (*dil. 1:1000*) rabbit antiserum was raised against (376–391) region of human protein, corresponding to the specific C-terminal sequence. CK2β (*Monoclonal, dil. 1:750, rabbit, Ref Ab76025*) and Phospho-Akt (S129) (*dil. 1:1000, rabbit, Ref 133458*) were purchased from Abcam (Cambridge, UK). β-actin (*dil.1:2000, mouse, Ref A2228*) and α-tubulin (*dil.1:2000, mouse, Ref A5441*) were obtained from Sigma-Aldrich, and β-tubulin (*dil. 1:1000, rabbit, Ref 2146*) and Akt1 (*dil 1:500, rabbit, Ref C3H10*) were purchased from Cell Signalling Technology (Beverly, MA, USA). Secondary antibodies towards rabbit and mouse IgG (*dil.1:2000*), conjugated to horse radish peroxidase, were purchased from PerkinElmer (Waltham, MA, USA).

4.4. Target Evaluation in GL261 Cultured Cells with CX-4945 Treatment

For the CK2 expression and activity studies, a total of 18 flasks (75 cm^2) of GL261 cells were cultured ($n = 3$ as controls, $n = 3$ as CX-4945 treatment during 1 h, 4 h, 8 h, 12 h and 24 h). Cells were cultured in flasks until 50% confluence and at that moment, CX-4945 was added to the "treatment" flasks, and an equal amount of the vehicle (DMSO) was added to the control cells. The CX-4945 concentration used was 67.2 μM (four times the EC_{50}, as stated by other authors [59]). Still, this concentration was included in the range of maximum CX-4945 effect as it can be seen in Figure 1. An in vitro dose-response study was also conducted in cultured GL261 cells in order to check for increasing target effects. For this, 300,000 cells/well were plated in 6-well plates and concentrations of CX-4945 of 0, 5, 10, 20, 30 and 60 μM were added. Treatments were performed during 8 and 24 h. Therapeutic agent preparations (CK2 inhibitors and TMZ) can be found in the Supplementary Materials file.

4.5. Animal Model for In Vivo Studies

A total of 60 C57BL/6 female wild type mice weighting 21.2 ± 1.3 g were used for this study. They were obtained from Charles River Laboratories (Charles River Laboratories International, L'Abresle, France) and housed in the animal facility of the Universitat AutÈnoma de Barcelona. All studies described in this paper were approved by the local ethics committee (Comissió d'ètica en Experimentació Animal i Humana (CEEAH), [60]), according to the regional and state legislation (protocol DMAH-8236/CEEAH-2785). Tumours were induced in C57BL/6 mice by intracranial stereotactic injection of 10^5 GL261 cells with 4 μL of RPMI (Roswell Park Memorial Institute) medium in the caudate nucleus, as previously described by us [61]. Mice were weighted every day or at alternated days (for metronomic treatments) and tumour volumes were followed using T$_2$-weighted MRI acquisition as in [5] the day 6 and 10-11 after implantation. Mice with most homogeneous weights and tumour sizes were chosen to make experimental groups after randomization (usually $n = 6$ per studied condition), and therapy started. The volume and weight averages did not show significant differences ($p > 0.05$) between the experimental groups (Tables S1–S4).

4.6. CX-4945 and TMZ Tolerability Assay

Two phases were performed for this study, based in the work described in [62]: in phase 1, $n = 1$ was used and the starting TMZ dose was the one described by us (60 mg/kg/day) [5], and for CX-4945, the dose was the one described in [22,59] (150 mg/kg/day), as no adverse effects have been observed with these doses. Administrations were performed with an oral gavage. Doses were increased (Table S5) until detection of toxicity symptoms (Table S6). Once MTD was estimated in this first phase, a second phase took place and a group of $n = 3$ mice were administered with the calculated

MTD. Mice follow-up (weight + welfare parameters for up to 30 days) was carried out every day (Figure S1).

4.7. Use of iCK2 in Tumour-Bearing Animals

4.7.1. Preliminary Studies of Target Validation

CX-4945 therapy was administered to tumour-bearing mice ($n = 2$) during three days (150 mg/kg split into two administrations per day). CX-4945 vehicle, phosphate buffer 25 mM pH 7.2 was administered to control mice ($n = 2$ per each experimental time). Administrations were performed with an oral gavage. Mice were euthanized at 2 h, 6 h and 24 h after the last administration for both treated and control mice to assess CK2 activity compared to control mice. Tumour samples were stored in liquid nitrogen until further processing.

4.7.2. Longitudinal Studies with iCK2 (alone or in combination)

CX-4945 therapy was administered to tumour-bearing mice, every day or in alternated days, 150 mg/Kg/day [23] (Figures S2A,B). CX-4945 total dose for every day or alternated days treatment administered was 150 mg/Kg/day, split into two times per day (75 mg/kg at 8 h, and 75 mg/kg at 16 h) and dissolved in vehicle administration, which was phosphate buffer 25 mM pH 7.2. For the combined CX-4945 + TMZ therapy (Figure S2C), CX-4945 was administered every day whereas TMZ (60 mg/Kg) was dissolved in 10% DMSO in saline solution (0.9% NaCl) prepared as described in [5]. CX-4945 therapy was given until the end point of animal survival, when animals were euthanized because of welfare parameters. For this, animals were euthanized by cervical dislocation, the brain was removed and tumour resected. Samples were stored in liquid nitrogen until further processing for CK2 activity analysis.

Regarding metronomic (every 6 days) administration protocol, eight doses of CX-4945 (150 mg/Kg; 75 mg/kg at 8 h and 75 mg/kg at 16 h) were administered to CX-4945 treated group (Figure S2D), eight doses of TMZ (60mg/Kg at 12 h) were administered to TMZ treated group (Figure S2E) and eight doses of CX-4945 (150 mg/Kg75 mg/kg at 8 h, and 75 mg/kg at 16 h) plus TMZ (60 mg/Kg at 12 h) were administered to CX and TMZ combined therapy group (Figure S2F). Control mice received TMZ and CX-4945 vehicles. In all cases, the maximum cumulative dose administered of CX-4945 was 1200 mg/Kg and of TMZ, 480 mg/kg.

All treatments were administered using an oral gavage and the administration volume for CX-4945 and TMZ was the same that has been used in our group for the TMZ administration (10 µL/g weight animal) [5].

4.8. CK2 Activity Assay

CK2 activity was measured in 1–2 µg of lysate proteins (total protein extract of cell lysates) and 5–10 µg (total protein extract of brain mice samples), previously incubated 10 min at 30 °C with 0.1 mM CK2-tide (specific CK2 substrate peptide), by means of radioactive assays with gamma-33P ATP, in the presence of phosphorylation reaction mixture as described in [34].

4.9. MRI Acquisition

Magnetic resonance studies were carried out at the joint NMR facility of UAB and CIBER-BBN, Unit 25 of NANBIOSIS, with a 7T horizontal magnet (BioSpec 70/30, Bruker BioSpin, Ettlingen, Germany). GL261 tumour-bearing mice were screened by acquiring high resolution coronal T_{2W} images (TR/TE$_{eff}$ = 4200/36 ms) using Rapid Acquisition with Relaxation Enhancement (RARE) sequence to detect brain tumour presence and monitor its evolution stage. The acquisition parameters were as follows: turbo factor, 8; field of view (FOV), 19.2 × 19.2 mm; matrix, 256 × 256 (75 × 75 µm/pixel); number of slices, 10; slice thickness (ST), 0.5 mm; inter-ST, 0.6 mm; number of averages (NA), 4; total acquisition time (TAT), 6 min and 43 s.

4.10. Tissue Homogenization and Protein Extraction/Western Blot Analysis

Detailed information of the experimental procedures can be found in the Supplementary Materials file.

4.11. Statistical Analysis

Variance homogeneity was assessed with the Levene's test. A two-tailed Student's t-test for independent measurements was used for comparisons, for samples of equal or different variances (depending on the Levene's test result). Dixon's and Grubb's tests were used to detect outliers. The global evolution of tumour growth curves or body weight control was evaluated with the UNIANOVA test. Comparisons of survival rates were performed with the Log-Rank test. The significance level for all tests was $p < 0.05$.

5. Conclusions

CX-4945 has a noticeable effect in decreasing GL261 GBM cell viability and CK2 activity in vitro. Additionally, CK2 activity analysis confirmed that CX-4945 reached the target tissue in vivo. Notable differences in mice outcome were obtained with CX-4945 every day/alternated days (alone or combined with 3 cycles of TMZ), in comparison with metronomic administration of CX-4945 and/or TMZ, the highest survival rates being obtained with the metronomic combining TMZ + CX-4945 every 6 days.

An appealing explanation for this fact would be related with the immune system role in tumour response and the possible impairment of cytotoxic T-cell maturation cycle due to continued administration of CX-4945, which was overcome by the 6-day schedule metronomic administration. Accordingly, due care should be exercised when treating immunocompetent mice harbouring preclinical tumours with CX-4945 to ensure optimal results.

Supplementary Materials: The following are available online at www.mdpi.com/1424-8247/10/1/24. Supplementary Materials and Methods S1.1: Cell Viability Assay, Supplementary Materials and Methods S1.2: Therapeutic Agent Preparations (CK2 Inhibitors and TMZ), Supplementary Materials and Methods S1.3: Tissue Homogenization and Protein Extraction, Supplementary Materials and Methods S1.4: Western Blot Analysis. Table S1: Tumor volume and body weight for mice before starting CX-4945 therapy every day, Table S2: Tumor volume and body weight for mice before starting CX-4945 therapy in alternated days, Table S3: Tumor volume and body weight for mice before starting combined TMZ+CX-4945 therapy, Table S4: Tumor volume and body weight for mice before starting metronomic therapy: CX-4945, TMZ, CX-4945 and TMZ, Table S5: Doses for CX-4945 and TMZ administration in MTD calculation experiments, Table S6: Symptoms and signals guidance to decide the MTD, Figure S1: Mice body weight (maximum tolerated dose (MTD) studies), Figure S2: Therapy administration scheme protocols, Figure S3: Weight averages of treated and control mice, Figure S4: MRI images of CX-4945 treated mice, Figure S5: Survival Kaplan-Meier curve for 3 cycles of TMZ vs. control.

Acknowledgments: Authors would like to thank Jordi Llorens from Department of Physiological Sciences, Faculty of Medicine and Health Sciences, Universitat de Barcelona, for initial guidance in the mice tolerability experiments. Laura Ferrer-Font held a PIF predoctoral fellowship from Universitat Autènoma de Barcelona. This work was funded by the Ministerio de Economía y Competitividad (MINECO) grant MOLIMAGLIO (SAF2014-52332-R). Also funded by Centro de Investigación Biomédica en Red—Bioingeniería, Biomateriales y Nanomedicina (CIBER-BBN, (http://www.ciber-bbn.es/en)), an initiative of the Instituto de Salud Carlos III (Spain) co-funded by EU Fondo Europeo de Desarrollo Regional (FEDER). Also funded by AIRC IG14180 to LAP.

Author Contributions: L.F.F. carried out most of the experimental studies and drafted the manuscript; LV elaborated the curve of GL261 dose-dependent to CX-4945 and the combined in vitro TMZ + CX-4945 studies; N.A.R. performed animal follow up in the in vivo experiments; J.V. was in charge of CK2 activity assays for the target confirmation in in vivo studies; M.P. oversee L.V. work; M.R. coordinated the CK2 expression and activity analysis and helped to draft the manuscript; L.A.P. and E.I. helped to draft the manuscript and to supervise CK2 related work; C.A. and A.P.C., participated in the study design and coordinated drafting of the manuscript. All authors read and approved the final text of the manuscript.

Conflicts of Interest: The authors declare no conflict of interest.

Abbreviation

APG	Apigenin
CK2	Protein Kinase CK2
CSCs	Cancer stem cells
CX-4945	5-(3-Chlorophenylamino)benzo[c][2,6] naphthyridine-8-carboxylic acid
CPA	Cyclophosphamide
DC_{50}	Half maximal cell death concentration
DMSO	Dimethyl sulfoxide
EC_{50}	Half maximal effective concentration,
GABRMN	Grup d'Aplicacions BiomÙdiques de la RMN
GBM	Glioblastoma
IC_{50}	Half maximal inhibitory concentration
iCK2	Protein Kinase CK2 inhibitors
JAK	Janus kinase
MGMT	O(6)-methylguanine-DNA methyltransferase
MTD	Maximum tolerated dose
p.i.	Post-inoculation
PIM-1	Proviral Integration of Moloney virus 1
STAT 3	Signal transducer and activator of transcription 3
TBB	4,5,6,7-Tetrabromobenzotriazole
TDB	Tetrabromodeoxyribofuranosyl-benzimidazole
TMZ	Temozolomide
WB	Western blot.

References

1. Buckner, J.C. Factors influencing survival in high-grade gliomas. *Semin. Oncol.* **2003**, *30*, 10–14. [CrossRef] [PubMed]
2. Ohgaki, H.; Kleihues, P. Genetic profile of astrocytic and oligodendroglial gliomas. *Brain Tumour Pathol.* **2011**, *28*, 177–183. [CrossRef] [PubMed]
3. Stupp, R.; Mason, W.P.; van den Bent, M.J.; Weller, M.; Fisher, B.; Taphoorn, M.J.B.; Belanger, K.; Brandes, A.A.; Marosi, C.; Bogdahn, U.; et al. Radiotherapy plus concomitant and adjuvant temozolomide for glioblastoma. *N. Engl. J. Med.* **2005**, *352*, 987–996. [CrossRef] [PubMed]
4. Yoshimoto, K.; Mizoguchi, M.; Hata, N.; Murata, H.; Hatae, R.; Amano, T.; Nakamizo, A.; Sasaki, T. Complex DNA repair pathways as possible therapeutic targets to overcome temozolomide resistance in glioblastoma. *Front. Oncol.* **2012**, *2*, 186. [CrossRef] [PubMed]
5. Delgado-Goni, T.; Julia-Sape, M.; Candiota, A.P.; Pumarola, M.; Arus, C. Molecular imaging coupled to pattern recognition distinguishes response to temozolomide in preclinical glioblastoma. *NMR Biomed.* **2014**, *27*, 1333–1345. [CrossRef] [PubMed]
6. Huang, Z.; Cheng, L.; Guryanova, O.A.; Wu, Q.; Bao, S. Cancer stem cells in glioblastoma—Molecular signaling and therapeutic targeting. *Protein Cell* **2010**, *1*, 638–655. [CrossRef] [PubMed]
7. Kaina, B.; Ochs, K.; Grösch, S.; Fritz, G.; Lips, J.; Tomicic, M.; Dunkern, T.; Christmann, M. BER, MGMT, and MMR in defense against alkylation-induced genotoxicity and apoptosis. *Prog. Nucleic Acid Res. Mol. Biol.* **2001**, *68*, 41–54. [PubMed]
8. Duncan, J.S.; Litchfield, D.W. Too much of a good thing: The role of protein kinase CK2 in tumourigenesis and prospects for therapeutic inhibition of CK2. *Biochim. Biophys.* **2008**, *1784*, 33–47. [CrossRef] [PubMed]
9. Ruzzene, M.; Pinna, L.A. Addiction to protein kinase CK2: A common denominator of diverse cancer cells? *Biochim. Biophys. Acta* **2010**, *1804*, 499–504. [CrossRef] [PubMed]
10. Münstermann, U.; Fritz, G.; Seitz, G.; Lu, Y.P.; Schneider, H.R.; Issinger, O.-G.G. Casein kinase II is elevated in solid human tumours and rapidly proliferating non-neoplastic tissue. *Eur. J. Biochem.* **1990**, *189*, 251–257.
11. Ortega, C.E.; Seidner, Y.; Dominguez, I. Mining CK2 in cancer. *PLoS ONE* **2014**, *9*, e115609. [CrossRef] [PubMed]

12. Dixit, D.; Sharma, V.; Ghosh, S.; Mehta, V.S.; Sen, E. Inhibition of Casein kinase-2 induces p53-dependent cell cycle arrest and sensitizes glioblastoma cells to tumour necrosis factor (TNFα)-induced apoptosis through SIRT1 inhibition. *Cell Death Dis.* **2012**, *3*, e271. [CrossRef] [PubMed]

13. Ji, H.; Lu, Z. The Role of Protein Kinase CK2 in Glioblastoma Development. *Clin. Cancer Res.* **2013**, *19*, 6335–6337. [CrossRef] [PubMed]

14. Ferrer-Font, L.; Alcaraz, E.; Plana, M.; Candiota, A.P.; Itarte, E.; Arús, C. Protein Kinase CK2 Content in GL261 Mouse Glioblastoma. *Pathol. Oncol. Res.* **2016**, *22*, 633–637. [CrossRef] [PubMed]

15. Tapia, J.C.; Torres, V.A.; Rodriguez, D.A.; Leyton, L.; Quest, A.F.G. Casein kinase 2 (CK2) increases survivin expression via enhanced beta-catenin-T cell factor/lymphoid enhancer binding factor-dependent transcription. *Proc. Natl. Acad. Sci. USA* **2006**, *103*, 15079–15084. [CrossRef] [PubMed]

16. Dixit, D.; Ahmad, F.; Ghildiyal, R.; Joshi, S.D.; Sen, E. CK2 inhibition induced PDK4-AMPK axis regulates metabolic adaptation and survival responses in glioma. *Exp. Cell Res.* **2016**, *344*, 132–142. [CrossRef] [PubMed]

17. Romieu-Mourez, R.; Landesman-Bollag, E.; Seldin, D.C.; Traish, A.M.; Mercurio, F.; Sonenshein, G.E. Roles of IKK Kinases and Protein Kinase CK2 in Activation of Nuclear Factor-{{kappa}}B in Breast Cancer. *Cancer Res.* **2001**, *61*, 3810–3818. [PubMed]

18. Das, A.; Banik, N.L.; Ray, S.K. Flavonoids activated caspases for apoptosis in human glioblastoma T98G and U87MG cells but not in human normal astrocytes. *Cancer* **2010**, *116*, 164–176. [CrossRef] [PubMed]

19. Zanin, S.; Borgo, C.; Girardi, C.; O'Brien, S.E.; Miyata, Y.; Pinna, L.A.; Donella-Deana, A.; Ruzzene, M. Effects of the CK2 inhibitors CX-4945 and CX-5011 on drug-resistant cells. *PLoS ONE* **2012**, *7*, e49193. [CrossRef] [PubMed]

20. Kim, J.; Hwan Kim, S. CK2 inhibitor CX-4945 blocks TGF-β1-induced epithelial-to-mesenchymal transition in A549 human lung adenocarcinoma cells. *PLoS ONE* **2013**, *8*, e74342.

21. Siddiqui-Jain, A.; Drygin, D.; Streiner, N.; Chua, P.; Pierre, F.; O'Brien, S.E.; Bliesath, J.; Omori, M.; Huser, N.; Ho, C.; et al. CX-4945, an orally bioavailable selective inhibitor of protein kinase CK2, inhibits prosurvival and angiogenic signaling and exhibits antitumour efficacy. *Cancer Res.* **2010**, *70*, 10288–10298. [CrossRef] [PubMed]

22. Pierre, F.; Chua, P.C.; O'Brien, S.E.; Siddiqui-Jain, A.; Bourbon, P.; Haddach, M.; Michaux, J.; Nagasawa, J.; Schwaebe, M.K. Pre-clinical characterization of CX-4945, a potent and selective small molecule inhibitor of CK2 for the treatment of cancer. *Mol. Cell. Biochem.* **2011**, *356*, 37–43. [CrossRef] [PubMed]

23. Zheng, Y.; McFarland, B.C.; Drygin, D.; Yu, H.; Bellis, S.L.; Kim, H.; Bredel, M.; Benveniste, E.N. Targeting protein kinase CK2 suppresses prosurvival signaling pathways and growth of glioblastoma. *Clin. Cancer Res.* **2013**, *19*, 6484–6494. [CrossRef] [PubMed]

24. Dose-escalation Study of Oral CX-4945. Available online: http://www.cancer.gov/clinicaltrials/search/view?cdrid=642699&version=HealthProfessional (accessed on 12 February 2017).

25. Cylene Presents Encouraging Clinical Data for Oral CK2 Inhibitor at ASCO. Available online: http://www.prnewswire.com/news-releases/cylene-presents-encouraging-clinical-data-for-oral-ck2-inhibitor-at-asco-123219423.html (accessed on 12 February 2017).

26. Nitta, R.T.; Gholamin, S.; Feroze, A.H.; Agarwal, M.; Cheshier, S.H.; Mitra, S.S.; Li, G. Casein kinase 2α regulates glioblastoma brain tumour-initiating cell growth through the β-catenin pathway. *Oncogene* **2015**, *34*, 3688–3699. [CrossRef] [PubMed]

27. Cozza, G.; Girardi, C.; Ranchio, A.; Lolli, G.; Sarno, S.; Orzeszko, A.; Kazimierczuk, Z.; Battistutta, R.; Ruzzene, M.; Pinna, L.A. Cell-permeable dual inhibitors of protein kinases CK2 and PIM-1: Structural features and pharmacological potential. *Cell. Mol. Life Sci.* **2014**, *71*, 3173–3185. [CrossRef] [PubMed]

28. Hanahan, D.; Bergers, G.; Bergsland, E. Less is more, regularly: Metronomic dosing of cytotoxic drugs can target tumour angiogenesis in mice. *J. Clin. Investig.* **2000**, *105*, 1045–1047. [CrossRef] [PubMed]

29. Gnoni, A.; Silvestris, N.; Licchetta, A.; Santini, D.; Scartozzi, M.; Ria, R.; Pisconti, S.; Petrelli, F.; Vacca, A.; Lorusso, V. Metronomic chemotherapy from rationale to clinical studies: A dream or reality? *Crit. Rev. Oncol. Hematol.* **2015**, *95*, 1–16. [CrossRef] [PubMed]

30. Wu, J.; Waxman, D.J. Metronomic cyclophosphamide schedule-dependence of innate immune cell recruitment and tumour regression in an implanted glioma model. *Cancer Lett.* **2014**, *353*, 272–280. [CrossRef] [PubMed]

31. Ausman, J.I.; Shapiro, W.R.; Rall, D.P. Studies on the chemotherapy of experimental brain tumours: Development of an experimental model. *Cancer Res.* **1970**, *30*, 2394–2400. [PubMed]
32. Szatmári, T.; Lumniczky, K.; Désaknai, S.; Trajcevski, S.; Hídvégi, E.J.; Hamada, H.; Sáfrány, G. Detailed characterization of the mouse glioma 261 tumour model for experimental glioblastoma therapy. *Cancer Sci.* **2006**, *97*, 546–553. [CrossRef] [PubMed]
33. Di Maira, G.; Salvi, M.; Arrigoni, G.; Marin, O.; Sarno, S.; Brustolon, F.; Pinna, L.A.; Ruzzene, M. Protein kinase CK2 phosphorylates and upregulates Akt/PKB. *Cell Death Differ.* **2005**, *12*, 668–677. [CrossRef] [PubMed]
34. Ruzzene, M.; Di Maira, G.; Tosoni, K.; Pinna, L.A. Assessment of CK2 constitutive activity in cancer cells. *Methods Enzymol.* **2010**, *484*, 495–514. [PubMed]
35. Kusabe, Y.; Kawashima, H.; Ogose, A.; Sasaki, T.; Ariizumi, T.; Hotta, T.; Endo, N. Effect of temozolomide on the viability of musculoskeletal sarcoma cells. *Oncol. Lett.* **2015**, *10*, 2511–2518. [CrossRef] [PubMed]
36. Bian, Y.; Han, J.; Kannabiran, V.; Mohan, S.; Cheng, H.; Friedman, J.; Zhang, L.; VanWaes, C.; Chen, Z. MEK inhibitor PD-0325901 overcomes resistance to CK2 inhibitor CX-4945 and exhibits anti-tumour activity in head and neck cancer. *Int. J. Biol. Sci.* **2015**, *11*, 411–422. [CrossRef] [PubMed]
37. Pierre, F.; Chua, P.C.; O'Brien, S.E.; Siddiqui-Jain, A.; Bourbon, P.; Haddach, M.; Michaux, J.; Nagasawa, J.; Schwaebe, M.K.; Stefan, E.; et al. Discovery and SAR of 5-(3-chlorophenylamino)benzo[c][2,6] naphthyridine-8-carboxylic acid (CX-4945), the first clinical stage inhibitor of protein kinase CK2 for the treatment of cancer. *J. Med. Chem.* **2011**, *54*, 635–654. [CrossRef] [PubMed]
38. McConville, P.; Hambardzumyan, D.; Moody, J.B.; Leopold, W.R.; Kreger, A.R.; Woolliscroft, M.J.; Rehemtulla, A.; Ross, B.D.; Holland, E.C. Magnetic resonance imaging determination of tumour grade and early response to temozolomide in a genetically engineered mouse model of glioma. *Clin. Cancer Res.* **2007**, *13*, 2897–2904. [CrossRef] [PubMed]
39. Plowman, J.; Waud, W.R.; Koutsoukos, A.D.; Rubinstein L, V.; Moore, T.D.; Grever, M.R. Preclinical antitumor activity of temozolomide in mice: Efficacy against human brain tumor xenografts and synergism with 1,3-bis(2-chloroethyl)-1-nitrosourea. *Cancer Res.* **1994**, *54*, 3793–3799. [PubMed]
40. Siddiqui-Jain, A.; Bliesath, J.; Macalino, D.; Omori, M.; Huser, N.; Streiner, N.; Ho, C.B.; Anderes, K.; Proffitt, C.; O'Brien, S.E.; et al. CK2 inhibitor CX-4945 suppresses DNA repair response triggered by DNA-targeted anticancer drugs and augments efficacy: mechanistic rationale for drug combination therapy. *Mol. Cancer Ther.* **2012**, *11*, 994–1005. [CrossRef] [PubMed]
41. Drablos, F.; Feyzi, E.; Aas, P.A.; Vaagbø, C.B.; Kavli, B.; Bratlie, M.S.; Peña-Diaz, J.; Otterlei, M.; Slupphaug, G.; Krokan, H.E. Alkylation damage in DNA and RNA-repair mechanisms and medical significance. *DNA Repair (Amst.)* **2004**, *3*, 1389–1407. [CrossRef] [PubMed]
42. Hegi, M.E.; Diserens, A.-C.; Godard, S.; Dietrich, P.-Y.; Regli, L.; Ostermann, S.; Otten, P.; Van Melle, G.; de Tribolet, N.; Stupp, R. Clinical trial substantiates the predictive value of O-6-methylguanine-DNA methyltransferase promoter methylation in glioblastoma patients treated with temozolomide. *Clin. Cancer Res.* **2004**, *10*, 1871–1874. [CrossRef] [PubMed]
43. Stupp, R.; Hegi, M.E.; Mason, W.P.; van den Bent, M.J.; Taphoorn, M.J.B.; Janzer, R.C.; Ludwin, S.K.; Allgeier, A.; Fisher, B.; Belanger, K.; et al. Effects of radiotherapy with concomitant and adjuvant temozolomide versus radiotherapy alone on survival in glioblastoma in a randomised phase III study: 5-year analysis of the EORTC-NCIC trial. *Lancet Oncol.* **2009**, *10*, 459–466. [CrossRef]
44. Zheng, Y.; Qin, H.; Frank, S.J.; Deng, L.; Litchfield, D.W.; Tefferi, A.; Pardanani, A.; Lin, F.-T.; Li, J.; Sha, B.; et al. A CK2-dependent mechanism for activation of the JAK-STAT signaling pathway. *Blood* **2011**, *118*, 156–166. [CrossRef] [PubMed]
45. Kohsaka, S.; Wang, L.; Yachi, K.; Mahabir, R.; Narita, T.; Itoh, T.; Tanino, M.; Kimura, T.; Nishihara, H.; Tanaka, S. STAT3 inhibition overcomes temozolomide resistance in glioblastoma by downregulating MGMT expression. *Mol. Cancer Ther.* **2012**, *11*, 1289–1299. [CrossRef] [PubMed]
46. Kim, H.; Choi, K.; Kang, H.; Lee, S.Y.; Chi, S.W.; Lee, M.S.; Song, J.; Im, D.; Choi, Y.; Cho, S. Identification of a novel function of CX-4945 as a splicing regulator. *PLoS ONE* **2014**, *9*, e94978. [CrossRef] [PubMed]
47. Vacchelli, E.; Aranda, F.; Eggermont, A.; Galon, J.; SautÙs-Fridman, C.; Cremer, I.; Zitvogel, L.; Kroemer, G.; Galluzzi, L. Trial Watch: Chemotherapy with immunogenic cell death inducers. *Oncoimmunology* **2014**, *3*, e27878. [CrossRef] [PubMed]

48. Wu, J.; Waxman, D.J. Metronomic cyclophosphamide eradicates large implanted GL261 gliomas by activating antitumour Cd8(+) T-cell responses and immune memory. *Oncoimmunology* **2015**, *4*, e1005521. [CrossRef] [PubMed]

49. Karman, J.; Ling, C.; Sandor, M.; Fabry, Z. Initiation of immune responses in brain is promoted by local dendritic cells. *J. Immunol.* **2004**, *173*, 2353–2361. [CrossRef] [PubMed]

50. Tabbekh, M.; Mokrani-Hammani, M.; Bismuth, G.; Mami-Chouaib, F. T-cell modulatory properties of CD5 and its role in antitumour immune responses. *Oncoimmunology* **2013**, *2*, e22841. [CrossRef] [PubMed]

51. Sestero, C.M.; McGuire, D.J.; De Sarno, P.; Brantley, E.C.; Soldevila, G.; Axtell, R.C.; Raman, C. CD5-dependent CK2 activation pathway regulates threshold for T cell anergy. *J. Immunol.* **2012**, *189*, 2918–2930. [CrossRef] [PubMed]

52. Alonso, M.N.; Wong, M.T.; Zhang, A.L.; Winer, D.; Suhoski, M.M.; Tolentino, L.L.; Gaitan, J.; Davidson, M.G.; Kung, T.H.; Galel, D.M.; et al. T(H)1, T(H)2, and T(H)17 cells instruct monocytes to differentiate into specialized dendritic cell subsets. *Blood* **2011**, *118*, 3311–3320. [CrossRef] [PubMed]

53. Ulges, A.; Witsch, E.J.; Pramanik, G.; Klein, M.; Birkner, K.; Bühler, U.; Wasser, B.; Luessi, F.; Stergiou, N.; Dietzen, S.; et al. Protein kinase CK2 governs the molecular decision between encephalitogenic TH17 cell and Treg cell development. *Proc. Natl. Acad. Sci. USA* **2016**, *113*, 10145–10150. [CrossRef] [PubMed]

54. Kim, T.-G.; Kim, C.-H.; Park, J.-S.; Park, S.-D.; Kim, C.K.; Chung, D.-S.; Hong, Y.-K. Immunological factors relating to the antitumour effect of temozolomide chemoimmunotherapy in a murine glioma model. *Clin. Vaccine Immunol.* **2010**, *17*, 143–153. [CrossRef] [PubMed]

55. Fritzell, S.; Sandén, E.; Eberstål, S.; Visse, E.; Darabi, A.; Siesjö, P. Intratumoural temozolomide synergizes with immunotherapy in a T cell-dependent fashion. *Cancer Immunol. Immunother.* **2013**, *62*, 1463–1474. [CrossRef] [PubMed]

56. Martins, L.R.; Lúcio, P.; Silva, M.C.; Anderes, K.L.; Gameiro, P.; Silva, M.G.; Anderes, K.L.; Gameiro, P.; Silva, M.G.; Barata, J.T. Targeting CK2 overexpression and hyperactivation as a novel therapeutic tool in chronic lymphocytic leukemia. *Blood* **2010**, *116*, 2724–2731. [CrossRef] [PubMed]

57. Simões R, V.; Delgado-Goñi, T.; Lope-Piedrafita, S.; Arús, C. 1H-MRSI pattern perturbation in a mouse glioma: the effects of acute hyperglycemia and moderate hypothermia. *NMR Biomed.* **2010**, *23*, 23–33. [CrossRef] [PubMed]

58. GraphPad. Available online: http://www.graphpad.com/ (accessed on 12 February 2017).

59. Martins, L.R.; Lúcio, P.; Melão, A.; Antunes, I.; Cardoso, B.; Stansfield, R.; Bertilaccio, M.T.S.; Ghia, P.; Drygin, D.; Silva, M.G.; et al. Activity of the clinical-stage CK2-specific inhibitor CX-4945 against chronic lymphocytic leukemia. *Leukemia* **2014**, *28*, 179–182. [CrossRef] [PubMed]

60. Web CEEAH. Available online: http://www.recerca.uab.es/ceeah (accessed on 12 February 2017).

61. Simões, R.V.; García-Martín, M.L.; Cerdán, S.; Arús, C. Perturbation of mouse glioma MRS pattern by induced acute hyperglycemia. *NMR Biomed.* **2008**, *21*, 251–264.

62. Saldaña-Ruíz, S.; Soler-Martín, C.; Llorens, J. Role of CYP2E1-mediated metabolism in the acute and vestibular toxicities of nineteen nitriles in the mouse. *Toxicol. Lett.* **2012**, *208*, 125–132. [CrossRef] [PubMed]

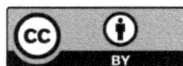

Chapter 3:
Structural insights

pharmaceuticals

MDPI

Article

Structural Hypervariability of the Two Human Protein Kinase CK2 Catalytic Subunit Paralogs Revealed by Complex Structures with a Flavonol- and a Thieno[2,3-d]pyrimidine-Based Inhibitor [†]

Karsten Niefind [1],*, Nils Bischoff [1], Andriy G. Golub [2], Volodymyr G. Bdzhola [3], Anatoliy O. Balanda [3], Andriy O. Prykhod'ko [3] and Sergiy M. Yarmoluk [3]

[1] Department für Chemie, Institut für Biochemie, Universität zu Köln, Otto-Fischer-Straße 12–14, D-50674 Köln, Germany; nils.bischoff@outlook.com

[2] Otava Ltd., 400 Applewood Crescent, Unit 100, Vaughan, ON L4K 0C3, Canada; andrew.golub@gmail.com

[3] Institute of Molecular Biology and Genetics, National Academy of Sciences of Ukraine, 150 Zabolotnogo Street, 03680 Kyiv, Ukraine; volodymyr_bdzhola@ukr.net (V.G.B.); b.anatolij@gmail.com (A.O.B.); a.o.prykhodko@gmail.com (A.O.P.); yarmolyuksm@gmail.com (S.M.Y.)

* Correspondence: Karsten.Niefind@uni-koeln.de; Tel.: +49-221-470-6444

† This publication is dedicated to Professor Dr. Olaf-Georg Issinger on the occasion of his 70th birthday.

Academic Editor: Mathias Montenarh

Received: 1 December 2016; Accepted: 5 January 2017; Published: 11 January 2017

Abstract: Protein kinase CK2 is associated with a number of human diseases, among them cancer, and is therefore a target for inhibitor development in industry and academia. Six crystal structures of either CK2α, the catalytic subunit of human protein kinase CK2, or its paralog CK2α' in complex with two ATP-competitive inhibitors—based on either a flavonol or a thieno[2,3-d]pyrimidine framework—are presented. The structures show examples for extreme structural deformations of the ATP-binding loop and its neighbourhood and of the hinge/helix αD region, i.e., of two zones of the broader ATP site environment. Thus, they supplement our picture of the conformational space available for CK2α and CK2α'. Further, they document the potential of synthetic ligands to trap unusual conformations of the enzymes and allow to envision a new generation of inhibitors that stabilize such conformations.

Keywords: protein kinase CK2; casein kinase 2; ATP-competitive inhibitors; halogen bond

1. Introduction

"The conformational plasticity of protein kinases" [1] and its correlation with regulation were described already in 2001. The authors of this review compared eukaryotic protein kinase (EPK) structures and identified significant local structural deviations. They emphasized in that context the activation segment and the long N-lobal helix αC as major flexible and thus regulatory key elements. At the same time the first complex structures of EPKs with pharmacologically relevant inhibitors were published [2,3] which demonstrated that the conformational plasticity of these enzymes is even higher than imagined before. The three inhibitors described in those studies bind their target kinases (c-Abl and p38 MAP kinase) in such a way that they address a region normally occupied by the phenylalanine side chain of the "DFG" sequence motif at the N-terminal end of the activation segment. Later these and similar local structural states were summarized as "DFG-out" conformations [4]. In subsequent years it was more and more realized that certain EPK inhibitors do not distort their target enzymes, but rather trap them in particular conformational states that are inherent parts of complex conformational equilibria [5]. Thus, besides their pharmaceutical relevance EPK inhibitors are tools to investigate the conformational space explored by the enzymes which is larger than assumed.

In this regard protein kinase CK2—a cell-stabilizing EPK [6] accumulating in cancer cells [7] that apparently exploit CK2 activity to escape apoptosis and to assist DNA repair [8]—seemed to be an exception. Since in all known CK2 crystal structures—irrespective of whether based on the isolated catalytic subunit CK2α or on the heterotetrameric CK2α$_2$β$_2$ holoenzyme—the activation segment and the helix αC obtain basically the same conformation which is characteristic for an active EPK [9]. Especially, conformations equivalent to the DFG-out states of other EPKs have never been observed with CK2α and are moreover unlikely because CK2α in all of its known ortho- and paralogs contains a DWG rather than a DFG motif at the beginning of the activation segment. The central tryptophan of this motif is stabilized by many more interactions than the DFG phenylalanine of other EPKs [10].

Thus, the classical conformational switches of EPKs are not used by CK2α which is consistent to its constitutively active nature [11]. However, gradually other parts of CK2α were found to be surprisingly structurally adaptable [12,13]. Primarily for the hinge/helix αD region of human CK2α two major conformations were described [14,15] which are in a dynamic equilibrium according to metadynamics simulations [16]. In crystal structures the occurrence of these hinge/helix αD conformations is not correlated to other local conformational flexibilities [17,18]; it depends on the nature of the ATP-site ligand and on the medium used for crystallization [19]. For the glycine-rich ATP-binding loop strong or even extreme distortions from the active conformation were found [20–22]. And in the β3/αC loop an absolutely conserved proline was detected that is able to switch to the *cis*-peptide configuration spontaneously [23].

Knowledge about the structural space the enzyme is able to explore and in particular about special local conformations in the proximity of its active site is relevant for ongoing efforts to develop highly potent and selective inhibitors of CK2 which might be beneficial to fight against hematological malignancies [24,25] as well as solid tumours [26,27]. Therefore, in this study we emphasize and extend those previous findings on local plasticities with a set of structures of both human CK2α paralogs showing partly extreme structural peculiarities. The structures were obtained by co-crystallization with two potent and selective (within a limited set of test EPKs [28,29]) ATP-competitive CK2 inhibitors: 4'-carboxy-6,8-dichloroflavonol (Figure 1a), a member of the flavonoid family of CK2 inhibitors [30] abbreviated as "FLC21" in the literature [28] and inhibiting the CK2α$_2$β$_2$ holoenzyme with an IC$_{50}$ of 40 nM and a K$_i$-value of 13 nM [28], and 3-{[5-(4-methylphenyl) thieno[2,3-d]pyrimidin-4-yl]thio}propanoic acid (Figure 1b)—referred to as "compound **6a**" in its original description [29] and "TTP22" in PUBCHEM (pubchem.ncbi.nlm.nih.gov/compound/ 1536915)—with an IC$_{50}$ of 100 nM and a K$_i$ of 40 nM [29].

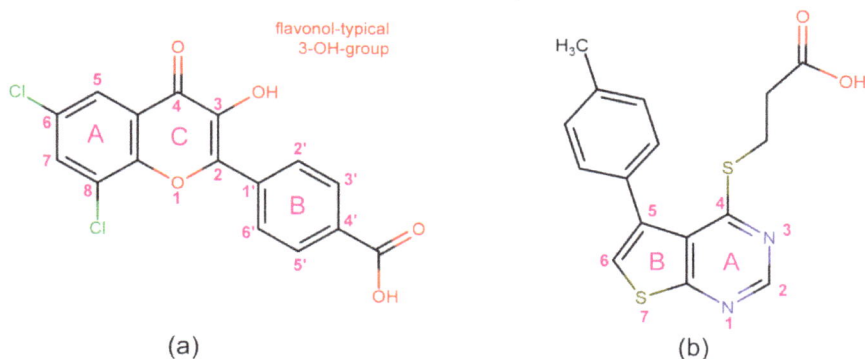

Figure 1. Structures of the ATP-competitive inhibitors FLC21 [28] (**a**); and TTP22 [29] (**b**) used for co-crystallization with human CK2α and/or CK2α′ constructs in this work. FLC26, the sister compound of FLC21 [22,28], which is used as a reference here (see Section 2.2), contains two bromo rather than chloro substituents at ring A attached to C-atoms 6 and 8.

2. Results and Discussion

2.1. Overview of the CK2α/CK2α′ Co-Crystal Structures

Six human CK2α/inhibitor crystal structures were determined (Table 1)—four with $CK2\alpha^{1-335}$, a recombinant C-terminally truncated version of the main paralog CK2α [31], and two with $CK2\alpha'^{Asp39Gly/Cys336Ser}$, a recombinant full-length construct of the isoform CK2α′ carrying an N-terminal (His)$_6$-tag and the two point mutations Asp39Gly and Cys336Ser [32] (it should be noted that Bischoff et al. [32] erroneously failed to mention the mutation Asp39Gly, i.e., the construct "*hs*CK2α′^{Cys336Ser}" referred to by Bischoff et al. [32] and tested in that work is identical with respect to the primary sequence to $CK2\alpha'^{Asp39Gly/Cys336Ser}$ used in this study). Notably, the two variants are unchanged in their active centre regions and in particular at the ATP cleft. Their K_M-values for ATP were reported to be 11.2 μM in the case of $CK2\alpha^{1-335}$ and 11.5 μM in the case of $CK2\alpha'^{Asp39Gly/Cys336Ser}$ [32]. For comparison: in an extensive review Tuazon and Traugh [33] collected K_M-values for ATP determined with 22 different non-recombinant CK2 or CK2α preparations from natural sources (mainly mammals, but in addition other vertebrates, insects, yeasts and plants); these K_M-values range from 2 to 31 μM with an average of 13.0 μM and a standard deviation of 8.0 μM. In other words: with respect to co-substrate affinity to ATP the recombinant and mutated CK2α/CK2α′ constructs used in this study are similar to wild-type CK2 and CK2α enzymes.

The two $CK2\alpha'^{Asp39Gly/Cys336Ser}$ structures and two of the $CK2\alpha^{1-335}$ structures contain FLC21 [28] (Figure 1a) as an ATP-site ligand which allows comparisons between the two human CK2α isoforms. Two further $CK2\alpha^{1-335}$ structures (No. 5 and 6 in Table 1) harbour TTP22 (Figure 1b) at the co-substrate binding site. Co-crystallization experiments of TTP22 were performed with $CK2\alpha'^{Asp39Gly/Cys336Ser}$ as well, but they did not provide crystals of sufficient quality for X-ray diffractometry.

The monoclinic $CK2\alpha'^{Asp39Gly/Cys336Ser}$/FLC21 complex crystals (No. 2 in Table 1) contain two independent copies of the enzyme per asymmetric unit while the five other structures consists of only one protomer. The structures are in general of high quality; in particular the bound inhibitor molecules are clearly defined by electron density. In all cases some N- and C-terminal residues which are not relevant for ligand binding at the ATP site are flexible and not visible in the electron density maps.

Table 1. Crystallization, X-ray diffraction data and refinement statistics.

Structure No.	1	2	3	4	5	6
PDB Code	5M4U	5M56	5M4F	5M4I	5M4C	5M44
Crystallization						
Crystallized complex	CK2α'$^{Asp39Gly/Cys336Ser}$ + FLC21	CK2α$^{1-335}$ + FLC21			CK2α$^{1-335}$ + TTP22	
Vapour diffusion reservoir composition	25% PEG5000 MME, 0.2 M ammonium sulphate, 0.1 M MES, pH 6.5	25% PEG4000, 15% glycerol, 0.17 M sodium acetate, 0.08 M Tris/HCl, pH 8.5	24% PEG3350, 0.2 M KCl	4.3 M NaCl, 0.1 M sodium citrate, pH 5.2	24% PEG8000, 0.2 M KCl	4.2 M NaCl, 0.1 M sodium citrate, pH 5.0
Sitting drop composition before equilibration	1 µL reservoir + 1 µL enzyme/FLC21 mixture (90 µL 5.5 mg/mL enzyme, 0.5 M NaCl, 25 mM Tris/HCl, pH 8.5, mixed and pre-equilibrated with 10 µL 10 mM FLC21 in DMSO)	1 µL reservoir + 1 µL enzyme/inhibitor mixture (90 µL 6 mg/mL enzyme, 0.5 M NaCl, 25 mM Tris/HCl, pH 8.5, mixed and pre-equilibrated with 10 µL 10 mM inhibitor in DMSO)				
X-ray Diffraction Data Collection						
Wavelength (Å)	1.0000	1.0000	0.91841	0.91841	1.0000	1.54179
Synchrotron (beamline)	SLS (X06DA)	SLS (X06DA)	HZB BESSY II (MX-14.1 [34])	HZB BESSY II (MX-14.1 [34])	SLS (X06DA)	Home source (rot. Cu anode)
Space group	P2$_1$2$_1$2$_1$	P2$_1$	P2$_1$2$_1$2$_1$	P4$_3$2$_1$2	P2$_1$2$_1$2$_1$	P4$_3$2$_1$2
Unit cell · a, b, c (Å)	46.85, 83.78, 142.34	69.34, 87.62, 72.98	48.03, 79.57, 82.14	72.59, 72.59, 133.25	48.10, 79.42, 82.34	72.06, 72.06, 131.58
Unit cell · α, β, γ (°)	90.0, 90.0, 90.0	90, 109.69, 90	90.0, 90.0, 90.0	90.0, 90.0, 90.0	90.0, 90.0, 90.0	90.0, 90.0, 90.0
Protomers per asymmetric unit	1	2	1	1	1	1
Resolution (Å) (highest res. shell)	44.50–2.195 (2.274–2.195) [1]	40.94–2.237 (2.317–2.237) [1]	41.12–1.519 (1.574–1.519) [1]	37.89–2.218 (2.297–2.218) [1]	41.14–1.935 (2.004–1.935) [1]	27.84–2.710 (2.807–2.710) [1]
R$_{sym}$ (%)	19.1 (118.5) [1]	9.3 (65.7) [1]	5.9 (78.7) [1]	11.1 (116.9) [1]	9.8 (73.1) [1]	13.1 (80.8) [1]
CC1/2	0.993 (0.684) [1]	0.996 (0.685) [1]	0.999 (0.661) [1]	0.999 (0.616) [1]	0.998 (0.758) [1]	0.996 (0.693) [1]
Signal-to-noise ratio (I/σ$_I$)	9.99 (1.72) [1]	9.76 (1.78) [1]	15.82 (1.89) [1]	15.35 (1.84) [1]	15.25 (2.26) [1]	15.75 (2.32) [1]
No. of unique refl.	29246 (2680) [1]	39,108 (3544) [1]	49,151 (4808) [1]	18,350 (1795) [1]	23,280 (1476) [1]	9935 (947) [1]
Completeness (%)	99.0 (93.0) [1]	98.0 (90.0) [1]	100.0 (99.0) [1]	100.0 (100.0) [1]	96.0 (62.0) [1]	100.0 (98.0) [1]
Multiplicity	6.4 (5.6) [1]	3.3 (2.9) [1]	4.1 (4.0) [1]	7.9 (7.9) [1]	6.3 (5.2) [1]	6.9 (5.9) [1]
Wilson B-fact (Å^2)	21.44	29.76	15.41	36.83	21.84	40.32
Structure Refinement and Validation						
No. of reflections for R$_{work}$/R$_{free}$	1142	37,938/1161	48,116/1031	17,314/1034	22,177/1104	8979/956
R$_{work}$/R$_{free}$ (%)	21.41/17.04	16.35/20.64	16.28/18.26	18.80/22.83	15.64/19.68	21.86/25.94
Number of non-H-atoms	3175	5987	3248	2936	3069	2820
Protein	2789	5537	2821	2798	2806	2782
Ligand/ion	71	72	43	28	35	27
Water	315	378	384	110	228	11
Aver. B-factor (Å^2)	28.61	38.76	20.89	52.22	28.55	52.32
Protein	27.33	38.57	19.30	52.64	28.01	52.52
Ligand/ion	43.49	40.20	26.19	45.09	27.14	44.05
water	36.62	41.20	31.95	43.45	35.37	22.12
RMS deviations						
Bond lengths (Å)	0.003	0.002	0.014	0.002	0.009	0.002
Bond angles (°)	0.570	0.50	1.28	0.46	0.96	0.45
Ramachandran plot						
favoured (%)	97.0	95.9	97.9	96.4	97.6	95.4
allowed (%)	2.7	3.8	1.8	3.6	2.1	4.0
outliers (%)	0.3	0.3	0.3	0.0	0.3	0.6

[1] Values in brackets refer to the highest resolution shell.

2.2. Complex Structures with FLC21

2.2.1. General Binding Mode of FLC21 to CK2α/CK2α'

For the binding of FLC21 to CK2α two types of advance information existed:

- Golub et al. [28] modelled FLC21 bound to CK2α as shown in Figure 2a. This CK2α/FLC21 complex model is based on a set of four predicted ionic, hydrogen bond and π/π interactions (Figure 2b). These interactions were assumed to be formed by the B and the C-ring of the flavone framework and its substituents whereas the A-ring with the two chloro atoms were supposed to be not involved.

- Guerra et al. [22] published two complex structures (PDB 4UBA and 4UB7) of CK2α[1–335] with FLC26 [28] which is the sister compound of FLC21 containing bromo rather than chloro substituents attached to the C-atoms 6 and 8 (Figure 1a). These structures revealed that the inhibitor was in fact bound to the enzyme in the predicted orientation and with exactly the set of non-covalent interactions suggested in Figure 2b.

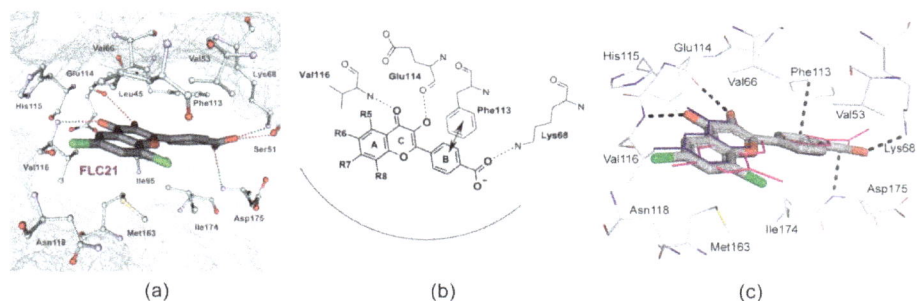

(a)	(b)	(c)

Figure 2. Binding mode of FLC21 to the ATP site of CK2α and CK2α'. (**a**) Section of a modelled CK2α/FLC21 complex as published by Golub et al. [28]. The picture is identical to Figure 6 in [28] © Springer Science + Business Media, LLC. 2011, and is reproduced with permission of Springer; (**b**) the four basic non-covalent interactions underlying the predicted model. The drawing is identical with Figure 1 in [28], © Springer Science+Business Media, LLC. 2011, reproduced with permission of Springer; (**c**) Section of a low-salt CK2α[1–335]/FLC21 complex (structure 3 in Table 1) drawn in an equivalent orientation and with a similar style as in Figure 2a in order to facilitate the comparison between the two pictures. The FLC21 ligands of structures 1, 2 and 4 (Table 1) were drawn with thin bonds after superimposition of the respective protein matrices.

In order to characterize the binding mode of FLC21 we superimposed the five protomers of structures 1 to 4 in Table 1. As illustrated in Figure 2c the FLC21 ligands bind in identical orientations and very similar conformations irrespective of the CK2α paralog used, the crystallization condition and the crystal packing. Merely, under high-salt conditions (structure 4) the carboxy group of FLC21 and its B ring are no longer nearly coplanar (as in the other structures) but rotated against one another by about 48 degrees (magenta-coloured ligand in Figure 2c). Taken together, as observed before for FLC26 [22] the principle position and orientation of FLC21 within the ATP site and its main interactions with the enzyme are identical to the predictions of Golub et al. [28] (Figure 2a,b).

2.2.2. A π-Halogen Bond Enabled by an Extremely Distorted ATP-Binding Loop

4'-Carboxyflavonol, the non-halogenated precursor compound of FLC21 and FLC26, is able to form all interactions indicated in Figure 2b and has an IC_{50} for CK2α$_2$β$_2$ holoenzyme inhibition of 1.3 μM [28]. The introduction of halogen substituents at positions 6 and 8 lowers this value significantly. The reported IC$_{50}$ data are 0.18 μM and 0.08 μM for the mono-halogenated compounds 6-chloro-4′-carboxyflavonol and 6-bromo-4′-carboxyflavonol as well as 0.04 μM and 0.008 μM for the di-halogenated inhibitors FLC21 and FLC26 [28]. In other words: to substitute the 6- and the 8-position with halogen atoms increases the inhibitory power although these halogen substituents point away from the hinge/helix αD region and are thus—unlike those of many typical halogenated EPK inhibitors [35]—unable to form halogen bonds with the peptide backbone (Figure 2a,b); a further conclusion from the inhibition data is that introducing bromine is more effective than chlorine.

For FLC26 these observations were rationalized with the two aforementioned complex structures 4UB7 and 4UBA [22]. One of these structures—obtained from high-salt crystallization conditions—showed a π-halogen bond between the Br8-atom and the aromatic ring of the Tyr50 which was only possible after a dramatic conformational change of the ATP-binding loop (Figure 3a). With low-salt crystallization conditions this π-halogen bond was absent in the crystalline state but kinetic studies [22] suggested that it nevertheless contributes to the inhibitory efficacy of FLC26 in the solute state.

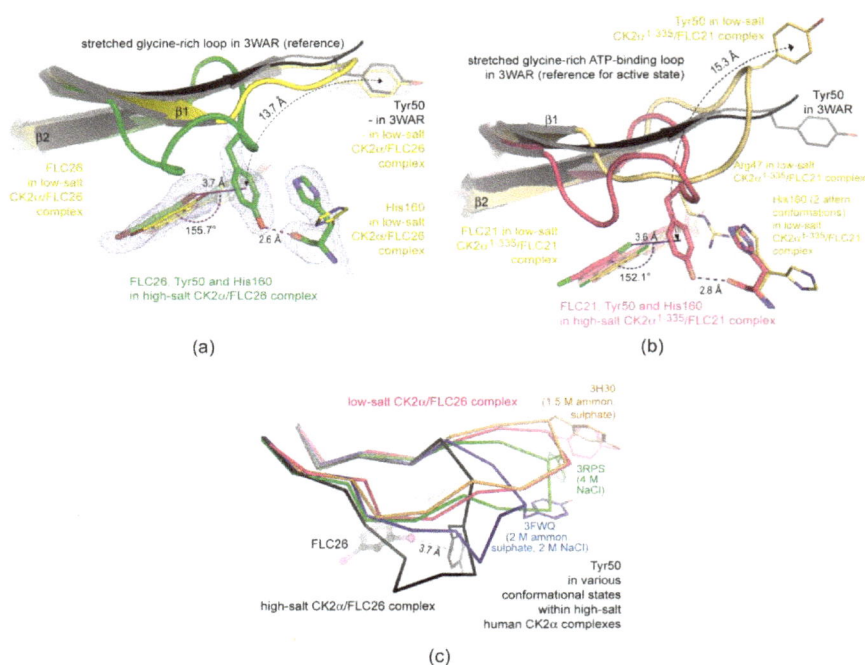

(a)

(b)

(c)

Figure 3. Formation of a kosmotropic-salt supported π-halogen bond between either FLC21 or FLC26 and CK2α$^{1-335}$. (**a**) FLC26: Under high-salt crystallization conditions Tyr50 at the tip of the ATP-binding loop bends down to the Br8 atom of FLC26 (π-halogen bond) and His160 (hydrogen bond); (**b**) In the case of FLC21 the same phenomenon is found under high-salt conditions (structure 4 of Table 1; parts with magenta-coloured C-atoms). Under low-salt conditions (structure 3 of Table 1; parts with yellow C-atoms) Arg47 replaces Tyr50 in the space between FLC21 and His160 which was not observed for FLC26; (**c**) ATP-binding loops in human CK2α structures obtained from various high-salt crystallization conditions. The strong distortion of the ATP-binding loop observed in the complexes with FLC26 and FLC21 is not exclusively caused by the high salt concentration since it was never found in any high-salt structure of CK2α published previously. Parts (**a**) and (**c**) of the figure are reprinted with kind permission from Guerra et al. [22]. Copyright (2015) American Chemical Society.

One aim of the study presented here was to test if FLC21 with its chloro instead of bromo substituents can form this remarkable π-halogen bond as well. An answer to this question is given in Figure 3: the high-salt CK2α$^{1-335}$/FLC21 structure (magenta-coloured structure in Figure 3b; No. 4 in Table 1) is very similar to the CK2α$^{1-335}$/FLC26 structure (green structure in Figure 3a) and contains in particular—and in contrast to its low-salt pendant (No. 3 in Table 1)—the π-halogen bond with Tyr50 in question. This π-halogen bond requires an extreme distortion of the ATP-binding loop (Figure 3c) which is found—with exception of the high-salt CK2α$^{1-335}$/FLC26 structure (Figure 3a)—in no other previously reported CK2α structure, in particular in none of the known high-salt structures (Figure 3c). Obviously, neither a properly located halogen substituent nor a high concentration of a kosmotropic salt alone is sufficient to establish this particular arrangement. Rather, both conditions must be matched simultaneously to capture this feature.

2.2.3. FLC21 Traps the Gly-Rich Loop Arginine of CK2α and CK2α' in a Non-Functional Conformation

While the high-salt CK2α$^{1-335}$ structures of FLC21 and FLC26 resemble each other right up to atomic details, there is a conspicuous local difference between the two low-salt structures: in the low-salt CK2α$^{1-335}$/FLC26 structure (yellow structure in Figure 3a) the glycine-rich ATP-binding loop adopts a stretched conformation resembling the atomic resolution CK2α apo structure 3WAR [36] (black structure in Figure 3a); in contrast in complex with FLC21 Arg47, a loop member flanked by two glycine residues and thus conferred with a significant adaptability, is bent down towards the C-terminal domain (Figures 3b and 4a) where it forms hydrogen bonds to His160 and Asn161 (Figure 4b).

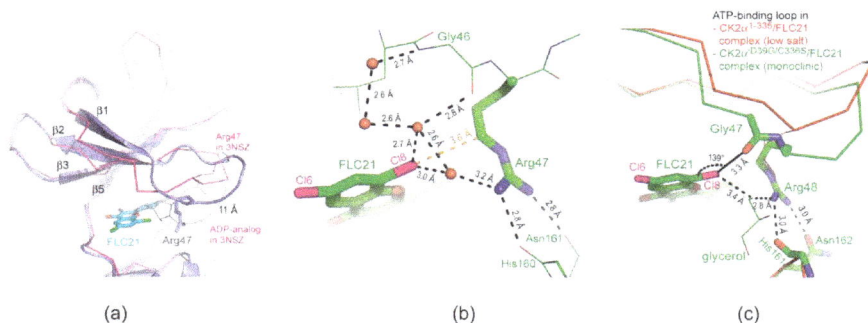

Figure 4. Arg47/48 and FLC21 stabilize a non-functional conformation of the ATP-binding loop. (**a**) The N-terminal domain of the low-salt CK2α$^{1-335}$/FLC21 complex (purple; structure 3 in Table 1) and for comparison (in order to illustrate the functional state of the ATP-binding loop) of PDB-file 3NSZ which contains human CK2α$^{2-331}$ in complex with an ADP-analog [37]; (**b**) More detailed and focused view of the low-salt CK2α$^{1-335}$/FLC21 complex in which the hydrogen-bonds of Gly46, Arg47 and the Cl8-atom of FLC21 are highlighted. The nearest atomic distance between FLC21 and Arg47 is indicated in orange colour. Four water molecules are drawn as red balls; (**c**) the equivalent region in protomer B of the monoclinic CK2α'$^{Asp39Gly/Cys336Ser}$/FLC21 complex structure (No. 2 in Table 1). For comparison the ATP-binding loop plus Arg47 side chain of the low-salt CK2α$^{1-335}$/FLC21 complex (structure 3 in Table 1) is drawn in red colour. Note that due to a one residue insertion near the N-terminus the sequence numbers in human CK2α' are shifted by +1 compared to human CK2α.

This is a non-functional state of the ATP-binding loop because the Arg47 side chain interferes with the ribose region of the canonical ATP site (Figure 4a). FLC21 seems to support this local conformation since it is present in the two FLC21 complex structures with CK2α'$^{Asp39Gly/Cys336Ser}$ (No. 1 and 2 in Table 1) as well albeit with more internal flexibility, i.e., less well defined electron densities. So far this "Arg47-down" conformation did not occur in complexes with FLC26; if this reflects a significant difference between FLC21 and FLC26 (which cannot be clarified currently due to the limited number of complex structures with FLC26), this would be surprising because it is the Cl8 atom of FLC21 that is in atomic contact to the Arg47 side chain (Arg48 in CK2α′) and because bromine—the Cl8 equivalent in FLC26—generally forms stronger halogen bonds than chlorine [38].

In fact, a closer inspection of the two best defined cases of the FLC21-Arg47/48 arrangement shows that halogen bonding plays a role as a stabilizing factor but that it is not the only one:

- In the low-salt CK2α$^{1-335}$/FLC21 structure a network of hydrogen bonds around the Cl8 atom stabilizes the conformation; the propensity to operate as hydrogen bond acceptor is for chloro in fact higher than for bromo substituents (Figure 4b).

- Figure 4c was drawn from one of the two protomers of the monoclinic CK2α′$^{Asp39Gly/Cys336Ser}$ complex structure with FLC21. Here, the Arg48 side chain is hydrogen-bonded to His161 and Asn162 (the CK2α′ equivalents of His160 and Asn161 in CK2α) similar to what is seen in Figure 4b. However, in addition the Cl8 atom forms a geometrically well-established halogen bond with a peptide oxygen of the ATP-binding loop, namely the peptide group connecting Gly47 and Arg48 (Figure 4c). There is no reason to believe that FLC26 binding cannot support such a particular state via a halogen bond as well; co-crystallization efforts of FLC26 with CK2α′$^{Asp39Gly/Cys336Ser}$ might clarify this.

A similar halogen bond, namely between an inhibitor and the backbone of the ATP-binding loop, was not observed in any CK2α/CK2α′ structure before.

2.2.4. Prolyl *cis/trans*-Isomerization at the β3/αC Loop

Just like the π-halogen bonds with FLC26 and FLC21 visible in Figure 3a,b, respectively, the unusual halogen bond illustrated in Figure 4c requires a strong deformation of the ATP-binding loop which is only possible if the β2-strand is partly resolved from the next strand (β3) of the canonical N-lobal β-sheet. This reduction of strands β1 and β2 and the inclination of the interconnecting ATP-binding loop away from the canonical β-sheet are illustrated in Figure 5a.

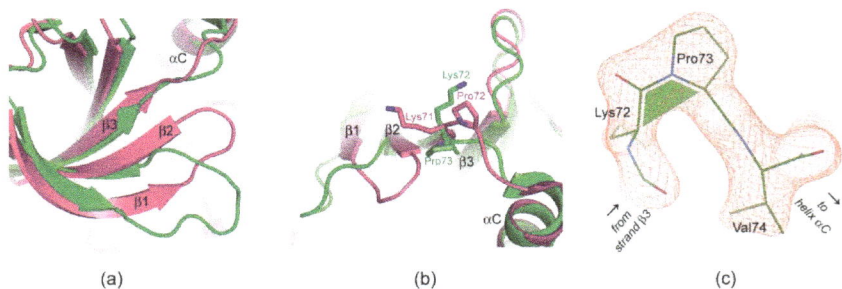

(a) (b) (c)

Figure 5. Strong deformations of the ATP-binding loop of CK2α/CK2α′ can be correlated with *cis*-peptide formation at the central proline residue of the β3/αC loop. (**a,b**) Overlay of protomer B of the monoclinic CK2α′$^{Asp39Gly/Cys336Ser}$/FLC21 complex structure (structure 2 in Table 1; green) and a high-resolution structure of human CK2α$^{2-331}$ in complex with an ADP-analogue (PDB 3NSZ [37]; magenta). The canonical β-sheet of the N-terminal domain is drawn in two different orientations; (**c**) the β3/αC loop in protomer B of the monoclinic CK2α′$^{Asp39Gly/Cys336Ser}$/FLC21 complex structure covered by electron density (cutoff level 1.5 σ).

In this context the C-terminal part of the neighbouring strand β3 is particularly critical. Here, the final residue Lys72 (Lys71 in CK2α) normally stabilizes the functional conformation of the ATP-binding loop first by a β-sheet-typical main chain/main chain hydrogen bond and second by stretching its side chain over the strand β2 as visible in Figure 5b. Without these contacts Lys71/72 is free for structural alternatives. It can even force its extended side chain into a completely different direction (Figure 5b) which is accomplished by a *cis*-peptide bond with the succeeding proline residue, the central residue of the β3/αC loop (Figure 5c). A cis-peptide bond at the equivalent position was observed only once before, namely in a CK2α[1-335] structure with a cyclic peptide bound to the CK2β interface [23]. Here, it occurs—well documented by electron density (Figure 5c)—in protomer B of the CK2α'[Asp39Gly/Cys336Ser]/FLC21 complex structure, i.e., for the first time with CK2α' and remarkably enough in correlation with a novel halogen bond (Figure 4c) and with the strongest ATP-binding loop deviation in any CK2α/CK2α' structure obtained so far under low-salt crystallization conditions.

In summary, the two halogenated flavonol compounds FLC21 and FLC26 [28] dispose of a remarkable potential to trap and stabilize CK2α/CK2α' in extraordinary conformations characterized by extreme deviations of the ATP-binding loop and by unusual halogen bonds between this loop and the inhibitor. So far, this was already known for the bromo compound FLC26 [22], but only for a single structure of human CK2α obtained from largely artificial high-salt crystallization conditions. The results reported here confirm this impression; more important, they extend it to the chloro compound FLC21 on the inhibitor side, to the paralog CK2α' on the protein side, to the structural environment of the ATP-binding loop (β3/αC-loop) and finally to low-salt crystallization conditions that are significantly closer to the physiological milieu.

2.2.5. The Hinge/Helix αD Region Harbours a Novel αD Site

A second remarkable detail of Figure 4c—apart from the novel FLC21/Gly47 halogen bond—is a glycerol molecule that acquires the role of a water molecule to form a hydrogen bond bridge between FLC21 and the side chain of Arg48. At a first glance this is not more than an artefact from the cryo solution used to prepare the monoclinic CK2α'[Asp39Gly/Cys336Ser]/FLC21 complex crystals for X-ray diffractometry. However, this observation gains stronger significance in the light of Figure 6a that is overtaken from a recent study by Brear et al. [39]. These authors crystallized a human CK2α construct (with an *N*-terminal extension which is not relevant in this context) together with the small benzene derivative 2-(3,4-dichlorophenyl)ethanamine. They found this fragment attached to several sites (Figure 6a), among them crystal contacts but also inherent binding sites of the enzyme.

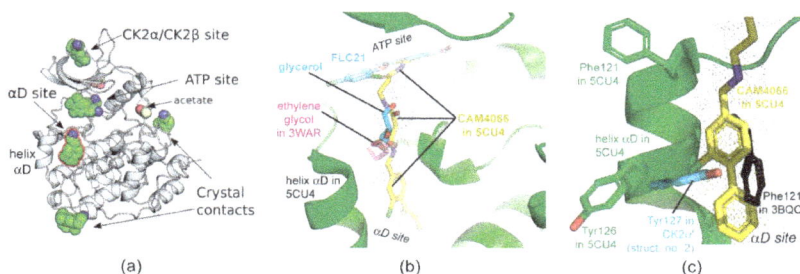

(a)   (b)   (c)

Figure 6. Molecular fragments at a novel αD site, at the ATP site and along the interconnecting path. (**a**) Brear et al. [39] found 2-(3,4-dichlorophenyl)ethanamine (green balls for carbon atoms) at several cavities of CK2α and identified in this way the αD site. The picture was taken and slightly modified from [39], published by The Royal Society of Chemistry; (**b**) Section of a complex structure of CK2α with the bivalent inhibitor CAM4066 (PDB 5CU4 [39], CAM4066 with yellow carbon atoms). After structural superimposition elements of PDB file 3WAR [36] (ethylene glycol, magenta coloured *C*-atoms) and of chain B of the monoclinic CK2α'[Asp39Gly/Cys336Ser]/FLC21 complex (light blue *C*-atoms) are drawn; (**c**) The αD site is occupied by Phe121 in CK2α structures with closed hinge/helix αD conformation (here represented by 3BQC; black) or partially by Tyr126 (Tyr127 in CK2α'; here drawn in light blue from structure 2 of Table 1) in structures with open hinge/helix αD conformation. αD site ligands like CAM4066 replace both of them.

Most interesting is a novel "αD site" behind the small helix αD (Figure 6a) and with access to the ATP site. Brear et al. [39] noticed that ethylene glycol can occupy the entrance region of the αD site (found in PDB 3WAR [36]) and exploited all findings about molecular fragments to design the bivalent CK2 inhibitor CAM4066. CAM4066 occupies the ATP site and the αD site simultaneously (Figure 6b). An overlay of a CK2α/CAM4066 co-crystal structure (PDB 5CU4) with chain B of the monoclinic CK2α$^{/Asp39Gly/Cys336Ser}$/FLC21 reveals that the aforementioned glycerol molecule is attached to the connecting path between the two sites (Figure 6b). Thus, it supplements the set of molecular fragments that can be combined to similar bivalent inhibitors.

The αD site is a consequence of a structural flexibility of the hinge/helix αD region that was noticed some years ago [9,12,15]. Two main local conformations were identified and interpreted in the light of the spine concept for EPK regulation [18,40], the less frequent "closed" conformation in which Phe121 is an integral part of a stack of hydrophobic residues called "catalytic spine" [41] and the predominant "open" conformation with Tyr126 (Tyr127 in CK2α') occupying at least partially the spine region (Figure 6c). Based on these crystallographic findings Klopffleisch et al. [19] anticipated that there is "a dynamic conformational equilibrium in solution that can be resolved by suitable ligands." Brear et al. [39] were the first now to identify such ligands and to demonstrate their potential for selective inhibition of CK2. In the sense of spine concept one can say: these compounds replace either Phe121 or Tyr126 from their catalytic spine locations, complete the catalytic spine themselves and create thus the αD site.

2.3. Complex Structures with TTP22

2.3.1. CK2α Binds TTP22 as Predicted under Low-Salt, but Differently under High-Salt Conditions

Like FLC21, TTP22 (Figure 1b) was theoretically docked to CK2α in the original description of the compound [29]. The carboxy group of the TTP22 molecule was assumed to form hydrogen bonds to Lys68 and to Asp175 (Figure 7a) in a similar way as FLC21 (Figure 2a). A further predicted anchor point was the N1-atom within the pyrimidine ring A which was supposed to be hydrogen bonded to the hinge backbone (Val116). The thienopropionic acid substituent has an optimal length to allow all three hydrogen bonds simultaneously [29]. In this orientation the aromatic substituent of the B-ring points to the solvent but is nevertheless flanked by some hydrophobic side chains as visible in Figure 7a.

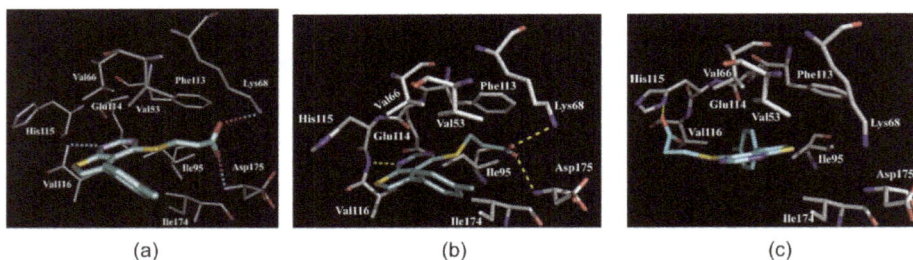

(a)   (b)   (c)

Figure 7. Comparison of modelled and experimental complex structures of TTP22 with CK2α. (a) In-silico model of a CK2α/TTP22 complex [29]. The picture was reproduced from Golub et al. [29] with kind permission by Elsevier B.V; (b) The same section and orientation as in (a), but now obtained from the experimental low-salt CK2α$^{1–335}$/TTP22 complex structure (No. 5 of Table 1); (c) The same section and orientation as in (a) and (b), but now obtained from the experimental high-salt CK2α$^{1–335}$/TTP22 complex structure (No. 6 of Table 1). Pictures (b) and (c) were designed in a similar style as panel (a) in order to enable easy comparisons.

A look at the low-salt $CK2\alpha^{1-335}$/TTP22 structure (No. 5 of Table 1) revealed that this prediction including all three hydrogen bonds was essentially correct. To illustrate this fact we designed a figure (Figure 7b) with the same orientation, structural elements and background as in Figure 7a. However, in contrast to FLC21 the binding mode of TTP22 changes dramatically under high-salt conditions (Figure 7c). Compared to the low-salt state the inhibitor turned by about 180 degrees around an axis perpendicular to the plane formed by rings A and B (Figure 8a). In this way the carboxy moiety is no longer in the proximity of Lys68, but now of the interdomain hinge member His115 (Figure 7c). Concerning the charges this makes sense because at the pH-value of the crystallization medium (about 5.0) the His115 side chain is protonated and positively charged while the carboxy group of TTP22 is still deprotonated. Vice versa, the methylphenyl substituent of ring B changes its direction from outside to inside. It is now (i.e., under high-salt conditions) perfectly embedded in a hydrophobic environment (Figure 8b). This observation fits nicely to the well-known fact that hydrophobic interactions are supported by kosmotropic salts that interact strongly with water and disturb thus the ordered water shell around hydrophobic patches in an aqueous environment.

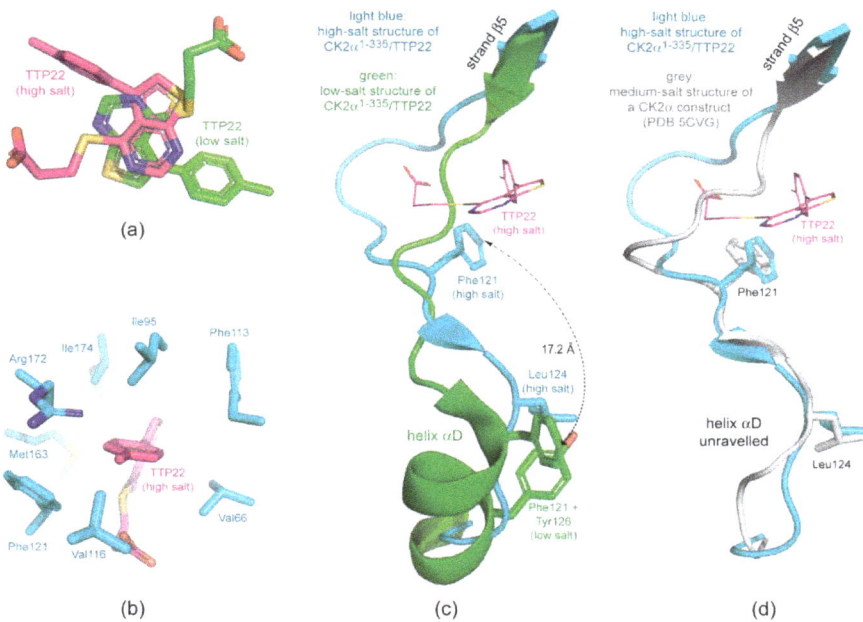

Figure 8. Structural differences between the high-salt and the low-salt $CK2\alpha^{1-335}$/TTP22 complex. (**a**) The inhibitor TTP22 bound to $CK2\alpha^{1-335}$ under low-salt conditions (structure 5 of Table 1; magenta-coloured C-atoms) and under high-salt conditions (structure 6 of Table 1; green C-atoms) after superimposition of the protein matrices; (**b**) Cage of hydrophobic side chains or side chains with an aliphatic part (Arg172) surrounding the methylphenyl moiety of TTP22 under high-salt conditions; (**c**) Comparison of the hinge/helix αD region of the low-salt (green) and the high-salt (light blue) $CK2\alpha^{1-335}$/TTP22 structure; (**d**) Comparison of the hinge/helix αD region of the high-salt $CK2\alpha^{1-335}$/TTP22 structure (light blue) and a recently published medium-salt CK2α structure with unraveled helix αD (PDB 5CVG [39]).

2.3.2. TTP22 Traps CK2α with an Unraveled Helix αD under High-Salt Conditions

A conspicuous feature in Figure 8b is the fact that Phe121 is part of the hydrophobic cage around the methylphenyl substituent of TTP22. This is quite surprising because it requires a movement of Phe121 by more than 17 Å compared to the low-salt CK2α^{1-335}/TTP22 complex (Figure 8c). In this low-salt structure Phe121 has its typical and well known position of an open hinge/helix αD conformation while Tyr126 occupies—also quite usual—the catalytic spine cavity (i.e., the αD site according to Brear et al. [39]). According to all experiences obtained so far (see in particular the analysis of Klopffleisch et al. [19]) a change to a high-salt medium should induce a switch to the closed hinge/helix αD conformation in which Phe121 completes the catalytic spine and harbours its side chain in the αD site (see black side chain in Figure 6c).

In the high-salt CK2α^{1-335}/TTP22 structure, however, something different happens: Phe121 moves as indicated in Figure 8c and gets in contact to the methylphenyl moiety of the inhibitor. Simultaneously Leu124 occupies the catalytic spine position (αD site) (Figure 8c). These drastic changes are only possible if the helix αD is completely unraveled as visible in Figure 8c. When we observed this instance of "hypervariability" of the hinge/helix αD region we first considered it as an interesting but completely artificial feature induced by the combination by the high salt concentration (>4 M NaCl) and a suitable ligand. However, in the recent publication by Brear et al. [39] a similar conformation with Phe121 and Leu124 at equivalent positions was reported (Figure 8d). This structure (PDB 5CVG) was obtained from crystals grown with a non-salt precipitant albeit with a significant addition (0.75 M) of ammonium acetate. Insofar it is possible, that such extreme conformations of the hinge/helix αD region belong to the normal conformational space explored by CK2α and that it just requires suitable ligands and crystallization conditions to trap them.

The hinge/helix αD region of CK2α was a discussion point already in the very first CK2 structure publication [42]. Since that time it has caused surprises repeatedly, and it seems as if it continues to do so. In particular, recent developments allow the vision that the unique nature of this region compared to other EPKs can be exploited to design CK2 inhibitors of high selectivity.

3. Materials and Methods

3.1. CK2 Inhibitors

The CK2 inhibitors FLC21 and TTP22 were synthesized as described previously [28,29].

3.2. Proteins

The two enzyme constructs CK2α^{1-335} and CK2$\alpha'^{Asp39Gly/Cys336Ser}$ were prepared as described previously [15,32]. In the case of CK2$\alpha'^{Asp39Gly/Cys336Ser}$ it should be noted that the point mutation Cys336Ser was planed to improve the protein solubility while the Asp39Gly mutation occurred unintendedly during PCR and was overlooked in spite of sequencing. Nevertheless the construct CK2$\alpha'^{Asp39Gly/Cys336Ser}$ was used here because it showed significant catalytic activity with a K_M-value for ATP of 11.5 µM [32] which is comparable to wild-type CK2 and CK2α preparations [33] and because the mutated position is remote from the ATP site and its environment (see more detailled discussion in Section 2.1). The proteins were stored in stock solutions containing 500 mM NaCl, 25 mM Tris/HCl, pH 8.5, as a background. The final protein mass concentrations (determined via UV-absorption at 280 nm) were 6.0 mg/mL for CK2α^{1-335} and 5.5 mg/mL for CK2$\alpha'^{Asp39Gly/Cys336Ser}$.

3.3. Crystallization

As indicated in Table 1 the crystallization efforts began in either case with mixing 90 µL protein solution with 10 µL 10 mM inhibitor (FLC21 or TTP22) solution in DMSO, incubating this mixture for at least 30 min at room temperature or—in the case of structure 3 of Table 1—on ice. After incubation precipitated material was removed by centrifucation. For crystallization according to the sitting drop variant of the vapour diffusion method 1 µL pre-incubated protein/inhibitor solution was mixed with 1 µL, respectively, of various reservoir solutions. All CK2α^{1-335} crystallization drops equilibrated at 20 °C and all CK2$\alpha'^{Asp39Gly/Cys336Ser}$ crystallization drops at 4 °C. Optimal crystal growth was observed with the reservoir compositions given in Table 1.

3.4. X-Ray Diffractometry

The CK2α^{1-335}/inhibitor and CK2$\alpha'^{Asp39Gly/Cys336Ser}$/inhibitor crystals were flash frozen in liquid nitrogen and mounted for X-ray diffractometry at 100 K. The CK2α^{1-335} crystals grown under high-salt conditions (structures 4 and 6 of Table 1) were directly transferred to liquid nitrogen without a special cryo colution. In the other four cases cryo solutions were prepared which were basically the reservoir solution, respectively, enriched with glycerol and through which the crystals were shortly drawn prior to the transfer to liquid nitrogen. The final glycerol concentrations of the cryo solutions were 20% (v/v) for structure 1 of Table 1, 25% (v/v) for structure 2 and 15% (v/v) for structures 3 and 5.

X-ray diffraction data were measured with a microfocus rotating copper anode X-ray diffractometer (MicroMax-007 from Rigaku, Tokyo, Japan) and with three synchrotron beamlines (beamline ID23-1 at the ESRF in Grenoble, France, beamline X06DA at the Swiss Light Source, Paul Scherrer Institut, in Villigen, Switzerland, and beamline MX-14.1 of HZB BESSY II, Helmholtz-Zentrum Berlin, Germany). Final diffraction data sets were collected as indicated in Table 1. All diffraction data sets were processed with XDS [43] for indexing and integration and with AIMLESS and CTRUNCATE of the CCP4 software package [44] for scaling and conversion to structure factor amplitudes.

3.5. Structure Solution, Refinement, Validation and Deposition

The structures were solved by molecular replacement with PHASER [45] and refined and validated with PHENIX [46]. The inhibitor ligands FLC21 and TTP22 were parameterised with PRODRG [47]. Manual corrections were performed with COOT [48]. The final structures were deposited at the Protein Data Bank and are available under the accession codes indicated in Table 1.

3.6. Illustration

Figure 5c was drawn with COOT [48]. All other illustrations—if not taken from the sources indicated in the respective figure legends—were prepared with PYMOL [49].

4. Conclusions

Previous analyses [9] have shown that CK2α—in spite of a conspicuous overall rigidity in comparison to other EPKs—has structurally rather variable regions. One of them—the ATP-binding loop—is well-known among EPKs for its conformational adaptability, another—the hinge/helix αD region—is in this respect unique for CK2α. The results presented here intensify this picture. They document structural snapshots reflecting, confirming and partially explaining a hypervariability in these two zones that only emerged in recent years. These findings are undoubtedly relevant for the development of CK2 inhibitors: they offer new strategies to improve selectivity by the combination of binding sites as already shown [39] or by stabilizing the enzyme in unique non-functional states and thus pave the way to a new generation of CK2 inhibitors.

Acknowledgments: We thank the staff of the synchrotron beamlines involved in the work (beamline ID23-1 at the ESRF in Grenoble, France, beamline X06DA at the Swiss Light Source, Paul Scherrer Institut, in Villigen, Switzerland, and beamline MX-14.1 of HZB BESSY II, Helmholtz-Zentrum Berlin, Germany) for support and assistance with X-ray data collection. We are grateful to Günter Schwarz and Ulrich Baumann (both University of Cologne, Germany) for access to protein crystallography equipment. The work was funded by the National Academy of Sciences of Ukraine (grants 0107U003345, 0107U003345 and 0112U004110) and the Deutsche Forschungsgemeinschaft (grants NI 643/4-1 and NI 643/4-2).

Author Contributions: K.N., N.B., A.G.G., V.G.B. and S.M.Y. conceived and designed the experiments; N.B. prepared the proteins and performed the crystallographic experiments; N.B. and K.N. analyzed the data; A.O.B. and A.O.P. contributed reagents and materials; K.N. wrote the paper.

Conflicts of Interest: The authors declare no conflict of interest.

References

1. Huse, M.; Kuriyan, J. The conformational plasticity of protein kinases. *Cell* **2002**, *109*, 275–282. [CrossRef]
2. Nagar, B.; Bornmann, W.G.; Pellicena, P.; Schindler, T.; Veach, D.R.; Miller, W.T.; Clarkson, B.; Kuriyan, J. Crystal structures of the kinase domain of c-Abl in complex with the small molecule inhibitors PD173955 and imatinib (STI-571). *Cancer Res.* **2002**, *62*, 4236–4243. [PubMed]
3. Pargellis, C.; Tong, L.; Churchill, L.; Cirillo, P.F.; Gilmore, T.; Graham, A.G.; Grob, P.M.; Hickey, E.R.; Moss, N.; Pav, S.; et al. Inhibition of p38 MAP kinase by utilizing a novel allosteric binding site. *Nat. Struct. Biol.* **2002**, *9*, 268–272. [CrossRef] [PubMed]
4. Bukhtiyarova, M.; Karpusas, M.; Northrop, K.; Namboodiri, H.V.; Springman, E.B. Mutagenesis of p38α MAP kinase establishes key roles of Phe169 in function and structural dynamics and reveals a novel DFG-OUT state. *Biochemistry* **2007**, *46*, 5687–5696. [CrossRef] [PubMed]
5. Shan, Y.; Seeliger, M.A.; Eastwood, M.P.; Frank, F.; Xu, H.; Jensen, M.; Dror, R.O.; Kuriyan, J.; Shaw, D.E. A conserved protonation-dependent switch controls drug binding in the Abl kinase. *Proc. Natl Acad Sci. USA* **2009**, *106*, 139–144. [CrossRef] [PubMed]
6. Ahmed, K.; Gerber, D.A.; Cochet, C. Joining the cell survival squad: An emerging role for protein kinase CK2. *Trends Cell Biol.* **2002**, *12*, 226–230. [CrossRef]
7. Ruzzene, M.; Tosoni, K.; Zanin, S.; Cesaro, L.; Pinna, L.A. Protein kinase CK2 accumulation in "oncophilic" cells: Causes and effects. *Mol. Cell. Biochem.* **2011**, *356*, 5–10. [CrossRef] [PubMed]
8. Rabalski, A.J.; Gyenis, L.; Litchfield, D.W. Molecular Pathways: Emergence of Protein Kinase CK2 (CSNK2) as a Potential Target to Inhibit Survival and DNA Damage Response and Repair Pathways in Cancer Cells. *Clin. Cancer Res.* **2016**, *22*, 2840–2847. [CrossRef] [PubMed]
9. Niefind, K.; Raaf, J.; Issinger, O.G. Protein kinase CK2 in health and disease: Protein kinase CK2: From structures to insights. *Cell. Mol. Life Sci.* **2009**, *66*, 1800–1816. [CrossRef] [PubMed]
10. Niefind, K.; Battistutta, R. Structural bases of protein kinase CK2 function and inhibition. In *Protein Kinase CK2*; Pinna, L.A., Ed.; John Wiley & Sons, Inc.: Hoboken, NJ, USA, 2012; pp. 1–75.
11. Niefind, K.; Yde, C.; Ermakova, I.; Issinger, O. Evolved to be active: Sulfate ions define substrate recognition sites of CK2α and emphasise its exceptional role within the CMGC family of eukaryotic protein kinases. *J. Mol. Biol.* **2007**, *370*, 427–438. [CrossRef] [PubMed]
12. Niefind, K.; Issinger, O.G. Conformational plasticity of the catalytic subunit of protein kinase CK2 and its consequences for regulation and drug design. *Biochim. Biophys. Acta* **2010**, *1804*, 484–492. [CrossRef] [PubMed]
13. Hochscherf, J.; Schnitzler, A.; Issinger, O.-G.; Niefind, K. Impressions from the Conformational and Configurational Space Captured by Protein Kinase CK2. In *Protein Kinase CK2 Cellular Function in Normal and Disease States*; Ahmed, K., Issinger, O.-G., Szyszka, R., Eds.; Springer International Publishing: New York, NY, USA, 2015; pp. 17–33.
14. Yde, C.W.; Ermakova, I.; Issinger, O.G.; Niefind, K. Inclining the purine base binding plane in protein kinase CK2 by exchanging the flanking side-chains generates a preference for ATP as a cosubstrate. *J. Mol. Biol.* **2005**, *347*, 399–414. [CrossRef] [PubMed]
15. Raaf, J.; Klopffleisch, K.; Issinger, O.G.; Niefind, K. The catalytic subunit of human protein kinase CK2 structurally deviates from its maize homologue in complex with the nucleotide competitive inhibitor emodin. *J. Mol. Biol.* **2008**, *377*, 1–8. [CrossRef] [PubMed]
16. Gouron, A.; Milet, A.; Jamet, H. Conformational flexibility of human casein kinase catalytic subunit explored by metadynamics. *Biophys. J.* **2014**, *106*, 1134–1141. [CrossRef] [PubMed]
17. Papinutto, E.; Ranchio, A.; Lolli, G.; Pinna, L.A.; Battistutta, R. Structural and functional analysis of the flexible regions of the catalytic α-subunit of protein kinase CK2. *J. Struct. Biol.* **2012**, *177*, 382–391. [CrossRef] [PubMed]
18. Battistutta, R.; Lolli, G. Structural and functional determinants of protein kinase CK2α: Facts and open questions. *Mol. Cell. Biochem.* **2011**, *356*, 67–73. [CrossRef] [PubMed]
19. Klopffleisch, K.; Issinger, O.G.; Niefind, K. Low-density crystal packing of human protein kinase CK2 catalytic subunit in complex with resorufin or other ligands: A tool to study the unique hinge-region plasticity of the enzyme without packing bias. *Acta Crystallogr. D Biol. Crystallogr.* **2012**, *68*, 883–892. [CrossRef] [PubMed]

20. Battistutta, R.; Sarno, S.; De Moliner, E.; Papinutto, E.; Zanotti, G.; Pinna, L.A. The replacement of ATP by the competitive inhibitor emodin induces conformational modifications in the catalytic site of protein kinase CK2. *J. Biol. Chem.* **2000**, *275*, 29618–29622. [CrossRef] [PubMed]

21. Raaf, J.; Issinger, O.G.; Niefind, K. First inactive conformation of CK2α, the catalytic subunit of protein kinase CK2. *J. Mol. Biol.* **2009**, *386*, 1212–1221. [CrossRef] [PubMed]

22. Guerra, B.; Bischoff, N.; Bdzhola, V.G.; Yarmoluk, S.M.; Issinger, O.G.; Golub, A.G.; Niefind, K. A Note of Caution on the Role of Halogen Bonds for Protein Kinase/Inhibitor Recognition Suggested by High- and Low-Salt CK2α Complex Structures. *ACS Chem. Biol.* **2015**, *10*, 1654–1660. [CrossRef] [PubMed]

23. Raaf, J.; Guerra, B.; Neundorf, I.; Bopp, B.; Issinger, O.G.; Jose, J.; Pietsch, M.; Niefind, K. First structure of protein kinase CK2 catalytic subunit with an effective CK2β-competitive ligand. *ACS Chem. Biol.* **2013**, *8*, 901–907. [CrossRef] [PubMed]

24. Gowda, C.; Sachdev, M.; Muthisami, S.; Kapadia, M.; Petrovic-Dovat, L.; Hartman, M.; Ding, Y.; Song, C.; Payne, J.L.; Tan, B.H.; et al. Casein kinase II (CK2) as a therapeutic target for hematological malignancies. *Curr. Pharm. Des.* **2016**, in press.

25. Martins, L.R.; Lúcio, P.; Melão, A.; Antunes, I.; Cardoso, B.A.; Stansfield, R.; Bertilaccio, M.T.; Ghia, P.; Drygin, D.; Silva, M.G.; et al. Activity of the clinical-stage CK2-specific inhibitor CX-4945 against chronic lymphocytic leukemia. *Leukemia* **2014**, *28*, 179–182. [CrossRef] [PubMed]

26. Guerra, B.; Rasmussen, T.D.; Schnitzler, A.; Jensen, H.H.; Boldyreff, B.S.; Miyata, Y.; Marcussen, N.; Niefind, K.; Issinger, O.G. Protein kinase CK2 inhibition is associated with the destabilization of HIF-1α in human cancer cells. *Cancer Lett.* **2015**, *356*, 751–761. [CrossRef] [PubMed]

27. Siddiqui-Jain, A.; Drygin, D.; Streiner, N.; Chua, P.; Pierre, F.; O'Brien, S.E.; Bliesath, J.; Omori, M.; Huser, N.; Ho, C.; et al. CX-4945, an orally bioavailable selective inhibitor of protein kinase CK2, inhibits prosurvival and angiogenic signaling and exhibits antitumor efficacy. *Cancer Res.* **2010**, *70*, 10288–10298. [CrossRef] [PubMed]

28. Golub, A.G.; Bdzhola, V.G.; Kyshenia, Y.V.; Sapelkin, V.M.; Prykhod'ko, A.O.; Kukharenko, O.P.; Ostrynska, O.V.; Yarmoluk, S.M. Structure-based discovery of novel flavonol inhibitors of human protein kinase CK2. *Mol. Cell. Biochem.* **2011**, *356*, 107–115. [CrossRef] [PubMed]

29. Golub, A.G.; Bdzhola, V.G.; Briukhovetska, N.V.; Balanda, A.O.; Kukharenko, O.P.; Kotey, I.M.; Ostrynska, O.V.; Yarmoluk, S.M. Synthesis and biological evaluation of substituted (thieno[2,3-d]pyrimidin-4-ylthio)carboxylic acids as inhibitors of human protein kinase CK2. *Eur. J. Med. Chem.* **2011**, *46*, 870–876. [CrossRef] [PubMed]

30. Lolli, G.; Cozza, G.; Mazzorana, M.; Tibaldi, E.; Cesaro, L.; Donella-Deana, A.; Meggio, F.; Venerando, A.; Franchin, C.; Sarno, S.; et al. Inhibition of protein kinase CK2 by flavonoids and tyrphostins. A structural insight. *Biochemistry* **2012**, *51*, 6097–6107. [PubMed]

31. Ermakova, I.; Boldyreff, B.; Issinger, O.G.; Niefind, K. Crystal structure of a *C*-terminal deletion mutant of human protein kinase CK2 catalytic subunit. *J. Mol. Biol.* **2003**, *330*, 925–934. [CrossRef]

32. Bischoff, N.; Olsen, B.; Raaf, J.; Bretner, M.; Issinger, O.G.; Niefind, K. Structure of the human protein kinase CK2 catalytic subunit CK2α' and interaction thermodynamics with the regulatory subunit CK2β. *J. Mol. Biol.* **2011**, *407*, 1–12. [CrossRef] [PubMed]

33. Tuazon, P.T.; Traugh, J.A. Casein kinase I and II—Multipotential serine protein kinases: Structure, function, and regulation. In *Advances in Second Messenger and Phosphoprotein Research*; Greengard, P., Robinson, G.A., Eds.; Raven Press, Ltd.: New York, NY, USA, 1991; Volume 23, pp. 123–164.

34. Gerlach, M.; Mueller, U.; Weiss, M.S. The MX beamlines BL14.1-3 at BESSY II. *J. Large Scale Res. Facil.* **2016**, *2*, A47. [CrossRef]

35. Grant, S.K.; Lunney, E.A. Kinase inhibition that hinges on halogen bonds. *Chem. Biol.* **2011**, *18*, 3–4. [CrossRef] [PubMed]

36. Kinoshita, T.; Nakaniwa, T.; Sekiguchi, Y.; Sogabe, Y.; Sakurai, A.; Nakamura, S.; Nakanishi, I. Crystal structure of human CK2α at 1.06 Å resolution. *J. Synchrotron Radiat.* **2013**, *20*, 974–979. [CrossRef] [PubMed]

37. Ferguson, A.D.; Sheth, P.R.; Basso, A.D.; Paliwal, S.; Gray, K.; Fischmann, T.O.; Le, H.V. Structural basis of CX-4945 binding to human protein kinase CK2. *FEBS Lett.* **2011**, *585*, 104–110. [CrossRef] [PubMed]

38. Politzer, P.; Lane, P.; Concha, M.C.; Ma, Y.; Murray, J.S. An overview of halogen bonding. *J. Mol. Model.* **2007**, *13*, 305–311. [CrossRef] [PubMed]

39. Brear, P.; De Fusco, C.; Georgiou, K.H.; Francis-Newton, N.J.; Stubbs, C.J.; Sore, H.F.; Venkitaraman, A.R.; Abell, C.; Spring, D.R.; Hyvönen, M. Specific inhibition of CK2α from an anchor outside the active site. *Chem. Sci.* **2016**, *7*, 6839–6845. [CrossRef]

40. Bischoff, N.; Raaf, J.; Olsen, B.; Bretner, M.; Issinger, O.; Niefind, K. Enzymatic activity with an incomplete catalytic spine: Insights from a comparative structural analysis of human CK2α and its paralogous isoform CK2α'. *Mol. Cell. Biochem.* **2011**, *356*, 57–65. [CrossRef] [PubMed]

41. Taylor, S.S.; Kornev, A.P. Protein kinases: Evolution of dynamic regulatory proteins. *Trends Biochem. Sci.* **2011**, *36*, 65–77. [CrossRef] [PubMed]

42. Niefind, K.; Guerra, B.; Pinna, L.A.; Issinger, O.G.; Schomburg, D. Crystal structure of the catalytic subunit of protein kinase CK2 from Zea mays at 2.1 A resolution. *EMBO J.* **1998**, *17*, 2451–2462. [CrossRef] [PubMed]

43. Kabsch, W. XDS. *Acta Crystallogr. D Biol. Crystallogr.* **2010**, *66*, 125–132. [CrossRef] [PubMed]

44. Winn, M.D.; Ballard, C.C.; Cowtan, K.D.; Dodson, E.J.; Emsley, P.; Evans, P.R.; Keegan, R.M.; Krissinel, E.B.; Leslie, A.G.; McCoy, A.; et al. Overview of the CCP4 suite and current developments. *Acta Crystallogr. D Biol. Crystallogr.* **2011**, *67*, 235–242. [CrossRef] [PubMed]

45. McCoy, A.J.; Grosse-Kunstleve, R.W.; Adams, P.D.; Winn, M.D.; Storoni, L.C.; Read, R.J. Phaser crystallographic software. *J. Appl Crystallogr.* **2007**, *40*, 658–674. [CrossRef] [PubMed]

46. Adams, P.D.; Afonine, P.V.; Bunkóczi, G.; Chen, V.B.; Davis, I.W.; Echols, N.; Headd, J.J.; Hung, L.W.; Kapral, G.J.; Grosse-Kunstleve, R.W.; et al. PHENIX: A comprehensive Python-based system for macromolecular structure solution. *Acta Crystallogr. D Biol. Crystallogr.* **2010**, *66*, 213–221. [CrossRef] [PubMed]

47. Schüttelkopf, A.W.; van Aalten, D.M. PRODRG: A tool for high-throughput crystallography of protein-ligand complexes. *Acta Crystallogr. D Biol. Crystallogr.* **2004**, *60*, 1355–1363. [CrossRef] [PubMed]

48. Emsley, P.; Lohkamp, B.; Scott, W.G.; Cowtan, K. Features and development of Coot. *Acta Crystallogr. D Biol. Crystallogr.* **2010**, *66*, 486–501. [CrossRef] [PubMed]

49. *The PyMol Molecular Graphics System*, Version 1.7; Schrödinger, LLC: New York, NY, USA, 2013.

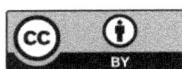

pharmaceuticals

MDPI

Review

The Development of CK2 Inhibitors: From Traditional Pharmacology to in Silico Rational Drug Design

Giorgio Cozza

Department of Molecular Medicine, University of Padova, 35131 Padova, Italy; giorgio.cozza@unipd.it;
Tel.: +39-049-827-6154

Academic Editor: Mathias Montenarh
Received: 15 December 2016; Accepted: 14 February 2017; Published: 20 February 2017

Abstract: Casein kinase II (CK2) is an ubiquitous and pleiotropic serine/threonine protein kinase able to phosphorylate hundreds of substrates. Being implicated in several human diseases, from neurodegeneration to cancer, the biological roles of CK2 have been intensively studied. Upregulation of CK2 has been shown to be critical to tumor progression, making this kinase an attractive target for cancer therapy. Several CK2 inhibitors have been developed so far, the first being discovered by "trial and error testing". In the last decade, the development of in silico rational drug design has prompted the discovery, de novo design and optimization of several CK2 inhibitors, active in the low nanomolar range. The screening of big chemical libraries and the optimization of hit compounds by Structure Based Drug Design (SBDD) provide telling examples of a fruitful application of rational drug design to the development of CK2 inhibitors. Ligand Based Drug Design (LBDD) models have been also applied to CK2 drug discovery, however they were mainly focused on methodology improvements rather than being critical for de novo design and optimization. This manuscript provides detailed description of in silico methodologies whose applications to the design and development of CK2 inhibitors proved successful and promising.

Keywords: CK2; inhibitors; structure based drug design; ligand based drug design; cancer; hit optimization

1. Introduction

CK2 (formerly called Casein Kinase II), was first detected, together with CK1, as early as in 1954 [1]. The conventional term "casein kinase" originally denoted a group of unrelated ser/thr protein kinases able to phosphorylate casein. Only one of these, Fam20C/G-CK (Golgi, or "genuine", casein kinase) is a bona fide casein kinase in vivo, while CK2 and CK1 share the ability to phosphorylate casein only in vitro. CK2 is an ubiquitous, highly pleiotropic and constitutively active enzyme, responsible for the generation of a significant proportion of the human phosphoproteome [2,3]. CK2 is active as catalytic subunit alone (α and α') or as tetrameric holoenzyme composed by two catalytic and two regulatory (β) subunits. The α subunit displays the common structural features of all the other member of the human kinome; to note that, unlike many other protein kinases, CK2 displays a constitutively active state, as its activation loop is frozen in an open and active conformation, independently of phosphorylation events [4,5]. CK2 has been linked to a number of human diseases, such as cancer [6], but also cardiac hypertrophy [7], multiple sclerosis [8], virus infections [9–11] and cystic fibrosis [12–14]. For this reason CK2 is intensively studied as a therapeutic target, especially in the treatment of cancer, and one CK2 inhibitor (CX-4945) is currently in Phase II clinical trials [15–17].

Several molecules, belonging to different chemical classes, have shown to inhibit CK2 during the last 20 years. Most of them have been isolated by traditional drug discovery methods, which rely on "trial and error testing" of molecules against the isolated enzyme (recombinant or purified from tissues). More recently many compounds have been discovered and optimized through rational drug design approaches, and in particular by computer aided drug design, combined with in vitro and in cell methodologies supported by crystallographic analysis. Two main groups of techniques should be mentioned, namely structure based and ligand based drug design approaches. Structure-Based Drug Design (SBDD) exploits the three dimensional structure of the biological target, obtained from X-ray crystallography or nuclear magnetic resonance (NMR) spectroscopy, more rarely through Homology modeling (Figure 1). The final goal of this approach is to predict whether chemical compounds are able to interact with a biological target and its affinity. The binding conformation of small molecules into their target, their intermolecular interactions and the structural changes of the drug/target complexes can be estimated through molecular mechanics and molecular dynamics. On the contrary Ligand-Based Drug Design (LBDD) exploits the knowledge of compounds able to interact with the biological target in order to identify a set of chemical features ensuring the molecules activities. This model can be used to design new potent drug-like entities; the pharmacophore approach and quantitative structure-activity relationship (QSAR) are the most used ligand-based methods (Figure 1).

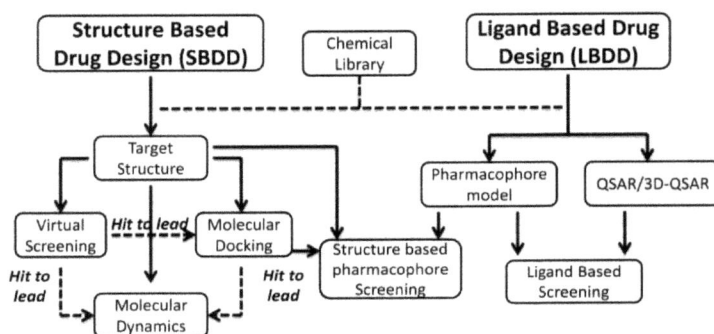

Figure 1. Schematic representation of in silico rational drug design techniques.

2. Structure and Biological Roles of CK2

The first crystal structure of human CK2 holoenzyme (Protein Data Bank (PDB) code: 1JWH) revealed a stable tetramer composed by two catalytic subunit (α and α'), belonging to the CMGC subfamily of the human kinome, and two regulatory β subunit (Figure 2). The two catalytic subunits differ only at the C-terminal domain, while sharing with all the other protein kinases, the main structural features (e.g., the P-loop or glycine-rich loop, the catalytic loop, the activation loop and the substrate binding site). Intriguingly, CK2 is considered a constitutive active enzyme, a rare property among protein kinases; this peculiarity is driven by its N-terminal domain, which is able to form a number of stable interactions with the activation loop [4], whose conformational changes are responsible for the active or non-active state of protein kinases. Normally, the activation loop of active conformer is triggered by single or multiple phosphorylation events. In the particular case of CK2 the N-terminal domain is able to block the activation loop in an open and full active conformation, by its own [4]. CK2 is an acidophilic kinase accepting substrates with the consensus sequence X_{n-1}-S/T-X_{n+1}-X_{n+2}-E/D/Sp/Yp (Figure 2). Even if an acidic residue at position +3 should be sufficient for being a CK2 substrate [18,19], at least five residues have been identified on average around its phosphorylable sites [2]. In fact, the CK2 substrate binding site is characterized by an unique amount of basic residues, in particular the basic stretch of the α-helix C (Lys74-Arg80) has been recognized to be important for substrate recognition, together with the amino acidic triplet, namely Arg191, Arg195 and Lys198 [20]. On the other hand, the mechanism by which the β subunit is able to regulate the activity of the catalytic subunit is still not clarified; however it is known that the β subunit can provide a recruitment surface for substrates, up- (e.g., HIV-rev [21] or eif2β [22]) or down-regulating (e.g., calmodulin [23]) their phosphorylation (Figure 2). Moreover, the autophosphorylation of the β subunit at the N-terminal domain MssSEE (Ser 2 and Ser 3) [24,25] has been suggested to be linked to the formation of multimers based on CK2 tetrameric units, which could play a role in the regulation of CK2 activity [26] (Figure 2).

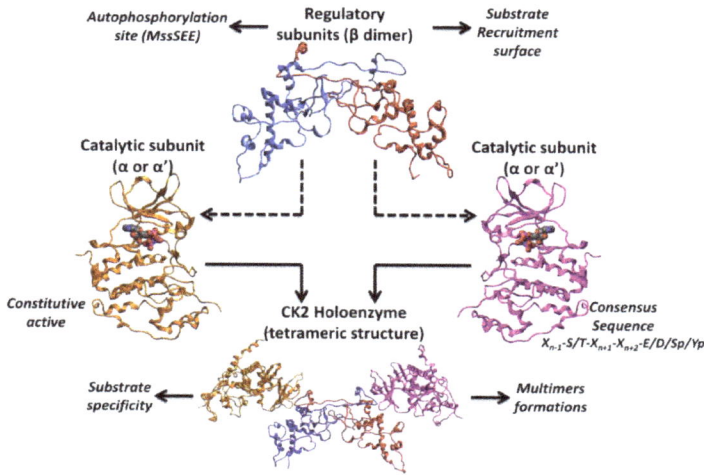

Figure 2. Representation of CK2 structure; catalytic subunits (α and α′), regulatory β dimer and the holoenzyme structure are highlighted.

Protein kinase CK2 is present in many cellular compartments, where it is able to phosphorylate hundreds of substrates. For this reason it has been linked to several cellular processes, being implicated in cell cycle, transcriptional control, neuronal function and response to cellular stress [27,28]. The role of CK2 in many pathologies is well known [27,28]; in particular it is implicated in cardiovascular pathology (hypoxia [29–32], atherosclerosis [33,34], cardiomyocyte hypertrophy [7]), neurodegeneration (Parkinson's [35–37] and Alzheimer's diseases [38–41]), inflammation (glomerulonephritis [42], experimental autoimmune encephalomyelitis, systemic lupus erythematosus [8,43,44], multiple sclerosis [8]), muscle diseases (cardiomyocyte hypertrophy [45,46]) as well as virus and parasite infections [9–11]. Moreover a role of CK2 in Cystic Fibrosis (CFTR) has been recently proposed [12–14,47]. The pathology where the role of CK2 is best documented and studied is cancer, where this kinase is almost invariably upregulated [6]; recent studies have clearly demonstrated that abnormally elevated CK2 level is required for tumor progression, due to its role in the regulation of almost all the processes essential for cancer development with special reference to the suppression of apoptosis [48]. This dependency of cancer cells to higher level of CK2 in comparison to normal cells, is called addiction, and provides a crucial argument for the development of selective CK2 inhibitors in cancer therapy [48].

A huge number of CK2 inhibitors are available, most of them belonging to the class I of kinase inhibitors, i.e., compounds able to directly target the ATP-binding site. Benzoimidazoles, anthraquinones, flavonoids, coumarins, and pyrazolotriazines are the most represented families of CK2 inhibitors [27,28] (Figure 3). Many members of these chemical classes were initially found by traditional pharmacology, exploiting trial-and error-testing against the isolated enzyme. With the increasing knowledge of CK2 structure, alone or in complex with different inhibitors, together with the circulation of novel, fast and optimized protocols for computer aided drug design, the rationalization of structural modification became of particular relevance in the design of CK2 inhibitors.

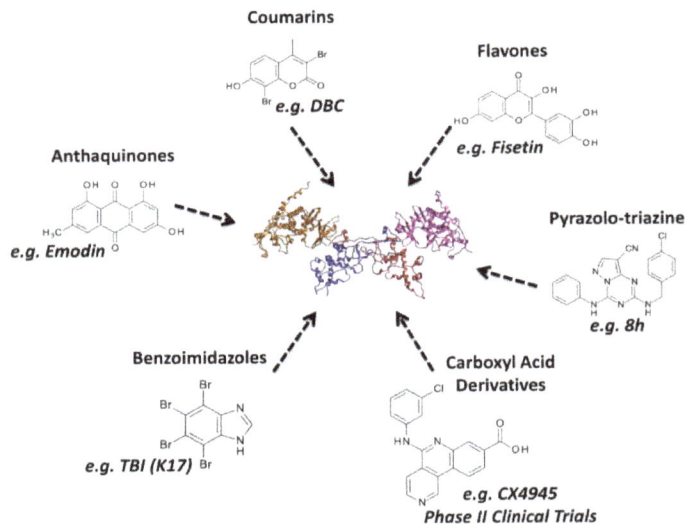

Figure 3. Schematic summary of the most representative families of CK2 inhibitors.

3. Rational Drug Design of CK2 Inhibitors: Structure Based Drug Design

The CK2 structure has been intensively studied through X-ray crystallography and homology modeling techniques. Currently a long and growing list of crystal structures is available from the Protein Data Bank (PDB); in particular, as summarized in the Supplementary (Table S1), a consistent group of structures is represented by the catalytic subunit α alone, both in its apo form or in complex with ATP analogs or inhibitors. On the contrary, only a couple of structure of the α′ (PDB codes: 3E2B, 3OFM) and of the entire tetramer are present in PDB (PDB codes: 1JWH, 4NH1, 4MD7, 4MD8, 4MD9, 4DGL). Noteworthy, among the species crystallized, CK2 from *Zea mays* was the most commonly deposited till 2010 (28/40); At a later time, human CK2 has represented the first choice for crystallization (63/75). This abundance of CK2 structures, represents an outstanding resource for in silico drug design and in particular structure based drug design. In fact, these structures provide: (a) high resolution representations of the active site of CK2, useful to design and optimize novel drug-candidates; (b) detailed information about the interactions between CK2 and its inhibitors, which have been demonstrated of particular significance in the training of in silico protocols and scoring functions. The most commonly used SBDD approaches are represented by virtual screening, molecular docking and molecular dynamics (Figure 1). Virtual screening and in particular structure based virtual screening is able to evaluate large libraries of compounds by directly docking the candidates against a structure of interest. Fast molecular docking algorithms are a central part of the procedure together with scoring function protocols able to extract the most promising molecules from the database of millions of compounds. To note that, despite the large number of compounds screened in silico, only a few of them (top selection) will be actually tested and even fewer will be able to achieve a reasonable affinity to the target molecule (see Section 3.2). More accurate molecular docking approaches are exploited in the optimization phase of hit compounds coming from in silico or in vitro screenings, better when combined with crystallographic data. Molecular dynamics simulations have been introduced at a later stage of in silico drug design, with aims of confirm the stability of ligand/target complexes generated from docking studies, and to estimate the free energy of binding between small molecules and their biological targets.

3.1. Protein and Ligand Preparation

SBDD approaches require on one side an accurate 3D structure of the target of intent and on the other a small set or a large library of compounds correctly prepared for in silico calculations. The preparation of the target structure generally starts with the addition of hydrogen atoms to the available 3D system [49,50]; this is particularly the case when crystallographic information is used to describe the biological target, while is not necessary in the case of NMR or homology models. Hydrogen atoms are consequently minimized to avoid contacts, keeping the heavy atoms fixed at their original positions [49,50]. This step can be performed using different types of Force Fields, which represent a set of parameters used to describe atoms and molecules properties (atom types, charges) and to calculate the potential energy of a system. The Force Fields commonly used during protein preparation and during SBDD calculations are generally based on molecular mechanics equations (e.g., Amber [51], CHARMM [52], MMFF [53], OPLS [54]) even if some examples of quantum mechanics or hybrid Force Fields are also available. Unwanted molecules (e.g., ions, ligands, water molecules) are generally excluded in the preparation process, but, in special cases, some of them are considered constitutive of the tridimensional system studied [49,50]. For example during CK2 protein structure preparation, a constitutive water molecule located in the ATP binding site is often maintained in all the in silico calculations [50,55]. Moreover, the selection of the most suitable CK2 crystal structure(s) for SBDD experiments strictly depends on several factors: first of all the SBDD technique applied, the in silico protocols involved, the crystal structure conformations, resolutions etc. In other words the target structure selection must be performed dependently to the computational problem addressed. However, based on the public materials available for SBDD studies on CK2, some general observations can be made. Even if crystal structures of both CK2 α and the tetramer are available, virtual screening and molecular docking procedures are generally based on the structures of the isolated catalytic subunits, because of a better crystallographic resolution and the presence of several inhibitor co-crystallized, missed, instead, in the crystal structures of the tetramer. To note that, even if recently several crystal structures of human CK2 α are available, earlier the in silico analysis on CK2 were exclusively based on *Zea mays* crystal structures. This lack in human CK2 tridimensional information was overtaken by building the human CK2 model through homology modeling technique, exploiting the high similarity between the ATP binding sites of *Zea mays* and *Homo sapiens* CK2 (>98%) [56]. Nowadays crystal structures of the human catalytic subunit are generally selected for virtual screening purpose; this can be done by testing the available protocols to isolate the most suitable structure(s) where the in silico algorithm is able to efficiently reproduce the compounds crystallographic pose. However, *Zea mays* structures remain important to retrieve the binding motif of several known inhibitors of CK2. In some cases, to address specific computational problems, the crystal structure of CK2 tetramer has been also considered. This is the case, for examples of protein-protein docking studies [22,57] or molecular dynamics simulation experiments [5].

On the other side, to optimize in silico processes, special care must be taken also to the preparation of chemical libraries; this event is primarily a manual process which starts from the direct building of 3D structure of molecules or from the 2D into 3D conversion of entire database of compounds [49,50]. Protonation states, tautomers and stereochemistry must be taken into account for all the molecules of the chemical library, as well as any desired geometric restraints (distances, angles, dihedrals), if necessary. Finally, partial charges are calculated and applied to the molecules together with an energy minimization protocol with a suitable force field [49,50]. At the end of the preparation process a database of potential candidates is ready to be tested in silico against a biological target. To note that the chemical library is commonly "contaminated" by compounds with known activity against the target of interest. This is of particular relevance during in silico screening campaigns, providing on one side an internal evaluation of the computational approach, on the other an idea of how a scoring function predicts the novel candidates activities in comparison to known ligands [49,50].

3.2. Virtual Screening Approach

Structural-based virtual screening approaches (also defined as high-throughput docking) exploit large libraries of compounds to identify those structures which are able to bind a biological target. The aim of this computational technique is not necessarily linked to the number of hits found during the process; on the contrary, the identification of novel interesting scaffolds is clearly preferable. For this reason two important and connected steps of virtual screening approach must be mentioned: the search algorithm and the scoring function (Figure 4) [58,59]. The search algorithm is able to explore all the possible orientations and conformations of a small molecule within a target binding site. Most of the protocols explore the conformational space of flexible ligands, while the protein structure remains fixed; each final ligand conformation docked inside the protein target is called "pose". Several search algorithms are available based on different principles: genetic algorithm (Autodock [60], Gold [61], MOE [62]), geometric matching (DOCK [63]), exhaustive search (Glide [64], FRED [65], eHits [66]), incremental search (FlexX [67]). However, defining the best search protocol for virtual screening in general, is not that easy; an evaluation of the available protocols for every case studied, instead, is a mandatory step to identify the best solution for the virtual screening procedure. Since search algorithms are potentially able to generate a huge number of conformations and poses, a procedure suitable to evaluate favorable and not favorable protein/inhibitor complex and to rank one ligand relative to another is required. This procedure is based on scoring function [58,59], which represent an approximate mathematical method used to predict and evaluate the strength of non-covalent interactions between small molecules and target proteins. During virtual screening, it is quite common to use more than one scoring function for the evaluation of the best candidates [49,50]; this procedure is known as "consensus scoring" and it is performed by combining different type of scoring functions in an intersection-based consensus approach. The main advantage of this method is to reduce the numbers of false positives identified by individual scoring functions and to increase the ability to discriminate between active and inactive ligands [49,50] (Figure 4).

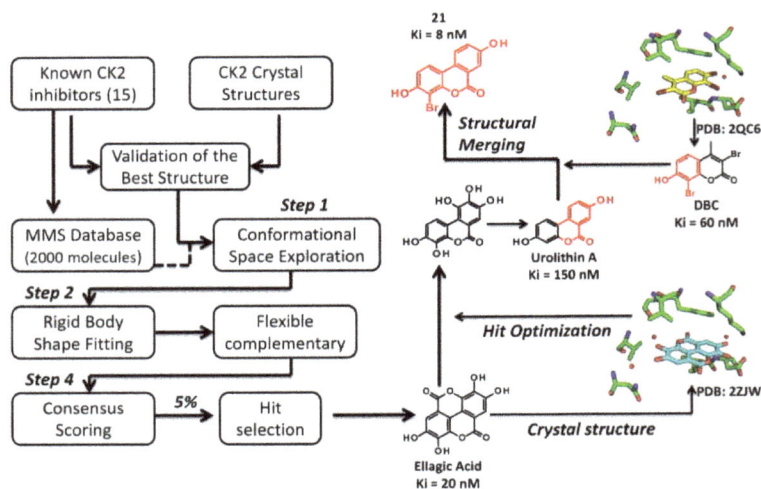

Figure 4. Schematic representation of the structure based virtual screening procedure leading to the discovery of ellagic acid (**left**); on the (**right**) hit optimization of ellagic acid. Inhibition constant (Ki) and PDB (Protein Data Bank) codes have been reported.

3.2.1. Virtual Screening Example 1: The Discovery of Ellagic Acid

A very first example of a structure based drug design technique used to identify novel inhibitors of CK2, was provided by the virtual screening process leading to the identification of the tannin derivative ellagic acid as the most potent CK2 inhibitor at that time [50] (Figure 4). Starting from a relatively small database of natural compounds (2000 molecules), enriched with 15 known CK2 inhibitors to calibrate the high-throughput screening protocol, the authors have set up a consensus screening procedure involving four principal steps (Figure 4). First of all the library was processed with OMEGA, adding hydrogen atoms/Gasteiger partial charges and generating the conformers for the second phase: the rigid body shape fitting. During this step FRED generates a pool of different rigid body poses able to interact with CK2 binding site without generating clashes; this poses were scored and ranked with a Gaussian shape function. Compounds, selected by FRED, that potentially fit CK2 catalytic cleft were subjected to a flexbile docking step, using three different program, namely MOE, Glide and Gold (third step). In the fourth and last phase, the poses generated from the docking procedure were ranked by five scoring function (MOE-Score, GlideScore, GoldScore, ChemScore and Xscore) [50]. A cut-off value for the top 5% compounds ranked by all possible combinations of flexible-docking/scoring functions was selected (consensus docking and scoring), prioritizing 73 molecules for biochemical evaluation [50] (Figure 4). Ellagic acid was selected, among others, as the best compound, resulting the most potent ATP-competitive inhibitor isolated at that time (Ki value of 0.020 µM) [50]. From a small selectivity panel, including 12 representative protein kinases, ellagic acid resulted to be quite selective [50]; this selectivity profile was recently enlarged by testing the residual activity of 70 protein kinases treated with 10µM ellagic acid (Table 1). At this concentration, ellagic acid is able to inhibit, more than 50%, the activity of 21 protein kinases, however only 9 are remarkably affected (residual activity <25%). Beside CK2 (13%), p38-regulated/ activated kinase (PRAK) is the most inhibited (3%) followed by Sphingosine kinase 1 (SPK1) and dual specificity tyrosine-phosphorylation-regulated kinase 3 (DYRK3) (9%), DYRK2 (12%), p21-activated kinase 4 (PAK4) (14%), maternal embryonic leucine zipper kinase 2 (MELK2) (17%), BR serine/threonine-protein kinase 2 (BRSK2) (18%) and Pim-3 proto-oncogene, serine/threonine kinase (PIM3) (21%). The moderate promiscuity of ellagic acid is not so rare among drug candidates from natural sources and could represent the driving force of their activity against diseases like cancer. Indeed, a cytotoxicity profile demonstrated that ellagic acid inhibited the growth of leukemic cells SUDHL1 and FEPD with a DC_{50} (Death Concentration 50) around 30–50 µM after 48-h exposure to the inhibitor [50].

Table 1. Selectivity profiles of ellagic acid on a 70 kinase panel. Residual Casein kinase II (CK2) activity (determined at 10 µM Ellagic Acid concentration) is expressed as a percentage of the control activity without inhibitor. Activities <25% of control are highlighted in grey. Conditions for the activity assays are described in [68].

Kinase	% Activity	Kinase	% Activity	Kinase	% Activity
PRAK	3	PDK1	66	Lck	101
SRPK1	9	PKC zeta	67	HIPK3	102
DYRK3	9	MSK1	68	ERK1	103
DYRK2	12	S6K1	68	PRK2	105
CK2	13	ROCK 2	68	JNK3	106
PAK4	14	PKA	69	P38b MAPK	107
MELK	17	PKBb	71	EFK2	111
BRSK2	18	CSK	73	CHK2	117
PIM3	21	PLK1	76	CAMKKa	118
DYRK1A	26	Src	76	SmMLCK	127
MAPKAP-K2	26	JNK1	78		
PAK5	29	SGK1	80		
CAMKKb	29	PKBa	80		
GSK3b	30	PKCa	81		

Table 1. *Cont.*

Kinase	% Activity	Kinase	% Activity	Kinase	% Activity
IKKb	36	CHK1	81		
MAPKAP-K3	39	NEK7	82		
PIM1	40	PHK	82		
PAK6	42	CAMK1	82		
ERK8	46	ERK2	84		
AURORA C	46	AMPK	86		
MARK3	47	JNK2	87		
PKD1	48	HIPK2	89		
PLK1	51	NEK6	91		
RSK2	51	MNK2	94		
CK1	58	p38s MAPK	98		
RSK1	58	p38a MAPK	100		
MKK1	62	MNK1	100		
AURORA B	64	p38g MAPK	101		
NEK2a	65	MST2	101		
PIM2	65	CDK2-Cyclin A	101		

3.2.2. Virtual Screening Example 2: The Discovery of Quinalizarin

An implementation of the virtual screening procedure adopted in the case of ellagic acid, led to the identification of quinalizarin as the best anthraquinone inhibitor of CK2 [49]. Starting from an enlarged molecular database (3000 molecules), implemented with 21 known CK2 inhibitors for the calibration phase, a flexible ligand-docking step with four different programs (MOE, Glide, Gold and FlexX) was performed in combination with the five scoring functions described above (cut-off for final selection: 10%) [49]. Quinalizarin, prioritized for biochemical evaluation, resulted to be an ATP competitive inhibitor with a Ki value of 0.052 µM (Figure 5), definitely lower as compared to other anthraquinone derivatives previously identified through traditional pharmacology, namely emodin (6-methyl-1,3,8-trihydroxyanthraquinone, Ki = 1.5 µM) [56], MNA (1,8-dihydroxy-4-nitro-anthracene-9,10-dione, Ki = 0.78 µM), MNX (1,8-dihydroxy-4-nitroxanthen-9-one, Ki = 0.80 µM), DAA (1,4-dihydroxy-5,8-diaminoanthracene-9,10-dione, Ki = 0.42 µM) [69]. Moreover, the first selectivity evaluation of quinalizarin against a panel of 70 protein kinases disclosed a promising specificity for CK2 [49], confirmed by a second assay against an enlarged panel of 140 protein kinases [70]. In particular, while CK2 residual activity, after treatment with 1 µM quinalizarin, resulted to be only 10%, none of the other 140 protein kinases displays a residual activity less than 50%, 132 of them being almost unaffected [70]. Several crystal structures of quinalizarin have been solved firstly by co-crystallization with *Zea mays* CK2 (PDB code: 3FL5 [10]), later with human CK2 (PDB codes: 3Q9Z and 3Q9Y [29]). These structural resources are exploited to disclose on one side the molecular features underlying quinalizarin selectivity and, on the other, its preference for CK2 holoenzyme over the CK2 α alone [70]. To note that, quinalizarin is readily cell permeable and very effective as pro-apoptotic agent, having been successfully used in many studies concerning CK2 physiological and pathological roles, as well to disclose proteomics perturbations caused by CK2 down regulation [71].

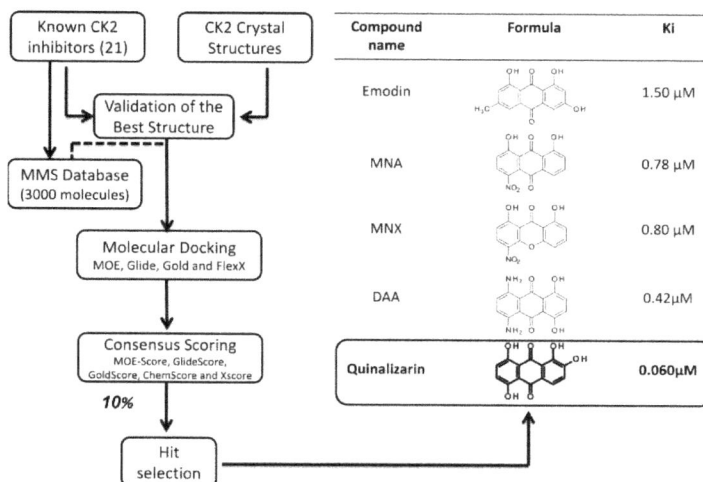

Figure 5. Schematic representation of the structure based virtual screening procedure leading to the discovery of quinalizarin (**left**); whose activity is shown in comparison with the previous discovered anthraquinone inhibitors (**right**).

3.2.3. Virtual Screening: Other Examples

One of the first examples of a successful virtual screening procedure applied to the identification of CK2 inhibitors was performed by Novartis Pharma: a fast high-throughput screening protocol (DOCK software), combined with a pharmacophore filter, was used to screen a database of 400,000 compounds. A dozen compounds were retrieved from the in silico procedure; of particular interest was a quinazoline derivative (compound **4**, 5-oxo-5,6-dihydroindolo- [1,2-a]quinazolin-7-yl, later named IQA), displaying an IC_{50} (half maximal inhibitory concentration) of 0.080 µM against CK2 and a good selectivity towards a small panel of 21 representative protein kinases [72]. Hereafter, IQA was profiled against 44 kinases, confirming its selectivity and prioritized for cell assays, showing remarkable efficacy in Jurkat cells [73]. The crystal structure of IQA and *Zea mays* CK2 was solved (PDB code: 1OM1), paving the way for further optimization of this promising scaffold [73].

Another example of a virtual screening application exploited the chemical structure of CX4945, the only CK2 inhibitor in clinical trials; a two-steps shape based virtual screening approach was used to retrieve novel compounds able to inhibit CK2 [74]. Firstly, a shape-based model derived from CX-4945 was built, and used to screen a database of molecules with the OMEGA/ROCS software, leading to the identification of one quinazoline derivative (SHP01, IC_{50} = 4.23 µM), whose interactions with CK2 active site were later clarified through molecular docking (GOLD software). Based on SHP01 scaffold, a second shape based model was built and a new set of compounds from the screening analysis have been prioritized for molecular docking and biochemical evaluation. The three best compounds SHP19, SHP26 and SHP27 (IC_{50} = 0.46 µM, 0.69 µM and 0.55 µM respectively) were also assayed for their cytotoxicity in several cell lines, displaying a DC_{50} values around 30 µM [74]. Although this strategy proved promising for the optimization of SHP01 inhibitory activity, it was not able to retrieve compounds as effective as CX4945. Moreover, the selectivity of the hit molecules identified in the virtual screening procedure remained undetermined, as well as the real contribution of CK2 to the cytotoxic effect of these chemical entities.

Finally an in silico screening application, called Cross-Docking-based Virtual Screening, was used to explore a database of over 300,000 compounds previously resized to around 80,000 using specific druglike property filter [75]. Ninety six compounds were retrieved from the screening procedure and submitted to a toxicity prediction procedure; only seven of them were assayed in vitro, compound **g** resulting to be the best inhibitor, with an activity in the micromolar range [75].

3.3. Molecular Docking, Molecular Dynamics and Hit Optimization (Hit to Lead)

Compounds selected from a virtual screening procedure (for example ellagic acid or quinalizarin) are generally defined as hits and evaluated by means of binding affinity for their biological target as well as for their selectivity toward unwanted off-targets. After their efficacy is validated in cell environment, to assess their cell permeability and ability to perturb biological functions. Co-crystallization of hits and the target protein is a crucial step in hit evaluation, since it provides significant information about the molecular interactions and may confirm or not the poses obtained from the in silico high-throughput screening procedure. Hit to lead represents a stage in early drug design where hits undergo a rational optimization of their chemical scaffold to improve, among others, chemical and metabolic stability, affinity and selectivity towards the biological target, as well as efficacy in cellular assays. Hit optimization is generally performed by exploiting optimized docking protocols as well as molecular dynamics simulations; these approaches are especially useful when coupled with crystallographic information about hit/target complexes. The design of novel compounds starting from existing hits can be evaluated through molecular docking which is able to predict the binding motif of optimized molecules and their affinity towards the biological target, using different scoring functions. The comparison between hit compounds binding affinity and the ones of novel designed candidates, helps to direct new synthesis of optimized molecules. On the other hand, molecular docking can be useful to determinate the Structure Activity Relationship (SAR) of a family of compounds variably active against a target. In fact the knowledge of the relationship between the chemical or 3D structure of a molecule and its biological activity, is critical to understand which kind of chemical substitutions are expected to improve the activity of hit compounds. Similarly, molecular dynamics simulation can be used to estimate the free binding energy of small ligands to biological macromolecules. In particular molecular dynamics calculations are used to study target/ligand complexes, to rationalize experimental findings and to improve the results of virtual screening and docking. Molecular mechanics (MM) energy coming from molecular dynamics experiments are coupled with PBSA and GBSA (Poisson Boltzmann or generalized Born and surface area continuum salvation) methods to estimate ligand binding affinities to the biological target [76]. To note that many attempts to improve these methodologies have been performed by exploiting for example Quantum Mechanics (QM) approaches. Liner Interaction Energy (LIE) is another method for hit optimization coupled with molecular dynamics simulations: it consists in a semiempirical approach that combines the advantages of Free Energy Perturbation (FEP) and Thermodynamic Integration (TI), by calculating binding free energies of the bound and the free state of ligands [77].

After hit optimization, the newly generated molecules are generally called lead compounds; they are further improved in a lead optimization phase, exploiting the acquisition of Adsorption, Distribution, Metabolism, Excretion, Toxicity (ADMET) properties, till the development of drug candidates ready for in vivo testing. This issue will not be considered in this paper because, although many inhibitors of CK2 have reached in vivo studies, in silico lead optimization of this molecules has not been performed.

3.3.1. Hit to Lead: Ellagic Acid

The optimization of the CK2 inhibitor ellagic acid is a telling example of a hit to lead strategy starting from a compound retrieved by a virtual screening technique. Starting from the crystallographic structures of ellagic acid and the cumarin derivative DBC (3,8-dibromo-7-hydroxy-4-methylchromen-2-one, Ki = 0.06 µM) in complex with the α-subunit of CK2 (PDB codes: 2ZJW and 2QC6, respectively [78,79]), an analysis of the interactions of the two compounds with CK2 catalytic site was performed (Figure 4). Ellagic acid and DBC display a similar binding mode; however, while ellagic acid is able to interact with both CK2 hinge region and the phosphate group binding area, DBC is able to directly bind only the hinge. To note that in 2008, a LIE model approach was performed on DBC and more than 60 coumarins derivatives, to define and understand the importance of different energy contributions to the binding free energy of this class of compounds [79].

From these observations, a molecular simplification of the ellagic acid scaffold has been proposed leading, among others, to an hydrolysable tannin, urolithin A (IC_{50} = 0.39 µM) [55] (Figure 4). Interestingly, the molecular docking experiments of urolithin A inside CK2 catalytic site, demonstrate that ellagic acid and urolithin A share the same binding motif characterized by the two crucial hydrogen-bonding interactions [55]. This was also confirmed by methylating, individually or together, the hydroxy groups at position 3 and 8, resulting in two molecules with low affinity (compound 9, IC_{50} = 3.5 µM) or completely inactive (compound 10, IC_{50} > 40 µM) [55]. Moreover, being urolithin A a benzocoumarin derivative, it was suggested to represent a bridging scaffold between ellagic acid and DBC (Figure 4). For this reason, the effect of electron-withdrawing substituents (nitro and bromine), was investigated through molecular docking approach [55]. Among various derivatives proposed in silico and prioritized for chemical synthesis and biochemical evaluation, 4-bromo-3,8-dihydroxy-benzo[c]chromen-6-one (compound 21, K_i = 0.007 µM) resulted to be even more efficacious than ellagic acid and DBC (Figure 4) [55].

3.3.2. Hit to Lead: Benzimidazole Scaffold

The optimization of chemical entities in drug discovery can be also performed starting from a scaffold recognized as a hit compound, even if not selected by high-throughput screening. One of the first family of compounds identified as inhibitors of CK2 is represented by polyhalogenated benzimidazole derivatives. DRB (5,6-dichloro-1-(β-D-ribofuranosyl)benzimidazole, K_i = 23 µM) [80], TBB (4,5,6,7-tetrabromobenzotriazole, K_i = 0.40 µM) [81], and the first generation of benzimidazole derivatives were discovered by traditional pharmacology ("trial and error testing") [82]. Several experimental data were collected for this first series of compounds, in particular focusing on the determination of their in vitro (e.g., K25 K_i = 0.04 µM) and in cell potency, their mechanism of action and their selectivity towards different kinases panels, as well as on the co-crystallization of some of them with CK2 catalytic subunit (Figure 6). Such as amount of data was essential to determinate a SAR for this starting group of compounds, and to perform additional modifications of the benzimidazole scaffold, exploiting the crystallographic informations available. First of all, the role of different halogen substitutions (Figure 6) was evaluated through molecular docking analysis combined with biochemical assays, proving that tetraiodined compounds present, on average, IC_{50} one of magnitude lower than the corresponding brominated ones (e.g., K88 K_i = 0.023 µM; K93 K_i = 0.019 µM; K100 K_i = 0.027 µM) [83].

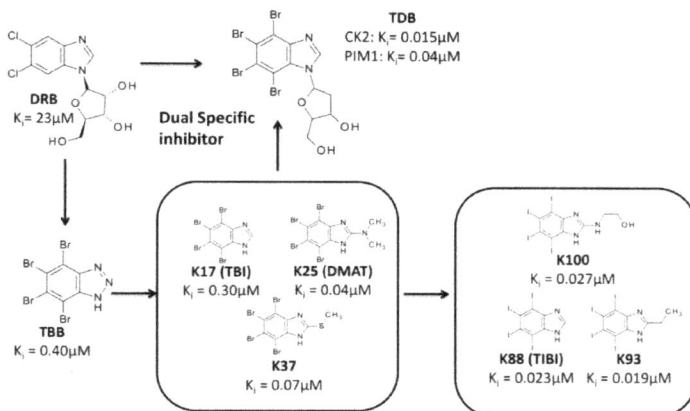

Figure 6. Schematic representation of the optimization of tetrabromobenzimidazoles.

Secondly, the benzimidazole scaffold was further optimized to design a molecule able to inhibit CK2 together with other protein kinases implicated in the same human disease [84] (Figures 6 and 7). The goal of such a strategy, called Multi Target Drug Design (MTDD), is to block redundant compensatory pathways in diseases like cancer or neurodegeneration, with consequently increase of efficacy and the reduction of drug resistance. Compounds able to target two or more protein kinases are called Multi Kinase Inhibitors (MKI); several example of MKI are present in literature, some of them have been also approved by FDA, like imatinib (Gleevec) [85] and lapatinib (Tykerb) [86,87]. The crosstalk between CK2 and PIM1 (kinase of the Proviral Integration of Moloney virus) [88] has been recognized in a number of tumors (e.g., prostate cancer, and hematologic malignancies) where they are implicated in the resistance to apoptosis [84]. The design of a specific dual and cell permeable inhibitor of CK2 and PIM1 was obtained through an in silico rational optimization of the benzimidazole scaffold, in particular by exploiting a structure based pharmacophore approach [84] (for details about pharmacophore model see Section 4). Even through this method can be used also with apo protein structures, in this case it was used to obtain pharmacophores from CK2 and PIM1 structures in complex with different inhibitors (Table 2). In fact, beside CK2, several co-crystal structures of PIM1 and its inhibitors are also available. Once collected, the structural data from both CK2 and PIM1 were divided into two groups; the first one representing the training set for the pharmacophore selection, the second one representing the test set to validate the pharmacophore model (Table 2). For both CK2 and PIM1, one single structure was chosen to generate the pharmacophore model taking into account all the interactions performed by CK2 and PIM1 ligands into the respective binding site, according to the training set. At the end of the procedure a set of chemical features was retrieved and clusterized into hydrogen donor, hydrogen acceptor, hydrophobic and aromatic features (Figure 7). Only the most recurring features retrieved from the protein ligand interaction pattern, were selected and included in the final generation of the pharmacophore models of CK2 and PIM1. These models were validated by using molecules from the test set; to note that all the inhibitors of CK2 and PIM1 present in the test set have not been used for the pharmacophore model determination, being, however, positively selected by the two final pharmacophore models, in the validation procedure. Couriously the pharmacophore models of CK2 and PIM1 resulted to be geometrically and qualitatively quite similar, being composed of two acceptor features, five hydrogen/aromatic feature, while four donor features were present in CK2 instead of three in PIM1 (Figure 7). Both the validated pharmacophore models were used as 3D queries in database searching. The chemical library represents a family of 350 tetrabromobenzimidazole derivatives built in silico through combinatory chemistry of small chemical fragments (Figure 7). Among others, TDB (1-β-D-2′-deoxyribofuranosyl-4,5,6,7- tetrabromo-1*H*-benzimidazole) resulted to be the most promising molecule retrieved from the screening procedure [84]. As expected TDB showed an ATP competitive inhibition with both CK2 and PIM1 (Ki values, 0.015 and 0.040 µM respectively), and a promising selectivity, being almost ineffective against a panel of 124 protein kinases, at 1 µM concentration [84]. The selectivity of TDB is also confirmed by the values for the Gini coefficient (0.553) and hit rate (0.14), denoting that TDB is one of the most specific inhibitors of CK2. Only two other protein kinase, DYRK1a and CLK2 have been shown to be affected by TDB ($IC_{50} = 0.4$ µM and 0.02 µM, respectively) [84]. To note that the overexpression of CLK2 is also implicated in many tumors, thus the triple specificity of TDB against CK2, CLK2 and PIM1, should be considered an advantage, rather than a weakness. The specificity of TDB towards CK2 and PIM1 was also demonstrated in living cells, where the compound was able to inhibit the endogenous activity of both protein kinases, and to reduce the phosphorylation level of specific substrates of CK2 and PIM1 (Akt Ser129 and Bad Ser112, respectively) [84]. To note that, the combined efficacy of TDB against CK2 and PIM1 was probably responsible of the remarkable cytotoxicity of the compound against cancer cells (CEM and HeLa) compared to non-tumor (cells CCD34Lu and heK-293t), showing that TDB was even better than CX-4945 in a comparative MTT test on CEM cells [84].

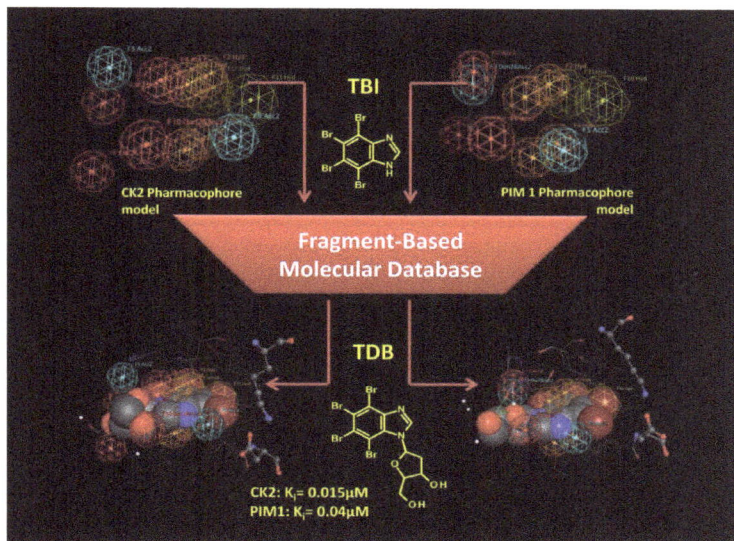

Figure 7. Structure based pharmacophore screening applied for the discovery of TDB (1-β-D-2′-deoxyribofuranosyl-4,5,6,7-tetrabromo-1H-benzimidazole), a CK2 and PIM1 dual inhibitor. Spheres represent chemical features: Red for donor, blue for acceptor, orange and yellow for hydrophobic/aromatic.

Table 2. List of CK2 and PIM1 crystal structures (PDB codes) used as training and test set for pharmacophore building.

CK2		PIM1	
Training Set	**Test Set**	**Training Set**	**Test Set**
3KXM	3KXN	4ENY	3UIX
3KXH	3KXG	4A7C	3T9I
3PVG	3PWD	3R00	3R01
3NGA	3Q9Y	3R02	3R04
3AMY	3OWK	3XJ1	3XJ2
4DGN	3MB7	3JPV	3DCV
3OWL	3OWJ	3C4E	3BGP
3MB6	3RPS	3BGQ	3BGZ
1ZOH	1ZOG	3UMX	4ENX
1M2R	1M2Q	4ALW	3UMW
2OXD	2OXY	4ALU	4ALV
1OM1	1M2P	4K18	4K1B

Another modification of the benzimidazole scaffold was rationalized starting from one of its ATP competitive derivative K137 (N1-(4,5,6,7-tetrabromo-1*H*-benzimidazol-2-yl)-propane- 1,3-diamine), with the aim to design a new family of bisubstrate inhibitors able to simultaneously interact with the ATP and the phosphoacceptor substrate binding sites [89] (Figure 8). To this purpose the extended knowledge acquired about the interactions between CK2 and its acidic peptide substrates (e.g., TS-Tide, RRRADDSDDDDD), together with the huge amount of crystallographic data for ATP competitive inhibitors, was transferred to a Molecular Dynamics guided Structure Based Docking procedure [89] (Figure 8). First of all the interaction pattern of K137 and of TS-Tide with CK2 ATP and substrate binding site respectively was acquired, through Docking and Molecular Dynamics simulations.

In particular K137 binding pose was retrieved through a genetic algorithm based molecular docking (Gold software, genetic algorithm), while the CK2-peptide substrate complex was obtained through a protein-protein docking procedure (PIPER software [90]). 1000 complexes were obtained from protein-protein docking algorithms and clusterized using the pairwise Root Mean Square Deviation (RMSD) into the six largest clusters. The final complex was chosen according to the energy scoring function. Both the docking experiments were submitted to a Molecular Dynamics protocol (NAMD 2.8 [91], 100 ns of NPT, 1 atm, 300 K) to optimize the interactions within the complexes. These data were used to propose a binding motif for K137, to identify the minimum interactions required to allocate the acidic peptide substrate in CK2 substrate binding site, and to design the best chemical spacer to connect the K137 moiety to the acidic peptide. From this procedure, a small group of molecules, was prioritized for biochemical evaluation [89]; the best compound resulted to be K137-E4 (IC_{50} = 0.025 μM) in which K137 was derivatized in position 3 by a chemical spacer connected to a peptidic fragment composed by 4 glutamic acid [89] (Figure 8). From the in silico analysis, K137-E4 was predicted to interact in the ATP binding site through the K137 moiety, and in the substrate binding region with the peptide portion (E4). Mixed competition kinetics and mutational analysis demonstrated in vitro that the compound is indeed able to interact simultaneously with both the ATP and substrate binding sites [89]. In addition to a highter potency as compared to K137 (IC_{50} = 0.13 μM), K137-E4 is more selective: while K137 is able to inhibit 35 out of 140 protein kinases more potently than CK2, K137-E4 is only active against CK2 [89]. This remarkable selectivity is also demonstrated by the value of the hit rate for K137-E4 (0.05) much lower than the one for K137 (0.27) [89].

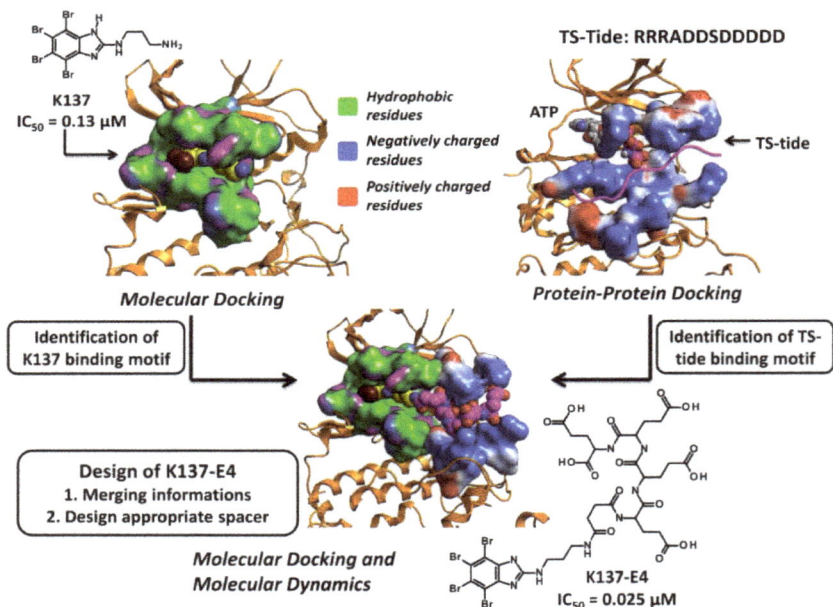

Figure 8. Schematic representation of the rational strategy leading to the design of bisubstrate inhibitors.

3.3.3. Hit to Lead: Other Examples

In the absence of crystallographic informations, molecular docking has been widely used to determine the binding motif of CK2 inhibitors. This technique was particularly useful to explain the SAR of several families of compounds, and to design optimized molecules starting from their docking pose. For example, a family of pyrimidine derivatives [92] was recently further optimized, generating a series of novel ATP-directed compounds with variable activities against CK2; one of them NHTP23 (3-(5-phenylthieno [2,3-d]pyrimidin-4-ylamino)benzoic acid) was extremely active (IC$_{50}$ = 0.01 μM) and selective against a small panel of eight protein kinases [93]. Likewise, a novel family of tetrabromobenzotriazole derivatives was studied for their inhibitory activity toward CK2 and rationalized through docking experiments. R-7b (IC$_{50}$ = 0.80μM) was the best hit compound obtained, being however effective in MCF7 adherent cells only at concentration between 50 and 100 μM [94]. To note that molecular docking was also used to clarify the binding mode of the promising peptide inhibitor Pc, able to interfere with the interaction surface between CK2 catalytic (α) and regulatory (β) subunits; this results could pave the way to the development of allosteric inhibitors of CK2 [95].

Many other computational studies have been performed on existing families of CK2 inhibitors. However, most of them have been dedicated to the development of new computational strategies and techniques, to clarify the SAR of existing families of compounds and their interaction with CK2, without leading to novel optimized chemical entities. For example, the tricyclic quinoline compound CX-4945, the only CK2 inhibitor in clinical trials, has been studied in silico, through molecular docking and dynamics, to clarify the role of its acidic portion, responsible for its marked activity [96]. In particular, the presence of non-R2 carboxylate function resulted in a different protein-ligand recognition, leading to unfavourable electrostatic interactions with the ATP binding site of CK2 [96]. Another example is provided by the exploration of interactions between a group of tetrabromobenzimidazole derivatives with CK2, exploiting a QM/MM-PB/SA method [97]. This approach was used to estimate the binding free energies of CK2-inhibitor complexes obtained through QM/MM molecular dynamics. The results demonstrated that the contribution of solvation (PB/SA) is essential to retrieve reliable results, that the hydrophobic contribution represents the driving force for the binding, while the electrostatic interactions are important for the correct orientation of benzimidazole inhibitors in the CK2 active site [97]. Moreover, the in silico methodology suggested modifications able to potentially increase the binding affinity, however no evaluation of these hypothetical molecules is actually available.

4. Rational Drug Design of CK2 Inhibitors: Ligand Based Drug Design

The huge number of crystallographic structures available for CK2, have tipped the balance of computational studies in favor of structure based drug design. However, some examples of efficient Ligand-Based Drug Design (LBDD) procedures applied to the development of CK2 inhibitors are also available in literature (discussed below). Instead of being focused on the biological target, like in the case of SBDD, LBDD exploits the knowledge of known active molecules to predict novel chemical entities able to affect the target of interest. To note that this approach, even if can be combined with SBDD techniques, it is born to be independent from the structure of the target, thus can prove extremely helpful to develop novel ligands against targets lacking tridimensional information. A huge amount of CK2 inhibitors (>200) are available in literature, belonging to several chemical class of compounds (e.g., anthraquinone, coumarin, flavone, quinoline) and characterized by a wide range of in vitro activities and selectivity (see specific reviews for detailed informations [27,28]). This structure diversity should be considered an advantage in the application of LBDD approaches for the developing and optimization of CK2 inhibitors. For this purpose, Pharmacophore screening [98] and Quantitative Structure–Activity Relationship (QSAR/3D-QSAR) [99,100] are the most used LBDD, the former mainly focused on the structural geometries and characteristics of known compounds, the latter on the correlation between calculated chemical properties of molecules and their experimentally determined activity.

4.1. The Pharmacophore Approach

A pharmacophore can be defined as an ensemble of chemical features, generally consisting of hydrogen bond acceptors/donors, electrostatic features and hydrophobic centroids, necessary to ensure the molecular recognition between a ligand and its biological target. A generated pharmacophore model could identify the minimum chemical features which different ligands should possess to bind a common binding site and can be used in a ligand-based virtual screening to identify new molecules with the same features [98]. It is normally built from a training set of diverse molecules active against the same biological target, whose low energy conformers are generated and superimposed. The 3D alignment of the ligands is used to extract chemical properties for the pharmacophore model, assigning the correct pharmacophoric features [98]. The final model must be validated with a set of known active compounds against the common biological target. It is fairly common for pharmacophore approach to be combined with SBDD techniques when tridimensional information for the biological target is available. For example, results from a ligand-based pharmacophore model are often confirmed through molecular docking before being validated by biochemical evaluation.

4.1.1. The Pharmacophore Approach: Applications

An interesting combination of pharmacophore hypothesis, the Bayesian model (LBDD technique) and molecular docking was recently performed [101]. Bayesian model, a probabilistic classifier based on applying Bayes' theorem, is one of the most versatile machine learning algorithms. It was used to distinguish active from non-active inhibitors of CK2, by training the protocol with a set 73 active and 29 inactive compounds. On the other side a pharmacophore model was developed using seven active CK2 inhibitors together with two non-active compounds; finally a docking protocol was used to confirm the data obtained from LBDD analysis. Bayesian model, pharmacophore model and molecular docking were sequentially used to filter more than one million molecules; 30 compounds were selected from the in silico analysis and one of them (compound **C1**) resulted to be structurally unrelated to the other known CK2 inhibitor and displayed an IC_{50} of 5.85 µM [101].

4.2. Quantitative Structure–Activity Relationship (QSAR)

Quantitative structure-activity relationships (QSAR) can be defined as regression or classification models used in several scientific applications. In computational chemistry and in drug design in general, QSAR have been applied to study the relationship between physicochemical properties of molecules and their biological activities; QSAR aims at building reliable statistical models to predict the activities of novel chemical entities [99,100]. The basic concept of QSAR is that structural properties of molecules are strictly connected with their biological activities; in other words inhibition constants, rate constants and affinities of compounds with their targets are correlated with chemical features like electronic and steric properties, lipophilicity, polarizability. 3D-QSAR has emerged as an optimized methodology for the design of new molecules, by exploiting the three-dimensional properties of known compounds to predict the biological activities of novel chemical entities through chemometric techniques such as Partial Least Squares (PLS), Principal Components Analysis (PCA), Comparative Molecular Field Analysis (CoMFA), Molecular Similarity Indices in a Comparative Analysis (CoMSIA).

4.2.1. The QSAR Approach: Applications

By exploiting a pool of 38 CK2/inhibitors complexes a QSAR model based on Multiple Linear Regression (MLR) was built in combination with a docking protocol (AutoDock) for the generation of energy-based descriptors. After a cross-validation procedure, 20 analogues of ellagic acid were subjected to the QSAR-Docking approach; intriguingly two compounds were predicted in silico to be more potent than ellagic acid, however these results were not validated in a biochemical assays [102]. On the other hand, CoMFA and CoMSIA methodologies, based on several CK2 inhibitors, were used in a 3D-QSAR study, generating a statistically solid model; unfortunately, the in silico analysis was not applied for the discovery of novel compounds, but only suggested plausible substitutions in the development of CK2 inhibitors [103]. CoMFA and CoMSIA descriptors were also applied to study 40 coumarin derivatives combined with molecular docking. The model was successfully validated using five known inhibitors of CK2 belonging to the coumarin family of compounds [104].

5. Discussion

CK2 is an ubiquitous and pleiotropic protein kinase, intensively studied for its biological roles and its implication in several human diseases in particular cancer, where its upregulation favours tumor progression. The search of CK2 inhibitors started several years ago and at the beginning it was grounded on "trial and error testing" against the purified enzyme. With the increasing number of crystallographic information about CK2 alone or in complex with the first isolated inhibitors, together with the availability of in silico protocols for the design and development of active ligands, several research groups started to merge the classical biochemical studies with computational methodologies able to rationalize the experimental data. Later on, in silico rational drug design became even more important for the discovery and optimization of CK2 inhibitors in particular exploiting Structure Based Drug Design (SBDD) techniques. The abundance of crystal structure of CK2 proved very helpful for the optimization of virtual screening and molecular docking algorithms, as well as for the building of solid free energy binding models. Several promising compounds have been obtained through virtual screening campaigns, like IQA, ellagic acid and quinalizarin. Moreover, rational hit optimization by means of molecular docking, pharmacophore approaches and molecular dynamics simulations has been shown to be able to retrieve novel potent inhibitors of CK2, with different mechanism of action and specificity.

Special reference needs to be made for Ligand-Based Drug Design (LBDD) techniques; despite the abundance of CK2 inhibitors available in the literature, the success of these approaches is very limited; in fact LBDD techniques were able to suggest new scaffolds, however characterized by poor potency and not further optimized. The general impression is that the development of CK2 inhibitors through LBDD techniques is still in an early phase, probably restrained by the presence of validated and efficacious SBDD protocols. This is confirmed also by the majority of published papers, where LBDD techniques are applied for the design of CK2 inhibitors. In these cases, indeed, calibration, validation and improvement of the methodologies are the main addressed aspects, rather than specific applications for the development of potent and selective inhibitors of CK2.

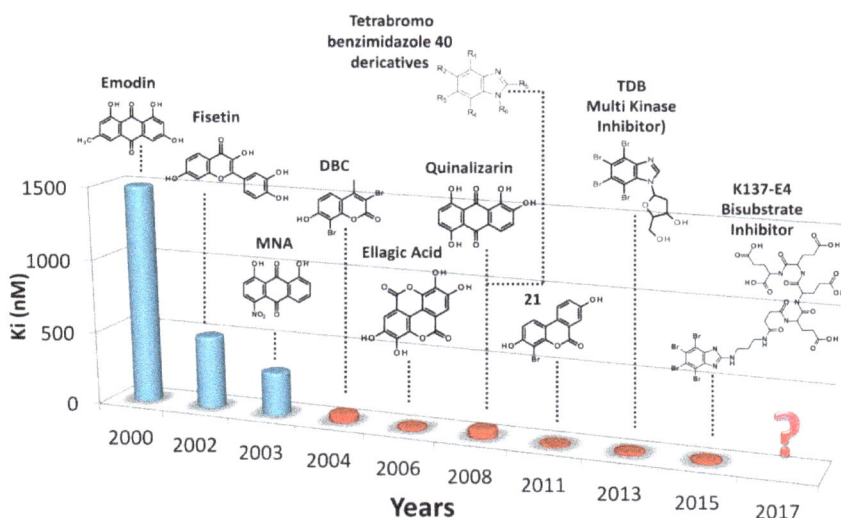

Figure 9. Activity of CK2 inhibitors over time expressed in Ki; blue bars represent the inhibition constant of compounds identified through random screen campaign of chemical compounds ("trial and error testing"), red bars the ones of compounds discovered through in silico rational drug design.

In conclusion, as summarized in Figure 9, the introduction of in silico rational drug design in the discovery and optimization of CK2 inhibitors was of invaluable usefulness to retrieve novel hit compounds by virtual screening and to focalize the synthesis of optimized molecules by molecular docking and dynamics. The combination of in silico techniques with biochemical, crystallographic, and in cell approaches has accelerated the discovery of more active and more selective inhibitors of CK2, as compared to the traditional trials and error testing. Moreover the increasing of computational power based not only on the Central Processing Unit (CPU) but also on the Graphics Processing Unit (GPU), gives a promising perspective on the development of even better computational algorithms for CK2 drug design, involving mechanics calculation in the quantum level based on larger databases of compounds.

Supplementary Materials: The following are available online at http://www.mdpi.com/1424-8247/10/1/26/s1, Table S1: Summary of all CK2 crystal structures deposited in the Protein Data Bank (PDB).

Acknowledgments: This work was supported by the University of Padova (Progetto Giovani Ricercatori) to G.C. The author gratefully acknowledge the Molecular Modeling Section coordinated by Stefano Moro, and the MRC Protein Phosphorylation Unit for ellagic acid selectivity profile. A special thanks to Prof. Lorenzo A. Pinna.

Conflicts of Interest: The author declares no conflict of interest.

References

1. Burnett, G.; Kennedy, E.P. The enzymatic phosphorylation of proteins. *J. Biol. Chem.* **1954**, *211*, 969–980.
2. Meggio, F.; Pinna, L.A. One-thousand-and-one substrates of protein kinase CK2? *FASEB J.* **2003**, *17*, 349–368. [CrossRef]
3. Salvi, M.; Sarno, S.; Cesaro, L.; Nakamura, H.; Pinna, L.A. Extraordinary pleiotropy of protein kinase CK2 revealed by weblogo phosphoproteome analysis. *Biochim. Biophys. Acta* **2009**, *1793*, 847–859. [CrossRef] [PubMed]
4. Sarno, S.; Ghisellini, P.; Pinna, L.A. Unique activation mechanism of protein kinase CK2. The n-terminal segment is essential for constitutive activity of the catalytic subunit but not of the holoenzyme. *J. Biol. Chem.* **2002**, *277*, 22509–22514. [CrossRef] [PubMed]
5. Cristiani, A.; Costa, G.; Cozza, G.; Meggio, F.; Scapozza, L.; Moro, S. The role of the n-terminal domain in the regulation of the "constitutively active" conformation of protein kinase CK2alpha: Insight from a molecular dynamics investigation. *ChemMedChem* **2011**, *6*, 1207–1216. [CrossRef]
6. Ortega, C.E.; Seidner, Y.; Dominguez, I. Mining CK2 in cancer. *PLoS ONE* **2014**, *9*, e115609. [CrossRef] [PubMed]
7. Murtaza, I.; Wang, H.X.; Feng, X.; Alenina, N.; Bader, M.; Prabhakar, B.S.; Li, P.F. Down-regulation of catalase and oxidative modification of protein kinase CK2 lead to the failure of apoptosis repressor with caspase recruitment domain to inhibit cardiomyocyte hypertrophy. *J. Biol. Chem.* **2008**, *283*, 5996–6004. [CrossRef] [PubMed]
8. Axtell, R.C.; Xu, L.; Barnum, S.R.; Raman, C. Cd5-CK2 binding/activation-deficient mice are resistant to experimental autoimmune encephalomyelitis: Protection is associated with diminished populations of il-17-expressing t cells in the central nervous system. *J. Immunol.* **2006**, *177*, 8542–8549. [CrossRef] [PubMed]
9. Ivanov, K.I.; Puustinen, P.; Gabrenaite, R.; Vihinen, H.; Ronnstrand, L.; Valmu, L.; Kalkkinen, N.; Makinen, K. Phosphorylation of the potyvirus capsid protein by protein kinase CK2 and its relevance for virus infection. *Plant Cell* **2003**, *15*, 2124–2139. [CrossRef] [PubMed]
10. Foka, P.; Dimitriadis, A.; Kyratzopoulou, E.; Giannimaras, D.A.; Sarno, S.; Simos, G.; Georgopoulou, U.; Mamalaki, A. A complex signaling network involving protein kinase CK2 is required for hepatitis c virus core protein-mediated modulation of the iron-regulatory hepcidin gene expression. *Cell. Mol. Life Sci.* **2014**, *71*, 4243–4258. [CrossRef] [PubMed]
11. Meggio, F.; Marin, O.; Boschetti, M.; Sarno, S.; Pinna, L.A. Hiv-1 rev transactivator: A beta-subunit directed substrate and effector of protein kinase CK2. *Mol. Cell. Biochem.* **2001**, *227*, 145–151. [CrossRef] [PubMed]
12. Pagano, M.A.; Arrigoni, G.; Marin, O.; Sarno, S.; Meggio, F.; Treharne, K.J.; Mehta, A.; Pinna, L.A. Modulation of protein kinase CK2 activity by fragments of CFTR encompassing f508 may reflect functional links with cystic fibrosis pathogenesis. *Biochemistry* **2008**, *47*, 7925–7936. [CrossRef] [PubMed]

13. Pagano, M.A.; Marin, O.; Cozza, G.; Sarno, S.; Meggio, F.; Treharne, K.J.; Mehta, A.; Pinna, L.A. Cystic fibrosis transmembrane regulator fragments with the phe508 deletion exert a dual allosteric control over the master kinase CK2. *Biochem. J.* **2010**, *426*, 19–29. [CrossRef] [PubMed]

14. Cesaro, L.; Marin, O.; Venerando, A.; Donella-Deana, A.; Pinna, L.A. Phosphorylation of cystic fibrosis transmembrane conductance regulator (CFTR) serine-511 by the combined action of tyrosine kinases and CK2: The implication of tyrosine-512 and phenylalanine-508. *Amino Acids* **2013**, *45*, 1423–1429. [CrossRef] [PubMed]

15. Siddiqui-Jain, A.; Drygin, D.; Streiner, N.; Chua, P.; Pierre, F.; O'Brien, S.E.; Bliesath, J.; Omori, M.; Huser, N.; Ho, C.; et al. Cx-4945, an orally bioavailable selective inhibitor of protein kinase CK2, inhibits prosurvival and angiogenic signaling and exhibits antitumor efficacy. *Cancer Res.* **2010**, *70*, 10288–10298. [CrossRef] [PubMed]

16. Pierre, F.; Chua, P.C.; O'Brien, S.E.; Siddiqui-Jain, A.; Bourbon, P.; Haddach, M.; Michaux, J.; Nagasawa, J.; Schwaebe, M.K.; Stefan, E.; et al. Pre-clinical characterization of cx-4945, a potent and selective small molecule inhibitor of CK2 for the treatment of cancer. *Mol. Cell. Biochem.* **2011**, *356*, 37–43. [CrossRef] [PubMed]

17. Ferguson, A.D.; Sheth, P.R.; Basso, A.D.; Paliwal, S.; Gray, K.; Fischmann, T.O.; Le, H.V. Structural basis of cx-4945 binding to human protein kinase CK2. *FEBS Lett.* **2011**, *585*, 104–110. [CrossRef] [PubMed]

18. Wilson, L.K.; Dhillon, N.; Thorner, J.; Martin, G.S. Casein kinase ii catalyzes tyrosine phosphorylation of the yeast nucleolar immunophilin fpr3. *J. Biol. Chem.* **1997**, *272*, 12961–12967. [CrossRef] [PubMed]

19. Marin, O.; Meggio, F.; Sarno, S.; Cesaro, L.; Pagano, M.A.; Pinna, L.A. Tyrosine versus serine/threonine phosphorylation by protein kinase casein kinase-2. A study with peptide substrates derived from immunophilin FPR3. *J. Biol. Chem.* **1999**, *274*, 29260–29265. [CrossRef] [PubMed]

20. Sarno, S.; Vaglio, P.; Meggio, F.; Issinger, O.-G.; Pinna, L.A. Protein kinase CK2 mutants defective in substrate recognition. Purification and kinetic analysis. *J. Biol. Chem.* **1996**, *271*, 10595–10601. [PubMed]

21. Marin, O.; Sarno, S.; Boschetti, M.; Pagano, M.A.; Meggio, F.; Ciminale, V.; D'Agostino, D.M.; Pinna, L.A. Unique features of hiv-1 rev protein phosphorylation by protein kinase CK2 ('casein kinase-2'). *FEBS Lett.* **2000**, *481*, 63–67. [CrossRef]

22. Poletto, G.; Vilardell, J.; Marin, O.; Pagano, M.A.; Cozza, G.; Sarno, S.; Falques, A.; Itarte, E.; Pinna, L.A.; Meggio, F. The regulatory beta subunit of protein kinase CK2 contributes to the recognition of the substrate consensus sequence. A study with an EIF2 beta-derived peptide. *Biochemistry* **2008**, *47*, 8317–8325. [CrossRef] [PubMed]

23. Meggio, F.; Boldyreff, B.; Marin, O.; Marchiori, F.; Perich, J.W.; Issinger, O.-G.; Pinna, L.A. The effect of polylysine on casein-kinase-2 activity is influenced by both the structure of the protein/peptide substrates and the subunit composition of the enzyme. *Eur. J. Biochem.* **1992**, *205*, 939–945. [CrossRef] [PubMed]

24. Boldyreff, B.; James, P.; Staudenmann, W.; Issinger, O.-G. Ser2 is the autophosphorylation site in the beta subunit from bicistronically expressed human casein kinase-2 and from native rat liver casein kinase-2 beta. *Eur. J. Biochem.* **1993**, *218*, 515–521. [CrossRef] [PubMed]

25. Litchfield, D.W.; Lozeman, F.J.; Cicirelli, M.F.; Harrylock, M.; Ericsson, L.H.; Piening, C.J.; Krebs, E.G. Phosphorylation of the beta subunit of casein kinase ii in human a431 cells. Identification of the autophosphorylation site and a site phosphorylated by p34cdc2. *J. Biol. Chem.* **1991**, *266*, 20380–20389. [PubMed]

26. Lolli, G.; Pinna, L.A.; Battistutta, R. Structural determinants of protein kinase CK2 regulation by autoinhibitory polymerization. *ACS Chem. Biol.* **2012**, *7*, 1158–1163. [CrossRef] [PubMed]

27. Cozza, G.; Pinna, L.A.; Moro, S. Kinase CK2 inhibition: An update. *Curr. Med. Chem.* **2013**, *20*, 671–693. [CrossRef] [PubMed]

28. Cozza, G.; Pinna, L.A. Casein kinases as potential therapeutic targets. *Expert Opin. Ther. Targets* **2015**, 1–22. [CrossRef] [PubMed]

29. Hubert, A.; Paris, S.; Piret, J.P.; Ninane, N.; Raes, M.; Michiels, C. Casein Kinase 2 inhibition decreases hypoxia-inducible factor-1 activity under hypoxia through elevated p53 protein level. *J. Cell Sci.* **2006**, *119*, 3351–3362. [CrossRef] [PubMed]

30. Hupp, T.R.; Meek, D.W.; Midgley, C.A.; Lane, D.P. Regulation of the specific DNA binding function of p53. *Cell* **1992**, *71*, 875–886. [CrossRef]

31. Mottet, D.; Ruys, S.P.; Demazy, C.; Raes, M.; Michiels, C. Role for casein kinase 2 in the regulation of HIF-1 activity. *Int. J. Cancer* **2005**, *117*, 764–774. [PubMed]

32. Pluemsampant, S.; Safronova, O.S.; Nakahama, K.; Morita, I. Protein kinase CK2 is a key activator of histone deacetylase in hypoxia-associated tumors. *Int. J. Cancer* **2008**, *122*, 333–341. [CrossRef] [PubMed]

33. Charo, I.F.; Taubman, M.B. Chemokines in the pathogenesis of vascular disease. *Circ. Res.* **2004**, *95*, 858–866. [CrossRef] [PubMed]

34. Harvey, E.J.; Li, N.; Ramji, D.P. Critical role for casein kinase 2 and phosphoinositide-3-kinase in the interferon-gamma-induced expression of monocyte chemoattractant protein-1 and other key genes implicated in atherosclerosis. *Arter. Thromb. Vasc. Biol.* **2007**, *27*, 806–812. [CrossRef]

35. Okochi, M.; Walter, J.; Koyama, A.; Nakajo, S.; Baba, M.; Iwatsubo, T.; Meijer, L.; Kahle, P.J.; Haass, C. Constitutive phosphorylation of the parkinson's disease associated alpha-synuclein. *J. Biol. Chem.* **2000**, *275*, 390–397. [CrossRef]

36. Lee, G.; Tanaka, M.; Park, K.; Lee, S.S.; Kim, Y.M.; Junn, E.; Lee, S.H.; Mouradian, M.M. Casein Kinase II-mediated phosphorylation regulates alpha-synuclein/synphilin-1 interaction and inclusion body formation. *J. Biol. Chem.* **2004**, *279*, 6834–6839. [CrossRef] [PubMed]

37. Ishii, A.; Nonaka, T.; Taniguchi, S.; Saito, T.; Arai, T.; Mann, D.; Iwatsubo, T.; Hisanaga, S.; Goedert, M.; Hasegawa, M. Casein kinase 2 is the major enzyme in brain that phosphorylates ser129 of human alpha-synuclein: Implication for alpha-synucleinopathies. *FEBS Lett.* **2007**, *581*, 4711–4717. [CrossRef] [PubMed]

38. Iimoto, D.S.; Masliah, E.; DeTeresa, R.; Terry, R.D.; Saitoh, T. Aberrant casein kinase II in alzheimer's disease. *Brain Res.* **1990**, *507*, 273–280. [CrossRef]

39. Aksenova, M.V.; Burbaeva, G.S.; Kandror, K.V.; Kapkov, D.V.; Stepanov, A.S. The decreased level of casein kinase 2 in brain cortex of schizophrenic and alzheimer's disease patients. *FEBS Lett.* **1991**, *279*, 55–57. [CrossRef]

40. Masliah, E.; Iimoto, D.S.; Mallory, M.; Albright, T.; Hansen, L.; Saitoh, T. Casein kinase ii alteration precedes tau accumulation in tangle formation. *Am. J. Pathol.* **1992**, *140*, 263–268. [PubMed]

41. Greenwood, J.A.; Scott, C.W.; Spreen, R.C.; Caputo, C.B.; Johnson, G.V. Casein kinase ii preferentially phosphorylates human tau isoforms containing an amino-terminal insert. Identification of threonine 39 as the primary phosphate acceptor. *J. Biol. Chem.* **1994**, *269*, 4373–4380. [PubMed]

42. Yamada, M.; Katsuma, S.; Adachi, T.; Hirasawa, A.; Shiojima, S.; Kadowaki, T.; Okuno, Y.; Koshimizu, T.A.; Fujii, S.; Sekiya, Y.; et al. Inhibition of protein kinase CK2 prevents the progression of glomerulonephritis. *Proc. Natl. Acad. Sci. USA* **2005**, *102*, 7736–7741. [CrossRef] [PubMed]

43. Maekawa, T.; Kosuge, S.; Karino, A.; Okano, T.; Ito, J.; Munakata, H.; Ohtsuki, K. Biochemical characterization of 60s acidic ribosomal p proteins from porcine liver and the inhibition of their immunocomplex formation with sera from systemic lupus erythematosus (sle) patients by glycyrrhizin in vitro. *Biol. Pharm. Bull.* **2000**, *23*, 27–32.

44. Caponi, L.; Anzilotti, C.; Longombardo, G.; Migliorini, P. Antibodies directed against ribosomal p proteins cross-react with phospholipids. *Clin. Exp. Immunol.* **2007**, *150*, 140–143. [CrossRef] [PubMed]

45. Hauck, L.; Harms, C.; An, J.; Rohne, J.; Gertz, K.; Dietz, R.; Endres, M.; von Harsdorf, R. Protein kinase CK2 links extracellular growth factor signaling with the control of p27(kip1) stability in the heart. *Nat. Med.* **2008**, *14*, 315–324. [CrossRef] [PubMed]

46. Tapia, J.C.; Bolanos-Garcia, V.M.; Sayed, M.; Allende, C.C.; Allende, J.E. Cell cycle regulatory protein p27kip1 is a substrate and interacts with the protein kinase CK2. *J. Cell. Biochem.* **2004**, *91*, 865–879. [CrossRef] [PubMed]

47. De Stefano, D.; Villella, V.R.; Esposito, S.; Tosco, A.; Sepe, A.; De Gregorio, F.; Salvadori, L.; Grassia, R.; Leone, C.A.; De Rosa, G.; et al. Restoration of CFTR function in patients with cystic fibrosis carrying the f508del-CFTR mutation. *Autophagy* **2014**, *10*, 2053–2074. [CrossRef] [PubMed]

48. Ruzzene, M.; Pinna, L.A. Addiction to protein kinase CK2: A common denominator of diverse cancer cells? *Biochim. Biophys. Acta Proteins Proteom.* **2010**, *1804*, 499–504. [CrossRef] [PubMed]

49. Cozza, G.; Mazzorana, M.; Papinutto, E.; Bain, J.; Elliott, M.; di Maira, G.; Gianoncelli, A.; Pagano, M.A.; Sarno, S.; Ruzzene, M.; et al. Quinalizarin as a potent, selective and cell-permeable inhibitor of protein kinase CK2. *Biochem. J.* **2009**, *421*, 387–395. [CrossRef] [PubMed]

50. Cozza, G.; Bonvini, P.; Zorzi, E.; Poletto, G.; Pagano, M.A.; Sarno, S.; Donella-Deana, A.; Zagotto, G.; Rosolen, A.; Pinna, L.A.; et al. Identification of ellagic acid as potent inhibitor of protein kinase CK2: A successful example of a virtual screening application. *J. Med. Chem.* **2006**, *49*, 2363–2366. [CrossRef] [PubMed]

51. Wang, J.; Wolf, R.M.; Caldwell, J.W.; Kollman, P.A.; Case, D.A. Development and testing of a general amber force field. *J. Comput. Chem.* **2004**, *25*, 1157–1174. [CrossRef] [PubMed]

52. Brooks, B.R.; Brooks, C.L., 3rd; Mackerell, A.D., Jr.; Nilsson, L.; Petrella, R.J.; Roux, B.; Won, Y.; Archontis, G.; Bartels, C.; Boresch, S.; et al. Charmm: The biomolecular simulation program. *J. Comput. Chem.* **2009**, *30*, 1545–1614. [CrossRef] [PubMed]

53. Halgren, T.A. Merck molecular force field. 1. Basis, form, scope, parameterization, and performance of mmff94. *J. Comput. Chem.* **1996**, *17*, 490–519. [CrossRef]

54. Harder, E.; Damm, W.; Maple, J.; Wu, C.J.; Reboul, M.; Xiang, J.Y.; Wang, L.L.; Lupyan, D.; Dahlgren, M.K.; Knight, J.L.; et al. Opls3: A force field providing broad coverage of drug-like small molecules and proteins. *J. Chem. Theory Comput.* **2016**, *12*, 281–296. [CrossRef] [PubMed]

55. Cozza, G.; Gianoncelli, A.; Bonvini, P.; Zorzi, E.; Pasquale, R.; Rosolen, A.; Pinna, L.A.; Meggio, F.; Zagotto, G.; Moro, S. Urolithin as a converging scaffold linking ellagic acid and coumarin analogues: Design of potent protein kinase CK2 inhibitors. *ChemMedChem* **2011**, *6*, 2273–2286. [CrossRef] [PubMed]

56. Sarno, S.; Moro, S.; Meggio, F.; Zagotto, G.; Dal Ben, D.; Ghisellini, P.; Battistutta, R.; Zanotti, G.; Pinna, L.A. Toward the rational design of protein kinase casein kinase-2 inhibitors. *Pharmacol. Ther.* **2002**, *93*, 159–168. [CrossRef]

57. Pagano, M.A.; Sarno, S.; Poletto, G.; Cozza, G.; Pinna, L.A.; Meggio, F. Autophosphorylation at the regulatory beta subunit reflects the supramolecular organization of protein kinase CK2. *Mol. Cell. Biochem.* **2005**, *274*, 23–29. [CrossRef] [PubMed]

58. Kroemer, R.T. Structure-based drug design: Docking and scoring. *Curr. Protein Pept. Sci.* **2007**, *8*, 312–328. [CrossRef] [PubMed]

59. Cavasotto, C.N.; Orry, A.J. Ligand docking and structure-based virtual screening in drug discovery. *Curr. Top. Med. Chem.* **2007**, *7*, 1006–1014. [CrossRef] [PubMed]

60. Morris, G.M.; Huey, R.; Lindstrom, W.; Sanner, M.F.; Belew, R.K.; Goodsell, D.S.; Olson, A.J. Autodock4 and autodocktools4: Automated docking with selective receptor flexibility. *J. Comput. Chem.* **2009**, *30*, 2785–2791. [CrossRef]

61. Jones, G.; Willett, P.; Glen, R.C.; Leach, A.R.; Taylor, R. Development and validation of a genetic algorithm for flexible docking. *J. Mol. Biol.* **1997**, *267*, 727–748. [CrossRef] [PubMed]

62. Vilar, S.; Cozza, G.; Moro, S. Medicinal chemistry and the molecular operating environment (moe): Application of qsar and molecular docking to drug discovery. *Curr. Top. Med. Chem.* **2008**, *8*, 1555–1572. [CrossRef] [PubMed]

63. Allen, W.J.; Balius, T.E.; Mukherjee, S.; Brozell, S.R.; Moustakas, D.T.; Lang, P.T.; Case, D.A.; Kuntz, I.D.; Rizzo, R.C. Dock 6: Impact of new features and current docking performance. *J. Comput. Chem.* **2015**, *36*, 1132–1156. [CrossRef] [PubMed]

64. Friesner, R.A.; Banks, J.L.; Murphy, R.B.; Halgren, T.A.; Klicic, J.J.; Mainz, D.T.; Repasky, M.P.; Knoll, E.H.; Shelley, M.; Perry, J.K.; et al. Glide: A new approach for rapid, accurate docking and scoring. 1. Method and assessment of docking accuracy. *J. Med. Chem.* **2004**, *47*, 1739–1749. [CrossRef] [PubMed]

65. McGann, M. Fred pose prediction and virtual screening accuracy. *J. Chem. Inf. Model.* **2011**, *51*, 578–596. [CrossRef] [PubMed]

66. Zsoldos, Z.; Reid, D.; Simon, A.; Sadjad, S.B.; Johnson, A.P. Ehits: A new fast, exhaustive flexible ligand docking system. *J. Mol. Graph. Model.* **2007**, *26*, 198–212. [CrossRef] [PubMed]

67. Rarey, M.; Kramer, B.; Lengauer, T.; Klebe, G. A fast flexible docking method using an incremental construction algorithm. *J. Mol. Biol.* **1996**, *261*, 470–489. [CrossRef] [PubMed]

68. Bain, J.; Plater, L.; Elliott, M.; Shpiro, N.; Hastie, C.J.; McLauchlan, H.; Klevernic, I.; Arthur, J.S.; Alessi, D.R.; Cohen, P. The selectivity of protein kinase inhibitors: A further update. *Biochem. J.* **2007**, *408*, 297–315. [CrossRef] [PubMed]

69. De Moliner, E.; Moro, S.; Sarno, S.; Zagotto, G.; Zanotti, G.; Pinna, L.A.; Battistutta, R. Inhibition of protein kinase CK2 by anthraquinone-related compounds. A structural insight. *J. Biol. Chem.* **2003**, *278*, 1831–1836. [CrossRef] [PubMed]

70. Cozza, G.; Venerando, A.; Sarno, S.; Pinna, L.A. The selectivity of CK2 inhibitor quinalizarin: A reevaluation. *Biomed. Res. Int.* **2015**, *2015*, 734127. [CrossRef] [PubMed]

71. Franchin, C.; Salvi, M.; Arrigoni, G.; Pinna, L.A. Proteomics perturbations promoted by the protein kinase CK2 inhibitor quinalizarin. *Biochim. Biophys. Acta* **2015**. [CrossRef] [PubMed]

72. Vangrevelinghe, E.; Zimmermann, K.; Schoepfer, J.; Portmann, R.; Fabbro, D.; Furet, P. Discovery of a potent and selective protein kinase CK2 inhibitor by high-throughput docking. *J. Med. Chem.* **2003**, *46*, 2656–2662. [CrossRef] [PubMed]

73. Sarno, S.; de Moliner, E.; Ruzzene, M.; Pagano, M.A.; Battistutta, R.; Bain, J.; Fabbro, D.; Schoepfer, J.; Elliott, M.; Furet, P.; et al. Biochemical and three-dimensional-structural study of the specific inhibition of protein kinase CK2 by [5-oxo-5,6-dihydroindolo-(1,2-a)quinazolin-7-yl]acetic acid (iqa). *Biochem. J.* **2003**, *374*, 639–646. [CrossRef] [PubMed]

74. Sun, H.; Xu, X.; Wu, X.; Zhang, X.; Liu, F.; Jia, J.; Guo, X.; Huang, J.; Jiang, Z.; Feng, T.; et al. Discovery and design of tricyclic scaffolds as protein kinase CK2 (CK2) inhibitors through a combination of shape-based virtual screening and structure-based molecular modification. *J. Chem. Inf. Model.* **2013**, *53*, 2093–2102. [CrossRef] [PubMed]

75. Sun, H.; Wu, X.; Xu, X.; Jiang, Z.; Liu, Z.; You, Q. Discovery of novel CK2 leads by cross-docking based virtual screening. *Med. Chem.* **2014**, *10*, 628–639. [CrossRef] [PubMed]

76. Genheden, S.; Ryde, U. The mm/pbsa and mm/gbsa methods to estimate ligand-binding affinities. *Expert Opin. Drug Discov.* **2015**, *10*, 449–461. [CrossRef] [PubMed]

77. Carlsson, J.; Boukharta, L.; Aqvist, J. Combining docking, molecular dynamics and the linear interaction energy method to predict binding modes and affinities for non-nucleoside inhibitors to hiv-1 reverse transcriptase. *J. Med. Chem.* **2008**, *51*, 2648–2656. [CrossRef] [PubMed]

78. Sekiguchi, Y.; Nakaniwa, T.; Kinoshita, T.; Nakanishi, I.; Kitaura, K.; Hirasawa, A.; Tsujimoto, G.; Tada, T. Structural insight into human CK2alpha in complex with the potent inhibitor ellagic acid. *Bioorg. Med. Chem. Lett.* **2009**, *19*, 2920–2923. [CrossRef] [PubMed]

79. Chilin, A.; Battistutta, R.; Bortolato, A.; Cozza, G.; Zanatta, S.; Poletto, G.; Mazzorana, M.; Zagotto, G.; Uriarte, E.; Guiotto, A.; et al. Coumarin as attractive casein kinase 2 (CK2) inhibitor scaffold: An integrate approach to elucidate the putative binding motif and explain structure-activity relationships. *J. Med. Chem.* **2008**, *51*, 752–759. [CrossRef] [PubMed]

80. Zandomeni, R.; Zandomeni, M.C.; Shugar, D.; Weinmann, R. Casein kinase type ii is involved in the inhibition by 5,6-dichloro-1-beta-d-ribofuranosylbenzimidazole of specific rna polymerase ii transcription. *J. Biol. Chem.* **1986**, *261*, 3414–3419. [PubMed]

81. Ruzzene, M.; Penzo, D.; Pinna, L.A. Protein kinase CK2 inhibitor 4,5,6,7-tetrabromobenzotriazole (TBB) induces apoptosis and caspase-dependent degradation of haematopoietic lineage cell-specific protein 1 (hs1) in jurkat cells. *Biochem. J.* **2002**, *364*, 41–47. [CrossRef] [PubMed]

82. Pagano, M.A.; Meggio, F.; Ruzzene, M.; Andrzejewska, M.; Kazimierczuk, Z.; Pinna, L.A. 2-dimethylamino-4,5,6,7-tetrabromo-1h-benzimidazole: A novel powerful and selective inhibitor of protein kinase CK2. *Biochem. Biophys. Res. Commun.* **2004**, *321*, 1040–1044. [CrossRef] [PubMed]

83. Gianoncelli, A.; Cozza, G.; Orzeszko, A.; Meggio, F.; Kazimierczuk, Z.; Pinna, L.A. Tetraiodobenzimidazoles are potent inhibitors of protein kinase CK2. *Bioorg. Med. Chem.* **2009**, *17*, 7281–7289. [CrossRef] [PubMed]

84. Cozza, G.; Girardi, C.; Ranchio, A.; Lolli, G.; Sarno, S.; Orzeszko, A.; Kazimierczuk, Z.; Battistutta, R.; Ruzzene, M.; Pinna, L.A. Cell-permeable dual inhibitors of protein kinases CK2 and pim-1: Structural features and pharmacological potential. *Cell. Mol. Life Sci.* **2014**, *71*, 3173–3185. [CrossRef] [PubMed]

85. Lorusso, P.M.; Eder, J.P. Therapeutic potential of novel selective-spectrum kinase inhibitors in oncology. *Expert Opin. Investig. Drugs* **2008**, *17*, 1013–1028. [CrossRef] [PubMed]

86. Lackey, K.E. Lessons from the drug discovery of lapatinib, a dual erbb1/2 tyrosine kinase inhibitor. *Curr. Top. Med. Chem.* **2006**, *6*, 435–460. [CrossRef] [PubMed]

87. Zhang, Y.M.; Cockerill, S.; Guntrip, S.B.; Rusnak, D.; Smith, K.; Vanderwall, D.; Wood, E.; Lackey, K. Synthesis and sar of potent egfr/erbb2 dual inhibitors. *Bioorg. Med. Chem. Lett.* **2004**, *14*, 111–114. [CrossRef] [PubMed]

88. Brault, L.; Gasser, C.; Bracher, F.; Huber, K.; Knapp, S.; Schwaller, J. Pim serine/threonine kinases in the pathogenesis and therapy of hematologic malignancies and solid cancers. *Haematologica* **2010**, *95*, 1004–1015. [CrossRef] [PubMed]

89. Cozza, G.; Zanin, S.; Sarno, S.; Costa, E.; Girardi, C.; Ribaudo, G.; Salvi, M.; Zagotto, G.; Ruzzene, M.; Pinna, L.A. Design, validation and efficacy of bisubstrate inhibitors specifically affecting ecto-CK2 kinase activity. *Biochem. J.* **2015**, *471*, 415–430. [CrossRef] [PubMed]

90. Kozakov, D.; Brenke, R.; Comeau, S.R.; Vajda, S. Piper: An fft-based protein docking program with pairwise potentials. *Proteins* **2006**, *65*, 392–406. [CrossRef] [PubMed]

91. Phillips, J.C.; Braun, R.; Wang, W.; Gumbart, J.; Tajkhorshid, E.; Villa, E.; Chipot, C.; Skeel, R.D.; Kale, L.; Schulten, K. Scalable molecular dynamics with namd. *J. Comput. Chem.* **2005**, *26*, 1781–1802. [CrossRef] [PubMed]

92. Golub, A.G.; Bdzhola, V.G.; Briukhovetska, N.V.; Balanda, A.O.; Kukharenko, O.P.; Kotey, I.M.; Ostrynska, O.V.; Yarmoluk, S.M. Synthesis and biological evaluation of substituted (thieno[2,3-d]pyrimidin-4-ylthio)carboxylic acids as inhibitors of human protein kinase CK2. *Eur. J. Med. Chem.* **2011**, *46*, 870–876. [CrossRef] [PubMed]

93. Ostrynska, O.V.; Balanda, A.O.; Bdzhola, V.G.; Golub, A.G.; Kotey, I.M.; Kukharenko, O.P.; Gryshchenko, A.A.; Briukhovetska, N.V.; Yarmoluk, S.M. Design and synthesis of novel protein kinase CK2 inhibitors on the base of 4-aminothieno[2,3-d]pyrimidines. *Eur. J. Med. Chem.* **2016**, *115*, 148–160. [CrossRef] [PubMed]

94. Borowiecki, P.; Wawro, A.M.; Winska, P.; Wielechowska, M.; Bretner, M. Synthesis of novel chiral tbbt derivatives with hydroxyl moiety. Studies on inhibition of human protein kinase CK2alpha and cytotoxicity properties. *Eur. J. Med. Chem.* **2014**, *84*, 364–374. [CrossRef] [PubMed]

95. Hochscherf, J.; Lindenblatt, D.; Steinkruger, M.; Yoo, E.; Ulucan, O.; Herzig, S.; Issinger, O.G.; Helms, V.; Gotz, C.; Neundorf, I.; et al. Development of a high-throughput screening-compatible assay to identify inhibitors of the CK2alpha/CK2beta interaction. *Anal. Biochem.* **2015**, *468*, 4–14. [CrossRef] [PubMed]

96. Zhou, Y.; Li, X.; Zhang, N.; Zhong, R. Structural basis for low-affinity binding of non-r2 carboxylate-substituted tricyclic quinoline analogs to CK2alpha: Comparative molecular dynamics simulation studies. *Chem. Biol. Drug Des.* **2015**, *85*, 189–200. [CrossRef] [PubMed]

97. Retegan, M.; Milet, A.; Jamet, H. Exploring the binding of inhibitors derived from tetrabromobenzimidazole to the CK2 protein using a qm/mm-pb/sa approach. *J. Chem. Inf. Model.* **2009**, *49*, 963–971. [CrossRef] [PubMed]

98. Langer, T.; Hoffmann, R.D. *Pharmacophores and pharmacophore searches*; Wiley-VCH ; [Chichester : John Wiley, distributor]: Weinheim, 2006.

99. Chirico, N.; Gramatica, P. Real external predictivity of qsar models. Part 2. New intercomparable thresholds for different validation criteria and the need for scatter plot inspection. *J. Chem. Inf. Model.* **2012**, *52*, 2044–2058. [CrossRef] [PubMed]

100. Chirico, N.; Gramatica, P. Real external predictivity of qsar models: How to evaluate it? Comparison of different validation criteria and proposal of using the concordance correlation coefficient. *J. Chem. Inf. Model.* **2011**, *51*, 2320–2335. [CrossRef]

101. Di-wu, L.; Li, L.L.; Wang, W.J.; Xie, H.Z.; Yang, J.; Zhang, C.H.; Huang, Q.; Zhong, L.; Feng, S.; Yang, S.Y. Identification of CK2 inhibitors with new scaffolds by a hybrid virtual screening approach based on bayesian model; pharmacophore hypothesis and molecular docking. *J. Mol. Graph. Model.* **2012**, *36*, 42–47. [CrossRef] [PubMed]

102. Srivastava, R.; Akthar, S.; Sharma, R.; Mishra, S. Identification of ellagic acid analogues as potent inhibitor of protein kinase CK2:A chemopreventive role in oral cancer. *Bioinformation* **2015**, *11*, 21–26. [CrossRef] [PubMed]

103. Morshed, M.N.; Muddassar, M.; Pasha, F.A.; Cho, S.J. Pharmacophore identification and validation study of CK2 inhibitors using comfa/comsia. *Chem. Biol. Drug Des.* **2009**, *74*, 148–158. [CrossRef] [PubMed]

104. Zhang, N.; Zhong, R. Docking and 3d-qsar studies of 7-hydroxycoumarin derivatives as CK2 inhibitors. *Eur. J. Med. Chem.* **2010**, *45*, 292–297. [CrossRef] [PubMed]

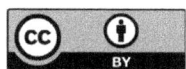

pharmaceuticals

MDPI

Article

Development of Pharmacophore Model for Indeno[1,2-*b*]indoles as Human Protein Kinase CK2 Inhibitors and Database Mining

Samer Haidar [1,2,*], **Zouhair Bouaziz** [3], **Christelle Marminon** [3], **Tuomo Laitinen** [4], **Antti Poso** [4,5], **Marc Le Borgne** [3] **and Joachim Jose** [1]

[1] Institut für Pharmazeutische und Medizinische Chemie, PharmaCampus, Westfälische Wilhelms-Universität Münster, Corrensstr. 48, 48149 Münster, Germany; joachim.jose@uni-muenster.de
[2] Faculty of Pharmacy, Damascus University, Damascus, P.O. Box 9411, Syria
[3] Université de Lyon, Université Claude Bernard Lyon 1, Faculté de Pharmacie—ISPB, EA 4446 Bioactive Molecules and Medicinal Chemistry, SFR Santé Lyon-Est CNRS UMS3453—INSERM US7, 8 Avenue Rockefeller, F-69373 Lyon CEDEX 8, France; zouhair.bouaziz@univ-lyon1.fr (Z.B.); christelle.marminon-davoust@univ-lyon1.fr (C.M.); marc.le-borgne@univ-lyon1.fr (M.L.B.)
[4] School of Pharmacy, Faculty of Health Sciences, University of Eastern, 70211 Kuopio, Finland; tuomo.laitinen@uef.fi (T.L.); antti.poso@uef.fi (A.P.)
[5] University Hospital Tübingen, Department of Internal Medicine VIII, Otfried-Müller-Straße 10, 72076 Tübingen, Germany
* Correspondence: shaid_01@uni-muenster.de; Tel.: +49-0-251-833-3154

Academic Editor: Lorenzo A. Pinna
Received: 13 December 2016; Accepted: 4 January 2017; Published: 9 January 2017

Abstract: Protein kinase CK2, initially designated as casein kinase 2, is an ubiquitously expressed serine/threonine kinase. This enzyme, implicated in many cellular processes, is highly expressed and active in many tumor cells. A large number of compounds has been developed as inhibitors comprising different backbones. Beside others, structures with an indeno[1,2-*b*]indole scaffold turned out to be potent new leads. With the aim of developing new inhibitors of human protein kinase CK2, we report here on the generation of common feature pharmacophore model to further explain the binding requirements for human CK2 inhibitors. Nine common chemical features of indeno[1,2-*b*]indole-type CK2 inhibitors were determined using MOE software (Chemical Computing Group, Montreal, Canada). This pharmacophore model was used for database mining with the aim to identify novel scaffolds for developing new potent and selective CK2 inhibitors. Using this strategy several structures were selected by searching inside the ZINC compound database. One of the selected compounds was bikaverin (6,11-dihydroxy-3,8-dimethoxy-1-methylbenzo[*b*]xanthene-7,10,12-trione), a natural compound which is produced by several kinds of fungi. This compound was tested on human recombinant CK2 and turned out to be an active inhibitor with an IC_{50} value of 1.24 µM.

Keywords: CK2; cancer; indeno[1,2-*b*]indoles; pharmacophore; MOE; ZINC database

1. Introduction

Cancer remains the leading cause of death in the world and around eight million deaths related to cancer were reported worldwide in 2012. The cancer cases are expected to increase sharply within the coming twenty years [1]. Different strategies for the treatment of cancer, including kinase inhibition [2] were employed and investigated to cure the disease or prolong life and increase its quality [3]. The first known protein kinase inhibitor was developed in the early 80s, and since then a large number of compounds has been described (for reviews see [3,4]). The first protein kinase inhibitor approved as drug was imatinib (Gleevec®, Novartis, Basel, Switzerland), which is used in the treatment of myelogenous leukemia [5]. To date, around one third of all drug discovery projects in pharmaceutical industry are related to protein kinase inhibitors [6]. Casein Kinase 2 (CK2) is a heterotetrameric enzyme which is ubiquitously expressed in mammalian cells [7]. CK2 enhances cancer phenotype by suppressing apoptosis and stimulating cell growth. Thus, inhibition of this enzyme can induce the physiological process of apoptosis, leading to tumor cell death [2]. Different backbones were used as skeleton for ATP competitive CK2 inhibitors, among them indeno[1,2-*b*]indoles have been identified as potent leads [8]. Several studies were published recently describing a large number of indeno[1,2-*b*]indoles and their activity as CK2 inhibitors [9–13]. Some of those compounds turned to be highly active with IC_{50} values in the low nanomolar range.

Molecular modeling is widely used for drug design and development, with the aim of finding new lead structures for the treatment of different diseases. Virtual screening or "mining" of databases is considered as an important tool in drug discovery. The aim in using in silico techniques is to reduce the costs and time to discover new active compounds, since reducing the period of a new drug from research laboratory to the market by one year can reduce the costs by millions of dollars. To develop a pharmacophore model is an important concept in computer-aided drug design (CADD), as this method can reduce the complexity of molecular interactions between compound and target to a set of few features. This method was successfully applied in drug discovery [14–19] and many molecular modeling software are available among them the Molecular Operating Environment (MOE). In this study a pharmacophore model for human protein kinase CK2 was constructed on the basis of 50 indeno[1,2-*b*]indoles and used to identify new hits by mining the ZINC compound database [20].

2. Results

In this work we used the inhibition data obtained with a set of 50 different indeno[1,2-*b*]indoles and human protein kinase CK2 [9,10,12,13]. We used these indeno[1,2-*b*]indoles, because they have all been tested on inhibition of human protein kinase CK2 in our lab with the same assay under identical conditions. We decided not to take any published inhibition data from other groups, because they were determined under different conditions (e.g., different assay, different ATP-concentration, substrate concentration, temperature etc.), and hence could lead to a blurred or less clear picture. The structures of the 50 compounds under investigation and their IC_{50} values are presented in Tables 1–3.

Table 1. Structures of the ketonic indeno[1,2-*b*]indoles and their IC_{50} values towards CK2, which were used for the training and test sets, data from Alchab et al. [9] and Gozzi et al. [13].

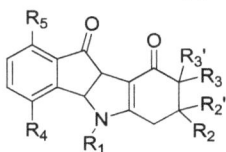

Code	R_1	R_2	$R_{2'}$	R_3	$R_{3'}$	R_4	R_5	IC_{50} (μM)
1	CH(CH$_3$)$_2$	H	H	H	H	O-CH$_2$CH=C(CH$_3$)$_2$	H	0.025
2	CH(CH$_3$)$_2$	CH$_3$	H	H	H	H	H	0.17
3	CH(CH$_3$)$_2$	H	H	H	H	H	H	0.36
5	CH(CH$_3$)$_2$	CH(CH$_3$)$_2$	H	H	H	H	H	0.61
8	CH$_2$CH$_2$(ortho-OMe)Ph	H	H	H	H	H	H	1.40
9		H	H	H	H	H	H	1.44
14	CH$_2$CH$_2$C$_6$H$_5$	CH$_3$	H	H	H	H	H	2.50
18	CH$_2$CH$_2$(para-OMe)Ph	H	H	H	H	H	H	4.10
22	CH$_2$CH$_2$(meta-OMe)Ph	H	H	H	H	H	H	5.10
23	CH$_2$CH$_2$ CH$_2$C$_6$H$_5$	H	H	H	H	H	H	6.00
24	CH$_2$CH$_2$C$_6$H$_5$	H	H	H	H	H	H	7.00
26	CH(CH$_3$)$_2$	H	H	CH$_3$	H	H	H	9.20
28	CH(CH$_3$)$_2$	H	H	(CH$_2$Ph)$_2$	CH$_2$Ph	H	H	>10
29	CH$_2$(para-OMe)Ph	H	H	H	H	H	H	>10

Table 1. *Cont.*

Code	R_1	R_2	$R_{2'}$	R_3	$R_{3'}$	R_4	R_5	IC_{50} (μM)
32	CH(CH$_3$)$_2$	H	H	H	H	H	O–CH$_2$CH=C(CH$_3$)$_2$	>10
37	CH(CH$_3$)$_2$	(*para*-F)Ph	H	H	H	H	H	>10
39	CH(CH$_3$)$_2$	furan-2-yl	H	H	H	H	H	>10
40	CH$_2$Ph	H	H	H	H	H	H	>10
41	CH$_2$CH$_2$Ph	Ph	H	H	H	H	H	>10
43	H	CH$_3$	H	COOCH$_3$	H	H	H	>10
44	H	H	H	H	H	H	H	>10
45	CH$_2$Ph	CH$_3$	H	COOCH$_3$	H	H	H	>10
46	CH(CH$_3$)$_2$	H	H	CH(CH$_3$)$_2$	H	H	H	>10
47	CH$_2$Ph	CH$_3$	CH$_3$	H	H	H	H	>10
48	CH$_2$Ph	CH$_3$	H	H	H	H	H	>10
49	CH(CH$_3$)$_2$	Ph	H	H	H	H	H	>10
50	CH$_2$Ph	Ph	H	H	H	H	H	>10

Table 2. Structures of the phenolic indeno[1,2-*b*]indoles and their IC_{50} values towards CK2, which were used for the training and test sets, data from Hundsdorfer et al. [10], and Gozzi et al. [12].

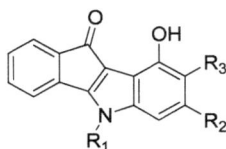

Code	R_1	R_2	R_3	IC_{50} (μM)
6	CH(CH$_3$)$_2$	CH$_3$	H	1.27
7	CH$_2$CH$_2$(*ortho*-OMe)Ph	H	H	1.30
10	CH(CH$_3$)$_2$	CH(CH$_3$)$_2$	H	1.65
12	CH(CH$_3$)$_2$	H	H	2.00
15	CH(CH$_3$)$_2$	(*para*-F)Ph	H	2.77
16	CH(CH$_3$)$_2$	furan-2-yl	H	3.63
25	CH$_2$CH$_2$C$_6$H$_5$	H	H	7.50
27	CH$_2$Ph	Ph	H	>10
30	CH$_2$CH$_2$C$_6$H$_5$	CH$_3$	H	>10
33	CH(CH$_3$)$_2$	H	CH$_3$	>10
38	CH(CH$_3$)$_2$	H	CH(CH$_3$)$_2$	>10
42	CH$_2$Ph	H	H	>10

Table 3. Structures of the quinonic indeno[1,2-*b*]indoles and their IC_{50} values towards CK2, which were used for the training and test sets, data from Alchab et al. [9], Gozzi et al. [12].

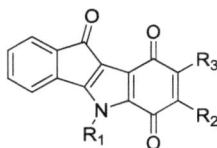

Code	R_1	R_2	R_3	IC_{50} (μM)
4	CH(CH$_3$)$_2$	CH$_3$	H	0.43
11	CH(CH$_3$)$_2$	furan-2-yl	H	1.65
13	CH$_2$C$_6$H$_5$	H	H	2.20
17	CH$_2$CH$_2$C$_6$H$_5$	CH$_3$,	H	4.10
19	CH(CH$_3$)$_2$	CH(CH$_3$)$_2$	H	4.76
20	CH(CH$_3$)$_2$	H	CH$_3$	4.90
21	CH(CH$_3$)$_2$	H	H	5.50
31	CH(CH$_3$)$_2$	H	CH(CH$_3$)$_2$	>10
34	CH(CH$_3$)$_2$	(*para*-F)Ph	H	>10
35	CH(CH$_3$)$_2$	Ph	H	>10
36	CH$_2$CH$_2$Ph	H	H	>10

MOE software (Chemical Computing Group, Montreal, Canada) package was used to perform this study [21]. MOE has been proved to be an effective tool for pharmacophore construction [22], other alternative software in this field might be Catalyst, LigandScout, and Phase, which are also effective for pharmacophore modeling.The resulting test set contained 524 conformations of these 50 compounds. Inhibitors with IC_{50} values of less than 10 μM were considered as moderate or highly active compounds. All others were designated as none active. This filter resulted in a number of 26 active and 24 non active compounds.

The pharmacophore model was developed by aligning the structures of the five most active compounds (training set), which were very well aligned as it is clear in Figure 1 were the backbones of the compounds fits very well above each other due to structure similarity.

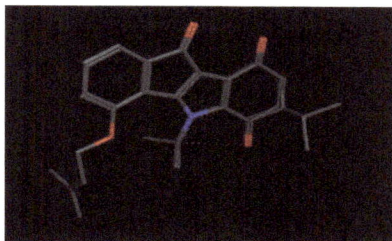

Figure 1. Alignment of compounds **1–5** from the training setof indeno [1,2-*b*]indole inhibitors of CK2, carbon atoms are in gray, oxygen atoms are in red, nitrogen atom in blue and intermolecular H-bond in dots.

The pharmacophore model derived thereof is shown in Figure 2. It is described by nine necessary features. In particular, a π ring center on the B ring, a hydrophobic centroid, two aromatic center/hydrophobic atoms on ring A and C, a π ring center/aromatic/hydrophobic centroid on ring D, and two hydrogen bond acceptors on rings B and D, together with two hydrogen acceptor projections, beside one excluded volume (no matching atom can be inside). Validity of the pharmacophore model was analyzed by its ability to identify the medium and highly active compounds only, which are represented by compounds **1–26**. It turned out that with this pharmacophore model it was possible to identify **22** out of the **26** designated as active compounds, which represents 85% of all. Compounds **9**, **13**, **17**, and **20** were not identified. Only four compounds out of the **24** non active compounds were selected and hence identified as false positive, which represents 17% of the non-active compounds. The compounds that were selected as false positives were compounds **29**, **31**, **36**, and **40**.

The nine features of this model as described were used to search in part of the ZINC database "All Now" (all purchasable in 2 weeks), with the aim of identifying an active CK2 inhibitor. However, by applying all the nine features of the developed pharmacophore model, it was not possible to identify any compound from the selected database. For that reason, the search was repeated using only eight out of nine features together with the excluding volume. The best result obtained was by omitting F2 (this feature is outside the main backbone of the indeno[1,2-*b*]indoles) and keeping all other features, which resulted in the selection of 57 compounds. The 57 compounds selected belong to different chemical backbones such as naphtho[2,3-*b*]furanedione, quino[2,3-*b*] acridinetetrone, naphthacenedione, and pyrazoloquinazoline. From this set of compounds, only two pyrrolizine based compounds were excluded from further observations, due to their inappropriate structure for enzyme inhibitors. They are rather fragment-like compounds according to "the role of three" filters (MW ≤ 300, cLogP ≤ 3, number of H-bond donors ≤ 3, number of H-bond acceptors ≤ 3) [23], which can be misleading for the development of active and selective inhibitors. The structures of the 55 selected compounds are shown in Supplementary Table S1. Surprisingly none of the selected compounds belonged to the indeno[1,2-*b*]indole group of compounds. As a control, the ZINC database was searched on the presence of indeno[1,2-*b*]indole like compounds and—to our surprise—it did not contain any.

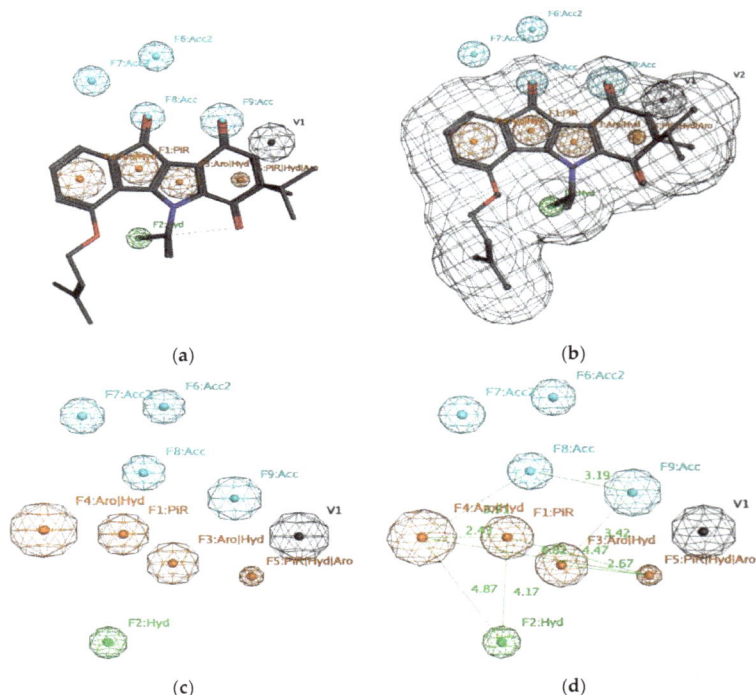

Figure 2. The developed pharmacophore model. (**a**) Alignment of common feature pharmacophore model with training set; (**b**) Alignment of common feature pharmacophore model with training set with occupied volume; (**c**) Common feature pharmacophore model of indeno[1,2-*b*]indole-type CK2 inhibitors; (**d**) Common feature pharmacophore model with the distance constraints. **Acc**: H-bond acceptor, **Acc 2**: H-bond acceptor projection, **Aro**: Aromatic center, **Hyd**: Hydrophobic centroid, **PiR**: π ring center.

In order to select the best candidates among the hit compounds, docking studies of the selected compounds against the ATP active site of the CK2 kinase were performed. A conformational search for the 55 selected compounds was carried out by MOE and all the resulting 777 conformations were used for the docking study. The conformations of all structures were docked in human CK2 enzyme using the MOE. For this purpose, the 3D X-ray crystal structure of the catalytic subunit of protein kinase CK2 (PDB ID: 3C13, resolution 1.95 Å [24]) was used. All conformations were sorted according to S score (energy-based scoring method implemented in MOE) to rank the best ligand in terms of orientation and binding to the active site, the top three ranking conformations with the minimum S score were selected after visual 2D inspection. Visual 2D inspection is a common additional tool in order to exclude "false positives due to assumptions and shortcomings in docking methods and scoring function" [25], where the active site is analyzed to determine protein-ligand interaction and show exactly which atoms have tether restraints [21]. It is important to note that scoring function values might not always correlated with biological activity. Compound ZINC35643753 was ranked as a top pose followed by compound ZINC44136135 and ZINC05765165 (bikaverin) with S scores of −24.0, −23.5, and −21.1, respectively. Beside the minimum S score, each pose for each compound was analyzed to find hydrogen binding and π-π interactions. 2D interactions between receptor and ligands for the three top ranked compounds were shown in Figure 3. The three best compounds fit well in the ATP binding site as it is shown in Figure 4.

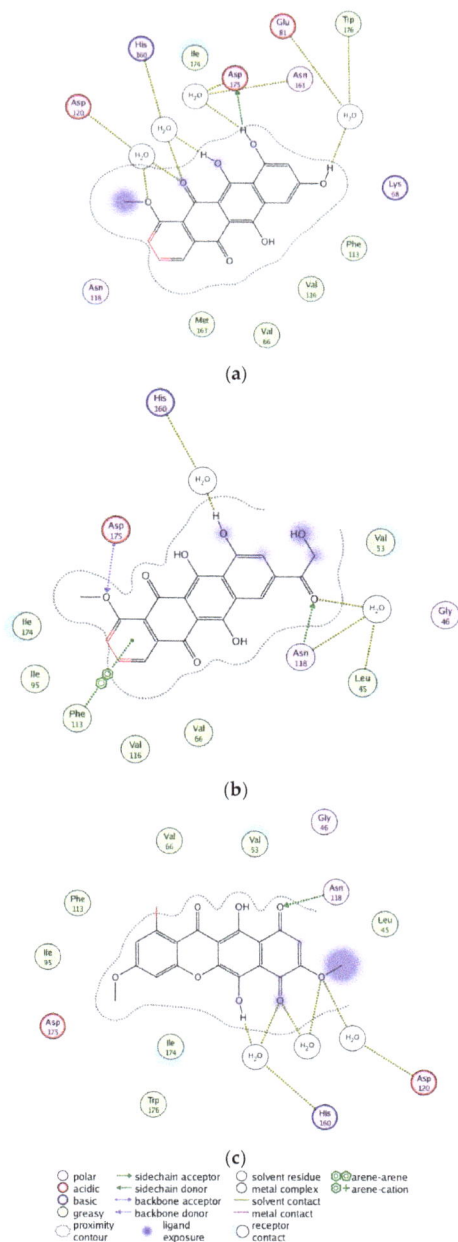

(a)

(b)

(c)

Figure 3. 2-D interactions between the three best selected compounds and the ATP binding site. (a) ZINC35643753; (b) ZINC44136135; (c) ZINC05765165.

(a)

(b)

(c)

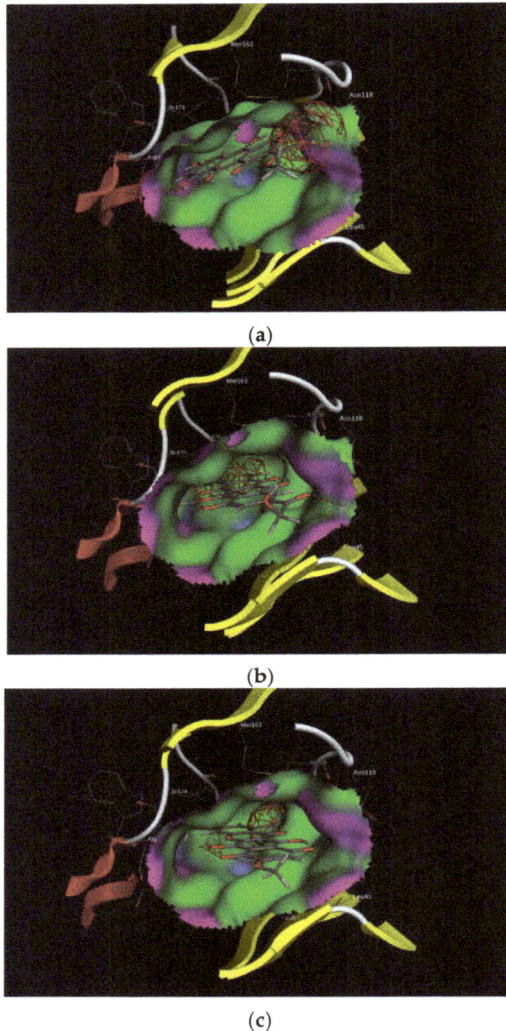

Figure 4. Binding mode of the selected ligands with the binding site of CK2. (**a**) ZINC35643753; (**b**) ZINC44136135; (**c**) ZINC05765165.

According to MOE docking, ZINC35643753 has direct bonding to Asp175, beside indirect bonding with His160, Asp120, Trp176, Glu81 and Asn161 via water molecules, Figure 3a, while ZINC44136135 shows direct interaction with Asp195 and Asn118, and arene-arene interaction with Phe113, as well as two indirect bonding with Leu45 and Asn118, via water molecules (Figure 3b). ZINC05765165 has interaction via hydrogen bonding with Asn118, as well as two indirect interactions with His160 and Asp120 via water molecules (Figure 3c). From the docking poses of the best selected compounds, it is clear that that docking strongly proposes the interaction between some functional groups of the compounds and some amino acid residues from the enzyme, and this is in line with known ATP kinase inhibitors. It might indicate that the compounds fit well in the ATP binding site of the enzyme.

Compound ZINC35643753 and compound ZINC44136135 are commercially available compounds as all compounds included in the ZINC database, both are anthracycline analogues. This group of compounds is among the most effective drugs used in chemotherapy for treatment of both solid tumors and leukemia in adults and children. Nevertheless those compounds suffer from several severe adverse effects, especially cardiotoxicity [26]. From the three compounds identified by ZINC database mining only bikaverin (6,11-dihydroxy-3,8-dimethoxy-1-methylbenzo[*b*]xanthene -7,10,12-trione, Figure 5) was chosen for further experiments. Compound ZINC35643753 and compound ZINC44136135 belong to a group of drugs known to have severe toxicities as it is mention above, while bikaverin is a natural compound with different biological activities. The fact that bikaverin is a natural compound with antitumor activity encourage us to investigate whether this activity might be related to CK2 inhibitory activity [27].

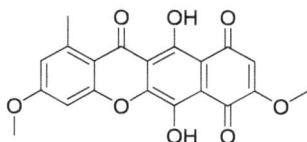

Figure 5. The chemical structure of bikaverin (6,11-dihydroxy-3,8-dimethoxy-1-methylbenzo[*b*]xanthene-7,10,12-trione), first isolated from the culture of *Fusarium vasinfectum* [28].

Bikaverin was tested on inhibition with purified human protein kinase CK2 expressed in *E. coli* as described before [29]. For this purpose eightconcentrations rangingfrom 0.001 μM to 100 μM of bikaverin were used in a capillary electrophoresis (CE)-based activity assay [30] in comparison the enzyme without inhibitor. The obtained dose-response curve is shown in Figure 6, and was used to determine the IC_{50} value of bikaverin, which turned out to be 1.24 μM. The IC_{50} value was determined in three independent biological replicates with basically similar results (1.29, 1.30 and 1.12 μM) the mean value was determined. It is important to note that all attempts to achieve 100% inhibition were not successful. This was not due to limited solubility of the compound. As it is shown in Figure 6, maximum activity with the highest concentration of bikaverin was 80%, and the relative IC_{50} value was 0.78 μM.

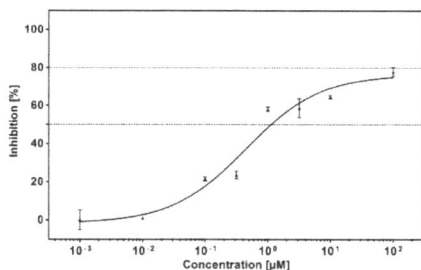

Figure 6. Determination of the IC_{50} value towards recombinant human CK2 of bikaverin (6,11-dihydroxy-3,8-dimethoxy-1-methylbenzo[*b*]xanthene-7,10,12-trione), the hit compound identified by ZINC database mining.CK2 holoenzyme was pre-incubated with different bikaverin concentrations (0.001–100 μM) and subsequently the in vitrophosphorylation of CK2 specificsubstrate peptide was determined by CE [30]. Relative CK2 activity at each inhibitor concentration is given in a dose-response diagram. IC_{50} values were determined in three independent replications and mean values with corresponding standard deviations are given.

3. Discussion

In this study a pharmacophore model for ATP-competitive inhibitors of human protein kinase CK2 was developed on the basis of known inhibitors with an indeno[1,2-*b*]indole scaffold. This model has been challenged against a set of compounds and was able to select most active compounds and excluded most nonactive ones, which indicate its validity. By using this model for database mining using the ZINC compound database, bikaverin ZINC05765165 was identified as a hit. By testing this natural compound with recombinant human CK2 it turned out to have an IC$_{50}$ value of 1.24 μM. Bikaverin, also known as lycopersin [31], is a reddish pigment produced by different fungal species. Chemically it is a polyketide with a tetracyclic benzoxanthone structure.It has been reported to possess diverse biological activities e.g., to have antibiotic, antifungal and anticancer properties [27]. Although the antitumoral activity of bikaverin has been reported, only few reports are focusing on its mode of action and up to know, no inhibition of CK2, as a possible target, was investigated. For these reasons we chose it for in vitro inhibition determination. Our in vitro test for this compound proved that it is active and can clearly inhibit the CK2, which is an evidence of the validity for the developed pharmacophore model.

In further studies bikaverin could be used for structural modification in order to improve its inhibitory towards CK2. Further studies are necessary to test the effects of some derivatives of this compound such as acetylated derivatives or dibromo-*O*-methylbikaverin, as those compounds were more cytotoxic than bikaverin in cell lines such as EAC cells [27,32]. Also further studies to test other selected structures from the 55 compounds and modify them accordingly is planned with the hope of finding new highly active and selective inhibitor of CK2. Actually, the aim of this study was to primary in silico filter the database and try to introduce new backbones serving as possible new hits for human CK2 which was performed by discovering that bikaverin is an active CK2 inhibitor with inhibitory activity comparable to other natural inhibitors of the target enzyme such as emodin which has an IC$_{50}$ value of 0.58 μM in our test system.

4. Materials and Methods

4.1. The Chemical Compounds

All compounds used in this study except bikaverin were described by us recently. The synthesis procedures to access to our target indeno[1,2-*b*]indoles have been published previously [9,10,12,13], bikaverin was purchased from Sigma-Aldrich (Munich, Germany).

4.2. In Vitro Assay

All indeno[1,2-*b*]indoles were tested for their inhibitory activity towards the human CK2 holoenzyme following the procedure described earlier [29]. The synthetic peptide RRRDDDSDDD was used as the substrate, which is reported to be most efficiently phosphorylated by CK2. The purity of the CK2 holoenzyme was superior to 99%. For initial testing, inhibition was determined relative to the controls at inhibitor concentrations of 10 μM in DMSO as a solvent. Therefore, 2 μL of the dissolved inhibitors (stock solution in DMSO) were mixed with 78 μL of CK2-supplemented kinase buffer which was composed of 1 μg CK2 holoenzyme, 50 mM Tris/HCl (pH 7.5), 100 mM NaCl, 10 mM MgCl$_2$ and 1 mM DTT. The reaction was started by the addition of 120 μL assay buffer, which was composed of 25 mM Tris/HCl (pH 8.5), 150 mM NaCl, 5 mM MgCl$_2$, 1 mM DTT, 100 μM ATP and 0.19 mM of the substrate peptide RRRDDDSDDD. The reaction was carried out for 15 minutes at 37 °C and stopped by the addition of 4 μL EDTA (0.5 M). Subsequently the reaction mixture was analyzed by a PA800 capillary electrophoresis from Beckman Coulter (Krefeld, Germany). Acetic acid (2 M, adjusted with conc. HCl to a pH of 2.0) was used as the electrolyte for electrophoretic separation. The separated substrate and product peptide were detected at 214 nm using a DAD-detector. Pure solvent was used as negative control (0% inhibition), assays without the enzyme were used as positive control (100% inhibition). Compounds with at least 50% inhibition at 10 μM were used for IC$_{50}$ determinations.

For the determination of IC_{50}, inhibition was determined using nine inhibitor concentrations ranging from 0.001 μM to 100 μM. IC_{50} were calculated from the resulting dose-response curves [30].

4.3. Computational Methods

4.3.1. Pharmacophore Generation

Molecular Operating Environment software package (MOE, Chemical Computing Group, Montreal, QC, Canada) was used to perform this study [21] running on an Intel Core, Duo based, 2.26 GHz processor. The molecular structures of the inhibitors were built with MOE and energy was minimized in the MMFF94x force field as implemented in the software. In order to develop a reliable pharmacophore model to identify new CK2 inhibitors, a database of known indeno[1,2-*b*]indole inhibitors was created. The structures of the inhibitors together with their inhibitory activity were published by us as mentioned above. In total this data base contained 50 compounds (Tables 1–3). The pharmacophore model was developed by aligning the minimized structures of the five most active compounds in the database namely compounds **1–5** with IC_{50} values of 25, 170, 360, 430, and 610 nM, respectively (training set). This alignment was obtained using MOE's flexible alignment and all conformations of the molecules were considered for the alignment [21]. Due to the relatively identical backbones of the compounds, the selected compounds were very well aligned (Figure 1). A conformational search was performed for each of the 50 compounds using the MMFF94x force field within the MOE to generate a multi-conformer database (test set). The search was performed using the default settings of MOE, and a query was developed based on the alignment of the five most active compounds (training set). The Consensus query of MOE was used to create all necessary features of the hypothetical pharmacophore model, tolerance was set at 1 and threshold was set at 80%. In order to optimize this multi features model, each individual pharmacophore feature was removed and the test set was scanned using the remaining features. Nine features were necessary as mentioned earlier (Figure 2), one Pi ring center on the B ring, one hydrophobic centroid, two aromatic center/hydrophobic atoms on ring A and C, one Pi ring center/aromatic/hydrophobic centroid on ring D, and two hydrogen bond acceptors on rings B and D, together with two hydrogen acceptor projections, beside one excluded volume. The radius of F1 and F3 were set at 0.8 A°, F2 was set at 0.6 A°, F4, F9 were set on 1 A°, F5 was set on 0.4 A°, F6 was set on 0.5 A°, F7 and F8 were set on 0.7 A°, and V1 was set on 1 A° (Figure 2). The pharmacophore search function of MOE was used to scan the test set using all default options of MOE.

4.3.2. Database Search

ZINC Database is a free database of commercially available compounds for virtual screening. It contains over 35 million purchasable compounds in ready-to-dock, 3D formats. ZINC is provided by Department of Pharmaceutical Chemistry at the University of California, San Francisco [20]. The compounds in the ZINC Database are organized in several categories namely, Standard: for delivery within 10 weeks, including in-stock and make on demand compounds; Clean: where stricter filtering rules have been applied, in stock: for immediate delivery; and Boutique: expensive selection of compounds not included in the former categories, and each of these categories is also redivided into Lead-like, Fragment-like, Drug-like and All. Since we are trying to find an active structure which can be directly purchasable, we chose in this work the "All Now" (all purchasable in 2 weeks) database which contains around 13 million compounds and was used to search for compounds that fit to most features of the developed pharmacophore. The compounds from the ZINC database were downloaded into MOE then used for the screening. The selected list of compounds from the database was docked against CK2 enzyme using the MOE software package.

4.3.3. Receptor Refinement

Three dimensional 3D structure of the CK2 complex with emodin was obtained from the Protein Data Bank (PDB) using PDB ID: (3C13) having a resolution of 1.95 Å. The structure was optimized by adding hydrogen atoms using the MOE software [21]. Then water molecules were removed from the structure and 3D protonation was done to change the state into ionization level. In the second step, energy minimization was performed using defaults parameters, where the force field was MMFF94x.

4.3.4. Database Generation

The selected compounds from the database were rebuilt with MOE building option implemented in the software. The compounds were optimized by adding hydrogen atoms using the option of MOE software. Energy of the compounds was minimized using the following parameters gradient: 0.05, Force Field: MMFF94X, Chiral constraint and Current Geometry. The conformation methodology was used to develop low energy conformations for each compound, applying the LowModMD method with RMS gradient of 0.05, all other parameters were used as default. All of the compounds and their conformations were saved in mdb database and later employed for docking studies.

4.3.5. Molecular Docking

The docking of the selected compounds from the database (compounds **1–55**) into the active site of CK2 enzyme (3C13) was achieved using MOE-Dock implemented on MOE. The docking parameters were set as Rescoring 1: London dG, Placement: triangle matcher, Retain 30, Refinement Force field, and Rescoring 2: London dG. Docking part of MOE can give correct conformation of the ligand to obtain minimum energy structure. The top conformation for each compound was selected based on the S score and visual inspection was carried out by Lgplot implemented in MOE. Compounds showing significant interaction with the residues of binding pocket of CK2 were picked as promising hits. Prior to dock, the initial ligand from the complex structure was extracted.For the scoring function, lower scores indicate more favorable poses. The unit for the scoring function is Kal/mol, and the S score refers to the final score, which is the score of the last stage that was not set to None. The Lig X function in MOE was used for conducting interactive ligand modification and energy minimization in the active site of the receptor.

5. Conclusions

In this study we were able to valorize the library of indeno[1,2-*b*]indoles designed for CK2 inhibition to determine the necessary ligand binding requirement for ATP binding CK2 inhibitors. We were also able to use the new model for searching in ZINC database. We discovered a potential inhibitor of CK2 and we experimentally confirmed its potency to inhibit CK2. Bikaverin can be regarded as a hit scaffold for designing CK2 inhibitors. It is also possible to use the pharmacophore model to further identify new inhibitors for the target enzyme from other databases, and modify the selected structures accordingly. Finally discovering that bikaverin is a CK2 inhibitor is an important finding and provides an important contribution toward finding active and selective CK2 inhibitors.

Supplementary Materials: The following is available online at http://www.mdpi.com/1424-8247/10/1/8/s1, Table S1.

Author Contributions: S.H. designed the virtual screening study, conducted most of the experiments, analyzed the data and wrote most parts of the manuscript. M.L.B., B.Z. and C.M. provided the compounds for the study, draw structures of compounds and critically read the manuscript, T.L. and A.P. helped with pharmacophore modeling, analyzed the data and critically read the manuscript, J.J. coordinated the project and wrote part of the manuscript.

Conflicts of Interest: The authors declare no conflict of interest.

References

1. WHO: Cancer Fact Sheet N°297. Available online: http://www.who.int/mediacentre/factsheets/fs297/en/ (accessed on 4 January 2017).
2. Ahmad, K.A.; Wang, G.; Slaton, J.; Unger, G.; Ahmed, K. Targeting CK2 for cancer therapy. *Anticancer Drugs* **2005**, *16*, 1037–1043. [CrossRef] [PubMed]
3. Cozza, G.; Pinna, L.A. Casein kinases as potential therapeutic targets. *Expert Opin. Ther. Targets* **2016**, *20*, 319–340. [CrossRef] [PubMed]
4. Cozza, G.; Pinna, L.A.; Moro, S. Protein kinase CK2 inhibitors: A patent review. *Expert Opin. Ther. Pat.* **2012**, *22*, 1081–1097. [CrossRef] [PubMed]
5. Druker, B.J.; Sawyers, C.L.; Kantarjian, H.; Resta, D.J.; Reese, S.F.; Ford, J.M.; Capdeville, R.; Talpaz, M. Activity of a specific inhibitor of the BCR-ABL tyrosine kinase in the blast crisis of chronic myeloid leukemia and acute lymphoblastic leukemia with the philadelphia chromosome. *N. Engl. J. Med.* **2001**, *344*, 1038–1042. [CrossRef] [PubMed]
6. Fabbro, D.; Cowan-Jacob, S.W.; Mobitz, H.; Martiny-Baron, G. Targeting cancer with small-molecular-weight kinase inhibitors. *Methods Mol. Biol.* **2012**, *795*, 1–34. [PubMed]
7. Faust, R.A.; Gapany, M.; Tristani, P.; Davis, A.; Adams, G.L.; Ahmed, K. Elevated protein kinase CK2 activity in chromatin of head and neck tumors: Association with malignant transformation. *Cancer Lett.* **1996**, *101*, 31–35. [CrossRef]
8. Rongved, P.; Kirsch, G.; Bouaziz, Z.; Jose, J.; le Borgne, M. Indenoindoles and cyclopentacarbazoles as bioactive compounds: Synthesis and biological applications. *Eur. J. Med. Chem.* **2013**, *69*, 465–479. [CrossRef] [PubMed]
9. Alchab, F.; Ettouati, L.; Bouaziz, Z.; Bollacke, A.; Delcros, J.G.; Gertzen, C.G.; Gohlke, H.; Pinaud, N.; Marchivie, M.; Guillon, J.; et al. Synthesis, biological evaluation and molecular modeling of substituted indeno[1,2-*b*]indoles as inhibitors of human protein kinase CK2. *Pharmaceuticals* **2015**, *8*, 279–302. [CrossRef] [PubMed]
10. Hundsdorfer, C.; Hemmerling, H.J.; Gotz, C.; Totzke, F.; Bednarski, P.; Le Borgne, M.; Jose, J. Indeno[1,2-*b*]indole derivatives as a novel class of potent human protein kinase CK2 inhibitors. *Bioorg. Med. Chem.* **2012**, *20*, 2282–2289. [CrossRef] [PubMed]
11. Hundsdorfer, C.; Hemmerling, H.J.; Hamberger, J.; le Borgne, M.; Bednarski, P.; Gotz, C.; Totzke, F.; Jose, J. Novel indeno[1,2-*b*]indoloquinones as inhibitors of the human protein kinase CK2 with antiproliferative activity towards a broad panel of cancer cell lines. *Biochem. Biophys. Res. Commun.* **2012**, *424*, 71–75. [CrossRef] [PubMed]
12. Gozzi, G.J.; Bouaziz, Z.; Winter, E.; Daflon-Yunes, N.; Honorat, M.; Guragossian, N.; Marminon, C.; Valdameri, G.; Bollacke, A.; Guillon, J.; et al. Phenolic indeno[1,2-*b*]indoles as ABCG2-selective potent and non-toxic inhibitors stimulating basal atpase activity. *Drug Des. Dev. Ther.* **2015**, *9*, 3481–3495.
13. Jabor Gozzi, G.; Bouaziz, Z.; Winter, E.; Daflon-Yunes, N.; Aichele, D.; Nacereddine, A.; Marminon, C.; Valdameri, G.; Zeinyeh, W.; Bollacke, A.; et al. Converting potent indeno[1,2-*b*]indole inhibitors of protein kinase CK2 into selective inhibitors of the breast cancer resistance protein ABCG2. *J. Med. Chem.* **2015**, *58*, 265–277. [CrossRef] [PubMed]
14. Tuccinardi, T.; Poli, G.; Corchia, I.; Granchi, C.; Lapillo, M.; Macchia, M.; Minutolo, F.; Ortore, G.; Martinelli, A. A virtual screening study for lactate dehydrogenase 5 inhibitors by using a pharmacophore-based approach. *Mol. Inform.* **2016**, *35*, 434–439. [CrossRef] [PubMed]
15. Patel, P.; Singh, A.; Patel, V.; Jain, D.K.; Veerasamy, R.; Rajak, H. Pharmacophore based 3D-qsar, virtual screening and docking studies on novel series of HDAC inhibitors with thiophen linker as anticancer agents. *Comb. Chem. High Throughput Screen.* **2016**, *1*, 1. [CrossRef]
16. Meetei, P.A.; Rathore, R.S.; Prabhu, N.P.; Vindal, V. In silico screening for identification of novel β-1,3-glucan synthase inhibitors using pharmacophore and 3D-QSAR methodologies. *Springerplus* **2016**, *5*, 965. [CrossRef] [PubMed]
17. Berinyuy, E.; Soliman, M.E. Identification of novel potential GP120 of HIV-1 antagonist using per-residue energy contribution-based pharmacophore modelling. *Interdiscip. Sci.* **2016**, *10*. [CrossRef] [PubMed]

18. Ugale, V.G.; Bari, S.B. Identification of potential GLY/NMDA receptor antagonists by cheminformatics approach: A combination of pharmacophore modelling, virtual screening and molecular docking studies. *SAR QSAR Environ. Res.* **2016**, *27*, 125–145. [CrossRef] [PubMed]

19. Cozza, G.; Bonvini, P.; Zorzi, E.; Poletto, G.; Pagano, M.A.; Sarno, S.; Donella-Deana, A.; Zagotto, G.; Rosolen, A.; Pinna, L.A.; et al. Identification of ellagic acid as potent inhibitor of protein kinase CK2: A successful example of a virtual screening application. *J. Med. Chem.* **2006**, *49*, 2363–2366. [CrossRef] [PubMed]

20. Irwin, J.J.; Sterling, T.; Mysinger, M.M.; Bolstad, E.S.; Coleman, R.G. Zinc: A free tool to discover chemistry for biology. *J. Chem. Inf. Model.* **2012**, *52*, 1757–1768. [CrossRef] [PubMed]

21. Molecular Operating Environment (MOE), C.C.G.I., 1010 Sherbooke St. West, Suite #910, Montreal, QC, Canada, H3A 2R7, 2013. Available online: https://www.chemcomp.com/MOE-Molecular_Operating_Environment.htm (accessed on 4 January 2017).

22. Sanders, M.P.; Barbosa, A.J.; Zarzycka, B.; Nicolaes, G.A.; Klomp, J.P.; de Vlieg, J.; del Rio, A. Comparative analysis of pharmacophore screening tools. *J. Chem. Inf. Model.* **2012**, *52*, 1607–1620. [CrossRef] [PubMed]

23. Congreve, M.; Chessari, G.; Tisi, D.; Woodhead, A.J. Recent developments in fragment-based drug discovery. *J. Med. Chem.* **2008**, *51*, 3661–3680. [CrossRef] [PubMed]

24. RCSB PDB-3C13: Low pH-Value Crystal Structure of Emodin in Complex with the Catalytic Subunit of Protein Kinase CK2. Available online: http://www.rcsb.org/pdb/explore/explore.do?structureId=3C13 (accessed on 4 January 2017).

25. Pauli, I.; dos Santos, R.N.; Rostirolla, D.C.; Martinelli, L.K.; Ducati, R.G.; Timmers, L.F.; Basso, L.A.; Santos, D.S.; Guido, R.V.; Andricopulo, A.D.; et al. Discovery of new inhibitors of mycobacterium tuberculosis inha enzyme using virtual screening and a 3D-pharmacophore-based approach. *J. Chem. Inf. Model.* **2013**, *53*, 2390–2401. [CrossRef] [PubMed]

26. Budman, D.R.; Berry, D.A.; Cirrincione, C.T.; Henderson, I.C.; Wood, W.C.; Weiss, R.B.; Ferree, C.R.; Muss, H.B.; Green, M.R.; Norton, L.; et al. Dose and dose intensity as determinants of outcome in the adjuvant treatment of breast cancer. The cancer and leukemia group B. *J. Natl. Cancer Inst.* **1998**, *90*, 1205–1211. [CrossRef] [PubMed]

27. Limon, M.C.; Rodriguez-Ortiz, R.; Avalos, J. Bikaverin production and applications. *Appl. Microbiol. Biotechnol.* **2010**, *87*, 21–29. [CrossRef] [PubMed]

28. Kreitman, G.; Nord, F.F. Lycopersin, a pigment from fusarium lycopersici. *Arch. Biochem.* **1949**, *21*, 457. [PubMed]

29. Olgen, S.; Gotz, C.; Jose, J. Synthesis and biological evaluation of 3-(substituted-benzylidene)-1,3-dihydro-indolin derivatives as human protein kinase CK2 and p60(c-SRC) tyrosine kinase inhibitors. *Biol. Pharm. Bull.* **2007**, *30*, 715–718. [CrossRef] [PubMed]

30. Gratz, A.; Gotz, C.; Jose, J. A ce-based assay for human protein kinase CK2 activity measurement and inhibitor screening. *Electrophoresis* **2010**, *31*, 634–640. [CrossRef] [PubMed]

31. Brase, S.; Encinas, A.; Keck, J.; Nising, C.F. Chemistry and biology of mycotoxins and related fungal metabolites. *Chem. Rev.* **2009**, *109*, 3903–3990. [CrossRef] [PubMed]

32. Fuska, J.; Proksa, B.; Fuskova, A. New potential cytotoxic and antitumor substances I. In vitro effect of bikaverin and its derivatives on cells of certain tumors. *Neoplasma* **1975**, *22*, 335–338. [PubMed]

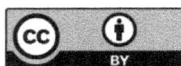

Chapter 4:
New inhibitors of human protein kinase CK2

pharmaceuticals

MDPI

Article

D11-Mediated Inhibition of Protein Kinase CK2 Impairs HIF-1α-Mediated Signaling in Human Glioblastoma Cells

Susanne Schaefer, Tina H. Svenstrup, Mette Fischer and Barbara Guerra *

Department of Biochemistry and Molecular Biology, University of Southern Denmark, 5230 Odense, Denmark; sschaefer@bmb.sdu.dk (S.S.); thl@bmb.sdu.dk (T.H.S.); mettefischer@outlook.com (M.F.)
* Correspondence: bag@bmb.sdu.dk; Tel.: +45-6550-2388; Fax: +45-6599-2640

Academic Editors: Joachim Jose, Marc Le Borgne, Lorenzo A. Pinna and Mathias Montenarh
Received: 1 November 2016; Accepted: 22 December 2016; Published: 1 January 2017

Abstract: Compelling evidence indicates that protein kinase CK2 plays an important role in many steps of cancer initiation and progression, therefore, the development of effective and cell-permeable inhibitors targeting this kinase has become an important objective for the treatment of a variety of cancer types including glioblastoma. We have recently identified 1,3-dichloro-6-[(E)-((4-methoxyphenyl)imino)methyl]dibenzo(b,d)furan-2,7-diol (D11) as a potent and selective inhibitor of protein kinase CK2. In this study, we have further characterized this compound and demonstrated that it suppresses CK2 kinase activity by mixed type inhibition (K_I 7.7 nM, K_I' 42 nM). Incubation of glioblastoma cells with D11 induces cell death and upon hypoxia the compound leads to HIF-1α destabilization. The analysis of differential mRNA expression related to human hypoxia signaling pathway revealed that D11-mediated inhibition of CK2 caused strong down-regulation of genes associated with the hypoxia response including *ANGPTL4*, *CA9*, *IGFBP3*, *MMP9*, *SLC2A1* and *VEGFA*. Taken together, the results reported here support the notion that including D11 in future treatment regimens might turn out to be a promising strategy to target tumor hypoxia to overcome resistance to radio- and chemotherapy.

Keywords: CK2; D11; HIF-1α; glioblastoma cells; gene expression profiling

---

1. Introduction

Glioblastoma is the most common primary tumor of the central nervous system and one of the most lethal types of human cancer. Patients with newly diagnosed glioblastoma have a median survival of approximately one year and respond poorly to all treatment modalities [1,2]. A comprehensive characterization of over 200 samples from patients diagnosed with glioblastoma has provided a detailed map of the many genomic and transcriptional alterations that occur in this type of malignancy and that contribute to its aggressive character [3–5]. Overexpression of the epidermal growth factor receptor (EGFR), which is linked to aberrant phosphoinositide 3-kinase (PI3K/AKT) pathway, is among the most frequent aberrations. However, cancer genomic studies have revealed that multiple components of the aforementioned pathway are frequently targeted by germline or somatic mutations contributing to tumor resistance to both radiotherapy and chemotherapy [5]. In this respect, glioblastoma has one of the highest incidence rates of phosphatase and tensin homolog (*PTEN*) mutation that has been strongly associated with a selective advantage for tumor expansion [6]. Loss of PTEN expression results in hyperactivation of the pro-survival PI3K/AKT pathway and increased resistance to apoptosis [7].

All tumors require active angiogenesis for expansion and glioblastoma is a highly vascularized type of cancer exhibiting increased expression of many pro-angiogenic genes such as vascular endothelial growth factor (*VEGF*) and fibroblast growth factor (*FGF*) [8]. Despite the extended vascularization, glioblastoma is highly heterogeneous and dominated by areas with low oxygen supply and compromised vascular integrity [9].

One of the major events in hypoxia adaptation is the induction of the hypoxia inducible factor 1 (HIF-1α) a transcription factor that regulates multiple intracellular processes including glycolysis, angiogenesis, immortalization, tissue invasion and metastasis, genetic instability and cell death (reviewed in [10]). From a therapeutic standpoint, hypoxia, genomic and tumor-tissue heterogeneity are a major clinical hurdle emphasizing the importance to set up tailored therapeutic strategies able to tackle the heterogeneous nature of brain cancer. Up-regulation of HIF-1α leads to a rapid response in hypoxic cells. Thus, identification of compounds able to block HIF-1α or its target genes for inhibiting tumor growth has become a top priority in many research laboratories.

We have recently identified 1,3-dichloro-6-[(E)-((4-methoxyphenyl)imino)methyl]dibenzo-(b,d)furan-2,7-diol (hereafter referred to as D11) as a potent and selective inhibitor of protein kinase CK2 [11,12]. CK2 is a highly conserved and constitutively active serine/threonine protein kinase whose expression levels have been found invariably elevated in highly proliferating cells. CK2 is implicated in multiple cellular functions as well as in cell transformation and tumorigenesis [13–17]. Recent data from our laboratory have demonstrated that D11 treatment induces apoptosis in brain and pancreatic cancer cells through a mechanism involving down-regulation of the PI3K/AKT and NF-κB signaling cascades [12]. Interestingly, inhibition of CK2 has been shown to decrease HIF-1α activity under hypoxia through elevated p53 expression levels [18].

Since the high incidence of PTEN mutation observed in glioblastoma cells has been strongly associated with stimulation of HIF-1α-mediated gene expression and increased apoptotic resistance [6], we investigated whether D11-mediated cell death induction was accompanied by destabilization and/or inhibition of HIF-1α transcription factor and, if so, how does D11 influence the expression of genes regulated by HIF-1α under hypoxic conditions. Results shown in this study suggest that D11 may exert anti-tumor activity by negatively affecting cellular pathways that are normally up-regulated under low oxygen tension and warrant in vivo studies for endorsing its efficacy in the treatment of multi-drug resistant human cancers.

2. Results

2.1. D11 is A CK2 Inhibitor That Leads to Cell Death in Glioblastoma Cells

D11 was identified employing the catalytic α-subunit of protein kinase CK2 following a screening of a small-molecule compound library of the Diversity Set III under the drug discovery and therapeutic program (DTP) of the National Cancer Institute (NCI, Rockville, MD, USA, [11]). Kinetic measurements revealed that this compound inhibits the catalytic activity of both CK2α and CK2 holoenzyme in the low nM range [11]. Furthermore, the screening of 354 protein kinases revealed that D11 is a selective inhibitor of CK2. By setting the threshold for inhibition to >98%, only three protein kinases were found inhibited to an extent observed with CK2 [11].

In this study, we carried out experiments in order to further characterize the type of inhibition exerted by D11 on CK2. Interestingly, increasing concentrations of co-substrate (i.e., ATP) tested with three different concentrations of inhibitor, respectively, resulted in decreased apparent maximum velocity (V^{app}_{max}) and increased apparent K_M (K^{app}_M) values suggesting a linear mixed-type inhibition against ATP as can be seen from the Michaelis-Menten plots (Figure 1A). Non-linear least-squares fits of the curves in Figure 1A to rectangular hyperbolas were used to determine the apparent K_M and V_{max} values resulting from the effect of different concentrations of inhibitor. From the estimated apparent K_M and V_{max} values we created re-plots for the determination of K_I (dissociation constant for binding of D11 to the free enzyme, 7.7 nM, Figure 1B) and K_I' (dissociation constant for binding of D11 to the enzyme-substrate complex, 42 nM, Figure 1C).

A

$$v_0 = \frac{V_{max}[ATP]}{\left(1 + \frac{[I]}{K_I}\right)K_M + \left(1 + \frac{[I]}{K_I'}\right)[ATP]}$$

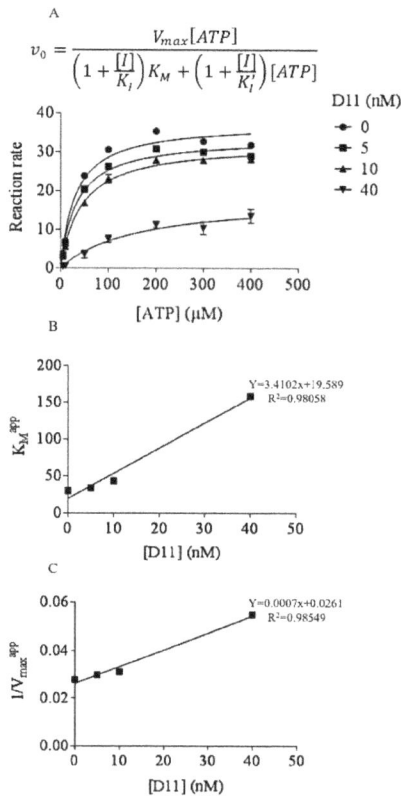

Figure 1. Kinetic mechanisms of CK2 inhibition. (**A**) Michaelis-Menten curves showing how velocity varies over a range of substrate concentrations for three different concentrations of inhibitor. The velocity equation relative to the hyperbolic curves of the graph for mixed inhibition is shown above the plots. I: inhibitor (D11), K_I: dissociation constant for binding of inhibitor to free enzyme, K_I': dissociation constant for binding of inhibitor to substrate-bound enzyme. (**B**) Apparent K_M (K_M^{app}) re-plotted against varying concentrations of inhibitor (used for the calculation of K_I). (**C**) Reciprocal apparent V_{max} ($1/V_{max}^{app}$) re-plotted against varying concentrations of inhibitor (employed for the calculation of K_I'). The reaction rate is expressed in pmol/min/ng. Experiments were repeated three times.

We previously showed that viability of the human glioblastoma cell line U-87 MG decreased by 50% following treatment with 25 µM D11 for 24 h [12]. Here, we carried out a cell cycle analysis by flow cytometry and asked the question whether D11 treatment induced cell death (Figure 2). Cells were treated with increasing concentrations of D11 for 24 h (Figure 2A, left bar graph) and 48 h (Figure 2A, right bar graph), respectively. As compared to control experiments, cells were not significantly affected by treatment with 50 µM D11 for 24 h (Figure 2A, left bar graph). However, incubation of cells with 50 µM D11 for 48 h was accompanied by a modest increase in the percentage of cells in sub-G1 phase indicative of cells that have undergone DNA degradation (Figure 2A, right bar graph). Next, Western blot analysis was carried out in order to determine the type of cell death. As shown in Figure 2B, treatment with 50 µM D11 for 48 h was necessary for inducing cleavage of full-length PARP, caspase 9 and caspase 3. However, a shorter incubation time (i.e., 24 h) was sufficient to induce increased LC3-II signal as compared to control cells suggesting induction of autophagy, in a time and concentration-dependent manner. The staining of cells with acridine orange (Figure 2C), a vital dye, which accumulates in acidic compartments emitting red fluorescence indicative of autophagic vacuoles formation, further confirmed results reported above.

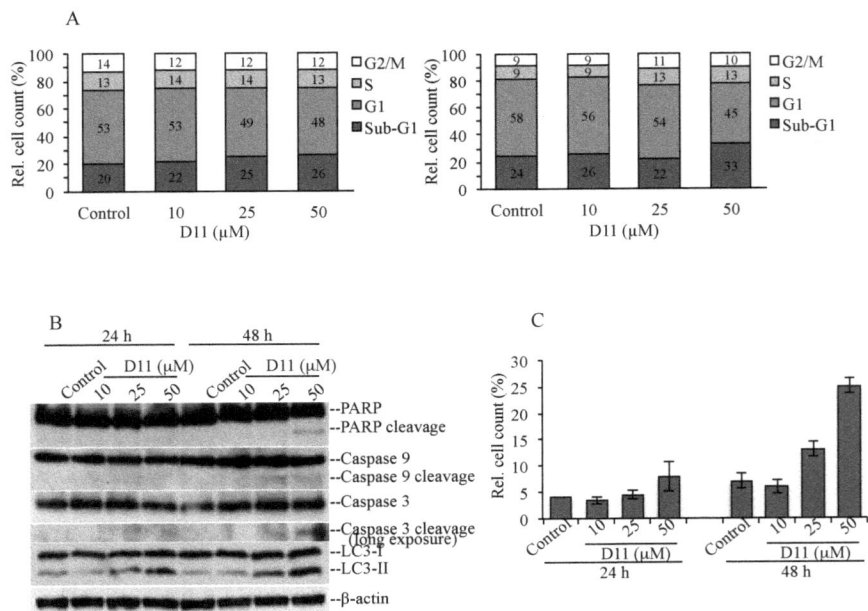

Figure 2. Anti-proliferative effects of D11 in human glioblastoma cells. (**A**) Flow cytometry analysis of cells vehicle-treated (Control, 0.1% DMSO) or incubated with increasing concentrations of D11 for 24 h (left bar graph) and 48 h (right bar graph), respectively. The relative amount of cells in the various phases of the cell cycle is shown in percentage. (**B**) Cells were treated as described above. Whole cell lysate was analyzed by western blot employing antibodies directed against the indicated proteins. β-actin detection was carried out as control for equal loading. (**C**) Flow cytometry analysis of cells treated as described in (**A**) stained with acridine orange for the determination of autophagic vacuoles formation. Number of red-positive cells is expressed in percentage. Experiments were performed three times obtaining similar results.

2.2. D11 Treatment Abolishes HIF-1α Transcriptional Activity and Results in Increased Activation of Autophagy under Hypoxia in Glioblastoma Cells

HIF-1 is a heterodimeric transcription factor consisting of two subunits; i.e., HIF-1β, which is constitutively expressed, and HIF-1α whose expression is regulated by oxygen levels. Stabilization of HIF-1α occurs under hypoxic conditions and leads to translocation into the nucleus where it induces the transcription of numerous genes as part to the hypoxia response (reviewed in [10]). Tumor suppressor genes encoding proteins such as the Von Hippel-Lindau (VHL) and PTEN have been reported to inhibit HIF-1α function. In particular, PTEN has been demonstrated to inhibit HIF-1α stabilization by antagonizing the PI3K pathway [6,19,20]. As U-87 MG cells contain mutant PTEN [21], we asked whether D11-mediated inhibition of CK2 resulted in HIF-1α destabilization and if this event had implications for the activation of cell death. To accomplish this, we compared the levels of expression of HIF-1α in cells treated with vehicle (0.1% DMSO), D11 or other known CK2 inhibitors under normoxia and hypoxia, respectively (Figure 3A). Under hypoxic conditions, U-87 MG cells showed induction of HIF-1α. Moreover, treatment with the indicated compounds resulted in inhibition of endogenous CK2 to various extents as indicated by decreased phosphorylation of NF-κB/p65 at S529 a known CK2 phosphorylation site [22]. Results shown in Figure 3A indicate that cell incubation with D11, E9 or CX-4945 resulted in destabilization of HIF-1α indicated by the reduced HIF-1α protein band intensity as compared to control experiments. Next, we analyzed whether D11 affected HIF-1α transcriptional activity employing a Luciferase reporter assay (Figure 3B).

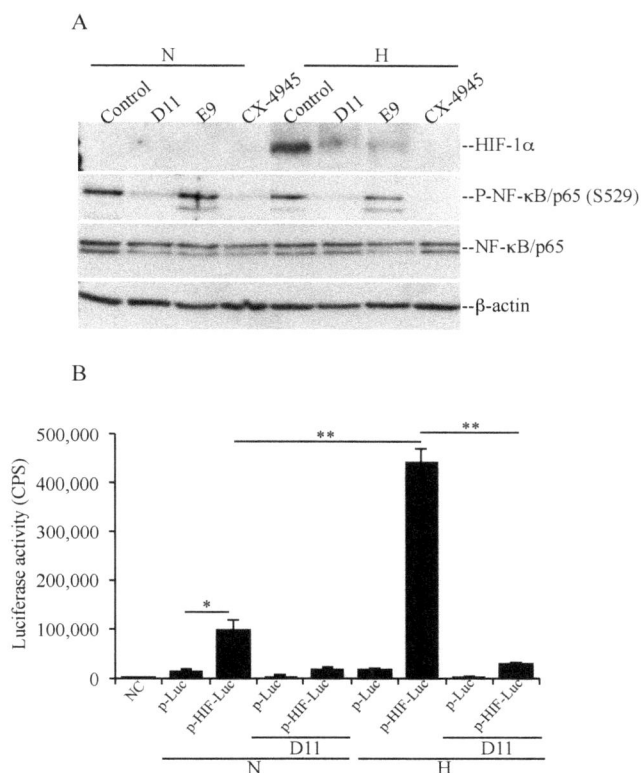

Figure 3. Stabilization and transcriptional activity of HIF-1α under hypoxia is impaired in cells treated with D11. (**A**) U-87 MG cells were treated with vehicle (Control), 50 µM D11, 50 µM E9 or 20 µM CX-4945 for 24 h under normoxia (N) and hypoxia (H), respectively. Whole cell lysate from cells treated as shown in the figure was subjected to western blot analysis and the expression and phosphorylation levels of the indicated proteins were analyzed. β-actin detection was used as loading control. Experiments were performed three times obtaining similar results. (**B**) Cells were transfected with a control plasmid (p-Luc) or a plasmid containing HIF-1α response element (p-HIF-Luc). 24 h from transfection, cells were added vehicle (0.1% DMSO) or 50 µM D11 and incubated under normoxic (N) or hypoxic (H) condition for the subsequent 24 h. HIF-1α transcriptional activity was analyzed employing a luciferase reporter gene assay. HIF-1α activity was measured testing the ability of the transcription factor to bind the HIF-1α response element that controls the expression of the luciferase reporter gene. HIF-1α transcription activity is expressed in counts/s (CPS). Experiments were repeated twice in triplicates obtaining similar results. * $p < 0.005$, ** $p < 0.0001$.

Cells were transfected with p-HIF1-Luc reporter vector able to express firefly luciferase under the control of a HIF-1-response element (p-HIF-Luc). As a negative control, cells were transfected with a vector lacking the specific response element (p-Luc). The transcription activity of HIF-1α increased dramatically under hypoxic conditions (i.e., 443128 CPS) as compared to its activity under normoxia (i.e., 98746 CPS). Upon treatment with 50 µM D11 for 24 h, luciferase activity induced by HIF-1α stabilization was drastically reduced (i.e., 31917 CPS) under hypoxia supporting the notion that D11 impairs the transcriptional activity of HIF-1α. In order to determine whether destabilization of HIF-1α had an influence on cell death, cells were incubated with D11 under normoxia and hypoxia, respectively. As shown in Figure 4, the exposure of cells to hypoxia did not result in higher PARP cleavage, however, it resulted in higher levels of autophagy induction as compared to cells grown under normoxia. Experiments carried out in the absence or presence of bafilomycin A$_1$, which blocks fusion of autophagosomes with lysosomes, revealed that D11 treatment leads to enhanced autophagic flux indicated by a further increase in LC3-II levels in the presence of bafilomycin A$_1$.

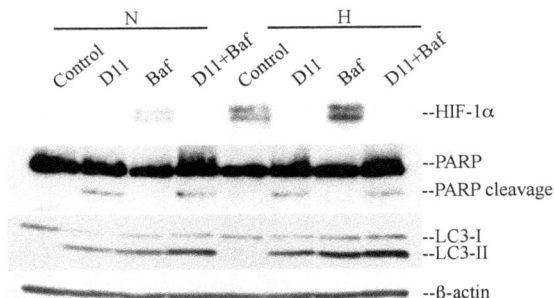

Figure 4. D11-mediated destabilization of HIF-1α under hypoxia is accompanied by higher levels of autophagy. Cells were incubated with 0.1% DMSO, 50 µM D11 alone or in combination with 100 nM bafilomycin A$_1$ (Baf) under normoxia and hypoxia, respectively. Cells were treated with D11 for 24 h while bafilomycin A$_1$ was added in the last 6 h of incubation time. Proteins were visualized by probing the western blot membranes with antibodies against the indicated proteins.

2.3. Cell Incubation with D11 Results in Altered Gene Expression Profile Induced by Hypoxia

Stabilization of HIF-1α in the absence of oxygen stimulates the expression of numerous hypoxia-response genes that promote the survival of cancer cells in an unfavorable environment. In order to investigate differential mRNA expression in glioblastoma cells resulting from D11 treatment under hypoxic conditions, we analyzed the expression of 84 genes that respond to low oxygen levels using the human hypoxia-signaling pathway RT^2 Profiler PCR array. Cells were grown under normoxic or hypoxic conditions for 24 h and incubated either with vehicle (0.1% DMSO) or 50 µM D11 for the same length of time. Based on scatter plot analysis (Figure 5B, upper plot), a number of known HIF-1α-target genes were found up-regulated in control cells in response to hypoxia (CT$_H$ vs. CT$_N$, fold-change $\geq$ 2, Table 1). In particular, the strongest up-regulation was observed in the case of angiopoietin-like 4 (*ANGPTL4*), Bcl2/adenovirus E1B 19 kDa interacting protein 3 (*BNIP3*), carbonic anhydrase IX (*CA9*), DNA-damage-inducible transcript 4 (*DDIT4*), coagulation factor III (*F3*), insulin-like growth factor binding protein 3 (*IGFBP3*), lysyl oxidase (*LOX*), matrix metallopeptidase 9 (*MMP9*), N-myc downstream regulated 1 (*NDRG1*), solute carrier family 2 member 1 (*SLC2A1*) and vascular endothelial growth factor A (*VEGFA*). In contrast, when we analyzed the genes that showed differential expression under hypoxic conditions and looked at their up- or down-regulation in response to D11 treatment (i.e., D11$_H$ vs. CT$_H$), we noticed that most of them failed to become up-regulated or appeared to be partially down-regulated (Figure 5B, lower plot and Table 1). However, strong down-regulation was observed in the case of *F3*, 6-phosphofructo-2-kinase/fructose-2,6-bisphosphatase 4 (*PFKFB4*), solute carrier family 16 member 3 (*SLC16A3*) and *VEGFA* (Table 1). HIF-1α protein expression levels increased under hypoxic conditions (Figure 5A). Conversely, consisting with data reported earlier [23,24], up-regulation of HIF-1α was not accompanied by a change in its mRNA levels in cells exposed to hypoxia as compared to cells incubated under normoxia. Interestingly, D11 treatment resulted in decreased expression of HIF-1α protein but not mRNA levels under hypoxia (results not shown) suggesting alternative D11-mediated mechanisms of regulation of HIF-1α.

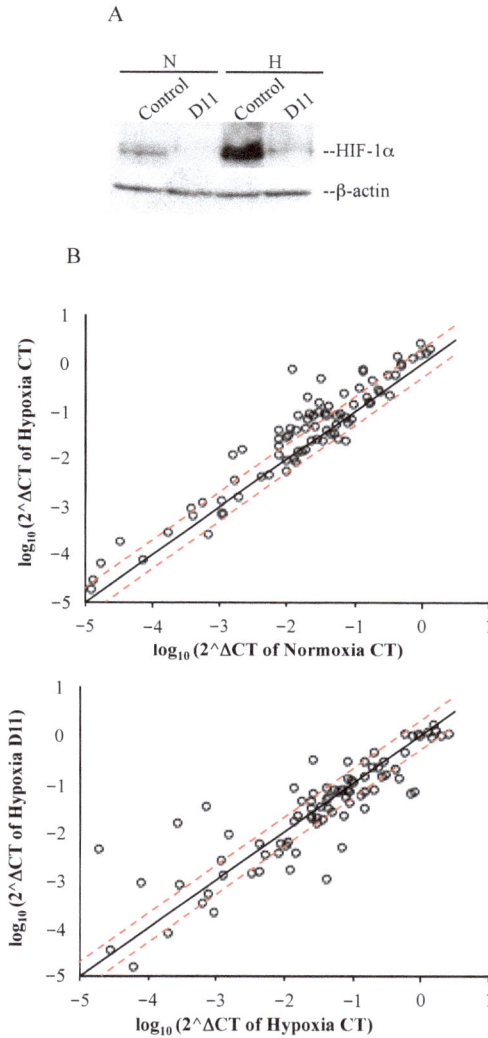

Figure 5. Genes differentially expressed in response to hypoxia and D11 treatment. (**A**) Western blot analysis of whole cell lysate from cells incubated with 0.1% DMSO or 50 μM D11 for 24 h under normoxia and hypoxia, respectively. Western blot membranes were employed for the detection of HIF-1α and β-actin expression levels, respectively. (**B**) Scatter plot of changes of expression of genes in glioblastoma cells. Upper panel: changes of gene expression between cells incubated under normoxia (control) and cells incubated under hypoxia for 24 h. Lower panel: changes of gene expression in the presence or absence of D11 under hypoxic conditions. The fold regulation cut-off (red dashed line) was set on 2.

Table 1. Gene expression analysis.

Protein	Gene Symbol	Fold-Change CT_H vs. CT_N	Fold-Change $D11_H$ vs. CT_H
Adrenomedullin	*ADM*	4.358	1.226
Angiopoietin-like 4	*ANGPTL4*	7.646	−7.888
Ankyrin repeat domain 37	*ANKRD37*	2.880	−2.106
Basic helix-loop-helix family member e40	*BHLHE40*	3.229	−2.275
Bloom syndrome, RecQ helicase-like	*BLM*	−1.904	−1.549
Bcl2 interacting protein 3	*BNIP3*	5.984	1.282
Bcl2 interacting protein 3-like	*BNIP3L*	3.364	−1.058
Carbonic anhydrase IX	*CA9*	10.768	−2.924
Cyclin G2	*CCNG2*	3.367	2.445
DNA-damage-inducible transcript 4	*DDIT4*	7.233	−4.314
Egl nine homolog 1 (*C. elegans*)	*EGLN1*	1.953	−2.032
Early growth response 1	*EGR1*	−2.474	54.951
Erythropoietin	*EPO*	2.150	1.275
ERO1-like (*S. cerevisiae*)	*ERO1A*	2.033	−1.566
Coagulation factor III	*F3*	5.802	−41.328
Glucan branching enzyme 1	*GBE1*	2.523	−2.082
Glycogen synthase	*GYS1*	2.051	−2.645
Hypoxia inducible factor 3 α subunit	*HIF3A*	3.719	−3.992
Hexokinase 2	*HK2*	3.152	1.100
Insulin-like growth factor binding protein 3	*IGFBP3*	67.054	−11.170
Lactate dehydrogenase A	*LDHA*	2.602	−2.361
Lectin, galactoside-binding, soluble, 3	*LGALS3*	2.363	−2.141
Lysyl oxidase	*LOX*	5.199	−4.730
Macrophage migration inhibitory factor	*MIF*	1.986	−1.040
Matrix Metallopeptidase 9	*MMP9*	6.044	−2.535
MAX interactor 1	*MXI1*	4.017	−1.462
N-myc downstream-regulated 1	*NDRG1*	15.150	−3.611
Ornithine decarboxylase 1	*ODC1*	−2.231	11.551
Prolyl 4-hydroxylase, α 1	*P4HA1*	3.362	1.053
Pyruvate dehydrogenase kinase	*PDK1*	2.946	−1.522
6-phosphofructo-2-kinase/fructose-2,6-bisphosphatase 3	*PFKFB3*	2.394	1.146
6-phosphofructo-2-kinase/fructose-2,6-bisphosphatase 4	*PFKFB4*	3.304	−14.057
Phosphofructokinase, liver	*PFKL*	2.452	−2.309
Placental growth factor	*PGF*	2.242	2.089
Phosphoglycerate kinase 1	*PGK1*	3.159	−1.581
Plasminogen activator, urokinase	*PLAU*	−2.926	1.674
Serpin peptidase inhibitor, clade E member 1	*SERPINE1*	1.911	1.744
Solute carrier family 16 member 3	*SLC16A3*	2.454	−4.346
Solute carrier family 2 member 1 (GLUT1)	*SLC2A1*	5.890	−1.162
Solute carrier family 2 member 3 (GLUT 3)	*SLC2A3*	2.462	2.460
Thioredoxin interacting protein	*TXNIP*	3.422	1.559
Vascular endothelial growth factor A	*VEGFA*	5.367	−11.028

CT_H: control cells (vehicle-treated) grown under hypoxia, CT_N: control cells (vehicle-treated) grown under normoxia, $D11_H$: D11-treated cells under hypoxia.

3. Discussion

Hypoxia is a critical condition for many types of cancers because it signals adaptation of cells to an anaerobic environment achieved by induction of gene expression. Limited oxygen diffusion is frequently observed in the glioma microenvironment and it has been associated with poor prognosis, increased metastasis, angiogenesis and resistance to radio- and chemotherapy. The stabilization of HIF-1α transcription factor is one of the most critical events occurring under hypoxia, as it is the primary factor responsible for many of the effects observed in aggressive tumors. Hence, it is not surprising that HIF-1α has become an important target for drug development in recent years as blocking HIF-1α activity would help starve growing tumors of oxygen and nutrients.

Our in vitro data show that treatment of cells with D11, a small-molecule inhibitor of protein kinase CK2, results in destabilization of HIF-1α protein under hypoxic conditions. Similar results were also reported in the case of other CK2 inhibitors (i.e., E9, CX-4945 and quercetin, [25]). It has been demonstrated that HIF-1α mRNA levels do not vary under hypoxic conditions [23,24]. Accordingly, the analysis of gene expression data did not reveal any significant differences in the expression of *HIF-1α* in cells growing under normoxia or exposed to hypoxia in the absence and presence of D11, respectively, suggesting that regulation of HIF-1α expression occurs at the post-translational level. Apart from CK2 inhibitors, other compounds can induce HIF-1α destabilization. The small molecule inhibitor YC-1 [3-(-5′-hydroxymethyl-2′-uryl)-1-benzylindazole] was shown to reduce HIF-1α levels and xenograft growth of various human tumors through mechanisms yet to be elucidated [26]. Under hypoxic conditions, HIF-1α stability is dependent on its interaction with the chaperone HSP-90 and cell incubation with the HSP-90 inhibitor 17-allylamino-17-demethoxygeldanamycin (17-AAG) has been shown to induce HIF-1α degradation in a VHL-independent manner [27–29].

The activity of chaperone proteins is dependent on their interaction with co-chaperone proteins and co-activators [30]. Compelling evidence has indicated that CK2-mediated phosphorylation of the co-chaperone CDC37 is essential for stabilization of HSP-90-CDC37 heterocomplex and its interaction with client protein kinases (reviewed in [31]). Hence, HIF-1α degradation observed in cells incubated with D11 under hypoxia might result from disruption of HSP-90-CDC37 interaction as cell treatment with this inhibitor has been reported to reduce CDC37 phosphorylation [11] and destabilize HSP-90-CDC37 heterocomplex [12].

Induction of autophagy was found significantly enhanced in U-87 MG cells following incubation with D11 for 24 and 48 h, respectively. At presence, it is not possible to assert whether induction of autophagy constitutes a stress adaptation conferring cytoprotection or an alternative cell death mechanism. However, the fact that PARP cleavage becomes visible after 48 h of incubation with D11 does not exclude that autophagy might develop as a primary response to stress stimuli in the first 24 h of incubation with the inhibitor and triggers apoptosis to kill cancer cells following a longer incubation time. This sequence of events has been shown to occur in the case of CD4/CXCR4-expressing T cells after binding of HIV-1 envelope proteins [32].

The hypoxic response includes the induction of a variety of pro-angiogenic genes. Specifically, the gene expression analysis identified strong up-regulation of *ADM*, *ANGPTL4* and *VEGFA* (Table 1). Conversely, the expression of these genes was found down-regulated in cells treated with D11 under hypoxia suggesting that D11 antagonizes the transcription of pro-angiogenesis genes through mechanisms that may be dependent or not on HIF-1α expression status.

Under hypoxic conditions, cells use glycolysis as a primary mechanism of ATP production. This metabolic switch is encouraged by stabilization of HIF-1α, which induces the expression of genes involved in metabolic adaptation including glucose uptake and the glycolytic pathway. Indeed, the expression of several of the genes involved in glucose metabolism (i.e., *HK1* and *-2*, *GLUT1* and *-3*, *GYS1*, *LDHA*, *PDK1*, *PFKFB3* and *-4*) was found up-regulated under hypoxia and marginally or largely down-regulated when cells were additionally treated with D11 (Table 1). This suggests that D11 treatment severely deprives cancer cells of oxygen and nutrient supply by suppressing the oxygen-independent metabolic pathway.

There is ample evidence that changes in metabolic activity observed in cancer cells influence the intracellular pH. Glycolysis is thought to be the major mechanism responsible for lowering the pH. Evidence indicates that the activity of carbonic anhydrase (*CA9*), which converts carbon dioxide and water to carbonic acid, is strongly induced in hypoxia contributing to low pH of the tumor. High expression levels of *CA9* have been associated with poor prognosis [33]. Our results are consistent with previous studies investigating gene expression in response to hypoxia. Accordingly, the expression of *CA9* was found largely up-regulated under hypoxia (i.e., 10.768 fold-change as compared to CT_N), however, treatment of cells with D11 resulted in a -2.924 fold-change of *CA9* with respect to CT_H suggesting that D11 compromises another important adaptation of tumor cells which seems to be essential for promoting tumor invasion. In this respect, it has been shown that many proteases are activated under acidic conditions promoting tumor invasion of surrounding tissue [34].

N-myc downstream-regulated gene 1 (NDRG1) is a member of the *NDRG* gene family, which is expressed ubiquitously in tissues in response to various stress conditions including cellular differentiation, tumor progression and metastasis, DNA damage and hypoxia. Expression of *NDRG1* in response to low oxygen concentrations is HIF-1α-regulated, as induction of *NDRG1* does not occur in HIF-1α$^{-/-}$ mouse embryo fibroblasts. However, an increase in intracellular Ca^{2+} seems to be sufficient to induce NDRG1 mRNA expression in HIF-1α-deficient cells under hypoxia (reviewed in [35]). A number of research groups have shown that NDRG1 over-expression decreases tumor growth, reduces invasion and suppresses metastasis [36,37]. However, Salnikow et al., demonstrated that NDRG1 expression is dramatically increased in aggressive prostate cancer cells [38]. In our study, *NDGR1* expression was found elevated (15.150 fold-change) under hypoxia while additional incubation with D11 resulted in a −3.6 fold-change (Table 1). There appears no clear connection in the effect of Ca^{2+} and HIF-1α on *NDRG1* induction in cancer cells. Hence, it is likely that when oxygen levels decrease, *NDRG1* induction is linked to intracellular mechanisms somewhat unrelated to metastasis and cell growth yet to be elucidated.

Finally, analysis of the gene expression array also revealed that two hypoxia-responsive genes involved in cell adhesion, invasion and vascular remodeling (i.e., *ANKRD37* and *MMP9*) were found largely down-regulated in D11 treated cells. Suppression of *ANKRD37* and *MMP9* expression may explain, at least in part, D11-mediated impaired migration of glioblastoma and pancreatic cancer cells reported previously [12] and indicates that treatment of glioblastoma cells with this compound compromises cell migration and invasion by suppressing the expression of proteins that are crucial in the metastatic process.

4. Materials and Methods

4.1. Cell Culture and Hypoxia

The human glioblastoma cell line U-87 MG was purchased from the American Type Culture Collection (ATCC, Rockville, MD, USA) and cultivated at 37 °C under a 5% CO$_2$ atmosphere in Dulbecco's modified Eagle's medium (DMEM, Invitrogen, Taastrup, Denmark) supplemented with 10% fetal bovine serum (FBS, Biochrom AG, Berlin, Germany). Cells were treated with 4-[(*E*)-(fluoren-9-ylidenehydrazinylidene)-methyl] benzoic acid (referred to as E9, [25]), D11 (both from DTP, NIH/NCI, Rockville, MD, USA) or CX-4945 (Selleck Chemicals, Houston, TX, USA) as indicated in the figure legends. Hypoxia (1% O$_2$) experiments were carried out according to [39]. Where indicated, cells were treated with 100 nM bafilomycin A$_1$ (Sigma-Aldrich, Brøndby, Denmark) for 6 h.

4.2. Radioactive Kinase Assay

The kinase activity of human recombinant CK2α$^{1-335}_2$β$_2$ was determined in the presence of the CK2 synthetic peptide RRRADDSDDDDD (100 μM), increasing concentrations of ATP (i.e., 5, 10, 50, 100, 200, 300 and 400 μM) and inhibitor as indicated in the figure legends and essentially as described elsewhere [40]. Kinetic parameters (i.e., K$_M$ and V$_{max}$) were calculated using GraphPad Prism version 6.0 computer software (GraphPad Software Inc., San Diego, CA, USA) based on the Michaelis-Menten plots. K$_I$ values were determined from the re-plots where apparent K$_M$ values and apparent V$_{max}$ values were plotted against inhibitor concentration, respectively.

4.3. Cell Cycle Analysis by Flow Cytometry

Propidium iodide staining of cells and flow cytometry analysis were performed essentially as previously described [41]. Autophagy was analyzed by staining cells with 1 μg/mL acridine orange (Sigma-Aldrich) for 15 min prior harvesting by trypsinization and flow cytometry analysis.

4.4. Preparation of Whole Cell Lysate, Western Blot Analysis and Antibodies

Western blot analysis of whole cell lysate was performed as reported in [41]. The following primary antibodies were employed in the study: rabbit monoclonal anti-NF-κB/RelA and rabbit monoclonal anti-LC3 (both from Cell Signaling Technology, Beverly, MA, USA); mouse monoclonal anti-β-actin (Sigma-Aldrich); rabbit polyclonal anti-phospho-NF-κB/p65 (S529, Abcam, Cambridge, MA, USA); mouse monoclonal anti-PARP and mouse monoclonal anti-HIF-1α (both from BD Biosciences, San Jose, CA, USA).

4.5. Luciferase Reporter Assay

Determination of the transcriptional activity of HIF-1α was carried out with whole cell lysate (10 μg) from cells transfected with a luciferase reporter vector (Panomics, Affymetrix, Santa Clara, CA, USA) carrying a control sequence or HIF-1α consensus element. Transfection of cells was performed with Lipofectamine 2000 according to the manufacturer's (Invitrogen) guidelines. After 24 h from transfection, cells were added 50 μM D11 for additional 24 h before harvesting. Cells were grown under normoxia or hypoxia in the last 24 h of incubation time as indicated in the figure legends. Determination of luciferase activity was performed employing the Luciferase Assay System kit (Promega, Stockholm, Sweden) according to the manufacturer's recommendations. Luminescence was measured with a Perkin Elmer Victor Light 1420 luminescence counter (Perkin Elmer, San Diego, CA, USA).

4.6. Gene Expression Analysis by Quantitative RT-PCR Array

Total RNA samples preparation from cells treated as described in the figure legends was carried out by phenol-chloroform extraction and subsequent silica-membrane-based purification in combination with on-column DNAse digestion with the miRNeasy kit (Qiagen, Hilden, Germany) following the manufacturer's instructions. RNA integrity was assessed by agarose gel analysis. The cDNA was prepared using the RT^2 First strand kit (Qiagen). The expression analysis of 84 genes associated with hypoxia was carried out with the Qiagen RT^2 Profiler PCR array according to the manufacturer's guidelines in 96-well plates with a StepOnePlus^{TM} real-time cycler (Applied Biosystems, Nærum, Denmark). Data were normalized to five housekeeping genes included in the kit. Normalized data were analyzed using the $\Delta\Delta C_t$ method with the equation $\Delta\Delta C_t = \Delta C_t$ (experimental sample group) $- \Delta C_t$ (control group), and the fold-change was calculated based on $\Delta\Delta C_t$ with $2^{-\Delta\Delta Ct}$ for positive changes or with $-1/2^{-\Delta\Delta Ct}$ for negative changes [42,43].

4.7. Statistical Analysis

Statistical significance of differences between means of two groups was determined by the two-tailed *t*-test (student's *t*-test). The levels of significance are indicated in the figure legends.

5. Conclusions

Hypoxic adaptation is a frequently occurring event in tumor growth and it is associated to a more invasive phenotype and resistance to conventional treatment. This has been unequivocally demonstrated in the case of brain cancer. Hence, the identification of new therapeutic strategies targeting HIF-1α represents an attractive alternative option to the current treatment modalities. Our data show that incubation of glioblastoma cells with D11 results in rapid HIF-1α destabilization and impaired transcriptional activity. Gene expression analysis show that reduced HIF-1α expression in response to D11 treatment is accompanied by down-regulation of genes involved in angiogenesis, glucose metabolism, pH regulation, cell adhesion and invasion. Collectively, these results suggest that the combination of D11, or more potent derivatives, with existing treatments may prove to be an effective strategy in the clinics for the cure of brain cancer in the future.

Acknowledgments: The authors wish to thank Olaf-Georg Issinger (University of Southern Denmark) for critically reading the manuscript and Lars Folke Olsen (University of Southern Denmark) for fruitful discussions and assisting with the kinetic analysis. We thank the Drug Synthesis and Chemistry Branch, Developmental Therapeutics Program, National Cancer Institute, USA, for providing us with vialed samples and the Danish Council for Independent Research-Natural Sciences (Grant 1323-00212A to Barbara Guerra).

Author Contributions: Susanne Schaefer performed a large part of the experiments and contributed to the data analysis. Tina H. Svenstrup carried out part of the kinetic analysis and Mette Fischer performed part of the experiments involving cell cycle and Western blot analysis. Barbara Guerra conceived the study, contributed to the data analysis and wrote the manuscript.

Conflicts of Interest: The authors declare no conflict of interest.

References

1. Louis, D.N.; Ohgaki, H.; Wiestler, O.D.; Cavenee, W.K.; Burger, P.C.; Jouvet, A.; Scheithauer, B.W.; Kleihues, P. The 2007 WHO classification of tumours of the central nervous system. *Acta Neuropathol.* **2007**, *114*, 97–109. [CrossRef] [PubMed]
2. Louis, D.N.; Perry, A.; Reifenberger, G.; von Deimling, A.; Figarella-Branger, D.; Cavenee, W.K.; Ohgaki, H.; Wiestler, O.D.; Kleihues, P.; Ellison, D.W. The 2016 World Health Organization Classification of Tumors of the Central Nervous System: A summary. *Acta Neuropathol.* **2016**, *131*, 803–820. [CrossRef] [PubMed]
3. Cancer Genome Atlas Research Network. Comprehensive genomic characterization defines human glioblastoma genes and core pathways. *Nature* **2008**, *455*, 1061–1068.
4. Verhaak, R.G.W.; Hoadley, K.A.; Purdom, E.; Wang, V.; Qi, Y.; Wilkerson, M.D.; Miller, C.R.; Ding, L.; Golub, T.; Mesirov, J.P.; et al. Integrated genomic analysis identifies clinically relevant subtypes of glioblastoma characterized by abnormalities in PDGFRA, IDH1, EGFR, and NF1. *Cancer Cell* **2010**, *17*, 98–110. [CrossRef] [PubMed]
5. Brennan, C.W.; Verhaak, R.G.W.; McKenna, A.; Campos, B.; Noushmehr, H.; Salama, S.R.; Zheng, S.; Chakravarty, D.; Sanborn, J.Z.; Berman, S.H.; et al. The somatic genomic landscape of glioblastoma. *Cell* **2013**, *155*, 462–477. [CrossRef] [PubMed]
6. Zundel, W.; Schindler, C.; Haas-Kogan, D.; Koong, A.; Kaper, F.; Chen, E.; Gottschalk, A.R.; Ryan, H.E.; Johnson, R.S.; Jefferson, A.B.; et al. Loss of PTEN facilitates HIF-1-mediated gene expression. *Genes Dev.* **2000**, *14*, 391–396. [PubMed]
7. Haas-Kogan, D.; Shalev, N.; Wong, M.; Mills, G.; Yount, G.; Stokoe, D. Protein kinase B (PKB/Akt) activity is elevated in glioblastoma cells due to mutation of the tumor suppressor PTEN/MMAC. *Curr. Biol.* **1998**, *8*, 1195–1198. [CrossRef]
8. Wesseling, P.; Ruiter, D.J.; Burger, P.C. Angiogenesis in brain tumors; pathobiological and clinical aspects. *J. Neurooncol.* **1997**, *32*, 253–265. [CrossRef] [PubMed]
9. Rong, Y.; Durden, D.L.; Van Meir, E.G.; Brat, D.J. "Pseudopalisading" necrosis in glioblastoma: A familiar morphologic feature that links vascular pathology, hypoxia, and angiogenesis. *J. Neuropathol. Exp. Neurol.* **2006**, *65*, 529–539. [CrossRef] [PubMed]
10. Harris, A.L. Hypoxia-a key regulatory factor in tumour growth. *Nat. Rev. Cancer* **2002**, *2*, 38–47. [CrossRef] [PubMed]
11. Guerra, B.; Hochscherf, J.; Jensen, N.B.; Issinger, O.-G. Identification of a novel potent, selective and cell permeable inhibitor of protein kinase CK2 from the NIH/NCI Diversity Set Library. *Mol. Cell. Biochem.* **2015**, *406*, 151–161. [CrossRef] [PubMed]
12. Guerra, B.; Fischer, M.; Schaefer, S.; Issinger, O.-G. The kinase inhibitor D11 induces caspase-mediated cell death in cancer cells resistant to chemotherapeutic treatment. *J. Exp. Clin. Cancer Res.* **2015**, *34*, 125. [CrossRef] [PubMed]
13. Guerra, B.; Issinger, O.-G. Protein kinase CK2 and its role in cellular proliferation, development and pathology. *Electrophoresis* **1999**, *20*, 391–408. [CrossRef]
14. Guerra, B.; Issinger, O.-G. Protein kinase CK2 in human diseases. *Curr. Med. Chem.* **2008**, *15*, 1870–1886. [CrossRef] [PubMed]
15. Duncan, J.S.; Litchfield, D.W. Too much of a good thing: The role of protein kinase CK2 in tumorigenesis and prospects for therapeutic inhibition of CK2. *Biochim. Biophys. Acta* **2008**, *1784*, 33–47. [CrossRef] [PubMed]
16. Trembley, J.H.; Wang, G.; Unger, G.; Slaton, J.; Ahmed, K. Protein kinase CK2 in health and disease: CK2: A key player in cancer biology. *Cell. Mol. Life Sci.* **2009**, *66*, 1858–1867. [CrossRef] [PubMed]

17. Ruzzene, M.; Pinna, L.A. Addiction to protein kinase CK2: A common denominator of diverse cancer cells? *Biochim. Biophys. Acta* **2010**, *1804*, 499–504. [CrossRef] [PubMed]

18. Hubert, A.; Paris, S.; Piret, J.-P.; Ninane, N.; Raes, M.; Michiels, C. Casein kinase 2 inhibition decreases hypoxia-inducible factor-1 activity under hypoxia through elevated p53 protein level. *J. Cell. Sci.* **2006**, *119*, 3351–3362. [CrossRef] [PubMed]

19. Mazure, N.M.; Chen, E.Y.; Laderoute, K.R.; Giaccia, A.J. Induction of vascular endothelial growth factor by hypoxia is modulated by a phosphatidylinositol 3-kinase/Akt signaling pathway in Ha-ras-transformed cells through a hypoxia inducible factor-1 transcriptional element. *Blood* **1997**, *90*, 3322–3331. [PubMed]

20. Jiang, B.H.; Jiang, G.; Zheng, J.Z.; Lu, Z.; Hunter, T.; Vogt, P.K. Phosphatidylinositol 3-kinase signaling controls levels of hypoxia-inducible factor 1. *Cell Growth Differ.* **2001**, *12*, 363–369. [PubMed]

21. Pore, N.; Liu, S.; Haas-Kogan, D.A.; O'Rourke, D.M.; Maity, A. PTEN mutation and epidermal growth factor receptor activation regulate vascular endothelial growth factor (VEGF) mRNA expression in human glioblastoma cells by transactivating the proximal VEGF promoter. *Cancer Res.* **2003**, *63*, 236–241. [PubMed]

22. Wang, D.; Westerheide, S.D.; Hanson, J.L.; Baldwin, A.S. Tumor necrosis factor α-induced phosphorylation of RelA/p65 on Ser529 is controlled by casein kinase II. *J. Biol. Chem.* **2000**, *275*, 32592–32597. [CrossRef] [PubMed]

23. Wenger, R.H.; Kvietikova, I.; Rolfs, A.; Gassmann, M.; Marti, H.H. Hypoxia-inducible factor-1 α is regulated at the post-mRNA level. *Kidney Int.* **1997**, *51*, 560–563. [CrossRef] [PubMed]

24. Huang, L.E.; Gu, J.; Schau, M.; Bunn, H.F. Regulation of hypoxia-inducible factor 1α is mediated by an O_2-dependent degradation domain via the ubiquitin-proteasome pathway. *Proc. Natl. Acad. Sci. USA* **1998**, *95*, 7987–7992. [CrossRef] [PubMed]

25. Guerra, B.; Rasmussen, T.D.L.; Schnitzler, A.; Jensen, H.H.; Boldyreff, B.S.; Miyata, Y.; Marcussen, N.; Niefind, K.; Issinger, O.-G. Protein kinase CK2 inhibition is associated with the destabilization of HIF-1α in human cancer cells. *Cancer Lett.* **2015**, *356*, 751–761. [CrossRef] [PubMed]

26. Yeo, E.-J.; Chun, Y.-S.; Cho, Y.-S.; Kim, J.; Lee, J.-C.; Kim, M.-S.; Park, J.-W. YC-1: A potential anticancer drug targeting hypoxia-inducible factor 1. *J. Natl. Cancer Inst.* **2003**, *95*, 516–525. [CrossRef] [PubMed]

27. Isaacs, J.S.; Jung, Y.-J.; Mimnaugh, E.G.; Martinez, A.; Cuttitta, F.; Neckers, L.M. Hsp90 regulates a von Hippel Lindau-independent hypoxia-inducible factor 1α-degradative pathway. *J. Biol. Chem.* **2002**, *277*, 29936–29944. [CrossRef] [PubMed]

28. Mabjeesh, N.J.; Post, D.E.; Willard, M.T.; Kaur, B.; Van Meir, E.G.; Simons, J.W.; Zhong, H. Geldanamycin induces degradation of hypoxia-inducible factor 1α protein via the proteosome pathway in prostate cancer cells. *Cancer Res.* **2002**, *62*, 2478–2482. [PubMed]

29. Zagzag, D.; Nomura, M.; Friedlander, D.R.; Blanco, C.Y.; Gagner, J.-P.; Nomura, N.; Newcomb, E.W. Geldanamycin inhibits migration of glioma cells in vitro: A potential role for hypoxia-inducible factor (HIF-1α) in glioma cell invasion. *J. Cell. Physiol.* **2003**, *196*, 394–402. [CrossRef] [PubMed]

30. Zuehlke, A.; Johnson, J.L. Hsp90 and co-chaperones twist the functions of diverse client proteins. *Biopolymers* **2010**, *93*, 211–217. [CrossRef] [PubMed]

31. Miyata, Y. Protein kinase CK2 in health and disease: CK2: The kinase controlling the Hsp90 chaperone machinery. *Cell. Mol. Life Sci.* **2009**, *66*, 1840–1849. [CrossRef] [PubMed]

32. Espert, L.; Denizot, M.; Grimaldi, M.; Robert-Hebmann, V.; Gay, B.; Varbanov, M.; Codogno, P.; Biard-Piechaczyk, M. Autophagy is involved in T cell death after binding of HIV-1 envelope proteins to CXCR4. *J. Clin. Investig.* **2006**, *116*, 2161–2172. [CrossRef] [PubMed]

33. Wykoff, C.C.; Beasley, N.; Watson, P.H.; Campo, L.; Chia, S.K.; English, R.; Pastorek, J.; Sly, W.S.; Ratcliffe, P.; Harris, A.L. Expression of the hypoxia-inducible and tumor-associated carbonic anhydrases in ductal carcinoma in situ of the breast. *Am. J. Pathol.* **2001**, *158*, 1011–1019. [CrossRef]

34. Verma, S.; Dixit, R.; Pandey, K.C. Cysteine Proteases: Modes of Activation and Future Prospects as Pharmacological Targets. *Front. Pharmacol.* **2016**, *7*, 107. [CrossRef] [PubMed]

35. Ellen, T.P.; Ke, Q.; Zhang, P.; Costa, M. NDRG1, a growth and cancer related gene: Regulation of gene expression and function in normal and disease states. *Carcinogenesis* **2008**, *29*, 2–8. [CrossRef] [PubMed]

36. Guan, R.J.; Ford, H.L.; Fu, Y.; Li, Y.; Shaw, L.M.; Pardee, A.B. Drg-1 as a differentiation-related, putative metastatic suppressor gene in human colon cancer. *Cancer Res.* **2000**, *60*, 749–755. [PubMed]

37. Bandyopadhyay, S.; Pai, S.K.; Gross, S.C.; Hirota, S.; Hosobe, S.; Miura, K.; Saito, K.; Commes, T.; Hayashi, S.; Watabe, M.; et al. The Drg-1 gene suppresses tumor metastasis in prostate cancer. *Cancer Res.* **2003**, *63*, 1731–1736. [PubMed]

38. Salnikow, K.; Costa, M.; Figg, W.D.; Blagosklonny, M.V. Hyperinducibility of hypoxia-responsive genes without p53/p21-dependent checkpoint in aggressive prostate cancer. *Cancer Res.* **2000**, *60*, 5630–5634. [PubMed]

39. Guerra, B.; Iwabuchi, K.; Issinger, O.-G. Protein kinase CK2 is required for the recruitment of 53BP1 to sites of DNA double-strand break induced by radiomimetic drugs. *Cancer Lett.* **2014**, *345*, 115–123. [CrossRef] [PubMed]

40. Sandholt, I.S.; Olsen, B.B.; Guerra, B.; Issinger, O.-G. Resorufin: A lead for a new protein kinase CK2 inhibitor. *Anticancer Drugs* **2009**, *20*, 238–248. [CrossRef] [PubMed]

41. Yde, C.W.; Olsen, B.B.; Meek, D.; Watanabe, N.; Guerra, B. The regulatory beta-subunit of protein kinase CK2 regulates cell-cycle progression at the onset of mitosis. *Oncogene* **2008**, *27*, 4986–4997. [CrossRef] [PubMed]

42. Livak, K.J.; Schmittgen, T.D. Analysis of relative gene expression data using real-time quantitative PCR and the 2(-Delta Delta C(T)) Method. *Methods* **2001**, *25*, 402–408. [CrossRef] [PubMed]

43. Schmittgen, T.D.; Livak, K.J. Analyzing real-time PCR data by the comparative C(T) method. *Nat. Protoc.* **2008**, *3*, 1101–1108. [CrossRef] [PubMed]

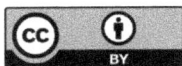

pharmaceuticals

MDPI

Article

Identification of a Potent Allosteric Inhibitor of Human Protein Kinase CK2 by Bacterial Surface Display Library Screening

Christian Nienberg [1,†]**, Claudia Garmann** [1,†]**, Andreas Gratz** [1]**, Andre Bollacke** [1]**, Claudia Götz** [2] **and Joachim Jose** [1,*]

[1] Institut für Pharmazeutische und Medizinische Chemie, PharmaCampus, Westfälische Wilhelms-Universität Münster, Corrensstraße 48, D-48149 Münster, Germany; christian.nienberg@uni-muenster.de (C.N.); claudia.reicheneder@gmx.de (C.G.); gratz.andreas@gmail.com (A.G.); andre.bollacke@uni-muenster.de (A.B.)

[2] Medizinische Biochemie und Molekularbiologie, Universität des Saarlandes, Kirrberger Str., Geb. 44, D-66421 Homburg, Germany; claudia.goetz@uks.eu

[*] Correspondence: joachim.jose@uni-muenster.de; Tel.: +49-251-833-2200

[†] These authors contributed equally to this work.

Academic Editor: Lorenzo A. Pinna
Received: 30 November 2016; Accepted: 27 December 2016; Published: 5 January 2017

Abstract: Human protein kinase CK2 has emerged as promising target for the treatment of neoplastic diseases. The vast majority of kinase inhibitors known today target the ATP binding site, which is highly conserved among kinases and hence leads to limited selectivity. In order to identify non-ATP competitive inhibitors, a 12-mer peptide library of 6×10^5 variants was displayed on the surface of *E. coli* by autodisplay. Screening of this peptide library on variants with affinity to CK2 was performed by fluorophore-conjugated CK2 and subsequent flow cytometry. Single cell sorting of CK2-bound *E. coli* yielded new peptide variants, which were tested on inhibition of CK2 by a CE-based assay. Peptide B2 (DCRGLIVMIKLH) was the most potent inhibitor of both, CK2 holoenzyme and the catalytic CK2α subunit (IC_{50} = 0.8 μM). Using different ATP concentrations and different substrate concentrations for IC_{50} determination, B2 was shown to be neither ATP- nor substrate competitive. By microscale thermophoresis (MST) the K_D value of B2 with CK2α was determined to be 2.16 μM, whereas no binding of B2 to CK2β-subunit was detectable. To our surprise, besides inhibition of enzymatic activity, B2 also disturbed the interaction of CK2α with CK2β at higher concentrations ($\geq$25 μM).

Keywords: autodisplay; human protein kinase CK2; non ATP-competitive inhibitor; peptide

1. Introduction

Human protein kinase CK2 is a heterotetrameric enzyme, consisting of two catalytic (CK2α or CK2α′) and two regulatory subunits (CK2β). The interaction between the CK2 subunits is highly dynamic and the balance between separation and interaction of the subunits to create a functional holoenzyme is crucial in the control of many cellular processes [1]. CK2 has a key role in cell signaling networks. It influences cell growth and proliferation, as numerous growth related proteins are substrates of CK2 [2]. The highly pleiotropic serine/threonine-kinase CK2 is constitutively active and present in nearly all tissues, cell types and most cell compartments. There is growing evidence for the involvement of deregulated CK2 activity in a variety of human cancers such as breast cancer [3], prostate cancer [4] and colorectal cancer [5]. Elevated CK2 activity has been associated with the malignant transformation of several tissues [6] and is supposed to serve as prognostic marker in several diseases such as acute myeloid leukemia [7] or Parkinson's disease [8]. Therefore CK2 has emerged as a potential therapeutic target for cancer treatment [9]. Drug discovery programs were launched aiming at the identification of specific inhibitors of CK2 reducing the elevated CK2 activity in cancer cells to a non-pathogenic level. To date, several lead structures of small molecule CK2 inhibitors are known, which in nearly all cases are competitive with respect to the co-substrate ATP [10]. One relevant representative is the halogenated benzimidazole derivative 4,5,6,7-tetrabromo-benzotriazole (TBB) with a K_i of 0.4 µM [11]. The flavonoid quercetin (IC_{50} = 0.55 µM) and the anthraquinone emodin (K_i = 1.85 µM) [10] are representatives of natural compounds which show CK2 inhibition. Other potent inhibitors with IC_{50} values in the nanomolar range have a pyrazolotriazine scaffold [12] or an indoloquinazoline scaffold such as IQA (IC_{50} = 0.39 µM) [13]. To date one inhibitor was able to complete successfully phase I clinical trials. Silmitasertib (CX-4945) is an oral small molecule inhibitor of CK2, showing a selective anti-proliferative activity [14]. Currently silmitasertib is in phase II clinical trials for the treatment of cholangiocarcinoma. The high degree of conservation of the ATP binding site throughout the human kinome [2] is often a disadvantage of ATP-competitive inhibitors. As a consequence, ATP competitive kinase inhibitors, including those targeting CK2, are poorly specific and also affect other kinases. The development of inhibitors with a different mode of action promises to impact CK2 activity more selectively. The first studies revealed CK2 inhibiting compounds not directly competing with ATP. By screening of highly diverse chemical libraries it was found that inorganic polyoxometalates (POMs) are nanomolar inhibitors of the CK2 holoenzyme and CK2α subunit [15]. However the active structure of the most potent POM with an IC_{50} of 5 nM) was not identified so far. The authors speculated that POMs target an exosite of the CK2α subunit as allosteric inhibitors. Other approaches are the development of inhibitors which interfere with the assembly of the subunits. It was found that—at least in vitro—the free catalytic subunit and the holoenzyme exhibit divergent substrate preferences [16]. The disassembly and reassembly of the CK2 holoenzyme seems to be a likely point of regulation of many cellular processes [16]. An inhibitor (W16) of the CK2 subunit interaction (IC_{50} = 40 µM) was found by screening a library of podophyllotoxin indole-analogs [17]. The kinase activity of the CK2 holoenzyme was not affected by W16, but the activity of CK2α (IC_{50} = 20 µM) was inhibited. The authors assumed that W16 docks to the CK2α/CK2β interface inducing an allosteric conformational change in CK2α that affects its activity. For azonaphthalene derivatives a non-ATP competitive inhibition of both the α-subunit and the heterotetrameric CK2 holoenzyme was shown (most potent inhibitor: IC_{50} = 0.4 µM) [18]. Azonaphthalene derivates were shown to decrease tumor genesis in vitro and in vivo. The exact binding site on CK2 is not known, but it was shown that the inhibitor caused a large conformational change of CK2α, thereby blocking the binding of substrates. A different class of emerging non-ATP competitive inhibitors is comprised of peptides. Among peptides a binding at the ATP cave is unlikely, taking into account the rigid structure of ATP-competitive inhibitors, usually consisting of heterocycles [19]. The Pc peptide is a cyclic 11-mer identified by a screening of conformational constrained peptides mimicking the binding interface of CK2β with CK2α. It is able to antagonize (IC_{50} = 3 µM) and to disassemble (IC_{50} = 6.5 µM) the formation of the CK2 holoenzyme complex [20]. In contrast to W16 the Pc peptide shows no inhibition of CK2α, but it acts as CK2β antagonist, inhibiting phosphorylation of CK2β dependent substrates. Another peptide-derived inhibitor is CIGB-300. It consists of two domains, the cyclic 9-mer P15, which inhibits CK2-catalyzed phosphorylation by blocking the interaction with the substrate and the Tat-peptide for enabling membrane translocation [21]. Antitumor effects were shown, among others, on patients with cervical malignancies [22] and meanwhile CIGB-300 has also entered phase II clinical trials. Nevertheless the interaction of CIGB-300 and CK2 is not understood on a molecular level. The 18-mer peptide P1 was isolated by screening of a combinatorial peptide aptamer library. It binds to an N-terminal domain on CK2β (K_D = 0.4 µM) [23]. The interaction of P1 with CK2β neither dissociates the CK2 holoenzyme complex nor prevents its formation and did not inhibit the phosphorylation of two protein substrates exclusively targeted by the CK2 holoenzyme. The authors assumed that binding of P1 to the N-terminal domain of CK2β compete for a common binding site on the protein for unknown endogenous ligands or protein kinase substrates that are essential for cell survival [24]. In different mammalian cell lines apoptosis through the recruitment of a p53-dependent apoptosis pathway was induced.

The aim of this study was to screen a surface displayed library of peptides for a non-ATP competitive CK2 inhibitor. A major advantage of screening randomized libraries is that new structures for specific targets can be identified without needing to know the exact peptide-surface interaction. Since the invention of phage display twenty years ago, display technologies have turned out to be a successful tool for broad biotechnology applications [25,26]. By surface display of libraries on cell surfaces the variants are available for screening without a purification step. It is possible to create a high number of cells with every single cell carrying a different peptide on the surface in high numbers. After selection the sequence of the peptide or protein can be easily determined, due to the fact that every cell carries an internal label, the DNA sequence. Surface display systems have shown to be a promising tool in the development of peptide inhibitors. They were used for identification of protease inhibitors [27,28], as also for discovery of antiviral peptides [29,30]. Autodisplay which was used in this study was shown to be a flexible surface display system for presenting polypeptide libraries on the surface of *E. coli* cells [31–33]. In combination with flow cytometry it yielded a new lead structure for human cathepsin G inhibitors (IC_{50} = 11.7 µM) [31]. Autodisplay based transport of peptides or proteins is facilitated by the natural autotransporter secretion mechanism of Gram negative bacteria [34] (Figure 1).

In the present study a 12-mer peptide library of up to 6×10^5 variants was displayed on the surface of *E. coli* cells via autodisplay. A flow cytometry-based screening based on the affinity of fluorescence coupled CK2 yielded a new allosteric inhibitor of CK2 with an IC_{50} value in the submicromolar range.

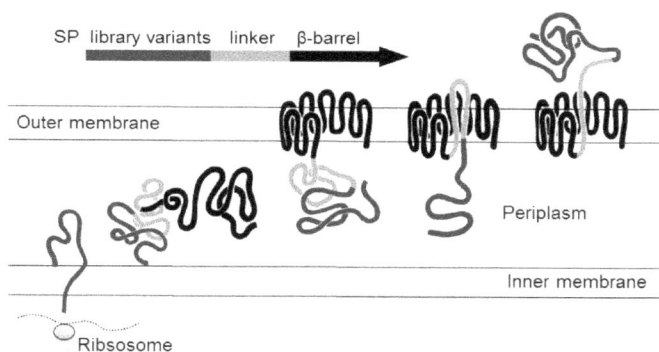

Figure 1. Secretion mechanism of library variants by autodisplay.The autotransporters are synthesized as precursor proteins containing all structural requirements for the transport to the cell surface. With the aid of the signal peptide, the polyprotein precursor is translocated across the inner membrane. Arriving at the periplasm, the precursor folds as a porin-like structure, the so called β-barrel within the outer membrane and the passenger is transmitted to the cell surface. To obtain full surface exposure, a linker region between the passenger and the β-barrel is required. SP: Signalpeptide.

2. Results

2.1. Autodisplay of Human α_{S1}-Casein and Cellular Labeling with CK2-FITC

Casein was one of the first substrates reported for CK2 [35]. Previous western blot experiments with an anti-phosphoserine antibody proved that human α_{S1}-casein is a substrate of CK2 (data not shown). Due to the fact that a target enzyme has affinity to its substrate it was expected that CK2 would show affinity to human α_{S1}-casein. The binding of surface displayed human α_{S1}-casein by fluorophore-coupled CK2 was supposed to be detectable in vitro via flow cytometry. Therefore,

α_{S1}-casein was inserted as passenger into an autotransporter-fusion protein and presented on the cell surface of *E. coli* (encoded by plasmid pKP10, Figure 2C).

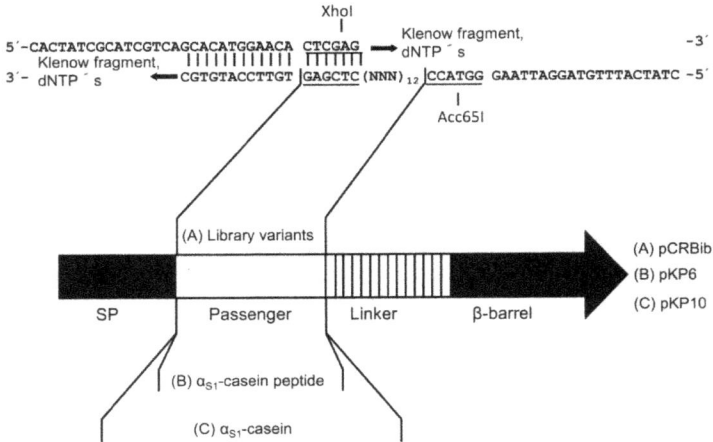

Figure 2. Structure of the autotransporter fusion proteins encoded by plasmid pCRBib (12mer peptide library, **A**), plasmid pKP6 (α_{S1}-casein peptide, **B**) and plasmid pKP10 (α_{S1}-casein, **C**) used for autodisplay. (**A**) The autodisplay passenger of plasmid pCRBib consists of 36 randomized nucleotides. The passenger region, the fusion sites to the signal peptide and the linker region of the autotransporter are given as DNA-sequences. The oligonucleotides CR21 and CR22 were hybridized and filled up to a double strand and then inserted by the underlined restriction sites. The fusion protein has a calculated molecular weight of 50.2 kDa after cleavage of the signal peptide. (**B**) Human α_{S1}-casein as autodisplay passenger of plasmid pKP10 has a length of 510 nt. (**C**) The autodisplay passenger of plasmid pKP6 is α_{S1}-casein peptide encoded by 48 nt. The passengers encoding sequences were inserted in frame into the autotransporter encoding gene. SP = signal peptide.

The surface display of α_{S1}-casein was proven by protease accessibility and immunofluorescence using a polyclonal rabbit serum against α_{S1}-casein [36]. The α_{S1}-casein displaying cells were incubated with fluorescein-isothiocyanate (FITC) coupled CK2 holoenzyme. The amount of bound CK2 determined the overall fluorescence intensity of α_{S1}-casein-displaying cells. Cells with increased fluorescence could be detected by flow cytometry indicating high affinity of CK2 to the surface presented α_{S1}-casein. As can be seen in Figure 3A, cells displaying human α_{S1}-casein on their surface (*E. coli* UT5600(DE3) pKP10) showed a tenfold higher fluorescence intensity than control cells (*E. coli* UT5600(DE3).

The tenfold higher amount of CK2 bound to surface displayed α_{S1}-casein cells indicated the affinity of human α_{S1}-casein to CK2. For the screening of a peptide library, it was indispensable to show that the affinity of CK2 to a surface-displayed peptide is detectable by flow cytometry as well. Therefore, as an additional control, a 16mer α_{S1}-casein derived peptide known to bind CK2 (α_{S1}-casein peptide) was surface displayed and analyzed by fluorescence labeled CK2 and flow cytometry as well (Figure 3B). For this purpose plasmid pKP6 was constructed (Figure 2B). After verification of expression and surface display (data not shown), cells of *E. coli* UT5600(DE3) pKP6 were incubated with fluorophore coupled CK2 and subjected to flow cytometry as done before for full-length α_{S1}-casein. As shown in Figure 3B, α_{S1}-casein peptide-displaying cells indeed had a significantly higher fluorescence than host cells without plasmid. This indicated that autodisplay of a peptide is sufficient for affinity labeling of cells by fluorophore coupled CK2.

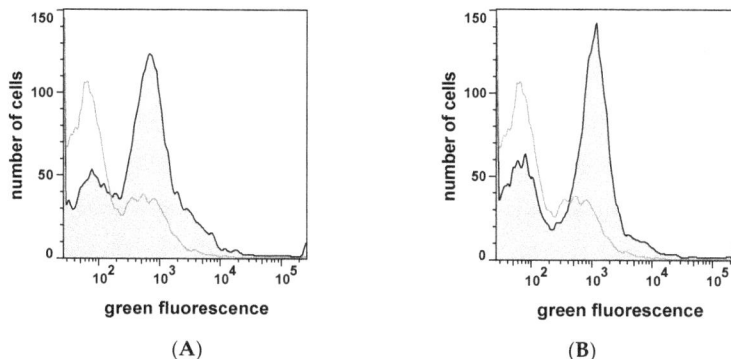

Figure 3. Flow cytometer analysis of *E. coli* cells displaying α_{S1}-casein (170 aa) (**A**) and α_{S1}-casein peptide (16 aa) (**B**) after incubation with fluorophore coupled CK2. By the use of a FACSAria flow cytometer 50,000 cells were analyzed with an exication wavelength of 488 nm and an emission wavelength between 527 and 530 nm. The host strain *E. coli* UT5600(DE3) was outlined in the same manner (grey line). (**A**): *E. coli* UT5600(DE3) pKP10; (**B**): *E. coli* UT5600(DE3) pKP6.

2.2. Design of a Bacterial Surface Display Library

For the construction of the peptide library, a PCR primer containing a fully random sequence of 12 codons was designed (Figure 2A). A 12-mer random peptide library was chosen, because the already known peptidic inhibitors of CK2 had a length of nine, eleven and eighteen amino acids. Beyond the random sequence the oligonucleotide primer of 82 nt length (CR22) contained a 5′- as well as a 3′-extension. The 3′-entension was complementary to a shorter oligonucleotide primer (CR21), which was used to fill up the random sequence of CR22 to a double strand by Klenow fragment DNA polymerization. The 5′-extension of CR22 finally led to a double stranded DNA fragment that could be easily identified in an agarose gel, to control the reaction. The XhoI/Acc65I restriction sites flanking the random sequence were used to insert the library cassette into the open reading frame of an autotransporter artificial gene construct in plasmid pCR19 (Figure 2A). *E. coli* UT5600(DE3) electrocompetent cells were transformed with the resulting plasmid library, yielding a library size of 6×10^5 colony forming units.

2.3. Selecting Peptides with Affinity towards CK2 by FACS

The *E. coli* surface display library was grown for 1 h after transformation in SOC-medium. Protein expression was induced with 1 mM IPTG. Subsequently, the complete library was incubated with fluorophore coupled CK2 and subjected to flow cytometry as described above. In the histogram plot of 10,000 cells analyzed, two populations were clearly visible, one with a strongly increased fluorescence and one with low fluorescence (Figure 4). A sorting gate was defined in order to isolate single cells with the highest values of increased fluorescence from the positive subpopulation, finally comprising 0.54% of all cells (Figure 4).

Using this sort gate 22 single cell variants were placed on an agar plate for further analysis. Out of this 22 variants, six variants (B1–B6) exhibited an increased affinity to fluorophore coupled CK2 when reanalysed by flow cytometry (Figure 5), indicating that 16 single cell variants appeared to be false positives.

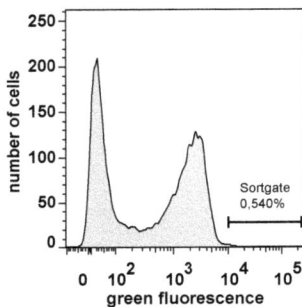

Figure 4. Flow cytometer analysis of *E. coli* cells displaying library peptides and sorting of cells with increased fluorescence. The analysis of 10,000 cells was accomplished with a FACSAria Cytometer with an integrated sorting module. The cells were incubated with fluorophore coupled CK2 and analyzed at a excitation wavelength of 488 nm and an emission wavelength between 527 and 530 nm. A sort gate was drawn around the population with an increased green fluorescence, which represent 0.54% of all events. These cells were selected out and grown on a agar plate for further analysis.

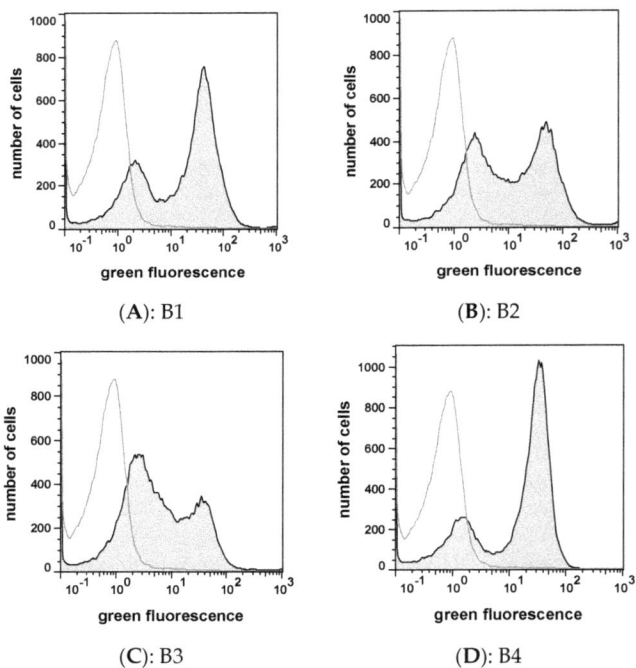

(**A**): B1

(**B**): B2

(**C**): B3

(**D**): B4

Figure 5. Flow cytometer based reanalysis of *E. coli* cells bearing library peptides (B1–B4) selected from the surface display library by FACS. The single cell variants, selected as single cell colonies, were incubated with fluorophore coupled CK2 as described. 50,000 cells were analyzed at a excitation wavelength of 488 nm and an emission wavelength between 527 and 530 nm by the use of a CyFlow Space (filled histograms). The host strain *E. coli* UT5600(DE3) was treated identically (unfilled histogram). (**A**): B1, *E coli* UT5600(DE3) pCR31; (**B**): B2, *E. coli* UT5600(DE3) pCR33; (**C**): B3, *E. coli* UT5600(DE3) pCR34; (**D**): B4; *E. coli* UT5600(DE3) pCR36.

2.4. Peptide Expression and Sequence Analysis

The peptide encoding sequence of the four variants (B1–B6) was subjected to DNA sequence analysis. The derived peptides all had different aa sequences with no apparent consensus motif, however, the peptide sequence of B5 and B6 contained stop codons. After growing the cells and induction of the protein expression with IPTG, bacterial outer membrane fractions containing the autotransporter fusion proteins were isolated and analyzed by SDS-PAGE. Whereas B5 showed expression of a protein of correct size, no protein expression was detectable in variant B6. In all other samples, a protein band with a molecular weight of 50.2 kDa—as expected—was detectable. Western blot with an AIDA-I-β-barrel specific antibody labelled the same band in all samples, indicating the successful expression the peptide autotransporter fusion protein.

In outer membrane fractions of *E. coli* UT5600(DE3) pCR31 (B1), UT5600(DE3) pCR33 (B2) and UT5600(DE3) pCR36 (B4) a protein band double the size of the expected molecular weight of the fusion protein could be recognized under non-reducing conditions. These three variants contained a cysteine residue (Table 1). The dimer band disappeared when reducing conditions in the SDS-PAGE sample buffer were used and an increase of the band corresponding to the monomer of the expected fusion protein was observed (data not shown). The β-barrel of the autotransporter is flexible within the outer membrane, hence a dimerization of passengers on the cell surface is possible and has been shown by many examples before [37].

Table 1. Inhibition of CK2 by peptides from bacterial surface display library screening.

Peptide	Sequence	Inhibition* (%)	IC$_{50}$ Value (μM)
B1	KHTKGPTAYCPL	< 5	n.d.
B2	DCRGLIVMIKLH	79	0.8
B3	YRKPHWFIHTRI	< 5	n.d.
B4	PCPAPRAPKLSI	29	n.d.

n.d. = not determined, * 10 μM final concentration.

2.5. CK2 Inhibitor Testing by Capillary Electrophoresis (CE)-Assay

Based on the aa sequences of variants B1–B4 (Table 1), the free peptides were synthesized and tested on inhibition of CK2 holoenzyme. For this purpose a CE-based CK2 inhibition assay was used as described before [38]. For initial testing CK2 was pre-incubated with the peptide in a final concentration of 10 μM for 10 min at 37 °C. After addition of the substrate and ATP, the reaction ran for 7 min and the amount of product was determined by CE. The amount of product obtained with inhibitor was set into relation to the amount obtained with the enzyme without inhibitor. At 10 μM, two of the peptides showed no inhibition (B1 and B3), one showed a weak inhibition of 29% (B4), whereas peptide B2 could be identified as a strong CK2 inhibitor with an inhibition of 79% (Table 1).

Apparently three of the peptides bound CK2 holoenzyme, but had no or almost no effect on enzymatic activity. For peptide B2 the IC$_{50}$ value was determined using different concentrations ranging from 0.001 μM to 100 μM for inhibition of CK2 holoenzyme, which turned out to be 0.8 μM (Figure 6A). The IC$_{50}$ value of B2 with the catalytic subunit CK2α alone was determined in a similar manner and turned out to be identical (0.8 μM, Figure 6B). This was a first indication that B2 interacted with CK2α directly and not via a conformational change of CK2β.

(A)

(B)

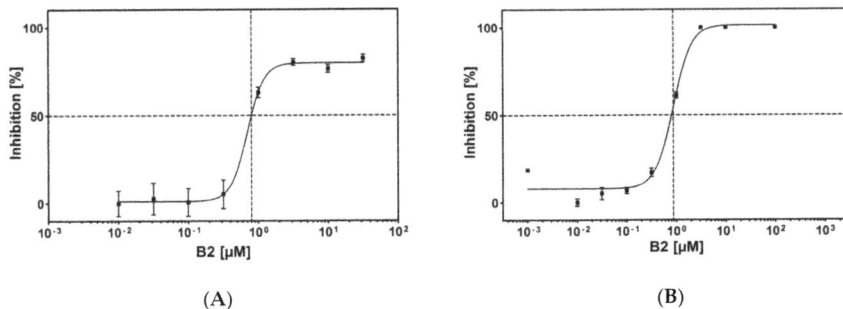

Figure 6. IC_{50} value determination of B2 by capillary electrophoresis measurements using CK2 holoenzyme (**A**) and the catalytic subunit CK2α (**B**). (**A**) Inhibition of recombinant CK2 holoenzyme by peptide B2 was measured after incubation with eight different compound concentrations ranging from 0.01 to 31.6 μM. (**B**) Inhibition of CK2α was tested using nine different inhibitor concentrations ranging from 0.001 μM to 100 μM. Samples were analyzed by CE. The resulting fractional inhibition values were plotted versus inhibitor concentrations in a semi-logarithmic diagram. The individual data points represent means of an experiment run in triplicates, the error bars indicate the standard deviation. In both cases an IC_{50} value of 0.8 μM was obtained by extrapolation the compound concentration at a residual CK2 activity of 50%. The dotted line marks the concentration at the midpoint (50%) of CK2 inhibition.

2.6. Mode of Inhibition

In order to investigate whether B2 is competitive or non-competitive with respect to ATP the IC_{50} values were determined using six different concentrations of ATP (1 mM to 100 mM) [39]. However, as shown in Figure 7A, there was no linear increase of the IC_{50} values in dependence of the ATP concentration detectable, indicating that B2 is non-competitive with respect to ATP.

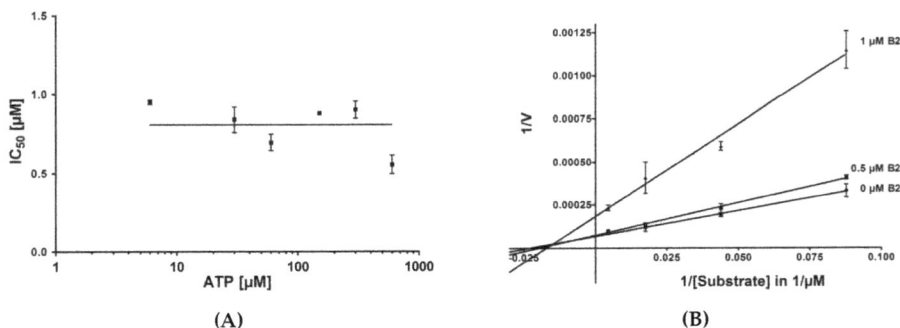

(A)

(B)

Figure 7. Graphical determination of the IC_{50} values of B2 in dependence of the ATP concentration and the substrate concentration. (**A**) Determination of IC_{50} values for the inhibition of CK2 by B2 with various concentrations of ATP. IC_{50} values were plotted against the corresponding ATP concentrations (ranging from 1 mM to 100 mM); the abscissa was plotted on a logarithmic scale. The individual data points represent means of an experiment run in triplicates, the error bars indicate the standard deviation. (**B**) Lineweaver-Burk inhibition plots of CK2 by B2 at different substrate concentrations. A double reciprocal plot of reaction velocity against the substrate concentration was done. CK2 kinase activity was determined in the absence (0 μM) or in the presence of 0.5 μM and 1 μM B2 with various concentration of peptide substrate. The individual data points represent means of an experiment run in triplicates, the error bars indicate the standard deviation.

In the next step it was investigated, whether B2 could have a substrate competitive mode of action. Therefore the reaction velocity for three different inhibitor concentrations (0 µM, 0.5 µM and 1 µM B2) and varying substrate concentrations (11.4 µM, 22.8 µM, 57 µM and 228 µM peptide RRRDDDSDDD) was determined. As shown in Figure 7B, the resulting diagram with the corresponding best-fit lines intersected at a single point left from the y-axes. This is characteristic for a non-competitive mode of inhibition [39]. The conclusion was that peptide B2 is non-competitive with respect to the substrate peptide RRRDDDSDDD and non-competitive with respect to ATP. In this situation two dissociation constants can be defined, one for the binary enzyme-inhibitor complex (K_i) and one for the ternary enzyme-substrate-inhibitor complex (αK_i). The best-fit lines in diagram 8 nearly converge at the x-axis. In this case both dissociation constants are equal, hence $\alpha = 1$. This means the inhibitor displays equal affinity for both, the free enzyme and the enzyme-substrate complex. According to the Cheng and Prusoff equation [40], in the case of non-competitive inhibition with $\alpha = 1$, the dissociation constant is equal to the IC_{50} value ($K_i = IC_{50}$) [39].

2.7. In Vitro Pull Down Assay

An in vitro pull down analysis with GST-tagged CK2α and in vitro translated [^{35}S]-labelled CK2β was performed in order to get a hint of whether B2 could disturb the interaction of both CK2 subunits. GST or GST-CK2α were expressed in *E. coli*, purified and immobilized on a GSH Sepharose resin. The GST tag without CK2α served as a control for unspecific binding. To analyze the effect of the B2 peptide on the assembly of the subunits to a holoenzyme, the catalytic α-subunit was pre-incubated with 25 or 100 µM peptide B2 before adding the labelled CK2β-subunit.

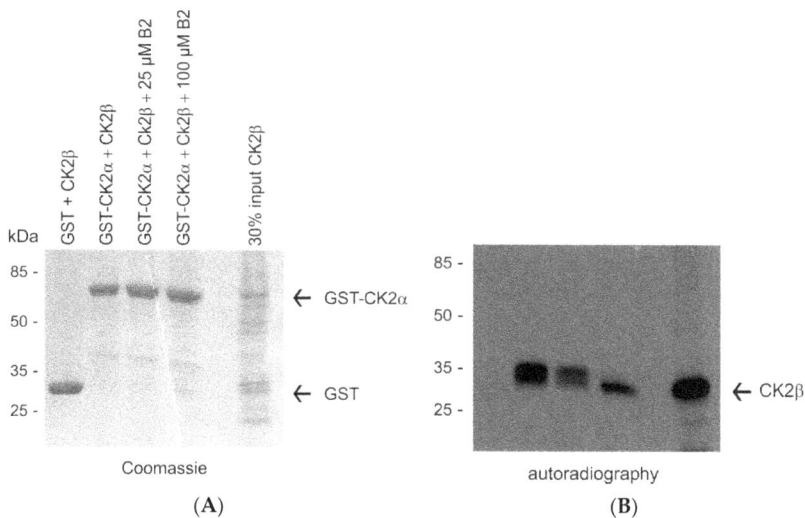

Figure 8. B2 interferes with the assembly of CK2α and CK2β. About 10 µg GST or GST-CK2α were incubated with 7.5 µL in vitro translated and [^{35}S]methionine labelled CK2β protein in the presence or the absence of 25 or 100 µM B2 peptide, respectively. The formed complex was coupled to GSH sepharose. Proteins eluted from the affinity resins were analyzed on a 12.5% SDS polyacrylamide gel, stained with Coomassie blue (**A**) and afterwards subjected to autoradiography (**B**).

Bound proteins were eluted subsequently with sample buffer and separated by SDS polyacrylamide gel electrophoresis. The gel was stained with Coomassie brilliant blue and afterwards subjected to autoradiography to visualize [^{35}S]-labelled CK2β. The Coomassie stained gel showed that equal amounts of GST-CK2α were applied in all lanes (Figure 8A). The autoradiography of the same gel also demonstrated that the GST control did not bind to the in vitro translated CK2β (Figure 8B, lane 1). GST-CK2α interacted effectively with CK2β. However, in case B2 peptide was added, the interaction was severely disturbed, resulting in significantly reduced amounts of CK2β eluted from the resin bound to GST-CK2α (compare lanes 3 and 4 with lane 2 in Figure 8B). Thus, it was concluded that the B2 peptide in concentrations of 25 µM and beyond interfered with the assembly of the holoenzyme.

2.8. MST Measurements

In order to support the idea that B2 binds to the catalytic CK2α subunit, the microscale thermophoresis (MST) method was applied [41]. Based on a different thermophoresis of a fluorescent protein after binding to an unlabeled interaction partner, it is possible to determine the dissociation constant (K_D). For this approach CK2α-pAzF, which exhibited the unnatural amino acid *p*-azidophenylalanine (pAzF), was purified and coupled to the fluorophore DBCO-Sulfo-Cy5 by click chemistry as described before [42].

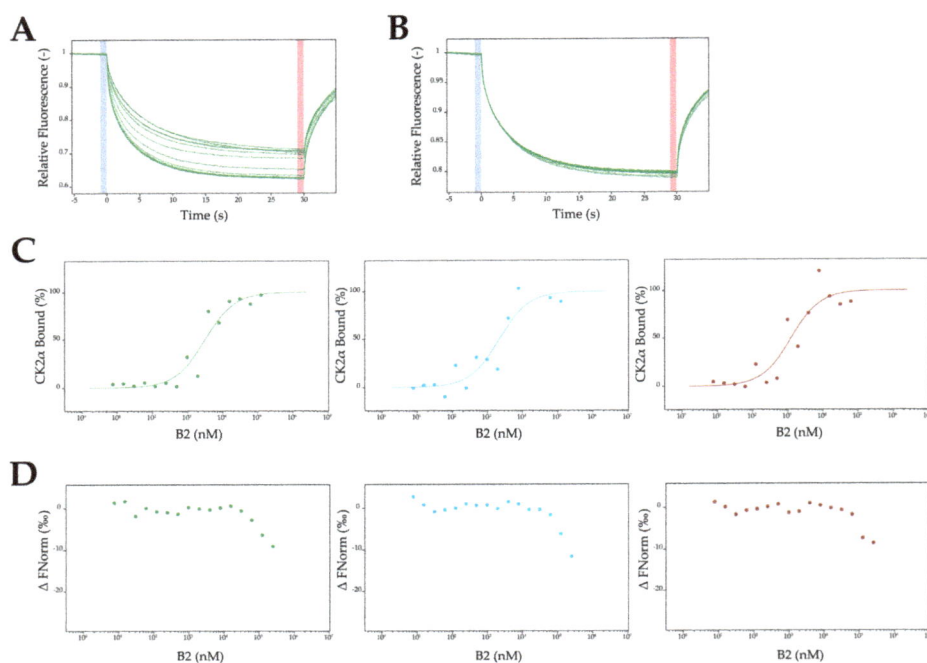

Figure 9. MST-measurements with B2 and CK2α or CK2β, respectively. For each subunit three independent measurements were performed and analyzed by the MO. Affinity Analysis v2.1.3 software (NanoTemper Technologies GmbH, München, Germany). (**A**) B2 was titrated in different concentrations ranging from 7.6 nM to 125 µM to a constant amount of CK2α (100 nM). The relative fluorescence signals of the thermophoresis of 15 different dilutions of B2 were recorded. (**B**) To a constant amount of CK2β (100 nM) concentrations of B2 ranging from 7.6 nM to 250 µM were added. A change in the relative fluorescence signals of the thermophoresis could only be detected in higher concentrations (above 62.5 µM). (**C**) The change in the thermophoresis led to a sigmoidal plot based on an unbound and a bound state of CK2α. This was done in three independent replicates. A mean K_D value of 2.16 ± 0.79 µM was determined. (**D**) The normalized fluorescence signals of the thermophoresis of CK2β[1-193]-Flu were plotted against the concentrations of B2 in three independent replicates.

Afterwards, different concentrations of B2 ranging from 7.6 nM to 125 µM were titrated to a constant amount of CK2α-DBCO-Sulfo-Cy5 (100 nM). A concentration dependent change in thermophoresis of CK2α was observed, which clearly indicated binding of B2 to CK2α (Figure 9A). The sigmoidal plot obtained by the differences in thermophoresis of the unbound state and the B2 bound state of CK2α was used to determine the K_D value, which turned out to be 2.16 ± 0.79 µM (Figure 9C). This was in good accordance with the inhibition of B2, either with CK2α or heterotetrameric CK2 holoenzyme ($\alpha_2\beta_2$). As a control the interaction between the regulatory CK2β subunit and B2 was investigated by MST. For this purpose a truncated version of CK2β (CK2β$^{1-193}$) was applied [43] and the unnatural amino acid pAzF was incorporated in CK2β$^{1-193}$ at position 174 instead of tyrosine, based on the method of Chin et al. [44]. Purification of CK2β$^{1-193}$-pAzF was performed according to the purification of CK2α-pAzF [42] and subsequently CK2β$^{1-193}$-pAzF was coupled to fluorescein (Flu) by click chemistry. B2 was added in concentrations ranging from 7.6 nM to 250 µM to constant a concentration of CK2β$^{1-193}$-Flu (100 nM) and applied to MST measurements. Only in very high concentrations (beyond 62.5 µM) a change in thermophoresis was detectable (Figure 9B,D). The determination of a K_D value was not possible by this strategy, and a K_D value, if any at all would be higher than 100 µM. In consequence the MST measurements clearly indicated the binding of B2 to CK2α and not to CK2β.

3. Discussion

By surface display library screening a potent peptidic inhibitor of CK2 holoenzyme and the α-subunit was identified. It was the 12-mer peptide B2, with the amino acid sequence DCRGLIVMIKLH. By a blast search in the UniProt protein database, no protein containing a similar sequence could be identified. B2 inhibited the catalytic activity of the α-subunit and the CK2 holoenzyme with an identical IC$_{50}$-value of 0.8 µM. By microscale thermophoresis measurements it was possible to determine the K_D value of B2 with the catalytic α-subunit experimentally and it turned out to be in the same order of magnitude. At higher concentrations beyond 25 µM, the peptide also disturbed the interaction of the catalytic α-subunit with the β-subunit of CK2 to form the holoenzyme. The question arises whether these two effects are facilitated by binding to the same allosteric binding site or by binding of two different sites at the α-subunit. Comparison of the dose-response curves used for the IC$_{50}$-value determination with the α-subunit and the holoenzyme (Figure 6A,B) reveals that—despite identical IC$_{50}$ values—complete inhibition was only obtained with the α-subunit, but not with the holoenzyme (max. 80% for the highest concentration of B2). This could be seen as an indication for a second binding site. Nevertheless, co-crystallization experiments of B2 with the α-subunit would help answering this question and are on the way at current.

The first step in the development of this new inhibitor was the surface display of a random 12-mer peptide library on the cell surface of *E. coli* by autodisplay. Beside the well-established phage-display, surface display on bacteria and yeast has emerged to a promising tool in drug discovery [45]. One advantage of bacteria in comparison to phage particles is that they are a big enough for flow cytometry analysis. The combination of library display on *E. coli* and subsequent fluorescence activated cell sorting is a powerful and rapid method, successfully applied in the development of new antibodies [46–48] and in the identification of high affinity peptides for different target proteins [49,50]. In this study the strategy for identifing new non-ATP competitive inhibitors of CK2 based on autodisplay, as autodisplay has been proven before suitable for the identification of new inhibitors of drug targets [31]. With the presented strategy, it was possible to create surface-displayed peptide libraries with up to 6×10^5 cell variants. After incubation with fluorescence-coupled CK2 the library could be directly used for a screening with whole cells by fluorescence activated cell sorting by which cells with increased green fluorescence were selected. After sorting, the coding sequences of the peptides presented on the cell surface could be easily determined by DNA sequence analyses of the co-selected plasmids. Within the selected variants, six peptide sequences were identified and four were tested on inhibition of the kinase activity of CK2 holoenzyme. Peptide B2 is a potent inhibitor of CK2 with a K_i value of 0.8 µM. The other peptides showed no inhibition or only weak inhibition. This was expectable, because the peptides were selected by their affinities towards CK2. Peptides binding to the target enzyme without influencing the activity of the enzyme can be selected by this way as well. Not expected was the high number of false positives selected by this strategy. False positives in this sense means that cells forming colonies on the agar plates after FACS selection, turned out to be negative after growing and re-labelling with CK2. This could have been due to several reasons and needs optimization. For example, a positive and a negative cell could have passed the laser beam in the detector so close that discrimination between the two was not possible, and both would have been selected. A mutant variant, not displaying any peptide could have been selected in one event with an active variant, and could have overgrown the peptide bearing strain during re-culturing. It could have been possible as well, that a peptide mutant selected had some extent of toxicity for the cells displaying it, again resulting in an overgrowing by cells not displaying it anymore. This will require systematic investigation and optimization, using mixtures of positive and negative variants with statistical analysis.

The ATP binding site is highly conserved throughout the human kinome. Thus most of the known ATP competitive inhibitors of CK2 exhibit a low selectivity across human protein kinases. By choosing a library of peptides, the development of a non-ATP competitive inhibitor was anticipated expecting a higher selectivity. Up to now three peptides interacting with CK2 are known, two of them are cyclic peptides, the Pc—peptide consist of 11 amino acids [20] and P15 is a 9-mer peptide [51] and one peptide (P1) which consists of 19 amino acids [23]. They all act as non-ATP competitive inhibitors thereby each showing a different mode of inhibition and inhibitory potency. Due to the fact that in the present study an inhibitor of the CK2 holoenzyme was identified, a comparison of effects of B2 to other described peptides with inhibitory activity towards CK2 is difficult. In the case of peptide P15 there are no in vitro data existing about the inhibition of the CK2 holoenzyme catalyzed phosphorylation of substrates [38] and it is not known if the inhibition is mediated by an interaction of the peptide with the CK2 or other effects in the cells. The Pc-peptide just inhibits the phosphorylation of CK2β-dependent substrates [17] and the peptide P1 shows no inhibition of CK2 holoenzyme activity at all [20]. In this study for the first time a potent peptidic inhibitor of the CK2 holoenzyme could be identified. The identified inhibitor B2 with a Ki value of 0.8 µM is the most potent peptidic non-ATP competitive inhibitor of CK2 known until now. Peptide B2 also inhibits the kinase activity of the alpha subunit with an IC_{50}-value of 0.8 µM, thus we concluded that B2 targets the alpha subunit. CK2 exhibits different exosites distinct from the catalytic cavity that may be targeted by small molecules [52]. Based on the fact that B2 inhibits the CK2 holoenzyme and the alpha subunit with the same IC_{50} value, it is rather unlikely that B2 targets the subunit interface in or near the CK2β binding pocket on CK2α. The existence of two different classes of compounds targeting the CKα/CKβ interface is described [53]. For the podophyllotoxine W16, targeting the CKα/β interface, an inhibition of the alpha subunit but no inhibition of the holoenzyme was observed. The authors assumed that unlike CK2β, docking of W16 into this binding site might induce an allosteric conformational change of CK2α thereby blocking a productive binding of substrates [17]. The Pc peptide is also targeting the CK2α/CK2β interface, but showing another mode of inhibition. It acts as CK2β antagonist thereby inhibiting the phosphorylation of CK2β dependent substrates by the holoenzyme [20]. Thus the Pc peptide is not influencing the catalytic activity of CK2α. By sequence comparison of B2 with Pc, a similarity of less than 30% was obtained. Based on these results it can be concluded, that B2 is belonging to neither of the two classes. It is more likely that B2 binds to an allosteric cavity of CK2α, thereby changing its conformation resulting in a decrease in activity of CK2α. This mode of inhibition was already described for azonaphthalene derivatives [18] and POMS [15], both small-molecule inhibitors of CK2. Azonaphthalene derivatives act as non-ATP competitive inhibitors, affecting the kinase activity of CK2 holoenzyme and the alpha subunit in each case with the same IC_{50} value (0.4 µM). The exact binding site of azonaphthalene derivatives is still unknown, but mutation analysis indicated that they induce a conformational change of CK2α, resulting in a non-productive binding of substrates.

POMs inhibit the kinase activity of CK2 holoenzyme and alpha subunit in the nanomolar range. The authors identified inhibitor-interacting domains consisting of key structural elements of CK2α, like the activation segment. They assume that by binding of the inhibitor the alpha subunit is locked in an inactive conformation. Regarding the results for the binding studies performed for azonaphthalene derivatives and POMs it can be hypothesized, that B2 docks to a similar exosite of CK2α. With B2 the first peptide could be identified which is supposed to bind to an allosteric binding site of CK2α, thereby showing a potent inhibition of the activity of catalytic CKα and also of the CK2 holoenzyme.

4. Materials and Methods

4.1. Chemicals and Reagents

Glycerol, sodium dodecyl sulfate (SDS), Tris, skimmed milk powder, Tween 20, tryptone, yeast extract and isopropyl β-D-1-thiogalactopyranoside (IPTG) were purchased from Roth (Karlsruhe, Germany), bromphenol blue, NaCl and acetic acid from Fisher Scientific (Schwerte, Germany), Coomassie brilliant blue R250 from Serva (Heidelberg, Germany), $MgCl_2$, NaOH, kanamycin and carbenicillin from Fluka (Buchs, Switzerland), polyvinylidene difluoride membranes from Schleicher & Schuell (Dassel, Germany) and 1,4-dithiothreitol and goat-anti-rabbit IgG secondary antibody (10.5 mg/mL) from Sigma (Deisenhofen, Germany). AIDA-I-β-barrel specific immune serum was purchased from Davids Biotechnology (Freiburg, Germany), PageRuler™ Prestained Protein Ladder and Klenow fragment from Fermentas (St. Leon-Rot, Germany), Mung-Bean-Nuclease, XhoI and KpnI from New England Biolabs (Frankfurt, Germany). Plasmid pET-11d and pCOLA-duet1™ were purchased from Merck KGaA (Darmstadt, Germany). Primers RM2, KP9, CR17 and CR18 were purchased from Sigma Aldrich (St. Louis, MO, USA) and primers CR21 and CR22 from Eurofins MWG Operon (Ebersberg, Germany). Peptides B1, B2, B3 and B4 for capillary electrophoresis (CE) measurements were ordered at JPT (Berlin, Germany). CK2 substrate peptide (RRRDDDSDDD) was synthesized by the biological medicinal research center Düsseldorf (Germany). Peptides had a purity >90% and were analyzed by HPLC & MS. The peptides delivered freeze dried and were resuspended in DMSO to a final concentration of 10 mM, subsequently they were stored at −20 °C. Human CK2α was prepared as described before [54].

4.2. Bacteria, Plasmids, and Culture Conditions

E. coli strain UT5600(DE3) [F⁻, ara-14, leuB6, secA6, lacY1, proC14, tsx-67, Δ(ompT-fepC)266, entA403, trpE38, rfbD1, rpsL109(Str), xyl-5, mtl-1, thi-1, λ(DE3)] was used for surface display of the peptide library, of $α_{S1}$-casein and the N-terminal shortened sequence of $α_{S1}$-casein ($α_{S1}$-casein peptide). *E. coli* strain BL21(D3) [B, F⁻, dcm, ompT, lon, hsdS(r_B⁻ m_B⁻), gal, λ(DE3)] was used for the recombinant expression of human CK2 holoenzyme. Plasmid pET-Adx encodes all AIDA-I autotransporter domains needed for surface display as described for plasmid pET-SH7 [55] and directs Adrenodoxin [37], the passenger domain to the cell surface. The backbone is based on pET-11d. Plasmid pKP10 was used for the autodisplay of $α_{S1}$-casein [36]. The autotransporter region of plasmid pCR3 derived from plasmid pET-Adx, the passenger was exchanged against the coding region for MS-S1 [56] and the backbone is based on pCOLA-duet1™.

The design and construction plasmid $pCK2α^{Y239Stop}$ encoding for CK2α-pAzF was described before [42]. For $pCK2β^{1-193,Y176Stop}$, the plasmid pT7-7CK2β was used as template in PCR. Site directed mutagenesis was performed by the use of the QuickChange protocol (Stratagene, San Diego, CA, USA). For the truncation of CK2β to $CK2β^{1-193}$ in order to avoid aggregation problems usually obtained with full length CK2β, the primers 5′-G-CTG-GTA-GGC-CAT-**TTA**-ATG-GAT-CTT-GAA-ACC-G-3′ and 5′-C-GGT-TTC-AAG-ATC-CAT-**TAA**-ATG-GCC-TAC-CAG-C-3′ were used (mutation in bold). For the incorporation of the stop codon at position 174 the primers 5′-GG-TCT-CTT-GGG-CCG-**CTA**-CTC-GGG-ATG-CAC-CAT-G-3′ and 5′-C-ATG-GTG-CAT-CCC-GAG-**TAG**-CGG-CCC-AAG-AGA-CC-3′ were applied (mutations in bold). Plasmid $pCK2β^{1-193,Y176Stop}$ as obtained after both sites directed mutagenesis was verified by DNA-sequence analysis (Seqlab, Göttingen, Germany). The plasmid pEVOL-pAzF (Addgene plasmid #31186) [44], which was used for the incorporation of the unnatural amino acid pAzF, was a gift from Peter G. Schultz (The Scripps Research Institute, La Jolla, CA, USA).

Bacteria were routinely cultivated at 37 °C in lysogeny broth (LB medium, 10 g tryptone, 5 g yeast extract, and 10 g NaCl per liter) with vigorous shaking (200 rpm). Depending on the vector backbone, the medium contained 30 mg/L kanamycin or 100 mg/L carbenicillin.

For flow cytometer experiments and outer membrane isolation cells were grown overnight and diluted 1:1000 in a freshly prepared medium. Cells were cultured at 37 °C with shaking at 200 rpm until the optical density (OD_{578}) reached 0.5–0.7. Protein expression was induced by the addition of 1 mM IPTG and subsequent incubation for 1 h at 30 °C with vigorous shaking (200 rpm).

4.3. Plasmid Construction Using Restriction Sites

For the construction of the plasmid directing α_{S1}-casein peptide to the cell surface the autotransporter framework of pET-Adx was used. The passenger was replaced by a 48 bp fragment coding for the α_{S1}-casein peptide. Plasmid pHaS1C2 [57] was amplified with primers KP9 (5'-GCC-TCG-AGC-CCA-CTG-CTC-ATG-AAA-ATT-ATG-3') and RM2 (5'-CGG-TAC-CCC-ACT-GTA-GCA-TGA-CG-3') which contained overlapping ends suitable for an insertion in a XhoI/KpnI digested pET-SH7 vector, the resulting plasmid was named pKP6.

4.4. Synthesis of Double Stranded DNA (dsDNA)

For generating artificial dsDNA two oligonucleotides were synthesized. The oligonucleotides CR17 (5'-CAT-TCC-ATG-GTT-AAA-TTA-AAA-TTT-GGT-GTT-TTT-TTT-ACA-GTT-TTA-CTA-TC-3') and CR18 (5'-TGC-CCT-CGA-GTG-TTC-CAT-GTG-CAT-ATG-CTG-AAG-ATA-GTA-AAA-CTG-TAA-AAA-AAA-C-3') were used for the construction of a shortened sequence between the restriction site of the signal peptide and the passenger. For creation of the library CR21 (5'-GCA-CTA-TCG-CAT-CGT-CAG-CAC-ATG-GAA-CAC-TCG-AG-3') and CR22 (5'-CTA-TCA-TTT-GTA-GGA-TTA-AGG-GTA-CC-$(NNN)_{12}$-CTC-GAG-TGT-TCC-ATG-TGC-TG-3') were used. The oligonucleotides were rehydrated (each 100 µM in water), mixed and hybridized by incubation at 95 °C for 5 min, followed by a cooling down to 36 °C within 10 min. Hydrogen bonds between 23 bp (CR17 and CR18) respectively 20 bp (CR21 and CR22) at the 3'-ends of the oligonucleotides were built. The overhanging ends were filled up with Klenow fragment and the resulting dsDNA was digested with NcoI/XhoI (CR17 and CR18) or by XhoI and Acc65I (CR21 and CR22).

4.5. Construction of the Plasmid Used for Surface Display of the Library

Plasmid pCR3 contained all structural elements for autodisplay. In order to remove seven dispensable amino acids between the cutting site of the signal peptidase and the passenger of plasmid pCR3, we used primers CR17 and CR18, which coded for the shortened sequence between a NcoI and a XhoI restriction site. In order to generate this artificial dsDNA, they were treated as described above and inserted into a NcoI/XhoI digested pCR3 vector. The resulting plasmid was named pCR13. The backbone of this plasmid is derived from pCOLA-duet1^{TM}. In the second multiple cloning site, the Acc65I restriction site was deleted by a restriction digest with BlpI/NotI, treatment with Mung-Bean-Nuclease and religation of the vector. The new created plasmid was named pCR18. The passenger DNA of pCR18, which could be replaced by the DNA encoding the library was too short (36 bp) to be analyzed by agarose gel electrophoresis before the following cloning reaction. In consequence it was replaced by the larger passenger sequence encoding for Adx (394 bp) by the use of the XhoI and Acc65I restriction site [36]. The resulting plasmid was named pCR19, which served as backbone for the peptide library.

4.6. Ligation

The ligation reaction contained T4-DNA ligase (1 Weiss unit/10 µL), the DNA fragments which should be ligated and $1 \times$ T4-DNA-ligase-puffer in water. The vector to insert molar ratio was 1:3 in a volume of 10 µL, thereby comprising 0.25 ng DNA. In the case of a ligation in library construction a vector: insert ratio of 7:1 was used in a volume of 90 µL, thereby comprising 2.5 µg DNA. The ligation reaction was incubated for 16 h at 16 °C and the reaction stopped by incubation at 65 °C for 10 min. The product of ligation was desalted via dialyses and used for transformation of electrocompetent *E. coli* strains. The ligation mixture of a library transformation was concentrated to a volume of 20 µL by the use of a rotational vacuum concentrator prior to transformation of cells.

4.7. Transformation of E. coli by Electroporation

Fifty µL of electrocompetent cells (2–3×10^{10} cells/mL) were used for transformation of 10 µL ligation product. The full reaction was placed into a chilled electroporation cuvette and exposed to a voltage of 1800 V by the use of electroporator 22510 (Eppendorf, Hamburg, Germany). Immediately after 1 mL of preheated SOC media (20 g/L Trypton, 5 g/L, Yeast extract, 0.5 g/L NaCl, 2.5 mM/L KCl, 20 mM D-Glucose, 10 mM $MgCl_2$) was added and the reaction was carried into a sterile micro reaction tube. Subsequently the transformation reaction was incubated for 60 min at 37 °C and 100 rpm. Respectively 1:50, 1:500 and 1:5000 dilutions in a volume of 100 µL LB media were platted on antibiotics containing agar plates for estimation of transformation efficiency.

4.8. Outer Membrane Preparation

Differential cell fractionation was performed according to the rapid isolation method of Hantke [58] using modifications by Schultheiss et al. [59] without resuspending in *N*-Lauryl sarcosine sodium salt and the following centrifugation step.

4.9. SDS-PAGE and Western Blot Analysis

For SDS-PAGE outer membrane preparations were diluted with sample buffer (100 mM Tris/HCl pH 6.8, 4% SDS, 0.2% bromphenol blue, 20% glycerol). If reducing conditions were used additional dithiothreitol (0.2 M) was added. Samples were boiled for 10 min, analyzed by SDS-PAGE and the proteins were visualized with Coomassie brilliant blue R250 staining. Prestained protein ladder was used to determine the apparent molecular weight of the separated proteins. For western blot analysis gels were electroblotted to polyvinylidene difluoride membranes and were blocked in TBS with 3% skimmed milk powder for 1 h. Membranes were incubated with the AIDA-I-β-barrel specific immune serum, diluted 1:500 in TBS with 3% skimmed milk powder, overnight at 4 °C. The blots were washed three times with TBST, the secondary antibody (10.5 mg/mL horseradish peroxidase linked goat-anti-rabbit IgG secondary antibody, diluted 1:10,000 in TBS with 3% dried milk powder) was added, and the blots were incubated for 1 h at room temperature. Proteins were visualized via chemiluminescence.

4.10. Preparation of Recombinant Human Protein Kinase CK2

Recombinant human CK2 holoenzyme was expressed and purified according to a protocol by Grankowski et al. [54] with modifications described in Gratz et al. [38]. CK2 activity was determined by radiometric filter assay as described earlier [60,61]. This protocol resulted in an amount of 50 mg CK2 holoenzyme with a concentration of 1 mg/mL. Fractions containing active CK2 were pooled and stored in aliquots at -70 °C.

4.11. Coupling of CK2 with Fluorescein Isothiocyanate (FITC)

Purified CK2 holoenzyme (1 mg/mL) was covalently coupled to 5(6)-fluorescein isothiocyanate (FITC) using the "FITC labeling Kit" from Calbiochem (San Diego, CA, USA) according to the instructions provided by the manufacturer. Before the labeling reaction CK2 solution was dialyzed against carbonate buffer which is recommended for the labeling reaction. The FITC labeled CK2 was stored in aliquots in PBS puffer with sodium azide (0.1%) at $-20\,^{\circ}\mathrm{C}$.

4.12. Flow Cytometer Analysis and Sorting

Cells were harvested and washed three times with reaction buffer (50 mM Tris/HCl, pH 7.4, 100 mM NaCl, 10 mM $MgCl_2$, 1 mM DTT) and resuspended in reaction buffer with 200 μm ATP to a final OD_{578} of 1. Subsequently, 40 μL of this solution were incubated with 10 μL Fluorescein-coupled CK2 (1 mg/mL) for 30 min at 37 $^{\circ}$C with exclusion of light. After adding reaction buffer (with 200 μM ATP) to a final volume of 500 μL, an additionally incubation for 5 min at 37 $^{\circ}$C occurred. Accordingly cells were sedimented and washed three times with 200 μL reaction buffer (with 200 μM ATP) and resuspended in 200 μL of this buffer for flow cytometer analysis. For each experiment at least 10,000 cells were analyzed with a FACSAria III instrument (Becton-Dickinson, Heidelberg, Germany) with a ACDV option for sorting experiments or with a CyFlow Space (Partec, Münster, Germany) for analysis. In all cases an excitation wavelength of 488 nm and a 527/30 nm filter for monitoring fluorescence was used. Cytometry data were visualized by FlowJow 9.4.10 (Tree Star, Ashland, OR, USA). In the case of sorting, single bacteria cells were deposited to LB agar plates containing 30 mg/L kanamycin and were grown over night.

4.13. Capillary Electrophoresis (CE)-based CK2 Assay

The inhibitory activity of the selected peptides on the CK2 holoenzyme and the CK2α subunit was determined using a non-radiometric capillary electrophoresis (CE) assay of Gratz et al. [38] with slight modifications. As substrate the common CK2 peptide RRRDDDSDDD was used. In the case of CK2α the amount of NaCl in the kinase and assay buffer was reduced to 20 mM, since the CK2α subunit without β is salt sensitive. The incubation time of CK2 holoenzyme reaction was reduced to 7 min, to keep the reaction within the linear range. Due to the reduced activity of the CK2α subunit and the different temperature optimum, the reaction of CKα was performed at 25 $^{\circ}$C for 30 min. A ProteomeLab PA800 System (Beckman, Coulter, Krefeld, Germany) was used for separation. Detection of the phosphorylated and the unphosphorylated peptide was possible by the absorption maximum of the peptide (195 nm) measured by its shoulder at 204 nm. The 32 karat 9.1 software (Beckman Coulter) served for operating the measurement and analyzing the results.

For determination of IC_{50} values a concentration-response analysis of the compound of interest was performed as described in Gratz et al. [38]. Concentrations ranging from 0.001 to 100 μM were used. The calculation of the date occurs by GraphPad Prism 5 (GraphPad, La Jolla, CA, USA). The IC_{50} value represents the concentration at the midpoint (50%) of CK2 inhibition on a semi logarithmic dose-response plot.

4.14. Mode of Inhibition

To figure out the mode of inhibition the previously described CK2 assay was used. For testing if the inhibitor is competitive with respect to ATP, IC_{50} values were estimated as described before and plotted versus the ATP concentration. Thereby measurements were performed using six different ATP concentrations, ranging from 1 mM to 100 mM.

For testing if the inhibitor is competitive with respect to the substrate peptide, the rate of the substrate peak at three different inhibitor concentrations (0 μM, 0.5 μM and 1 μM) were measured. The reaction time of CK2 was reduced from 7 to 6 min, so the reaction is within the linear range for substrate concentrations, which are lower than under standard conditions (114 μM). These data were plotted in a Lineweaver-Burk diagram against four varied substrate concentrations (11.4 μM, 22.8 μM, 57 μM and 228 μM) [39].

4.15. Expression and Purification of GST-CK2α

The cDNA of human CK2α was cloned in frame in the BamH1 site of pGEX4-T-1 (GE Healthcare, Freiburg, Germany). GST-CK2α was expressed in *E. coli* XL1Blue according to the protocol of Aberle et al. [62]. Bacteria were harvested by centrifugation at $5000 \times g$ and 4 °C for 10 min. The bacterial pellet from 500 mL culture was resuspended in 25 ml buffer R1 (100 mM Tris-HCl, pH 7.8, 100 mM NaCl, 10 mM $MgCl_2$, 0.1% Tween 20) supplemented with protease inhibitor (Complete®, Roche Diagnostics, Mannheim, Germany) and 1 mg/mL lysozyme. Cells were lysed on ice by stirring for 15 min, followed by subsequent sonification. After centrifugation at $20,000 \times g$ and 4 °C for 10 min, the supernatant was subjected to affinity purification with 300 µL glutathione sepharose beads (GE Healthcare) pre-equilibrated with cold Buffer R1. The cell lysate was incubated with the beads under slight agitation at 4 °C for 90 min. The resin was washed with at least 30 beads volumes of Buffer R1. For pull-down experiments immobilized GST-fusion protein was left on the resin.

4.16. In Vitro Translation of CK2β

The cDNA of human CK2β in a pRSET A plasmid [63] was used for the T7-polymerase dependent in vitro translation by a reticulocyte lysate. CK2β was in vitro translated in the presence of [^{35}S]methionine according to the manufacturer's recommendations (TNT T7 coupled reticulocyte lysate system, Promega GmbH, Mannheim, Germany).

4.17. Pull Down Assay with Recombinant Proteins

The pull down assay was essentially done as described by Sun et al. [64]. Purified GST or GST-CK2α (10 µg) were immobilized on GSH-sepharose and equilibrated with PBS-T binding buffer (PBS, pH 7.4, 1% Tween 20). Immobilized proteins were pre-incubated with 25 or 100 µM B2 peptide for 1 h at 4 °C under slight agitation. Then 7.5 µL of in vitro translated CK2β was added to the mixture and incubation was continued over night at 4 °C. After washing three times with cold PBS-T, bound proteins were eluted with SDS sample buffer (65 mM Tris-HCl, pH 6.8, 2% SDS, 5% β-mercaptoethanol, 10% glycerol, 0.01% bromophenol blue) and analysed by SDS polyacrylamide gel electrophoresis, followed by protein staining with Coomassie blue and autoradiography.

4.18. Click Reaction of CK2α-pAzF and CK2β$^{1-193}$-pAzF

The biosynthesis and purification of CK2α-pAzF was performed as described before [42]. For the recombinant expression of CK2β$^{1-193}$-pAzF, plasmids pCK2β$^{1-193,Y176Stop}$ and pEVOL-pAzF were used to transform *E. coli* BL21(DE3). CK2β$^{1-193}$-pAzF was obtained and purified referring to the process of CK2α-pAzF [42] with the exception that before purification the cell lysate was stirred overnight at 4 °C in order to extract CK2β$^{1-193}$-pAzF [54].

Purified CK2α-pAzF (130 µg/mL) in buffer P50 (25 mM Tris/HCl (pH 8.5), 50 mM NaCl) was incubated with 50 µM DBCO-Sulfo-Cy5 (Jena Bioscience, Jena, Germany) for 1 h in the dark at room temperature (RT). By SPAAC reaction the specific labeled CK2α-DBCO-Sulfo-Cy5 was obtained. For the site-specific labeling of CK2β$^{1-193}$, purified CK2β$^{1-193}$-pAzF in buffer P100 (25 mM Tris/HCl (pH 8.5), 100 mM NaCl) was treated with fluorescein alkyne (0.25 mM), TCEP (Tris(2-carboxyethyl)phosphine, 1 mM), TBTA (Tris(benzyltriazolylmethyl)amine, 0.17 mM) and $CuSO_4$ (1 mM) for for 1 h in the dark at RT. By CuAAC reaction the specific labeled CK2β$^{1-193}$-Flu was obtained. For MST measurements an additional ultrafiltration step using vivaspin500 columns (Sartorius, Göttingen, Germany) was used to remove unbound fluorophore and additives of the click reaction.

4.19. MST Measurements

For MST measurements CK2α-DBCO-Sulfo-Cy5 and CK2β$^{1-193}$-Flu were applied to the Monolith NT.115 (NanoTemper Technologies GmbH, München, Germany). The concentration of the proteins were determined in triplicate by NanoPhotometer Pearl (Imlpen, München, Germany). For K_D value determination, 10 µL of CK2α-DBCO-Sulfo-Cy5 (100 nM) or CK2β$^{1-193}$-Flu (100 nM) in kinase buffer (50 mM Tris/HCl (Ph 7.5), 25 mM NaCl, 20 mM MgCl$_2$) supplemented with 0.1% Tween-20 were mixed with 10 µL B2 (50 mM Tris/HCl (pH 7.5), 25 mM NaCl, 20 mM MgCl$_2$, 5% DMSO) in different concentrations. Fluorescence (red filter (CK2α-DBCO-Sulfo-Cy5), blue filter (CK2β$^{1-193}$-Flu)) and thermophoresis (MST power 60%) were recorded at 37 °C for 30 s. The K$_D$ value was determined from three independent measurements using MO.Affinity Analysis v2.1.3 software (NanoTemper Technologies GmbH).

5. Conclusions

Human protein kinase CK2 plays an important role in the genesis of cancer. Up to date several CK2 inhibitors were developed. Most of them target the highly conserved ATP cavity and show a weak selectivity throughout human protein kinases. Hence, there is increasing interest in the development of inhibitors with a different mode of inhibition. In the present study a potent peptidic non-ATP competitive inhibitor (B2) of CK2 holoenzyme and the α-subunit was identified with an IC$_{50}$ value of 0.8 µM. At higher concentrations ($\geq$ 25 µM) it disturbed also the interaction between the α-subunit and the β-subunit of CK2 to form the holoenzyme. No peptidic inhibitor of CK2 has been described before exhibiting these characteristics. B2 could serve as starting point in the design of new libraries in order to find a lead structure for the development of a new class of CK2 inhibitors.

Author Contributions: Christian Nienberg identified the binding mode of B2, performed the MST measurements and contributed to the manuscript. Claudia Garmann constructed the libraries, analyzed the selected clones and contributed to the manuscript. Andreas Gratz performed the flow cytometer experiments, measured inhibition of CK2α, and contributed to the manuscript. Andre Bollacke measured the inhibition of CK2 holoenzyme. Claudia Götz performed the pull down assays and contributed to the manuscript. Joachim Jose designed the study, guided its coordination and wrote the manuscript. All authors analyzed and discussed the data.

Conflicts of Interest: The authors declare no conflict of interest.

References

1. Filhol, O.; Martiel, J.L.; Cochet, C. Protein kinase CK2: A new view of an old molecular complex. *EMBO Rep.* **2004**, *5*, 351–355. [CrossRef] [PubMed]
2. Litchfield, D.W. Protein kinase CK2: Structure, regulation and role in cellular decisions of life and death. *Biochem. J.* **2003**, *369*, 1–15. [CrossRef] [PubMed]
3. Landesman-Bollag, E.; Romieu-Mourez, R.; Song, D.H.; Sonenshein, G.E.; Cardiff, R.D.; Seldin, D.C. Protein kinase CK2 in mammary gland tumorigenesis. *Oncogene* **2001**, *20*, 3247–3257. [CrossRef] [PubMed]
4. Laramas, M.; Pasquier, D.; Filhol, O.; Ringeisen, F.; Descotes, J.L.; Cochet, C. Nuclear localization of protein kinase CK2 catalytic subunit (CK2α) is associated with poor prognostic factors in human prostate cancer. *Eur. J. Cancer* **2007**, *43*, 928–934. [CrossRef] [PubMed]
5. Zou, J.; Luo, H.; Zeng, Q.; Dong, Z.; Wu, D.; Liu, L. Protein kinase CK2α is overexpressed in colorectal cancer and modulates cell proliferation and invasion via regulating emt-related genes. *J. Transl. Med.* **2011**, *9*, 97. [CrossRef] [PubMed]
6. Duncan, J.S.; Litchfield, D.W. Too much of a good thing: The role of protein kinase CK2 in tumorigenesis and prospects for therapeutic inhibition of CK2. *Biochim. Biophys. Acta* **2008**, *1784*, 33–47. [CrossRef] [PubMed]
7. Kim, J.S.; Eom, J.I.; Cheong, J.W.; Choi, A.J.; Lee, J.K.; Yang, W.I.; Min, Y.H. Protein kinase CK2α as an unfavorable prognostic marker and novel therapeutic target in acute myeloid leukemia. *Clin. Cancer Res.* **2007**, *13*, 1019–1028. [CrossRef] [PubMed]
8. Ryu, M.Y.; Kim, D.W.; Arima, K.; Mouradian, M.M.; Kim, S.U.; Lee, G. Localization of CKII β subunits in lewy bodies of parkinson's disease. *J. Neurol. Sci.* **2008**, *266*, 9–12. [CrossRef] [PubMed]
9. Trembley, J.H.; Chen, Z.; Unger, G.; Slaton, J.; Kren, B.T.; Van Waes, C.; Ahmed, K. Emergence of protein kinase CK2 as a key target in cancer therapy. *Biofactors* **2010**, *36*, 187–195. [CrossRef] [PubMed]
10. Sarno, S.; Salvi, M.; Battistutta, R.; Zanotti, G.; Pinna, L.A. Features and potentials of ATP-site directed CK2 inhibitors. *Biochim. Biophys. Acta Proteins Proteom.* **2005**, *1754*, 263–270. [CrossRef] [PubMed]

11. Pagano, M.A.; Andrzejewska, M.; Ruzzene, M.; Sarno, S.; Cesaro, L.; Bain, J.; Elliott, M.; Meggio, F.; Kazimierczuk, Z.; Pinna, L.A. Optimization of protein kinase CK2 inhibitors derived from 4,5,6,7-tetrabromobenzimidazole. *J. Med. Chem.* **2004**, *47*, 6239–6247. [CrossRef] [PubMed]

12. Nie, Z.; Perretta, C.; Erickson, P.; Margosiak, S.; Almassy, R.; Lu, J.; Averill, A.; Yager, K.M.; Chu, S. Structure-based design, synthesis, and study of pyrazolo[1,5-a][1,3,5]triazine derivatives as potent inhibitors of protein kinase CK2. *Bioorg. Med. Chem. Lett.* **2007**, *17*, 4191–4195. [CrossRef] [PubMed]

13. Sarno, S.; de Moliner, E.; Ruzzene, M.; Pagano, M.A.; Battistutta, R.; Bain, J.; Fabbro, D.; Schoepfer, J.; Elliott, M.; Furet, P.; et al. Biochemical and three-dimensional-structural study of the specific inhibition of protein kinase CK2 by [5-oxo-5,6-dihydroindolo-(1,2-a)quinazolin-7-yl]acetic acid (IQA). *Biochem. J.* **2003**, *374*, 639–646. [CrossRef] [PubMed]

14. Siddiqui-Jain, A.; Drygin, D.; Streiner, N.; Chua, P.; Pierre, F.; O'Brien, S.E.; Bliesath, J.; Omori, M.; Huser, N.; Ho, C.; et al. Cx-4945, an orally bioavailable selective inhibitor of protein kinase CK2, inhibits prosurvival and angiogenic signaling and exhibits antitumor efficacy. *Cancer Res.* **2010**, *70*, 10288–10298. [CrossRef] [PubMed]

15. Prudent, R.; Moucadel, V.; Laudet, B.; Barette, C.; Lafanechère, L.; Hasenknopf, B.; Li, J.; Bareyt, S.; Lacôte, E.; Thorimbert, S.; et al. Identification of polyoxometalates as nanomolar noncompetitive inhibitors of protein kinase CK2. *Chem. Biol.* **2008**, *15*, 683–692. [CrossRef] [PubMed]

16. Allende, C.C.; Allende, J.E. Promiscuous subunit interactions: A possible mechanism for the regulation of protein kinase CK2. *J. Cell. Biochem. Suppl.* **1998**, *30–31*, 129–136. [CrossRef]

17. Laudet, B.; Moucadel, V.; Prudent, R.; Filhol, O.; Wong, Y.S.; Royer, D.; Cochet, C. Identification of chemical inhibitors of protein-kinase CK2 subunit interaction. *Mol. Cell. Biochem.* **2008**, *316*, 63–69. [CrossRef] [PubMed]

18. Moucadel, V.; Prudent, R.; Sautel, C.F.; Teillet, F.; Barette, C.; Lafanechere, L.; Receveur-Brechot, V.; Cochet, C. Antitumoral activity of allosteric inhibitors of protein kinase CK2. *Oncotarget* **2011**, *2*, 997–1010. [CrossRef] [PubMed]

19. Knight, Z.A.; Shokat, K.M. Features of selective kinase inhibitors. *Chem. Biol.* **2005**, *12*, 621–637. [CrossRef] [PubMed]

20. Laudet, B.; Barette, C.; Dulery, V.; Renaudet, O.; Dumy, P.; Metz, A.; Prudent, R.; Deshiere, A.; Dideberg, O.; Filhol, O.; et al. Structure-based design of small peptide inhibitors of protein kinase CK2 subunit interaction. *Biochem. J.* **2007**, *408*, 363–373. [CrossRef] [PubMed]

21. Perea, S.E.; Reyes, O.; Baladron, I.; Perera, Y.; Farina, H.; Gil, J.; Rodriguez, A.; Bacardi, D.; Marcelo, J.L.; Cosme, K.; et al. CIGB-300, a novel proapoptotic peptide that impairs the CK2 phosphorylation and exhibits anticancer properties both in vitro and in vivo. *Mol. Cell. Biochem.* **2008**, *316*, 163–167. [CrossRef] [PubMed]

22. Perea, S.E.; Baladron, I.; Garcia, Y.; Perera, Y.; Lopez, A.; Soriano, J.L.; Batista, N.; Palau, A.; Hernández, I.; Farina, H.; et al. CIGB-300, a synthetic peptide-based drug that targets the CK2 phosphoaceptor domain. Translational and clinical research. *Mol. Cell. Biochem.* **2011**, *356*, 45–50. [CrossRef] [PubMed]

23. Martel, V.; Filhol, O.; Colas, P.; Cochet, C. P53-dependent inhibition of mammalian cell survival by a genetically selected peptide aptamer that targets the regulatory subunit of protein kinase CK2. *Oncogene* **2006**, *25*, 7343–7353. [CrossRef] [PubMed]

24. Bibby, A.C.; Litchfield, D.W. The multiple personalities of the regulatory subunit of protein kinase CK2: CK2 dependent and CK2 independent roles reveal a secret identity for CK2β. *Int. J. Biol. Sci.* **2005**, *1*, 67–79. [CrossRef] [PubMed]

25. Smith, G.P. Filamentous fusion phage: Novel expression vectors that display cloned antigens on the virion surface. *Science* **1985**, *228*, 1315–1317. [CrossRef] [PubMed]

26. Wernerus, H.; Stahl, S. Biotechnological applications for surface-engineered bacteria. *Biotechnol. Appl. Biochem.* **2004**, *40*, 209–228. [PubMed]

27. Szabo, A.; Heja, D.; Szakacs, D.; Zboray, K.; Kekesi, K.A.; Radisky, E.S.; Sahin-Toth, M.; Pal, G. High affinity small protein inhibitors of human chymotrypsin C (CTRC) selected by phage display reveal unusual preference for p4' acidic residues. *J. Biol. Chem.* **2011**, *286*, 22535–22545. [CrossRef] [PubMed]

28. de Marco, R.; Azzolini, S.S.; Lovato, D.V.; Torquato, R.J.; Amino, R.; de Miranda, A.; Tanaka, A.S. Validation of phage display method for protease inhibitor selection using synthetic hybrid peptides. *Comb. Chem. High. Throughput Screen.* **2010**, *13*, 829–835. [CrossRef] [PubMed]

29. Rajik, M.; Jahanshiri, F.; Omar, A.R.; Ideris, A.; Hassan, S.S.; Yusoff, K. Identification and characterisation of a novel anti-viral peptide against avian influenza virus H9N2. *Virol J.* **2009**, *6*, 74. [CrossRef] [PubMed]

30. Welch, B.D.; VanDemark, A.P.; Heroux, A.; Hill, C.P.; Kay, M.S. Potent D-peptide inhibitors of HIV-1 entry. *Proc. Natl. Acad. Sci. USA* **2007**, *104*, 16828–16833. [CrossRef] [PubMed]

31. Jose, J.; Betscheider, D.; Zangen, D. Bacterial surface display library screening by target enzyme labeling: Identification of new human cathepsin g inhibitors. *Anal. Biochem.* **2005**, *346*, 258–267. [CrossRef] [PubMed]

32. Gratz, A.; Jose, J. Protein domain library generation by overlap extension (PDLGO): A tool for enzyme engineering. *Anal. Biochem.* **2008**, *378*, 171–176. [CrossRef] [PubMed]

33. Gratz, A.; Jose, J. Focussing mutations to defined domains: Protein domain library generation by overlap extension (PDLGO). In *Cdna Libraries: New Techniques and Applications*; Lu, C., Browse, J., Wallis, J.G., Eds.; Humana Press: London, UK, 2011; Volume 279, pp. 153–166.

34. Jose, J.; Jähnig, F.; Meyer, T.F. Common structural features of IGA1 protease-like outer membrane protein autotransporters. *Mol. Microbiol.* **1995**, *18*, 378–380. [CrossRef] [PubMed]

35. Burnett, G.; Kennedy, E.P. The enzymatic phosphorylation of proteins. *J. Biol. Chem.* **1954**, *211*, 969–980. [PubMed]

36. Petermann, K.; Vordenbaumen, S.; Maas, R.; Braukmann, A.; Bleck, E.; Saenger, T.; Schneider, M.; Jose, J. Autoantibodies to α_{s1}-casein are induced by breast-feeding. *PLoS ONE* **2012**, *7*, e32716. [CrossRef] [PubMed]

37. Jose, J.; Bernhardt, R.; Hannemann, F. Cellular surface display of dimeric adx and whole cell p450-mediated steroid synthesis on E. coli. *J. Biotechnol.* **2002**, *95*, 257–268. [CrossRef]

38. Gratz, A.; Götz, C.; Jose, J. A ce-based assay for human protein kinase CK2 activity measurement and inhibitor screening. *Electrophoresis* **2010**, *31*, 634–640. [CrossRef] [PubMed]

39. Copeland, R.A. Evaluation of enzyme inhibitors in drug discovery: A guide for medicinal chemists and pharmakologists. John Wiley & Sons, Inc.: Hoboken, NJ, USA, 2005.

40. Cheng, Y.; Prusoff, W.H. Relationship between the inhibition constant (K1) and the concentration of inhibitor which causes 50 per cent inhibition (I50) of an enzymatic reaction. *Biochem. Pharmacol.* **1973**, *22*, 3099–3108. [PubMed]

41. Jerabek-Willemsen, M.; Wienken, C.J.; Braun, D.; Baaske, P.; Duhr, S. Molecular interaction studies using microscale thermophoresis. *Assay Drug Dev. Technol.* **2011**, *9*, 342–353. [CrossRef] [PubMed]

42. Nienberg, C.; Retterath, A.; Becher, K.S.; Saenger, T.; Mootz, H.D.; Jose, J. Site-specific labeling of protein kinase CK2: Combining surface display and click chemistry for drug discovery applications. *Pharmaceuticals* **2016**, *9*, 36. [CrossRef] [PubMed]

43. Raaf, J.; Brunstein, E.; Issinger, O.G.; Niefind, K. The interaction of CK2α and CK2β, the subunits of protein kinase CK2, requires CK2β in a preformed conformation and is enthalpically driven. *Protein Sci.* **2008**, *17*, 2180–2186. [CrossRef] [PubMed]

44. Chin, J.W.; Santoro, S.W.; Martin, A.B.; King, D.S.; Wang, L.; Schultz, P.G. Addition of p-azido-L-phenylalanine to the genetic code of escherichia coli. *J. Am. Chem. Soc.* **2002**, *124*, 9026–9027. [CrossRef] [PubMed]

45. Georgiou, G.; Stathopoulos, C.; Daugherty, P.S.; Nayak, A.R.; Iverson, B.L.; Curtiss, R., 3rd. Display of heterologous proteins on the surface of microorganisms: From the screening of combinatorial libraries to live recombinant vaccines. *Nat. Biotechnol.* **1997**, *15*, 29–34. [CrossRef] [PubMed]

46. Boder, E.T.; Midelfort, K.S.; Wittrup, K.D. Directed evolution of antibody fragments with monovalent femtomolar antigen-binding affinity. *Proc. Natl. Acad. Sci. USA* **2000**, *97*, 10701–10705. [CrossRef] [PubMed]

47. Daugherty, P.S.; Chen, G.; Olsen, M.J.; Iverson, B.L.; Georgiou, G. Antibody affinity maturation using bacterial surface display. *Protein Eng.* **1998**, *11*, 825–832. [CrossRef] [PubMed]

48. Christmann, A.; Wentzel, A.; Meyer, C.; Meyers, G.; Kolmar, H. Epitope mapping and affinity purification of monospecific antibodies by *Escherichia coli* cell surface display of gene-derived random peptide libraries. *J. Immunol. Methods* **2001**, *257*, 163–173. [CrossRef]

49. Bessette, P.H.; Rice, J.J.; Daugherty, P.S. Rapid isolation of high-affinity protein binding peptides using bacterial display. *Protein Eng. Des. Sel.* **2004**, *17*, 731–739. [CrossRef] [PubMed]

50. Kenrick, S.A.; Daugherty, P.S. Bacterial display enables efficient and quantitative peptide affinity maturation. *Protein Eng. Des. Sel.* **2010**, *23*, 9–17. [CrossRef] [PubMed]

51. Perea, S.E.; Reyes, O.; Puchades, Y.; Mendoza, O.; Vispo, N.S.; Torrens, I.; Santos, A.; Silva, R.; Acevedo, B.; Lopez, E.; et al. Antitumor effect of a novel proapoptotic peptide that impairs the phosphorylation by the protein kinase 2 (casein kinase 2). *Cancer Res.* **2004**, *64*, 7127–7129. [CrossRef] [PubMed]

52. Prudent, R.; Cochet, C. New protein kinase CK2 inhibitors: Jumping out of the catalytic box. *Chem. Biol.* **2009**, *16*, 112–120. [CrossRef] [PubMed]

53. Prudent, R.; Sautel, C.F.; Cochet, C. Structure-based discovery of small molecules targeting different surfaces of protein-kinase CK2. *Biochim. Biophys. Acta Proteins Proteom.* **2010**, *1804*, 493–498. [CrossRef] [PubMed]

54. Grankowski, N.; Boldyreff, B.; Issinger, O.G. Isolation and characterization of recombinant human casein kinase II subunits α and β from bacteria. *Eur. J. Biochem.* **1991**, *198*, 25–30. [CrossRef] [PubMed]

55. Petermann, K.; Vordenbäumen, S.; Pyun, J.C.; Braukmann, A.; Bleck, E.; Schneider, M.; Jose, J. Autodisplay of 60-kDa Ro/SS-A antigen and development of a surface display enzyme-linked immunosorbent assay for systemic lupus erythematosus patient sera screening. *Anal. Biochem.* **2010**, *407*, 72–78. [CrossRef] [PubMed]

56. Zuo, R.; Ornek, D.; Wood, T.K. Aluminum- and mild steel-binding peptides from phage display. *Appl. Microbiol. Biotechnol.* **2005**, *68*, 505–509. [CrossRef] [PubMed]

57. Kim, Y.K.; Chung, B.H.; Yoon, S.; Lee, K.K.; Lönnerdal, B.; Yu, D.Y. High-level expression of human αs1-casein in *Escherichia coli*. *Biotechnol. Tech.* **1997**, *11*, 675–678. [CrossRef]

58. Hantke, K. Regulation of ferric iron transport in *Escherichia coli* K12: Isolation of a constitutive mutant. *Mol. Gen. Genet.* **1981**, *182*, 288–292. [CrossRef] [PubMed]

59. Schultheiss, E.; Paar, C.; Schwab, H.; Jose, J. Functional esterase surface display by the autotransporter pathway in *Escherichia coli*. *J. Mol. Catal.* **2002**, *18*, 89–97. [CrossRef]

60. Hastie, C.J.; McLauchlan, H.J.; Cohen, P. Assay of protein kinases using radiolabeled ATP: A protocol. *Nat. Protoc.* **2006**, *1*, 968–971. [CrossRef] [PubMed]

61. Schneider, C.C.; Hessenauer, A.; Gotz, C.; Montenarh, M. Dmat, an inhibitor of protein kinase CK2 induces reactive oxygen species and DNA double strand breaks. *Oncol. Rep.* **2009**, *21*, 1593–1597. [PubMed]

62. Aberle, H.; Butz, S.; Stappert, J.; Weissig, H.; Kemler, R.; Hoschuetzky, H. Assembly of the cadherin-catenin complex in vitro with recombinant proteins. *J. Cell. Sci.* **1994**, *107*, 3655–3663. [PubMed]

63. Spohrer, S.; Dimova, E.Y.; Kietzmann, T.; Montenarh, M.; Gotz, C. The nuclear fraction of protein kinase CK2 binds to the upstream stimulatory factors (USFS) in the absence of DNA. *Cell. Signal.* **2016**, *28*, 23–31. [CrossRef] [PubMed]

64. Sun, Q.; Yu, X.P.; Degraff, D.J.; Matusik, R.J. Upstream stimulatory factor 2, a novel foxa1-interacting protein, is involved in prostate-specific gene expression. *Mol. Endocrinol.* **2009**, *23*, 2038–2047. [CrossRef] [PubMed]

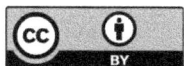

pharmaceuticals

MDPI

Article

In Search of Small Molecule Inhibitors Targeting the Flexible CK2 Subunit Interface

Benoît Bestgen [1,2,3,4,5], Zakia Belaid-Choucair [6], Thierry Lomberget [5], Marc Le Borgne [5], Odile Filhol [1,2,3] and Claude Cochet [1,2,3,*]

[1]   Biology of Cancer and Infection, INSERM, U 1036, 38054 Grenoble, France; benoit.bestgen@gmail.com (B.B.); odile.filhol-cochet@cea.fr (O.F.)
[2]   Biology of Cancer and Infection, University Grenoble-Alpes (UGA), 38000 Grenoble, France
[3]   Commissariat à l'Energie Atomique et aux Energies Alternatives (CEA), Direction de Recherche Fondamentale (DRF), Biosciences and Biotechnology Institute of Grenoble (BIG), Biology of Cancer and Infection (BCI), 38054 Grenoble, France
[4]   Pharmaceutical and Medicinal Chemistry, Saarland University, Campus C2.3, 66123 Saarbrücken, Germany
[5]   Faculté de Pharmacie—ISPB, EA 4446 Bioactive Molecules and Medicinal Chemistry, SFR Santé Lyon-Est CNRS UMS3453—INSERM US7 Université Lyon 1, 8 avenue Rockefeller, F-69373 Lyon CEDEX 8, France; thierry.lomberget@univ-lyon1.fr (T.L.); marc.le-borgne@univ-lyon1.fr (M.L.B.)
[6]   INSERM U 1163 / CNRS ERL 8254, Institut IMAGINE, Université Paris Descartes, 75015 Paris, France; zbelaidchoucair@gmail.com
*   Correspondence: claude.cochet@cea.fr; Tel.: +33-438-78-42-04

Academic Editor: Joachim Jose
Received: 25 November 2016; Accepted: 22 January 2017; Published: 3 February 2017

Abstract: Protein kinase CK2 is a tetrameric holoenzyme composed of two catalytic (α and/or α') subunits and two regulatory (β) subunits. Crystallographic data paired with fluorescence imaging techniques have suggested that the formation of the CK2 holoenzyme complex within cells is a dynamic process. Although the monomeric CK2α subunit is endowed with a constitutive catalytic activity, many of the plethora of CK2 substrates are exclusively phosphorylated by the CK2 holoenzyme. This means that the spatial and high affinity interaction between CK2α and CK2β subunits is critically important and that its disruption may provide a powerful and selective way to block the phosphorylation of substrates requiring the presence of CK2β. In search of compounds inhibiting this critical protein–protein interaction, we previously designed an active cyclic peptide (Pc) derived from the CK2β carboxy-terminal domain that can efficiently antagonize the CK2 subunit interaction. To understand the functional significance of this interaction, we generated cell-permeable versions of Pc, exploring its molecular mechanisms of action and the perturbations of the signaling pathways that it induces in intact cells. The identification of small molecules inhibitors of this critical interaction may represent the first-choice approach to manipulate CK2 in an unconventional way.

Keywords: protein kinase CK2; subunit interface; cyclic peptides; protein–protein interaction; cell death

1. Introduction

Protein Kinase CK2 exhibits a heterotetrameric quaternary structure composed of two catalytic (α and/or α') subunits linked to a stable dimer of two regulatory (β) subunits. In contrast to other multi-subunit protein kinases, the free catalytic α/α' subunits are constitutively active, and the regulatory β subunits act as targeting subunits controlling the substrate specifity and cellular localization of the holoenzyme complex. As a pro-survival kinase, CK2 has emerged as a relevant therapeutic target being dysregulated in various cancers and several human pathologies, therefore supporting the development of chemical inhibitors as promising drug candidates [1–4]. Most CK2 inhibitors identified during the last two decades are ATP-competitive molecules [5,6] with one of them, CX-4945, being investigated in phase I and II clinical trials [7–9]. CK2 is endowed with a peculiar molecular architecture suggesting the existence of different exosites distinct from the catalytic cavity that can be targeted by small molecules to achieve functional effects [10]. The inter-subunit flexibility suggested by X-ray crystallography studies [11] and live-cell fluorescent imaging [12], together with the imbalance in the expression of CK2 subunits in various tumors [13], suggest that their interaction is a key point of regulation. This offers attractive opportunities for the identification of small molecules that modulate this interaction. Therefore, we focused our attention on the CK2α/CK2β interface [11,12], which is relatively small (832 Å^2), and harboring a suitable binding pocket for small molecules [14]. In the CK2 holoenzyme structure, a segment located in the CK2β tail points away from the protein core and forms a β-hairpin loop that inserts deep into a shallow hydrophobic groove present in the β4/β5 sheets of CK2α [11] (Figure 1A). Notably, the sequence of this C-terminal hairpin loop of CK2β is highly conserved in different species (Figure 1B). Site-directed mutagenesis and functional assays have revealed that only a small set of primary hydrophobic residues (Tyr188 and Phe190) present in this CK2β hairpin loop dominates affinity [15]. Further characterization of these hotspots led to the structure-based design of CK2β-derived peptides that were cyclized through two cysteines forming one disulfide bridge. One of these conformationally constrained cyclic peptides, initially termed Pc, was able to efficiently antagonize the assembly of the CK2 holoenzyme complex and to strongly affect its substrate preference [15], indicating that this peptide adopts an energetically favorable state. This 13-mer peptide (GCRLYGFKIHGCG) was the first small antagonist that binds to the CK2 interface and inhibits its high affinity subunit interaction. Based on CK2β sequence, alanine scanning mutagenesis of Pc revealed a cluster of residues (Tyr188 and Phe190) essential for its bioactivity [15]. Moreover, a structural rationalization of the CK2β-competitive potential of Pc was provided by the X-ray structure of a Pc-CK2α complex [16]. Recently, comparative molecular dynamics simulations performed on this complex highlighted, among the hydrophobic residues, the prominent role of Phe190 for a stable and active conformation of Pc [17]. Thus, as a high affinity subunit interaction inhibitor, Pc is a promising CK2 antagonist candidate. However, structural modifications of this cyclic peptide, such as attachment to cell-permeant adducts, head-to-tail cyclization or biotin conjugation, are respectively required to confer in vivo activity or for its detection in cell extracts. We performed these studies with the aim to characterize the molecular mechanisms of action of Pc in intact cells and to investigate how this different mode of CK2 inhibition, through the perturbation of signaling pathways, will translate into phenotypes.

2. Results and Discussion

2.1. Structure and Mode of Binding of CK2β on CK2α

The high-resolution structure of the CK2 holoenzyme has revealed that the subunit interface is composed of: (1) hydrophobic residues in a groove located N-terminally at the outer surface formed by the juxtaposition of the antiparallel β4/β5 sheets of CK2α and (2) a cluster of well-defined hydrophobic residues present on the CK2β chain. This cluster, which contains highly conserved residues (R$_{186}$LYGFKIH$_{193}$) in different species (Figure 1B), exhibits a specific structural feature: it points away from the protein core and forms a 90° β-hairpin loop with Tyr188 at its top, which binds into a shallow hydrophobic groove present in the β4/β5 sheets of CK2α [11]. The interface relies on the steric complementarity between this CK2α groove and the hydrophobic face of the CK2β hairpin loop and, in particular, on a triad of CK2β amino acids, Tyr188, Gly189 and Phe190, which inserts deep into the CK2α groove (Figure 1A). The existence of this potential druggable pocket within the interface area of CK2 was corroborated by a structural study showing that a CK2 inhibitor, 5,6-dichloro-1-β-D-ribofuranosylbenzimidazole (DRB), binds, in addition to the canonical ATP cleft, to the CK2α/CK2β interface [14].

A

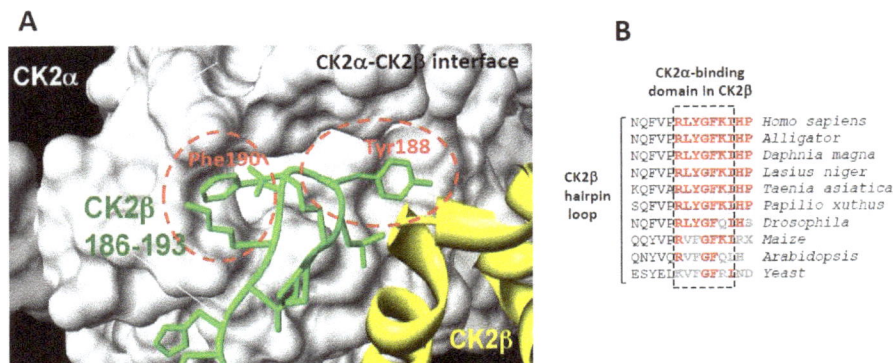

B

CK2α-binding
domain in CK2β

CK2β hairpin loop	NQFVPRLYGFKIHP	*Homo sapiens*
	NQFVPRLYGFKIHP	*Alligator*
	NQFVPRLYGFKIHP	*Daphnia magna*
	NQFVPRLYGFKIHP	*Lasius niger*
	KQFVARLYGFKIHP	*Taenia asiatica*
	SQFVPRLYGFKIHP	*Papilio xuthus*
	NQFVPRLYGFQIHS	*Drosophila*
	QQYVPRVFGFKIRX	*Maize*
	QNYVQRVFGFQIH	*Arabidopsis*
	ESYELKVTGFRIND	*Yeast*

Figure 1. (**A**) surface representation of the binding pocket of CK2α interacting with a short C-terminal hairpin loop of CK2β adapted from [15]. Crystal structure of the CK2 holoenzyme shows that a C-terminal fragment of the CK2β1chain encompasing residues 186–193 (green) forms a loop inserting into a deep hydrophobic pocket of CK2α [11]. Surface representation of the CK2α cleft in grey highlights its pocket-like characteristics. The phenol and phenyl rings of the two non-polar and aromatic CK2β residues Tyr188 and Phe190, respectively, (red) are in quasi-planar opposite orientation and fit tightly into it; and (**B**) a highly conserved cluster in the C-terminal domain of CK2β in different species.

2.2. Rational Design of CK2β-Derived Cyclic Peptides

In a previous study, we used the X-ray structure of CK2β in the holoenzyme complex as a template for the design of a conformationally constrained 13-mer peptide (Pc 13) derived from the CK2β C-terminal domain and centred around the Tyr188 and Phe190 hotspots. Pc 13 is an eight-residue peptide (Arg186–His193) that contains a cluster of hydrophobic residues (Leu187, Tyr188 and Ile192) and three additional glycine residues, cyclized via two cysteine residues to 'staple' its conformation and to mimic the binding face of CK2β with CK2α [15]. A comparative analysis of the effect of varying the length from 11 to eight amino acids in a series of cyclized peptide analogues was performed by testing their effect on the phosphorylation of a peptide substrate (eIF2β peptide) whose phosphorylation relies on the holoenzyme formation [18]. Although most length variants inhibited the CK2β-dependent phosphorylation of this peptide to the same extent ($IC_{50} = 1–3$ μM), the 8-residue peptide (Pc 8 (CC)) was inactive (Figure 2A). Noteworthy, a linear form of Pc 11 (CC) or an inverted sequence were without effect (not shown), indicating that both the sequence and the constrained conformation of the peptide are essential for its antagonist activity. The cyclized structure of Pc 11 (CC) peptide that was used in the following experiments is shown in Figure 2B. A functional assay of the Pc 11 (CC) peptide was also performed testing its effect on the phosphorylation of the Olig-2 transcription factor, which relies exclusively on the tetrameric form of CK2 [19]. Figure 2C shows that the presence of Pc 11 (CC) led to a strong decrease of the original Olig-2 phosphorylation. Similarly, the phosphorylation of CK2β in the holoenzyme, an indicator of CK2 oligomerization [20], was significantly affected by the presence of Pc 11 (CC), reflecting a Pc-induced dissociation of the catalytically active CK2 holoenzyme complex.

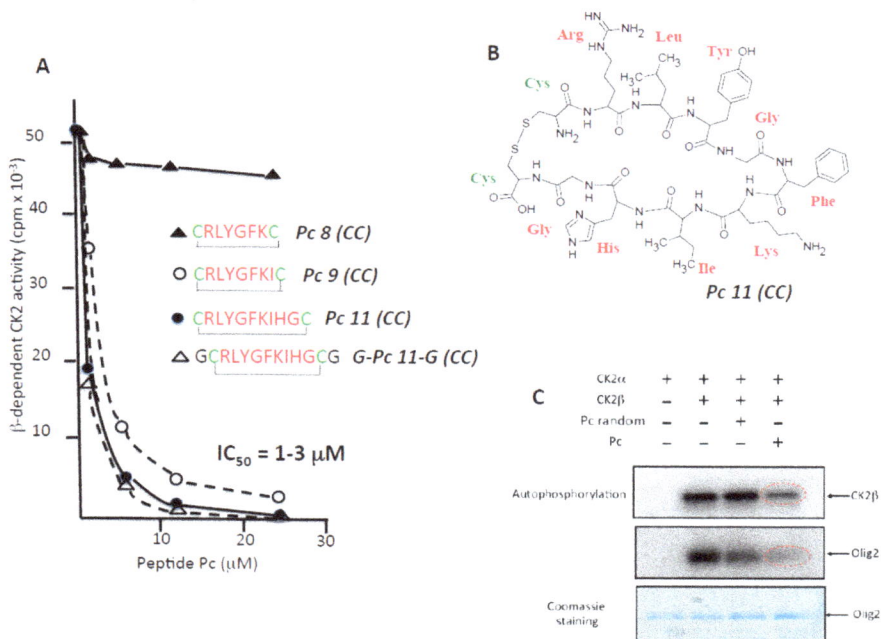

Figure 2. CK2β-derived cyclic peptides inhibit CK2 activity in vitro. (**A**) a series of cyclized CK2β-derived peptide analogues varying in length from eight to 11 amino acids were tested for their effect on the phosphorylation of eIF2β-derived peptide substrate whose phosphorylation relies on the holoenzyme formation. Representative data shown from two independent experiments; (**B**) structure of Pc 11 (CC); (**C**) antagonist effect of Pc 11 (CC) on CK2-mediated phosphorylation of the CK2β-dependent substrate Olig2. CK2α was incubated alone or with CK2β in the absence or presence of 25 μM random Pc 11 (CC) or Pc 11 (CC) for 15 min at 4 °C, followed by the addition of GST (Gluthatione *S*-Transferase)-Olig2 (5 μg) and 25 μM [γ-^{32}P]ATP/MgCl$_2$ for 5 min at room temperature. Phosphorylated proteins were separated by SDS/PAGE (Sodium dodecylsulfate/ Polyacrylamide gel electrophoresis) and analyzed by autoradiography. The gel was stained with coomassie blue to visualize GST-Olig2.

2.3. Pc Binds to CK2β in CK2β-Deficient Cell Extracts

We designed a covalent head-to-tail cyclic Pc 11 analogue linked to biotin through a 4-bAla linker to circumvent any sterical hindrance. This Biot-(bAla)$_4$-Pc 11 analogue was suitable for a pull-down assay using streptavidin-coated beads (Figure 3A). Recombinant CK2α was incubated with increasing concentrations of bead-bound Biot-(bAla)$_4$-Pc 11 and after several washes, CK2 activity associated with the beads was determined. Figure 3B shows that, in this pull-down assay, the immobilized Pc peptide was efficient for a productive high-affinity interaction with CK2α. This interaction was strongly impaired by the presence of increasing concentrations of CK2β, showing that Pc 11 binds tightly to CK2α and behaves as an antagonist of the CK2 subunits interaction (Figure 3C). We then incubated Biot-(bAla)$_4$-Pc 11-coated beads with WT (Wild Type) or CK2β-depleted MCF-10A cell extracts (Figure 3D upper panel). Western blot analysis showed that the free CK2α/α' subunits present in CK2β-depleted MCF-10A cell extracts were recovered associated with the beads indicating a tight binding. In contrast, CK2 was not detected on beads incubated with WT cell extracts in which CK2β behaves as a Pc antagonist (Figure 3D lower panel).

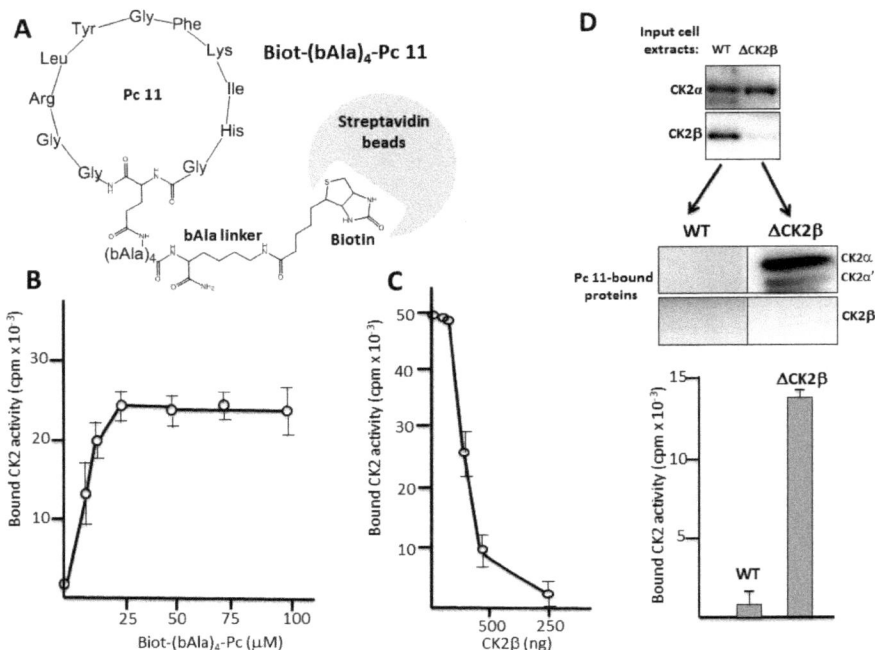

Figure 3. Pc binds to CK2α. (**A**) Biot-(bAla)$_4$-Pc: Head-to-tail cyclic Pc 11 analogue linked to biotin through a 4-Ala linker; (**B**) aliquots of streptavidin-agarose beads were incubated with increasing concentrations of Biot-(bAla)$_4$-Pc 11 in the presence of CK2α (100 ng) for 2 h at 4 °C. After three washes, CK2 activity assays were carried out for 5 min on the beads pellets. Representative data shown from two independent experiments. Results are presented as mean ± s.d. of triplicates; (**C**) aliquots of streptavidin-agarose beads were loaded with 25 μM Biot-(bAla)$_4$-Pc 11 and incubated with CK2α (100 ng) in the presence of increasing amounts of CK2β for 2 h at 4 °C. After three washes, CK2 activity assays were carried out for 10 min on the beads pellets; (**D**) CK2α in cell extracts. Aliquots of streptavidin-agarose beads loaded with 25 μM Biot-(bAla)$_4$-Pc 11 were incubated with WT or CK2β-depleted MCF-10A cell extracts (upper panel) for 2 h at 4 °C. After three washes, CK2 subunits retained on the beads were determined by Western blot (middle panel). CK2 activity was also determined in the bead pellets with the CK2β-independent peptide substrate (lower panel).

2.4. Design and Characterization of a TAT-Conjugated Pc Analogue

The successful transport of peptides/proteins to intracellular targets was accomplished by the use of a sequence derived from the HIV transactivator of transcription protein (TAT), which, when fused to cargo, facilitates receptor- and energy-independent transport across cell membranes [21]. As disulfide bonds are very sensitive to intracellular reductive conditions, head-to-tail cyclization is intuitively expected to improve bioactivities by increasing stability and lowering flexibility as well as sensitivity to proteolytic attack. Therefore, we fused the TAT sequence to the N-terminus of a covalent head-to-tail cyclized Pc 13 analogue (TAT-Pc 13, Figure 4). The biological properties of this peptide were first evaluated in vitro in a kinase assay using two different CK2 peptide substrates. As shown in Figure 4A, the CK2β-dependent phosphorylation of the eIF2β-derived peptide was strongly inhibited by increasing concentrations of TAT-Pc 13 (IC$_{50}$ = 5 μM), whereas, as previously described [16], the CK2β-independent peptide phosphorylation was significantly stimulated at high TAT-Pc 13 concentrations. The bioactivity of TAT-Pc 13 was also tested in a CK2 subunit interaction assay. At a 50 μM concentration of TAT-Pc 13, the subunit interaction was inhibited by 80%. Interestingly, the addition of TAT-Pc 13 to a pre-formed α/β complex led to a significant reduction of CK2α binding (by more than 40%), suggesting a partial dissociation of the complex. In this assay, a TAT-conjugated random Pc 13 was without effect (Figure 4B). Thus, the TAT-conjugated Pc peptide retains inhibitory binding activity in vitro.

TAT-Pc 11   GRKKRRQRRRPPQ-KGGRLYGFKIHGG

TAT-Pc 11 random   GRKKRRQRRRPPQ-KGYGRHLKGIGFG

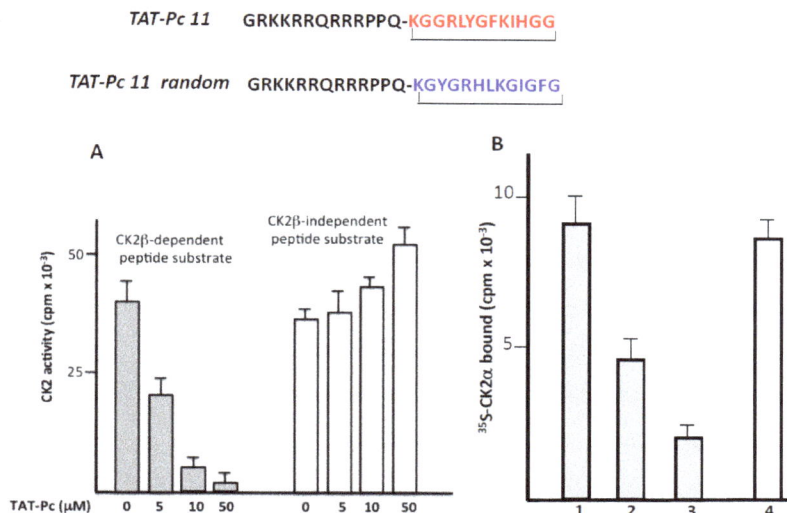

Figure 4. Inhibitory activity of a TAT-Pc analogue in vitro. (**A**) CK2 holoenzyme (100 nM) was incubated in the presence of increasing concentrations of TAT-Pc 13 for 15 min at 4 °C. CK2 activity was then determined with CK2β-dependent or independent peptide substrates; (**B**) [^{35}S]-labeled CK2α was incubated with biotinylated MBP-CK2β immobilized on streptavidin coated plates (preformed complex) in the absence (1) or presence (2) of TAT-Pc 13. Alternatively, [^{35}S]-labeled CK2α was incubated with TAT-Pc 13 (3) or random TAT-Pc 13 (4) and then with immobilized biotinylated MBP-CK2β. After washing, the amount of [^{35}S]-labeled CK2α remaining in the complex was determined by radioactivity counting. Representative data shown from two independent experiments. Results are presented as mean ± s.d. of triplicates.

2.5. Bioactivity of TAT-Pc 13 in Cell Extracts

Thermal shift assay (TSA) is based on the biophysical principle of ligand-induced thermal stabilization of target proteins. This assay can be used to detect protein–ligand interactions in complex cell extracts. Therefore, we have generated thermal melting curves from cell extracts, in which the extent of CK2 unfolding was measured. The assays were performed on WT or CK2β-depleted MCF-10A cell extracts incubated with 50 μM of TAT or TAT-Pc 13 and exposed to increasing temperatures. Figure 5A shows that an obvious shift (4 °C) in the melting curves was detected in CK2β-depleted cell extracts incubated with TAT-Pc 13. Similarly, a significant shift (3 °C) was observed in cell extracts incubated with recombinant CK2β as compared to controls (Figure 5B). Of note, in extracts from WT MCF-10A cells expressing stoechiometric amount of CK2β, no thermal shift was observed upon incubation with TAT-Pc 13 (not shown). Thus, the ligand-induced stabilization of CK2α shows its engagement as a target for TAT-Pc 13 or CK2β in CK2β-depleted cell extracts.

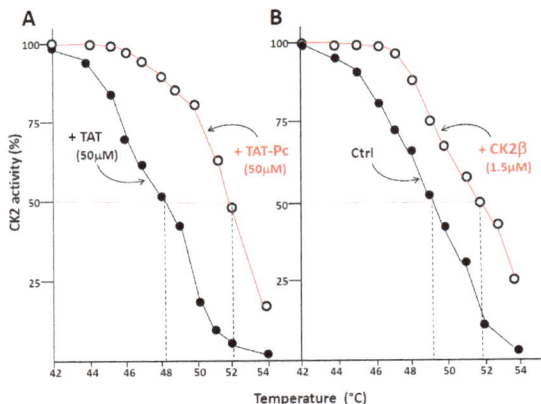

Figure 5. Thermal shift assay in cell lysates. CK2β-depleted MCF-10A cell lysates were treated with 50 μM TAT or TAT-Pc 13 (**A**), or with PBS (Phosphate-buffered saline) or CK2β (**B**) for 30 min at room temperature. The respective lysates were divided into 20 μL aliquots and heated individually at different temperatures for 3 min. After centrifugation, the supernatants were assayed for CK2 activity with the CK2β-independent peptide substrate. Representative data shown from two independent experiments in duplicate.

In a second set of experiments, WT or CK2β-depleted MCF-10A cell extracts incubated with 50 μM of TAT or TAT-Pc 13 were immunoprecipitated with a TAT antibody and the presence of CK2α in the immunoprecipitates was evaluated by both Western blotting and CK2 kinase assays. In CK2β-depleted MCF-10A cell extracts, a higher amount of CK2α protein (Figure 6A) or CK2 activity (Figure 6B) were found associated with immunoprecipitated TAT-Pc 13 compared to TAT immunoprecipitates. In WT MCF-10A cell extracts, CK2α present in TAT-Pc 13 immunoprecipitates was not significantly different compared to TAT immunoprecipitates.

Altogether, these experiments show that TAT-Pc 13 can form a stable complex with CK2α in CK2β-depleted MCF-10A cell extracts, whereas, in WT cell extracts, this interaction was hampered by the presence of endogenous CK2β.

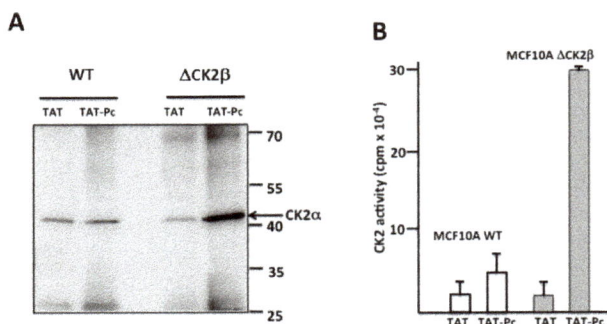

Figure 6. Physical binding of CK2α to TAT-Pc 13 in cell extracts. WT or CK2β-depleted MCF-10A cell lysates were incubated with 50 μM TAT or TAT-Pc 13 for 30 min at room temperature and immunoprecipitated with a TAT antibody. CK2α protein and CK2 activity were evaluated by Western blot (**A**) and CK2 kinase assay (**B**), respectively. Representative data for CK2 activity shown from two independent experiments. Results are presented as mean ± s.d. of triplicates.

2.6. Uptake and Cellular Effects of TAT-Pc

To assess the cell-penetrating properties of TAT-Pc 13, we used a tetramethylrhodamine-conjugated TAT-Pc 13 analogue (TAMRA-TAT-Pc 13). The cellular uptake of this fluorescently labeled peptide was very rapid: only 2 min after incubation, the peptide was detectable in MCF-10A cells and plateauing after 5 min (Figure 7A). The impact of TAT-Pc 13 cell uptake on the expression of the CK2 subunits in WT and CK2β-depleted MCF-10A cells was evaluated by Western blot. This analysis showed that, after an 8 h-treatment with TAT-Pc 13, the level of CK2 subunits was not significantly changed in both cell types (Figure 7B). We next evaluated the effect of TAT-Pc 13 on the CK2 subunit association using two independent strategies. First, CK2β was immunoprecipitated in extracts of MCF-10A cells treated with TAT or TAT-Pc 13 and the amount of CK2α recovered in the immunoprecipitates was analyzed by Western blot. Figure 7C shows that CK2β immunoprecipitates from cells incubated with TAT-Pc 13 contained significantly less CK2α than cells treated with TAT, thus demonstrating that TAT-Pc 13 impaired CK2α/CK2β interaction in living cells.

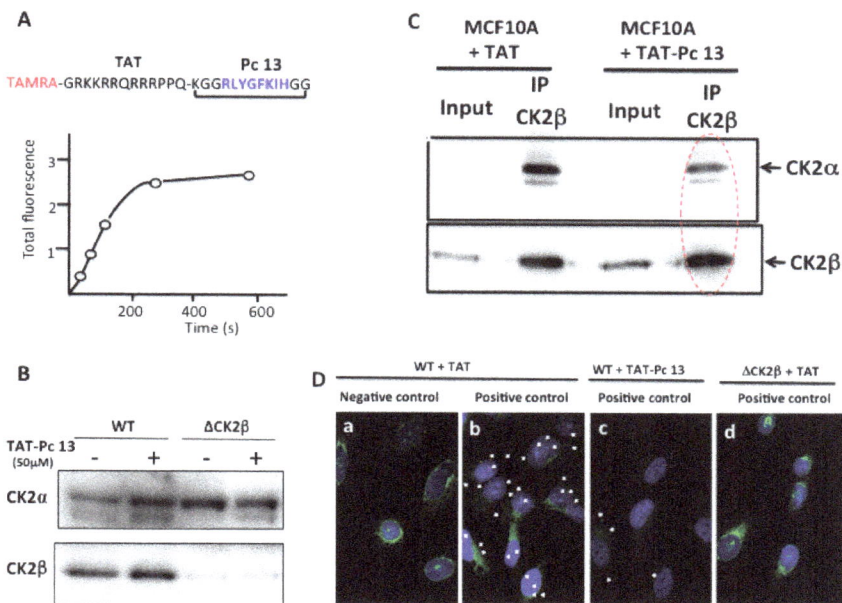

Figure 7. Uptake and cellular effects of TAT-Pc 13. (**A**) kinetic of TAMRA-TAT-Pc 13 uptake in MCF-10A cells; (**B**) WT or CK2β-depleted MCF-10A cells were incubated with 50 μM TAT or TAT-Pc 13 for 8 h and the expression of CK2 subunits was evaluated by Western blot; (**C**) anti-CK2β immunoprecipitates were prepared from WT MCF-10A cells incubated with 50 μM TAT or TAT-Pc 13 for 2 h. Presence of CK2 subunits in the corresponding immunoprecipitates was determined by Western blot; (**D**) in situ proximity ligation images of MCF-10A cells incubated with 50 μM TAT (a,b,d) or TAT-Pc 13 (c) for 6 h. WT cells were incubated with CK2α antibody alone (a) or CK2α and CK2β antibodies (b,c). CK2β-depleted cells (ΔCK2β) were incubated with 50 μM TAT and then with CK2α and CK2β antibodies (d). Actin staining in green, scale bar 10 μm.

To confirm these results, the effect of TAT-Pc was evaluated in MCF-10A cells, using the in situ proximity ligation assay (PLA). PLA is an antibody-based method representing a reliable readout of molecular proximity of two antigens located on two distinct proteins. In this method, two different proteins of interest are recognized by their respective specific primary antibody and then with a corresponding pair of secondary antibodies conjugated to complementary oligonucleotides. In close proximity (<40 nm), the oligonucleotides hybridize and are ligated and amplified. The fluorescent signal from each pair of PLA probes confirms a close proximity and not simply subcellular colocalization and can then be detected and quantified as fluorescent spots in microscopic images of the cells [22]. Our results illustrated in Figure 7D indicate a clear proximity between CK2α and CK2β subunits, attested by several fluorescent interaction dots in cells incubated with antibodies against both proteins (panel b, positive control, 4.8 ± 1.5 dots/cell), but not in a negative control sample (panel a) in which the CK2β primary antibody has been omitted. The specificity of the signal was also confirmed by turning down the expression of CK2β through RNA interference (see Figure 3D, upper panel). No signal was detected in CK2β-depleted cells (panel d). Remarkably, incubation of the cells with TAT-Pc 13 for 6 h strongly reduced the number of interaction dots (panel c, 2.2 ± 1.1 dots/cell). Collectively, these results show that TAT-Pc 13 has suitable properties to gain intracellular access and to disrupt the dynamic CK2 subunit interaction in living cells.

2.7. Inhibition of Cell Viability by TAT-Pc 13

TAT-Pc 13 was found to be an unusually rapid inducer of cell death. Three hours after TAT-Pc 13 was introduced into the cultures, more than 50% of the cells rounded up and shrank, suggesting cell death (Figure 8A upper panel). This was confirmed using the LIVE&DEAD^{TM} cell viability assay that provides a visual readout of cell integrity (Figure 8A lower panel). This cellular effect was also analyzed after treatment of WT or CK2β-depleted MCF-10A cells with increasing concentrations of TAT-Pc 13. TAT-Pc 13 caused a cell death in both cell types, which was already detectable at a concentration of 25 μM and became massive at 50–60 μM (Figure 8B). Compared to WT cells, CK2β-depleted MCF-10A cells were more sensitive to cell death (IC$_{50}$ = 60 μM and 48 μM, respectively) suggesting that TAT-Pc 13-induced cell death is partially antagonized by CK2β present in WT cells. Notably, this cell death was insensitive to the pan-caspase inhibitor, z-VAD-FMK, indicating that the cytotoxic effect of TAT-Pc 13 relies on the induction of a caspase-independent cell death irrelevant to cell apoptosis (Figure 8C). Moreover, TAT-Pc 13 was found to induce cell death of various cancerous cell lines (HeLa, MDA MB-231, 786-0) indicating activity across a wide variety of cell lines (Supplementary Materials Figure S1). In order to investigate the intracellular events induced by TAT-Pc 13, MCF-10A cells were incubated with increasing concentrations of TAT-Pc 13 and analyzed by Western blot. Figure 8D shows no sign of AKT activation, whereas TAT-Pc 13 induced the phosphorylation of the tumor suppressor p21 on Thr145 and a decrease of survivin expression in a dose-dependent manner (EC$_{50}$ = 15 μM). In contrast, phosphorylation of p21 was strongly inhibited in presence of CX-4945 (Supplementary Materials Figure S1).

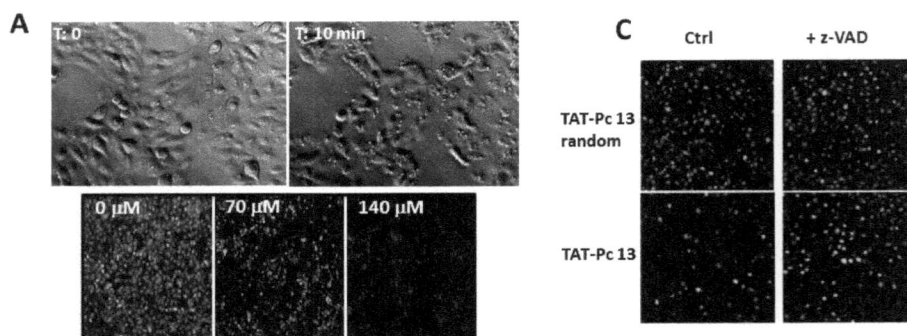

Figure 8. *Cont.*

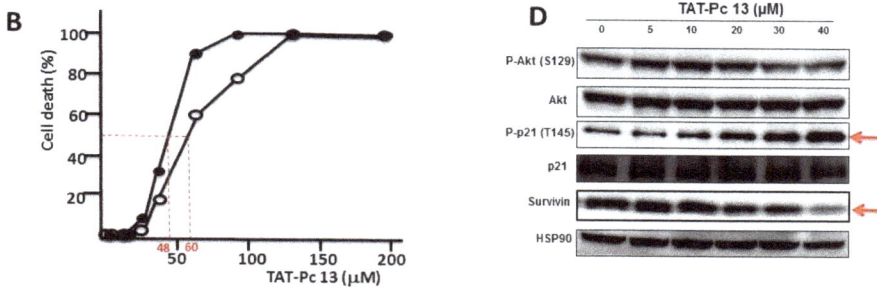

Figure 8. Cellular effects of TAT-Pc 13. (**A**) MCF-10A cells were incubated with 25 μM of TAT-Pc 13 for 3 h and imaged with phase microscopy (upper panel) or with increasing concentrations of TAT-Pc 13 for 2 h and cell viability was evaluated using the LIVE&DEAD™ assay. Live cells fluoresce bright green (530 nm), whereas dead cells fluoresce red-orange (645 nm) (lower panel, scale bare: 100 μm); (**B**) WT (○-○) or CK2β-depleted (●-●) MCF-10A cells were incubated for 4 h with increasing concentrations of TAT-Pc 13 and cell death was evaluated using the LIVE&DEAD™ assay recording fluorescence at 645 nm. Representative data shown from two independent experiments in duplicate; (**C**) MCF-10A cells were pre-treated in the absence or presence of 20 μM z-VAD for 5 h and then incubated for 4 h with 25 μM random TAT-Pc 13 or TAT-Pc 13 and cell viability was evaluated as in (A) (scale bare: 100 μm); and (**D**) intracellular events induced by increasing concentrations of TAT-Pc 13. After 12 h of treatment, 786-O cells were lysed and analyzed by Western blot.

3. Materials and Methods

3.1. Materials

The antibodies used for Western blotting were: rabbit anti-Akt and rabbit anti-anti-HSP90 (Cell Signaling Technology, Danvers, MA 01923, USA), rabbit anti-phospho-Akt (Ser129) from Abgent (San Diego, CA 92121, USA), rabbit anti-p21 and mouse anti-TAT were from Santa Cruz Biotechnologies (Dallas, Texas 75220, USA), rabbit anti-phospho-p21 (Thr145) from Abcam (Paris, 75010, France), and rabbit anti-Survivin (Novus Biologicals, Littleton, CO 80120, USA). Mouse anti-CK2β and rabbit anti-CK2α were previously described [13,23].

HRP (Horse Raddish Peroxidase)-conjugated secondary goat anti-rabbit IgG antibodies were from Jackson Immunoresearch (West Grove, PA 19390, USA). Wild type (WT) MCF-10A cells were obtained from ATCC (Middlesex, TW11, UK). Stable CK2β silencing in MCF-10A cells (ΔCK2β) was accomplished by transduction with pLKO1 lentivirus (Sigma-Aldrich, St. Louis, MO 63178, USA), followed by puromycin selection as previously described [13]. The cells tested negative from mycoplasma contamination were grown as described [24].

3.2. Peptide Synthesis

Cystein-bridged cyclic peptides and biotinylated cyclic peptides were obtained from Genosphere Biotechnologies (Paris, France). TAT-Pc 13 was obtained from GeneCust (Dudelange, Luxembourg). TAMRA-TAT-Pc 13 was synthesized by VCPBIO (Shenzhen, China).

3.3. Proteins

Production and purification of recombinant CK2α and CK2β proteins were described previously [25–27].

3.4. In Vitro Kinase Assays

CK2 kinase assays were performed in a phosphorylation buffer containing recombinant CK2α (36 ng) or recombinant CK2 holoenzyme (50 ng) and a mixture containing 10 mM MgCl$_2$ and 1 µCi of [γ-32P]ATP and 0.15 M NaCl in the presence of 0.2 mM of the CK2β-independent substrate RRREDEESDDEE [28] or the CK2β-dependent substrate MSGDEMIFDPTMSKKKKKKKKP [18]. The final concentration of ATP was 100 µM and assays were performed under linear kinetic conditions for 5–10 min at room temperature. Kinase reactions were terminated by the addition of 60 µL of 4% trichloroacetic acid and sample adsorption on phosphocellulose P81 paper, which were washed in 0.5% phosphoric acid and counted in a scintillation counter.

3.5. In Vitro Pull-Down Assay

Streptavidin-agarose beads (Fluka #85881) were equilibrated in binding buffer A (50 mM Tris-HCl pH 7.5, 0.2 M NaCl, 0.1% Tween 20) containing 1 mg/mL BSA. After several washes in buffer B (50 mM Tris-HCl pH 7.5, 0.4 M NaCl, 0.1% Tween 20), beads were incubated with 10–100 µM Biot-(bAla)$_4$-Pc 11 for 1 h at room temperature and washed twice in buffer B. Beads were then incubated with 100 ng recombinant CK2α in 100 µL of buffer A for 2 h at 4 °C . After three washes in 250 µL of buffer B, CK2 associated with Biot-(bAla)$_4$-Pc 11 beads was evaluated using the CK2 kinase assay. Alternatively, Biot-(bAla)$_4$-Pc 11 beads were incubated with extracts from WT or CK2β-depleted MCF-10A cells for 1 h at 4 °C. After 3 washes, beads were used in the CK2 kinase assay or analyzed by Western blot to detect the CK2 subunits.

3.6. In Vitro CK2α–CK2β Interaction Assay

The CK2α–CK2β interaction assay involved competition between plate-bound biotinylated MBP–CK2β and various cyclic peptides for binding to [^{35}S] methionine-labelled CK2α. The assay was performed as previously described in [15].

3.7. Thermal Shift Denaturation Assay

CK2β-depleted MCF-10A cell lysates prepared in 50 mM Tris-HCl pH 7.5, 150 mM NaCl, and 2% glycerol supplemented with Complete Protease Inhibitor Cocktail (Sigma, #P8340) were divided into four aliquots with two being treated with 50 µM TAT or TAT-Pc 11 and the other two aliquots with CK2β or PBS (control). After 30 min incubation at room temperature, the respective lysates were divided into small (20 µL) aliquots in 0.2 mL microtubes and heated individually at different temperatures for 3 min (Thermocycler, Biometra) followed by cooling for 3 min in ice. WT MCF-10A cell lysates were heat-treated similarly. The heated lysates were centrifuged at 14,000× g for 20 min at 4 °C in order to separate the soluble fractions from precipitates. The supernatants were assayed for CK2 activity with the CK2β-independent peptide substrate.

3.8. Proximity Ligation Assay

In situ PLAs were performed using a Duolink kit (Olink Bioscience, Uppsala, Sweden) according to the manufacturer's instructions with some modifications. MCF-10A cells were fixed in 4% paraformaldehyde for 10 min. The cells were then permeabilized with 0.1% Triton in Tris-buffered saline (TBS; 50 mM Tris, pH 7.6, 150 mM NaCl) and incubated with 100 mM glycine in phosphate-buffered saline (137 mM NaCl, 2.7 mM KCl, 10 mM Na$_2$HPO$_4$, and 1.8 mM KH$_2$PO$_4$, pH 7.4) for 20 min. Permeabilized cells were incubated overnight at 4 °C with primary antibodies diluted as follows: mouse CK2α 1:250 and rabbit CK2β 1:50. Cells were washed three times in TBS with 0.05% Tween-20 for 5 min each with gentle agitation. Secondary antibodies conjugated with oligonucleotides, PLA probe anti-mouse MINUS and PLA probe anti-rabbit PLUS, were added to the cells and incubated for 90 min at 37 °C in a humidity chamber. Finally, after ligation and amplification steps, cells were counterstained with the DNA-binding dye Hoechst and Phaloïdine-488 for actin staining (Molecular Probes, Thermo Fisher Scientific, Courtaboeuf, France). Images were observed using a Zeiss Apotome microscope and analyzed using a Zen Pro imaging software (Zeiss, Oberkochen, Germany). Quantification was performed using the BlobFinder software (V3.2, Swedish University of Agricultural Sciences, Uppsala University) [29]. Negative controls were one primary antibody with both of the secondary antibodies.

3.9. Cell Viability Assay

Cells were seeded in 96-well microtiter plates at a concentration of 1×10^5 cells/mL and were allowed to attach for 24 h at 37 °C in 5% CO_2. Cells were then exposed to different concentrations of TAT-Pc 13 for the indicated time. Cell viability was evaluated using the fluorescence-based LIVE&DEAD™ assay (Molecular Probes, Thermo Fisher Scientific, Courtaboeuf, France) according to the manufacturer. Images were taken with an Apotome-equipped Zeiss Axioimager microscope (Zeiss, Oberkochen, German) recording the fluorescence at 530 nm (Live cells) and 645 nm (dead cells) respectively using a FluoStar Optima plate reader (BMG LabTech, Ortenberg, Germany).

Alternatively, cell viability was measured using the PrestoBlue® assay (Invitrogen, Carlsbad, CA, USA). The microtiter plates containing the treated cells were incubated for 1 h with 10 μL PrestoBlue. The fluorescence was recorded at 580 nm using a FluoStar Optima plate reader (BMG LabTech, Ortenberg, Germany).

4. Conclusions

The irreversible nature of the CK2 holoenzyme formation has been challenged by both its crystal structure [11] and live-cell imaging studies [12]. In addition, free populations of each CK2 subunit have been identified in several organs [30], and differential subcellular localizations have also been reported for CK2α and CK2β. Since the free catalytic subunit and the holoenzyme exhibit divergent substrate preferences, it could be predicted that such a balance is crucial to control the numerous cellular processes that are governed by this multifaceted enzyme [31]. The ability to interfere with specific protein–protein interactions has already provided powerful means of influencing the functions of selected proteins within the cell [32]. Consequently, it is expected that perturbating the CK2α/CK2β interface with artificial ligands might suppress specific CK2 holoenzyme functions providing a less toxic approach than total CK2 enzymatic inhibition. In a previous study, the presence within this interface of a small hydrophobic cavity on CK2α led us to a structure-based design of a CK2β-derived Pc peptide that can efficiently antagonize in vitro the high-affinity CK2 subunit interaction. To evaluate the potency and impact of the selective disruption of CK2α/CK2β interaction in a biologically relevant context, we describe here a cell-permeable version of Pc (TAT-Pc 13), exploring its molecular mechanisms of action and the perturbations of the signaling pathways that it induces in intact cells. Our study shows that TAT-Pc 13 rapidly accumulates into living cells, promoting the disruption of the CK2 subunit interaction, thereby antagonizing specific functions of CK2β. Intriguingly, cell treatment with TAT-Pc 13 rapidly induces dramatic cellular perturbations leading to caspase-independent cell death. In particular, we observed that TAT-Pc 13 induced a phosphorylation on Thr145 of the p21 protein, associated with its nuclear accumulation. It has been reported that p21 is regulated by phosphorylation and several protein kinases such as AKT [33], Pim1 [34] or the death-associated protein kinase DAPK3 [35,36] have been shown to stabilize p21 through phosphorylation of Thr145. A functional relationship between CK2 and the Pim1 kinase has not been reported yet. Moreover, since we could not detect any AKT activation, this kinase is probably not implicated in TAT-Pc 13-induced p21 phosphorylation. DAPK3, also called ZIP kinase (ZIPK), has been implicated in interferon γ-and TNFα/Fas-induced cell death [37] and low ZIPK expression was correlated with increased migration and invasion in breast cancer cells [38]. Interestingly, a potential link between CK2 and the ZIPK has been established. The transcription and splicing factor CDC5 was shown to be an interacting partner of ZIPK and both proteins co-localize with CK2 in speckle-like structures. Moreover, CDC5 is associated with and efficiently phosphorylated by CK2 suggesting a potential CK2-CDC5-ZIPK-p21 axis in triggering cell death [39]. Nevertheless, further investigations in this direction will be beneficial in understanding the implication of p21 in the specific cellular mechanisms leading to cell death upon TAT-Pc 13 treatment. Unexpectedly, in contrast to the cytotoxic effect of CX-4945, TAT-Pc 13-induced cell death did not require caspase activation. Therefore, future studies will focus on defining the cell death modality activated following disruption of the CK2 subunit interaction. As a preliminary clue, the results illustrated in Supplementary Materials Figure S2 show that TAT-Pc 13-induced cell death was prevented by Necrostatin-1, a selective small molecule inhibitor of necroptosis [40].

In summary, TAT-Pc 13 can significantly facilitate functional studies, in particular to identify CK2β-targeted CK2 substrates in living cells using phosphoproteomic approaches. Selective disruption of CK2α/CK2β interaction could also find important applications to pharmacologically test the importance of this interaction in normal and tumor cell biology. With the help of structure-based rational design, TAT-Pc 13 may also serve as a lead for the rational design of function-specific drugs that disrupt some actions of CK2. It is expected that such compounds will be substrate selective, inhibiting through an unconventional way the activity of the kinase against a subset of its substrates but leaving others intact.

Supplementary Materials: The following are available online at http://www.mdpi.com/1424-8247/10/1/16/s1, Figure S1: Cellular effects of TAT-Pc 13, Figure S2: Inhibition of TAT-Pc-induced cell death.

Acknowledgments: We thank Justine Hua for excellent technical assistance. This work was supported by grants from the Institut National de la Santé et de la Recherche Médicale (INSERM), Commissariat à l'Energie Atomique et aux Energies Alternatives (CEA), Ligue Nationale et Régionale contre le Cancer (Isère), and Université Grenoble-Alpes (UGA). We gratefully acknowledge the financial support given by "Région Rhône-Alpes" (grant "ARC 1 Santé" 12-008707-01). M. Benoît Bestgen would like to thank the "Cancéropôle Lyon Rhône-Alpes Auvergne (CLARA)" for a fellowship "Mobilité Jeunes Chercheurs" (Institut National du Cancer (INCa) Grant No. 2011-097). Prof. M. Le Borgne would like to acknowledge CLARA, "Université France Allemagne" (UFA) and "Région Rhône-Alpes" for the emergence of the ChemBioInteract network. We thank Ministère de l'Education Nationale de la Recherche et de Technologie (MENRT) and Ecole Doctorale Interdisciplinaire Sciences-Santé (EDISS) for the PhD fellowship of Benoît Bestgen in collaboration between University Lyon 1 and Saarland University as well as Institut des Sciences Pharmaceutiques et Biologiques (ISPB) for an Attaché Temporaire d'Enseignement et de Recherche (ATER) year contract for Benoît Bestgen.

Author Contributions: Odile Filhol and Claude Cochet conceived and designed the experiments; Benoît Bestgen performed the experiments and Zakia Bellaid-Choucair carried out the PLA; Benoît Bestgen, Thierry Lomberget, Marc Le Borgne, Odile Filhol and Claude Cochet analyzed the data; and Odile Filhol and Claude Cochet wrote the paper.

Conflicts of Interest: The authors declare no conflict of interest.

References

1. Guerra, B.; Issinger, O.G. Protein kinase CK2 in human diseases. *Curr. Med. Chem.* **2008**, *15*, 1870–1886. [CrossRef] [PubMed]

2. Ahmed, K.; Gerber, D.A.; Cochet, C. Joining the cell survival squad: An emerging role for protein kinase CK2. *Trends Cell Biol.* **2002**, *12*, 226–230. [CrossRef]

3. Filhol, O.; Giacosa, S.; Wallez, Y.; Cochet, C. Protein kinase CK2 in breast cancer: The CK2beta regulatory subunit takes center stage in epithelial plasticity. *Cell. Mol. Life Sci.* **2015**, *72*, 3305–3322. [CrossRef] [PubMed]

4. Cozza, G.; Pinna, L.A.; Moro, S. Protein kinase CK2 inhibitors: A patent review. *Expert Opin. Ther. Patents* **2012**, *22*, 1081–1097. [CrossRef] [PubMed]

5. Sarno, S.; Papinutto, E.; Franchin, C.; Bain, J.; Elliott, M.; Meggio, F.; Kazimierczuk, Z.; Orzeszko, A.; Zanotti, G.; Battistutta, R.; et al. ATP site-directed inhibitors of protein kinase CK2: An update. *Curr. Top. Med. Chem.* **2011**, *11*, 1340–1351. [CrossRef] [PubMed]

6. Cozza, G.; Pinna, L.A.; Moro, S. Kinase CK2 inhibition: An update. *Curr. Med. Chem.* **2013**, *20*, 671–693. [CrossRef] [PubMed]

7. Pierre, F.; Chua, P.C.; O'Brien, S.E.; Siddiqui-Jain, A.; Bourbon, P.; Haddach, M.; Michaux, J.; Nagasawa, J.; Schwaebe, M.K.; Stefan, E.; et al. Discovery and sar of 5-(3-chlorophenylamino)benzo[c][2,6]naphthyridine-8-carboxylic acid (CX-4945), the first clinical stage inhibitor of protein kinase CK2 for the treatment of cancer. *J. Med. Chem.* **2010**, *54*, 635–654. [CrossRef] [PubMed]

8. Siddiqui-Jain, A.; Drygin, D.; Streiner, N.; Chua, P.; Pierre, F.; O'Brien, S.E.; Bliesath, J.; Omori, M.; Huser, N.; Ho, C.; et al. CX-4945, an orally bioavailable selective inhibitor of protein kinase CK2, inhibits prosurvival and angiogenic signaling and exhibits antitumor efficacy. *Cancer Res.* **2010**, *70*, 10288–10298. [CrossRef] [PubMed]

9. Marschke, R.F.; Borad, M.J.; McFarland, R.W.; Alvarez, R.H.; Lim, J.K.; Padgett, C.S.; Von Hoff, D.D.; O'Brien, S.E.; NorthfeltFront, D.W. Findings from the phase I clinical trials of CX-4945, an orally available inhibitor of CK2. *J. Clin. Onc.* **2011**, *29*, 3087.

10. Prudent, R.; Cochet, C. New protein kinase CK2 inhibitors: Jumping out of the catalytic box. *Chem. Biol.* **2009**, *16*, 112–120. [CrossRef] [PubMed]

11. Niefind, K.; Guerra, B.; Ermakowa, I.; Issinger, O.G. Crystal structure of human protein kinase CK2: Insights into basic properties of the CK2 holoenzyme. *EMBO J.* **2001**, *20*, 5320–5331. [CrossRef] [PubMed]

12. Filhol, O.; Nueda, A.; Martel, V.; Gerber-Scokaert, D.; Benitez, M.J.; Souchier, C.; Saoudi, Y.; Cochet, C. Live-cell fluorescence imaging reveals the dynamics of protein kinase CK2 individual subunits. *Mol. Cell. Biol.* **2003**, *23*, 975–987. [CrossRef] [PubMed]

13. Deshiere, A.; Duchemin-Pelletier, E.; Spreux, E.; Ciais, D.; Combes, F.; Vandenbrouck, Y.; Coute, Y.; Mikaelian, I.; Giusiano, S.; Charpin, C.; et al. Unbalanced expression of CK2 kinase subunits is sufficient to drive epithelial-to-mesenchymal transition by snail1 induction. *Oncogene* **2013**, *32*, 1373–1383. [CrossRef] [PubMed]

14. Raaf, J.; Brunstein, E.; Issinger, O.G.; Niefind, K. The CK2 alpha/CK2 beta interface of human protein kinase CK2 harbors a binding pocket for small molecules. *Chem. Biol.* **2008**, *15*, 111–117. [CrossRef] [PubMed]

15. Laudet, B.; Barette, C.; Dulery, V.; Renaudet, O.; Dumy, P.; Metz, A.; Prudent, R.; Deshiere, A.; Dideberg, O.; Filhol, O.; et al. Structure-based design of small peptide inhibitors of protein kinase CK2 subunit interaction. *Biochem. J.* **2007**, *408*, 363–373. [CrossRef] [PubMed]

16. Raaf, J.; Guerra, B.; Neundorf, I.; Bopp, B.; Issinger, O.G.; Jose, J.; Pietsch, M.; Niefind, K. First structure of protein kinase CK2 catalytic subunit with an effective CK2beta-competitive ligand. *ACS Chem. Biol.* **2013**, *8*, 901–907. [CrossRef] [PubMed]

17. Zhou, Y.; Zhang, N.; Chen, W.; Zhao, L.; Zhong, R. Underlying mechanisms of cyclic peptide inhibitors interrupting the interaction of CK2alpha/CK2beta: Comparative molecular dynamics simulation studies. *Phys. Chem. Chem. Phys.* **2016**, *18*, 9202–9210. [CrossRef] [PubMed]

18. Poletto, G.; Vilardell, J.; Marin, O.; Pagano, M.A.; Cozza, G.; Sarno, S.; Falques, A.; Itarte, E.; Pinna, L.A.; Meggio, F. The regulatory beta subunit of protein kinase CK2 contributes to the recognition of the substrate consensus sequence. A study with an eIF2beta-derived peptide. *Biochemistry* **2008**, *47*, 8317–8325. [CrossRef] [PubMed]

19. Buchou, T.; Vernet, M.; Blond, O.; Jensen, H.H.; Pointu, H.; Olsen, B.B.; Cochet, C.; Issinger, O.G.; Boldyreff, B. Disruption of the regulatory beta subunit of protein kinase CK2 in mice leads to a cell-autonomous defect and early embryonic lethality. *Mol. Cell. Biol.* **2003**, *23*, 908–915. [CrossRef] [PubMed]

20. Schnitzler, A.; Olsen, B.B.; Issinger, O.G.; Niefind, K. The protein kinase CK2 (andante) holoenzyme structure supports proposed models of autoregulation and trans-autophosphorylation. *J. Mol. Biol.* **2014**, *426*, 1871–1882. [CrossRef] [PubMed]

21. Frankel, A.D.; Pabo, C.O. Cellular uptake of the tat protein from human immunodeficiency virus. *Cell* **1988**, *55*, 1189–1193. [CrossRef]

22. Weibrecht, I.; Leuchowius, K.J.; Clausson, C.M.; Conze, T.; Jarvius, M.; Howell, W.M.; Kamali-Moghaddam, M.; Soderberg, O. Proximity ligation assays: A recent addition to the proteomics toolbox. *Expert Rev. Proteom.* **2010**, *7*, 401–409. [CrossRef] [PubMed]

23. Laramas, M.; Pasquier, D.; Filhol, O.; Ringeisen, F.; Descotes, J.L.; Cochet, C. Nuclear localization of protein kinase CK2 catalytic subunit (CK2alpha) is associated with poor prognostic factors in human prostate cancer. *Eur. J. Cancer* **2007**, *43*, 928–934. [CrossRef] [PubMed]

24. Debnath, J.; Muthuswamy, S.K.; Brugge, J.S. Morphogenesis and oncogenesis of MCF-10A mammary epithelial acini grown in three-dimensional basement membrane cultures. *Methods* **2003**, *30*, 256–268. [CrossRef]

25. Heriche, J.K.; Lebrin, F.; Rabilloud, T.; Leroy, D.; Chambaz, E.M.; Goldberg, Y. Regulation of protein phosphatase 2A by direct interaction with casein kinase 2alpha. *Science* **1997**, *276*, 952–955. [CrossRef] [PubMed]

26. Leroy, D.; Alghisi, G.C.; Roberts, E.; Filhol-Cochet, O.; Gasser, S.M. Mutations in the C-terminal domain of topoisomerase II affect meiotic function and interaction with the casein kinase 2 beta subunit. *Mol. Cell. Biochem.* **1999**, *191*, 85–95. [CrossRef] [PubMed]

27. Chantalat, L.; Leroy, D.; Filhol, O.; Nueda, A.; Benitez, M.J.; Chambaz, E.M.; Cochet, C.; Dideberg, O. Crystal structure of the human protein kinase CK2 regulatory subunit reveals its zinc finger-mediated dimerization. *EMBO J.* **1999**, *18*, 2930–2940. [CrossRef] [PubMed]

28. Songyang, Z.; Lu, K.P.; Kwon, Y.T.; Tsai, L.H.; Filhol, O.; Cochet, C.; Brickey, D.A.; Soderling, T.R.; Bartleson, C.; Graves, D.J.; et al. A structural basis for substrate specificities of protein ser/thr kinases: Primary sequence preference of casein kinases I and II, NIMA, phosphorylase kinase, calmodulin-dependent kinase II, CDK5, and ERK1. *Mol. Cell. Biol.* **1996**, *16*, 6486–6493. [CrossRef] [PubMed]

29. Allalou, A.; Wahlby, C. Blobfinder, a tool for fluorescence microscopy image cytometry. *Comput. Methods Programs Biomed.* **2009**, *94*, 58–65. [CrossRef] [PubMed]

30. Guerra, B.; Siemer, S.; Boldyreff, B.; Issinger, O.G. Protein kinase CK2: Evidence for a protein kinase CK2beta subunit fraction, devoid of the catalytic CK2alpha subunit, in mouse brain and testicles. *FEBS Lett.* **1999**, *462*, 353–357. [CrossRef]

31. Filhol, O.; Martiel, J.L.; Cochet, C. Protein kinase CK2: A new view of an old molecular complex. *EMBO Rep.* **2004**, *5*, 351–355. [CrossRef] [PubMed]

32. Fry, D.C. Protein-protein interactions as targets for small molecule drug discovery. *Biopolymers* **2006**, *84*, 535–552. [CrossRef] [PubMed]

33. Li, Y.; Dowbenko, D.; Lasky, L.A. AKT/PKB phosphorylation of p21Cip/WAF1 enhances protein stability of p21Cip/WAF1 and promotes cell survival. *J. Biol. Chem.* **2002**, *277*, 11352–11361. [CrossRef] [PubMed]

34. Wang, Z.; Bhattacharya, N.; Mixter, P.F.; Wei, W.; Sedivy, J.; Magnuson, N.S. Phosphorylation of the cell cycle inhibitor p21Cip1/WAF1 by PIM-1 kinase. *Biochim. Biophys. Acta* **2002**, *1593*, 45–55. [CrossRef]

35. Burch, L.R.; Scott, M.; Pohler, E.; Meek, D.; Hupp, T. Phage-peptide display identifies the interferon-responsive, death-activated protein kinase family as a novel modifier of MDM2 and p21WAF1. *J. Mol. Biol.* **2004**, *337*, 115–128. [CrossRef] [PubMed]

36. Fraser, J.A.; Hupp, T.R. Chemical genetics approach to identify peptide ligands that selectively stimulate DAPK-1 kinase activity. *Biochemistry* **2007**, *46*, 2655–2673. [CrossRef] [PubMed]

37. Cohen, O.; Inbal, B.; Kissil, J.L.; Raveh, T.; Berissi, H.; Spivak-Kroizaman, T.; Feinstein, E.; Kimchi, A. DAP-kinase participates in TNF-alpha- and FAS-induced apoptosis and its function requires the death domain. *J. Cell Biol.* **1999**, *146*, 141–148. [CrossRef] [PubMed]

38. Wazir, U.; Sanders, A.J.; Wazir, A.M.; Ye, L.; Jiang, W.G.; Ster, I.C.; Sharma, A.K.; Mokbel, K. Effects of the knockdown of death-associated protein 3 expression on cell adhesion, growth and migration in breast cancer cells. *Oncol. Rep.* **2015**, *33*, 2575–2582. [PubMed]

39. Engemann, H.; Heinzel, V.; Page, G.; Preuss, U.; Scheidtmann, K.H. DAP-like kinase interacts with the rat homolog of *Schizosaccharomyces pombe* CDC5 protein, a factor involved in pre-mRNA splicing and required for G2/M phase transition. *Nucleic Acids Res.* **2002**, *30*, 1408–1417. [CrossRef]

40. Degterev, A.; Huang, Z.; Boyce, M.; Li, Y.; Jagtap, P.; Mizushima, N.; Cuny, G.D.; Mitchison, T.J.; Moskowitz, M.A.; Yuan, J. Chemical inhibitor of nonapoptotic cell death with therapeutic potential for ischemic brain injury. *Nat. Chem. Biol.* **2005**, *1*, 112–119. [CrossRef]

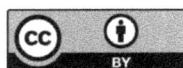

Chapter 5:
New insights into the physiological role of CK2: the clue to therapeutic intervention

pharmaceuticals

MDPI

Review

Drosophila Protein Kinase CK2: Genetics, Regulatory Complexity and Emerging Roles during Development

Mohna Bandyopadhyay, Scott Arbet, Clifton P. Bishop and Ashok P. Bidwai *

Department of Biology, West Virginia University, Morgantown, WV 26506, USA; mohnab04@gmail.com or bandyopadhyaym@hollins.edu (M.B.); sarbet@mix.wvu.edu (S.A.); cbishop@wvu.edu (C.P.B.)
* Correspondence: abidwai@wvu.edu; Tel: +1-304-293-5233

Academic Editor: Mathias Montenarh
Received: 29 November 2016; Accepted: 19 December 2016; Published: 29 December 2016

Abstract: CK2 is a Ser/Thr protein kinase that is highly conserved amongst all eukaryotes. It is a well-known oncogenic kinase that regulates vital cell autonomous functions and animal development. Genetic studies in the fruit fly Drosophila are providing unique insights into the roles of CK2 in cell signaling, embryogenesis, organogenesis, neurogenesis, and the circadian clock, and are revealing hitherto unknown complexities in CK2 functions and regulation. Here, we review Drosophila CK2 with respect to its structure, subunit diversity, potential mechanisms of regulation, developmental abnormalities linked to mutations in the gene encoding CK2 subunits, and emerging roles in multiple aspects of eye development. We examine the Drosophila CK2 "interaction map" and the eye-specific "transcriptome" databases, which raise the prospect that this protein kinase has many additional targets in the developing eye. We discuss the possibility that CK2 functions during early retinal neurogenesis in Drosophila and mammals bear greater similarity than has been recognized, and that this conservation may extend to other developmental programs. Together, these studies underscore the immense power of the Drosophila model organism to provide new insights and avenues to further investigate developmentally relevant targets of this protein kinase.

Keywords: CK2; Drosophila; Notch; eye development; neurogenesis

1. General Overview

Protein phosphorylation is recognized to be a fundamental and evolutionarily conserved regulatory mechanism that controls virtually all aspects of cell and developmental biology. Despite knowledge of the existence of phospho-proteins, the nature of the participatory enzymes remained unknown until the early 1950s, when the laboratory of Eugene Kennedy described, for the first time, the presence of an enzyme, which they called a protein "phosphokinase" [1]. This enzyme possessed the capacity to transfer a phosphate group from ATP to proteins and resulted in the formation of phospho-serine, known to be highly enriched in casein. In addition, they demonstrated that this enzyme preferentially phosphorylated α-casein, as compared to β-casein. In a sense, these seminal studies of Burnett and Kennedy not only revealed the enzymatic basis for the covalent attachment of phosphate to proteins, but also raised the possibility that this type of enzyme exhibited substrate-specificity, now acknowledged to be a fundamental and defining feature of all members of the protein kinase family. Despite the profound implications of their findings, further studies on this "phosphokinase" were not pursued. Just four years later, Edwin Krebs and Edmond Fischer reported the seminal and landmark discovery that phosphorylation controls enzymatic activity [2], subsequently recognized by the Nobel Prize in 1992 [3]. Recalling the decision to not pursue further studies on "phosphokinases", and in a perspectives article in 1992, Eugene Kennedy stated that "*I dropped the study of protein kinases, and like the base Indian, cast a pearl away, else richer than all his tribe*" [4]. The identity of the protein kinase(s) described by Burnett and Kennedy remained unknown. Subsequent purification and identification of the participatory enzymes resulted in their naming as "casein kinase(s)", a misnomer because these enzymes do not reside in the Golgi apparatus, a prerequisite for phosphorylation of the secreted protein casein. These aspects will not be discussed here, given the detailed and excellent historical perspectives (for reviews on CK2, see References [5–9]). The casein-modifying activity has now been definitively linked to the Fam20C protein kinase, that not only phosphorylates casein but is also responsible for the generation of most of the secreted phospho-proteome [10,11]. To remove confusion, the two enzymes Casein Kinase I and II were renamed protein kinase CK1 and CK2. We use this more recent nomenclature, but note that many reports and genome/proteome databases still use the old name.

This review focuses on protein kinase CK2 from the fruit fly *Drosophila melanogaster*, a preeminent animal model, which has illuminated many fundamental principles underlying cell signaling, regulation of gene expression and animal development. We review the subunit composition of Drosophila CK2, the complexity of its gene structure, the multiplicity of its physiological targets that are supported by genetic analyses, physiological/developmental processes revealed by analysis of CK2 mutant flies, large scale screens that have identified proteins that interact with individual CK2 subunits, and conclude with its emerging roles in multiple aspects of eye development.

2. Biochemical Properties and Regulation of Dm-CK2

Drosophila CK2 (henceforth abbreviated as Dm-CK2) was first purified to homogeneity by Glover and co-workers, who demonstrated that the enzyme purified from 0 to 18 h old embryos, like its mammalian counterpart [12–14], is composed of two catalytic Dm-CK2-α and two regulatory Dm-CK2-β subunits that form a hetero-tetrameric ($\alpha 2\beta 2$) holoenzyme. This enzyme utilizes ATP or GTP with almost equal efficiency, appears to be messenger-independent, auto-phosphorylates Dm-CK2-β, modifies Ser or Thr residues in its targets, and is inhibited by Heparin [15,16]. In addition, Dm-CK2 modifies hyper-acidic regions in target proteins, a property that was first described for the mammalian enzyme from various sources [17–20]. However, unlike mammalian CK2, which contains two distinct catalytic subunits (α and α' [21,22]), Dm-CK2 contains a single α isoform. In contrast, metazoan organisms generally contain a single isoform of CK2-β, which was thought to also be the case with Dm-CK2 purified from embryos [15]. However, more recent studies are revealing that the Drosophila genome encodes for the greatest diversity of CK2-β subunit isoforms (see below). These features are also associated with CK2 purified from the yeast *Saccharomyces cerevisiae* [14,16,23–29]. The first evidence that CK2 is conserved through evolution came from the findings that antibodies raised against mammalian (bovine) CK2 strongly cross-reacted with the corresponding subunits of Dm-CK2 [30]. The cloning of cDNAs encoding Dm-CK2-α and CK2-β subunits by the laboratory of Claiborne Glover [31] revealed the primary sequences of these two subunits, thereby enabling the characterization of the cDNAs of the corresponding subunits from diverse species including budding yeast [32,33], fission yeast [34], nematodes [35–37], plants [38], amphibians [39], and mammals [40–43]. Together, these studies not only reinforced the high conservation of CK2 throughout eukaryotic evolution, but revealed subunit heterogeneity that is unique to each taxonomic group.

Despite a search for regulation through second messengers, small ligands, or phosphorylation, the mechanisms influencing CK2 activity have remained unknown. Consequently, CK2 is generally regarded as a second-messenger independent and constitutively active protein kinase. Regulation through holoenzyme ($\alpha 2\beta 2$ tetramer) dissociation seems unlikely, because monomeric Dm-CK2-α (generated by biochemical or recombinant approaches) displays approximately 25% of the activity seen with the holoenzyme [44–46], and addition of CK2-β stimulates activity four-fold concomitant with reconstitution of the tetrameric holoenzyme. Similar findings have been reported for monomeric CK2-α subunits from other sources [27,47]. Regulation through polyamines has been well described [48–52]; these compounds affect Dm-CK2 activity against specific target proteins in vitro, generally act through interactions with the CK2-β subunits [44], and have now been proposed to link CK2 activity to the

EGFR/MAPK signaling pathway [53]. However, the broader implications of these findings and their physiological relevance remain unresolved. The findings that CK2 levels and activity respond to mitogen signaling, e.g., Epidermal Growth Factor [54,55], led to broad interest because CK2 functions could be linked to EGFR signaling, a pathway known to be intricately linked to cancer and animal development [56–58]. However, a detailed reevaluation reveals that these earlier findings on induction by mitogens were artefactual [59]. Further interest stemmed from the findings that CK2 levels/activity correlate to leukemic transformations [60,61], and other cancers, but whether this involves aberrant CK2 regulation remains unknown.

A novel regulatory mechanism has been recently proposed, and extends an observation, first reported by Claiborne Glover, that Dm-CK2 undergoes polymerization involving an ordered but reversible association of the tetrameric holoenzyme into a filamentous state [62]. Filament formation is favored at physiological ionic strengths, and the filaments dissociate into the tetrameric holoenzyme at ionic strengths that are optimal for CK2 activity in vitro. This property is not seen with the monomeric Dm-CK2-α subunit either expressed in bacteria, yeast or insect cell culture (Bidwai, unpublished), suggesting that tetramer–tetramer associations involve the regulatory CK2β subunit. Indeed, it has recently been demonstrated that human CK2 also undergoes polymerization [63] in a CK2β subunit-dependent manner, raising the prospect that the earlier findings on Dm-CK2 may have broader impact. CK2 filaments do not appear to involve structural rearrangements akin to a "prion-type" polymerization, and the filamentous state is proposed to down-regulate CK2 activity. However, the biological relevance of the CK2 filaments in their native (in vivo) milieu remains to be investigated. A robust in vivo evaluation of this property is now possible given the availability of null and hypomorphic mutants for the *Dm-CK2-α/β* genes (see below) and the identification of interfacial residues that mediate filament formation.

3. Substrates of Dm-CK2

The first substrate for Dm-CK2 to be identified was DNA Topoisomerase II [64,65], whose activity was stimulated three-fold upon phosphorylation. This post translational modification (PTM) occurs in vitro and in vivo (Drosophila embryonic Kc cells in culture), findings that have been corroborated for DNA Topoisomerase II from the yeast *S. cerevisiae* [66–68]. The application of high throughput whole cell proteomic strategies has enabled detailed analysis of the CK2-dependent cellular phospho-proteome. This approach has successfully been applied to mammalian cells or yeast expressing heterologous proteins upon treatment with high-affinity and -specificity inhibitors of CK2 [69,70], and reveals a multitude of proteins whose phosphorylation is stimulated as well as inhibited, and includes many proteins with cell-autonomous roles. While such information can illuminate the extent of the CK2 phospho-proteome, analyses of cell lines do not reveal targeting of developmentally important genes, whose expression is often restricted to a specific cell-type, a region of the developing embryo/animal, or is under temporal control. Accordingly, Giot and coworkers used the yeast two hybrid strategy to evaluate Drosophila protein–protein interactions at a global level [71], but these interactions have not been subject to follow-up studies. These latter two aspects have restricted our understanding of the CK2 "phospho-proteome" relevant to animal (Drosophila) development, and much of our knowledge of specific targets has emerged on a case-by-case basis (see below).

Compared to mammalian cell-based strategies, studies in Drosophila have identified a smaller cohort of CK2 substrates, and many of these have revealed important roles in development. We used the Drosophila database (Flybase, release date of 18 October 2016), and identified proteins whose interaction with CK2 was revealed by studies that combined direct biochemical with reverse-genetic approaches. We note that the role of Dm-CK2 has also been inferred based on genetic screens using RNAi against Dm-CK2-α/β subunits or via dominant-negative (DN) constructs against Dm-CK2-α, and these studies implicate roles in cell signaling, development, tissue morphogenesis and organogenesis. However, we have excluded these from consideration in this review, because molecular target(s) cannot be discerned solely by "reverse-genetic" approaches. We correlated known targets to the Drosophila-Protein-Interaction-Map (DPIM) database [72,73], an LC-MS based approach in which Dm-CK2 interacting proteins were identified following its expression and co-immunoprecipitation from Drosophila S2 cells (see below). It should, however, be noted that follow-up studies to identify which of these proteins is an interacting partner and/or a substrate for phosphorylation are generally lacking, and therefore only those proteins for which direct biochemical evidence has been reported are included in Table 1.

Table 1. CK2 targets from FlyBase (November 2016).

Protein	Function	Effect of Phosphorylation
Ankyrin-2	Cytoskeletal Adaptor	Maintenance of synaptic stability
Antennapedia	Transcription Factor	Spatial restriction of activity
Armadillo	Transcription Factor	Phosphorylation triggers degradation
Cactus	Transcription Factor	Required for activity during axis formation
Clock	Transcription Factor	Stabilizes Clock
CREB2	Transcription Factor	Inhibits DNA binding
Dishevelled (dsh)	Transcription Factor	Influences Wg/Wnt signaling
dMi-2 (DPIM)	Chromatin Structure	Inhibits nucleosome-stimulated ATPase
E(spl)-M8/M5/M7	Transcription Factor	Phosphorylation required for repressor activity
Engrailed	Transcription Factor	Phosphorylation enhances DNA-binding
Enhancer of Rudimentary	Transcription Factor	Promotes and inhibits activity
FMR1 (DPIM)	RNA-Binding	Affects dimerization and RNA-binding
GAGA factor (519)	Transcription Factor	Reduced DNA binding affinity
Groucho	Transcription Factor	Stimulates short range repression
Hairy	Transcription Factor	Promotes repressor activity
Heterochromatin protein HP1	Chromatin Structure	Stimulates DNA binding
mushroom body miniature	Ribosome Biogenesis	Promotes nucleolar localization
NAP1	Chromatin Structure	Affects degradation and cellular locale
Odd	Transcription Factor	Inhibits Groucho binding and repression
Orb (CPEB-family)	RNA-Binding	Promotes Orb activity
P element Somatic Inhibitor (PSI)	Splicing factor	Modulates interactions with splicing factors
Period	Circadian Clock	Promotes nuclear entry
Raf	Protein Kinase	Required for ERK activation
Ribosomal S6 kinase	Protein Kinase	Required for activity
RPL-22	Ribosome Structure	Unknown
Smoothened	Signaling	Stabilizes and promotes Hedgehog signaling
Syntaxin-1	Membrane Protein	Stimulates interaction with Dopamine Transporter
Timeless	Circadian Clock	Promotes nuclear entry
Topoisomerase II (DPIM)	DNA-replication	Stimulates activity
Warts	Protein Kinase	Indirectly promotes Warts suppression of Yorkie

DPiM (in red) denotes proteins identified in the Drosophila Protein Interaction Map.

As shown in Table 1, this list of bona fide Dm-CK2 target proteins is not as extensive as that in mammals. Nevertheless, this list includes numerous developmentally important transcription factors, proteins involved in regulation of cytoskeletal and chromatin structure, ribosome structure and biogenesis, DNA-replication, circadian rhythms, etc. With few exceptions (such as CREB2 [74], Raf [53], Topo-II [64], and rPL22 [75]), most of the proteins in this list serve well-established roles in development. Examples are, Ankyrin-2 [76], Antennapedia [77], Armadillo [78], Cactus [79],

Clock [80], Dishevelled [81], dMI-2 [82], E(spl)-M5/M7/M8 [83,84], Engrailed [85], Enhancer of Rudimentary [86], FMR1 [87], GAGA factor-519 [88], Groucho [89], Hairy [90], Heterochromatin protein HP1 [91], mushroom body miniature [92], NAP1 [93], Odd [94], Orb [95], P element Somatic Inhibitor [96], Ribosomal S6 kinase [97], Smoothened [98], Syntaxin-1 [99], and Warts [100]. Remarkably, only three proteins from this list, dMi-2, FMR1 and DNA-Topo-II, have been also identified in the DPiM database (Table 1 and see below). The low overlap between genetically analyzed proteins targeted by CK2 to those identified in the DPiM database reveals limitations inherent to cell-based assays. Although the S2-cell line is of embryonic origin, it does not fully recapitulate gene expression patterns across a developing embryo/animal. Consequently, many genes whose expression is controlled in a spatially and/or temporally restricted manner are not captured in S2-based assays. For example, although the Notch effector proteins E(spl)-M8/M5/M7 were identified in a yeast two-hybrid screen of a Drosophila (0–18 h) embryo cDNA library [101], and the consequences of CK2-mediated phosphorylation of E(spl)-M8 during neurogenesis (eye and bristle development) are well understood [83], these proteins appear to not be endogenously expressed in S2 cells. This is, perhaps, the greatest weakness of high-throughput proteomic methods to reveal the extent of the CK2 "interactome" that regulates animal development.

4. Drosophila Genes Encoding Catalytic (α) and Regulatory (β) Subunits

Unlike most metazoan organisms, Drosophila harbors a single *Dm-CK2-α* gene [31]. On the other hand, and unique to Drosophila, is the presence of multiple genes, both X-linked and autosomal, that encode proteins with high homology with metazoan CK2-β subunits (Table 2), which are functionally non-redundant (see below). These are the X-linked *Dm-CK2-β* [102] and *Stellate (Ste)* genes [103–105], and the autosomal genes *Dm-CK2-β'* [106] and *Suppressor of Stellate Like (SSL,* also called Dm-CK2-β^{Tes}) [107,108]. The *Stellate* locus is unusual in that it harbors multiple copies of the *Ste* gene; this appears to vary between strains, with perhaps the highest number (~200) in the *D. melanogaster* strain Oregon R. This multi copy *Ste* locus, located in a heterochromatic region of the X-chromosome, is unique in that its expression is testis-specific and normally repressed through the action of a Y-linked *Su(Ste)* gene cluster [109]. Consequently, in X/O males (those lacking the Y chromosome), *Ste* undergoes massive de-repression and the Ste protein accumulates at levels sufficient to form crystalline aggregates that disrupt spermatocyte maturation resulting in loss of fertility. *Ste* gene copy number seems to influence the type of crystals; needle-shaped crystals in strains with low copy number but star-shaped crystals in strains with high copy number. The reasons underlying these differences are unresolved, and it is also unknown if sterility in XO males involves Ste-dependent impairment of endogenous Dm-CK2. In a similar manner, *SSL/Dm-CK2-β^{Tes}* was thought to be testis-specific [110]. However, *SSL* transcripts are present in the embryo, although levels markedly increase in a male-specific manner in third-instar-larvae, pupae, and adults [107]. These results demonstrate that *SSL/Dm-CK2-β^{Tes}* expression encompasses a greater developmental window, and raise the possibility that this alternative Dm-CK2 subunit may confer distinct functions to CK2 in a sex-specific manner.

Table 2. Subunit diversity and non-redundancy of Dm-CK2β isoforms.

Genes Encoding CK2 Subunits in Drosophila			
Gene (Chromosome)	**Isoforms**	**Alleles**	**Nature**
CK2α (III)	Single	*CK2α-Tik* *CK2α-TikR* *CK2α-MB00477* *CK2α-G703* *CK2α-H3091*	M161K + E165D Loss of Function Hypomorphic W279G D212N
CK2β (X)	Multiple	*CK2βAndante* *CK2βmbuP1* *CK2βmbuΔA26-2L*	M166I Hypomorphic Loss of Function
Stellate (X)	Single	None	N/A
CK2β' (II)	Single	None	N/A
SSL/CK2-βTes (II)	Single	None	N/A
Phenotypes of Ectopic Expression			
Isoform	**Tissue**	**Overexpression Phenotype**	
CK2α-WT	Proneural cluster	No Effect	
CK2α-Tik	Proneural cluster	Impaired Notch Signaling (eye & bristle)	
CK2α-M161K	Proneural cluster	Impaired Notch Signaling (eye & bristle)	
CK2α-E165D	Proneural cluster	Impaired Notch Signaling (eye & bristle)	
CK2β-VII-a	Ubiquitous	No Effect	**Rescues *CK2β^{ΔA26}***
CK2β-VII-b	Ubiquitous	Dominant Lethal	**Rescues *CK2β^{ΔA26}***
CK2β-VII-c	Ubiquitous	No Effect	**Rescues *CK2β^{ΔA26}***
CK2β-VII-d	Ubiquitous	Dominant Lethal	No rescue of *CK2β^{ΔA26}*
CK2β-VII-d-VI	Ubiquitous	No Effect	No rescue of *CK2β^{ΔA26}*
Stellate	Not Tested	N/A	Not tested
CK2β'	Ubiquitous	Dominant Lethal	No rescue of *CK2β^{ΔA26}*
SSL/CK2-βTes	Ubiquitous	Dominant Lethal	No rescue of *CK2β^{ΔA26}*

Yellow box highlights ability to complement the lethality of *CK2β^{ΔA26}* mutants. CK2-β isoforms that fail to rescue loss of the X-linked CK2-β gene are indicated in red.

In contrast to *Dm-CK2-β'*, *Ste*, and *SSL/CK2-β^{Tes}*, all of which encode for a single protein isoform, the *Dm-CK2-β* gene encodes for multiple isoforms due to alternative transcription and splicing. These include five transcripts named CK2-β type-VIIa, -VIIb, -VIIc, -VIId and -VII-VI (Table 2, and see References [102,111]). This diversity of transcript types has so far not been reported for other metazoan organisms. All five transcripts encode the highly conserved core of CK2-β, which includes the well characterized (N-terminal) auto-phosphorylation site and the zinc-finger [112], but differ in the length and sequence heterogeneity of ~15–20 C-terminal residues [111]. Consequently, these variations do not affect interaction with Dm-CK2-α, but significantly impact in vivo activities of the encoded proteins (see below). In a similar vein, *Dm-CK2-β'*, *Ste*, *SSL/CK2-β^{Tes}* also interact with Dm-CK2-α and appear competent for forming the tetrameric holoenzyme in vitro, but these alternative *Dm-CK2-β* proteins do not act in a functionally redundant manner with the X-linked *Dm-CK2-β* gene (see below).

5. Mutations in Catalytic (α) and Regulatory (β) Subunits

Mutations in *Dm-CK2-α* were isolated in a genetic screen for dominant modifiers of the circadian clock and resulted in the identification of the first mutant allele called *Timekeeper* (*Tik*). Specifically, *Tik/+* animals display an aberrant circadian clock, whereas *Tik*-homozygotes (*Tik/Tik*) die at the first larval stage ([113], and see Figure 1). A spontaneous and partial revertant of the clock phenotype was also identified; this allele called *TikR* is also lethal at the first larval stage in the homozygous state (Figure 1). The *Tik* allele harbors two missense mutations, $M^{161}K+E^{165}D$, and encodes an inactive form of Dm-CK2-α, which retains proper folding because its ability to interact with Dm-CK2-β is indistinguishable from wild-type Dm-CK2-α. In addition, Rasmussen and coworkers have reported that, compared to the wild type enzyme, human CK2-α containing the $M^{161}K + E^{165}D$ mutations exhibits a ~40-fold reduction of activity towards exogenous substrates [47]. The *Tik* mutation thus acts as a CK2 dominant-negative (CK2-DN) allele, and its ability to perturb the circadian clock reflects incorporation into and downregulation of the $\alpha2\beta2$ holoenzyme [114]. In addition to the $M^{161}K + E^{165}D$ mutations, the *TikR* protein harbors an in-frame deletion of nine amino acids that are invariant between Drosophila and human CK2-α (Figure 1) and localize to a highly structured region of the protein [115,116]. This deletion compromises folding and abrogates interaction with Dm-CK2-β, consequently preventing incorporation of the TikR protein into the $\alpha2\beta2$ holoenzyme. This is supported by the identical *"effective lethal phase"* of *Tik/Tik*, *TikR/TikR* or *Tik/TikR* flies (see Figure 1). Thus, the partial reversion of the clock phenotype by the *TikR* mutation does not reflect restored CK2 activity, but instead reflects an inability of the mis-folded TikR protein to act as a CK2-DN. In line with this interpretation, over-expression of the Tik mutant (in otherwise wild-type flies) elicits defects in the clock, and perturbs development of the eye and bristles, a characteristic of impaired Notch signaling (see Table 2 and Reference [83]). A similar impairment of Notch signaling manifests upon targeted over-expression of the single mutants, CK2α-$M^{161}K$ or CK2α-$E^{165}D$; the former acts as a CK2-DN, whereas the latter through its ability to elicit a gain in activity of the phosphatase PP2A. Tik should therefore be considered a "double hit" with respect to Notch signaling. It remains to be clarified if this applies to CK2 functions in other developmental programs. No eye/bristle defects manifest upon overexpression of TikR protein or wild-type Dm-CK2-α (Bidwai, unpublished, and see below).

Other than defects in the circadian clock, neither *Tik/+* nor *TikR/+* flies display any other developmental abnormalities (Figure 1). The normal development of *Tik/+* animals is surprising, given the DN nature of this allele and the large number of targets of this protein kinase (Table 1). These findings raise the prospect that the circadian clock is more sensitive to levels of CK2 activity, i.e., a 50% reduction in *TikR/+* animals elicits minor defects, whereas further reductions in *Tik/+* (<50%) become rate-limiting. The absence of overt phenotypes in *TikR/+* animals could be reconciled with the findings that only a few developmental processes are haplo-insufficient, and because development is often "buffered" against fluctuations in gene-dosage (see below).

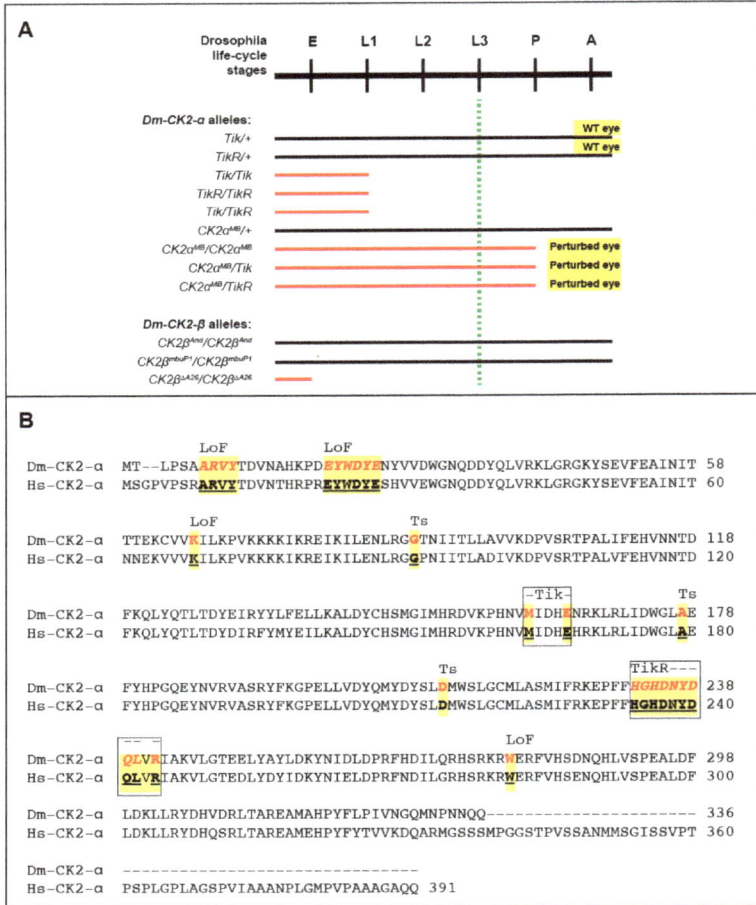

Figure 1. (**A**) Drosophila life cycle stages and effective lethal phase of CK2 mutants. Abbreviations are; E, Embryo; L1, 1st larval stage; L2, 2nd larval stage; L3, 3rd larval stage; P, pupal stage; A, adult. Note that *Dm-CK2-α* mutants *Tik* and *TikR* arrest at the L1 stage, whereas *CK2α^MB* mutants die at the P-to-A transition. In contrast, *CK2β^And* and *CK2β^mbuP1* are viable, whereas *CK2β^ΔA26* die during embryogenesis. Dashed green line denotes stage of life cycle when eye development initiates; black lines denote normal development, whereas red lines denote effective lethal phases of indicated mutant combinations; (**B**) Alignment of CK2-α from *D. melanogaster* (Dm) and *H. sapiens* (Hs). LoF denotes loss-of-function, whereas Ts denotes Temperature-sensitive. The locations of the Tik and TikR mutations are boxed and yellow highlighting denotes conservation of residues between Dm and Hs CK2α subunits.

Additional mutations such as *CK2-α-G703* and *CK2-α-H3091* have also been identified, but analysis of these alleles in eye/bristle development or clock functions has not been reported. It is of interest to note that the *CK2-α-H3091* allele replaces a highly conserved Asp^{212} with Asn (Figure 1). Remarkably, the first temperature-sensitive (ts) alleles of CK2, which were isolated in the laboratory of Claiborne Glover, include a D^{220}N mutation in the *CKA2* gene encoding the yeast CK2-α' subunit [117]. Asp^{220} of yeast *CKA2* corresponds to Asp^{212} in Dm-CK2-α (and Asp^{214} in Hs-CK2-α, see Figure 1), and the targeted introduction of a D^{212}N mutation also engenders a ts-behavior upon Dm-CK2-α in a yeast complementation assay [118]. The $D^{220/212}$ site resides in the C-lobe of CK2-α, is close to the active site, and points towards the core of this region, making it likely that this is a permissive site for destabilizing CK2 structure, thereby rendering the mutant protein temperature-sensitive in yeast as well as flies. Additionally, as seen in Figure 1, many of the mutations that abrogate CK2-α activity or perturb its structure appear to reside in highly structured regions. Recent advances in evolutionary statistical coupling [119] may offer a route to better understand the clustering of these mutations, and provide new insights into the evolutionary relationships between CK2-α subunits across the tree of life. Given these findings, it will be of interest to determine if *CK2-α-H3091* mutant flies display overt developmental defects (such as defects in embryogenesis, or eye/bristle development) in a temperature-sensitive manner. If so, it will provide the first bona fide ts-allele of *Dm-CK2-α*, which should enhance our ability to better define the Dm-CK2 dependent phospho-proteome, and the multitude of developmental programs that are controlled by this protein kinase. In contrast, the *CK2-α-G703* allele harbors a $W^{279}G$ mutation, affecting a residue conserved in both yeast CK2-α genes (*CKA1/CKA2* [32]) as well as Hs-CK2-α (Figure 1, and not shown); but the mechanism underlying the lethality of this allele remains unclear. The only hypomorphic allele that has been identified to date is *CK2α-MB00477* (*CK2α^MB^*). This allele results from the insertion of a P-element (a transposon) in the 5′ control region. Consequently, *CK2α^MB^* is lethal when homozygous, and these animals die at the pupal-to-adult transition (see Figure 1A). Importantly, pupal lethality is also seen in *CK2α^MB^/Tik* or *CK2α^MB^/TikR* animals, confirming that *CK2α^MB^* is a new unique hypomorphic mutation in *Dm-CK2-α*. As expected, *CK2α^MB^/+* animals display normal eye development. However, unlike *Tik* or *TikR* homozygotes, which die prior to the onset of retinal development (dashed green line in Figure 1A), *CK2α^MB^* homozygotes progress normally through the third larval stage, which is a critical juncture marking the onset of retinal neurogenesis and eye development. We discuss the nature of this allele and highlight its utility to better understand the roles of CK2 in eye development later in this review (see below).

The first mutant of *Dm-CK2-β* was the *Andante* allele (see Table 2), originally identified by Ron Konopka [120,121]. This mutation, which was mapped to the 10E1-E7 region of the X-chromosome, is in close proximity to the *Dm-CK2-β* gene [102] and was characterized by the lengthening of the circadian period and locomotor activity rhythms by 1.5–2.0 h. The nature of the mutation and the affected gene remained unknown until the laboratory of F. Rob Jackson identified it as a mis-sense mutation in *Dm-CK2-β*. This mutation called *Dm-CK2-β^And^* [122] replaces $M^{166}I$, a residue that lies in helix α-F [112], which is positioned close to the interface between CK2-α and CK2-β. Consequently, it was thought that *CK2-β^And^* is impaired for proper assembly into the α2β2 holoenzyme or destabilizes this ternary state. However, human CK2-β with the $M^{166}I$ mutation interacts with CK2-α as efficiently as wild-type CK2-β and forms the holoenzyme with normal activity [47], raising questions on its proposed relevance to the clock defects of *CK2-β^And^* flies. Consistent with these latter findings, *CK2-β^And^* flies are viable as hemizygous males or homozygous females. A second hypomorphic allele, *CK2-β^mbuP1^*, was reported by the laboratory of Thomas Raabe. Remarkably, Jauch and co-workers demonstrated that *CK2-β^mbuP1^* impairs proliferation of Kenyon cells thus affecting development of the mushroom body, a structure key to learning and memory. Their studies also identified an excision allele, *Dm-CK2-β^mbuΔA26^*, that disrupts the *CK2-β* coding region and results in embryonic lethality when homozygous. Together with earlier findings from the mouse model [123], these studies demonstrate that *CK2-β* is an essential gene in Drosophila.

It is currently unclear why loss of the *Dm-CK2-α* gene results in lethality at the first larval stage, whereas that of *Dm-CK2-β* is embryonic lethal (see Figure 1). Maternal contribution of Dm-CK2 could account for the larval lethality of *Dm-CK2-α* mutants, but how does one reconcile the earlier lethality of *Dm-CK2-β* mutants. One possibility is differential half-life of individual subunits or their mRNAs, such that Dm-CK2-β protein/transcripts have a higher turnover-rate compared to Dm-CK2-α. This issue is unlikely to be resolved by pulse-chase analysis in S2-cells, because free subunits have not been detected in this embryonic cell type [46], and factors that regulate differential turnover and/or holoenzyme assembly might well be present only in an intact developing embryo. An alternative possibility is that differential turnover is spatially and/or temporally controlled. Current technologies do not allow us to evaluate/distinguish between these possibilities. However, the development and refinement of genome editing technologies may allow the differential tagging of Dm-CK2-β protein or transcripts to resolve these issues.

6. Multiple Non-Redundant Variants Encoded by the Dm-CK2-β Gene

As mentioned above, the *Dm-CK2-β* coding region encodes for five distinct protein isoforms, some of which reflect distinct splicing events and are likely produced in a tissue-specific manner. In all cases, the isoforms differ only in their C-terminal tail, which becomes appended with ~15–20 amino acids unique to each isoform. In the crystal structure of the human CK2 holoenzyme (PDB code 1 JWH, [115]), the CK2-β subunit is truncated such that it lacks the penultimate 10 amino acids. Consequently, the structural constraints on the C-terminus of CK2-β are unclear. Nevertheless, the region preceding these missing residues is a well-defined helix, which does not contribute to the CK2-β/CK2-α interaction interface, but projects away from the core holoenzyme structure. Given that CK2-β subunits generally display length and sequence heterogeneity in their C-terminal tail, one might expect that these would have minimal impact on CK2 functions. To the contrary, the laboratory of Thomas Raabe has individually tested all five Dm-CK2-β variants in an exceptionally robust in vivo functional complementation assay, i.e., their ability to rescue the lethality of the $Dm\text{-}CK2\text{-}\beta^{mbu\Delta A26}$ mutation. Remarkably, only three out of five Dm-CK2-β isoforms (CK2-β-VIIa, -VIIb, -VIIc) rescue lethality [111], leading to the view that these alternative C-termini alter in vivo functionality of Dm-CK2-β variants (see Table 2). In addition, they also conducted tests for phenotypic outcomes of ubiquitous expression of each isoform in otherwise wild-type flies using the *tubulin* (*tub*) promoter, and find that only two Dm-CK2-β isoforms, VIIb and VIId, elicit dominant lethality. The dominant lethality of these two isoforms may reflect competition for limiting amounts of Dm-CK2-α that is available to form the holoenzyme. Together, these in vivo results are strong indicators that these variants bias the Dm-CK2-β "interactome", perhaps by regulating target protein specificity, cellular locale, turnover rates, etc. Alternatively, these C-terminal variations may result in holoenzyme isoforms that differ in their ability to form ternary complexes. As shown by the laboratory of Roberto Battistutta, the C-terminus of CK2-β impacts the ability of CK2 tetramers to form ternary complexes, i.e., filaments [63]. In a new trimeric ring-like structure, which they call $\alpha 2\beta 2^{new}$, the C-terminus of CK2-β competes with ATP for binding to CK2-α, and appears to stabilize a nonproductive conformation upon insertion into the ATP-binding pocket. Additionally, they demonstrate that this interaction impairs pairing of residues in CK2-α that are critical for catalysis and are a generally conserved feature of protein kinases. If so, this could represent a novel structural basis for CK2 downregulation. Given these findings, it is likely that CK2 holoenzymes containing Dm-CK2-β isoforms with alternative C-terminal sequences differ in their propensity to form trimeric ring-like structures. The possibility thus arises that the dominant lethality of the alternative Dm-CK2-β isoforms (VIIb and VIId) revealed by the studies of Jauch and coworkers [111] may, in fact, involve aberrant in vivo regulation of Dm-CK2. It would hence be worthwhile to investigate which of the five Dm-CK2-β isoforms favor or disfavor the formation of ring-like states.

In the same study, Raabe and coworkers also tested and demonstrated that neither Dm-CK2-β′ nor $SSL/CK2\text{-}\beta^{Tes}$ rescue the lethality of the $Dm\text{-}CK2\text{-}\beta^{mbu\Delta A26}$ mutation, and both elicit dominant lethality upon ubiquitous expression in wild type flies (Table 2). These findings are of interest, because even though Dm-CK2-β′ and SSL/CK2-β^{Tes} are structurally similar to Dm-CK2-β, they exhibit two differences. (1) Unlike the auto-phosphorylation site in Dm-CK2-β (M^{1}SSSEE), Dm-CK2-β′ harbors the motif M^{1}TDSDE, whereas it is M^{1}SCPRS in SSL. Consequently, Dm-CK2-β′ may resemble a constitutively phosphorylated protein, while SSL would be refractory; (2) The acidic micro-domain is also different such that the rank order of acidity is Dm-CK2-β > SSL/CK2-β^{Tes} > Dm-CK2-β′. Given the findings of Jauch and coworkers, it will be of interest to determine if rescue of the $Dm\text{-}CK2\text{-}\beta^{mbu\Delta A26}$ mutation by Dm-CK2-β requires an intact auto-phosphorylation site and/or acidic micro-domain.

As of the writing of this review, no mutants of the $Dm\text{-}CK2\text{-}\beta'$ or $SSL/CK2\text{-}\beta^{Tes}$ genes are available, precluding predictions of their biological functions. In a yeast-based assay, these two proteins appear to partially compensate for phenotypes elicited by loss of the yeast CK2-β genes [107], but this may not be an appropriate assay for in vivo functions. However, considering their tissue-specificity and/or male-specificity and dominant lethality, it is reasonable to speculate that if these isoforms were to downregulate CK2 activity, alter its target specificity, or impact formation of trimeric rings, these functions may be tied to male development. Nevertheless, the studies of the Raabe laboratory make it likely that the diverse CK2-β like proteins in Drosophila (splice variations and distinct genes) serve unique tissue, developmental stage, or sex-specific functions or confer unique regulation upon the enzyme itself. To our knowledge, this level of complexity in CK2-β subunits has not been described for any metazoan organism, but is not without precedence. For example, the laboratory of Marc Vidal has reported that the "interactome" of a protein is significantly altered by splicing variations, almost as if the alternative products are encoded by distinct genes [124]. It would hence be worthwhile to determine the extent of overlap and non-overlap of proteins that interact with alternative isoforms that are encoded by the Dm-CK2-β gene versus those that interact with $Dm\text{-}CK2\text{-}\beta'$ or $SSL/CK2\text{-}\beta^{Tes}$.

7. The DPiM Database Provides New Insights into the Dm-CK2 Interactome and Subunit Specific Interactions

Whole cell proteomics affords an unbiased route to identify interacting partners. Such an approach has been taken using Drosophila S2 cells [72,73]. In this comprehensive study, Guruharsha and coworkers expressed ≥5000 individual FLAG-HA epitope-tagged Drosophila proteins, which was followed by co-affinity purification coupled to mass spectrometry analysis. This study has enabled the determination of a vast number of protein complexes, which they call the 'Drosophila protein interaction map (DPiM, https://interfly.med.harvard.edu). Given the structural and functional diversity of CK2-β isoforms, we analyzed the DPiM database for all five Dm-CK2 subunits, i.e., CK2-α, CK2-β, CK2-β', Stellate, and SSL/CK2-β^{Tes} (see Table 3). Although the DPiM database includes analysis of only three, CK2-α, CK2-β, CK2-β', new insights nevertheless emerge.

Table 3. The DPiM database reveals novel insights into the Dm-CK2 interactome.

Dm-CK2-α Interactors in Drosophila S2-Cells (DPiM)			
Protein	**Function**	**Protein**	**Function**
CK2-α	CK2 Catalytic Subunit	Lasp	Cytoskeletal organization
CK2-β	CK2 Regulatory Subunit	Rump	RNA-binding
AGO2	RNA-binding	Ran	Small GTPase
pAbp	Poly-A binding protein	Rack1	Receptor for activated PKC
glo	mRNA binding	Topo2 (Genetic)	DNA Topoisomerase 2
FMR1 (Genetic)	Fragile-X syndrome	p38b	MAP-kinase
Dek (CK2-β)	Homeodomain	Wmd	Wing morphogenesis
Rasputin	RNA-binding	Mts	PP2A catalytic subunit
Dre4 (CK2-β)	Chromatin-binding	Scf (CK2-β)	Chromatin Organization
Vig2	RNA-binding	Su-var(3)9	Chromatin regulator
Ssrp	HMG Box Domain	14-3-3	pSer binding
Interactions between Dm-CK2-α, Dm-CK2-β and Dm-CK2-β'			
FLAG-HA-Fusion (Bait)	**Interacting Proteins**	**Interactions Not Detected**	
CK2-α	CK2-α, CK2-β	CK2-β'	
CK2-β	CK2-α, CK2-β	CK2-β'	
CK2-β'	CK2-α, CK2-β'	CK2-β	

Interactions shared with CK2-β in the DPiM database or those revealed by genetic studies are highlighted in red.

7.1. Interactions between Dm-CK2 Subunits

As expected (see Table 3), these studies identified the canonical interactions between CK2-α + CK2-β and CK2-α + CK2-β′, consistent with previous studies using the yeast two hybrid approach [101,106,125]. Given the tetrameric structure of the human/Drosophila CK2 holoenzyme, the co-purification of CK2-α using FLAG-HA-CK2-α is unlikely to reflect direct interactions, but instead "bridged" by CK2-β. Surprisingly, even though S2-cells endogenously express both CK2-β and CK2-β′, the only interactions that were detected were CK2-β + CK2-β and CK2-β′ + CK2-β′ (Table 3). The absence of cross-CK2-β subunit interactions in S2 cells suggests that the CK2-holoenzyme cannot be generated using mixed CK2-β dimers, such as CK2-β + CK2-β′. Whether this also applies to the Stellate, and SSL/CK2-β^{Tes} proteins remains unknown. The CK2-β-vs.-CK2-β′ subunit-specific bias (for dimerization) makes it likely that sector analysis [126,127] may provide new insights into the evolution and diversity of the CK2-β family in Drosophila. The possibility that this aspect of CK2 structure impacts in vivo functionality is exciting, and may represent a unique mode of regulation, which has remained the most elusive aspect of CK2 functions across all eukaryotes.

7.2. Dm-CK2-α Interactors

In large part, the proteins that interact with Dm-CK2-α are unique, and encompass a multitude of functions. Notably absent from this list are proteins whose targeting by CK2 has been confirmed by combined biochemical and genetic studies (see Table 1). The only proteins for which such evidence exists are Topo-II and FMR1. Interestingly, four of the interacting proteins, Dek, Dre4, Scf, and Ssrp, were also identified as interactors of Dm-CK2-β (see below). It is of interest that the DPiM database reveals interactions of CK2-α with Mts, the catalytic subunit of the phosphatase PP2A [128]. This phosphatase plays multiple essential roles in metazoan cell/organismal biology; it is a known tumor suppressor that is involved in oncogenesis [129,130], and regulates the Notch and Hedgehog signaling pathways [131–133], autophagy [134] and the cell-cycle [133,135]. Consequently, loss of Mts activity is lethal in Drosophila. Of interest, the CK2-α + PP2A interaction was originally reported for the human proteins, and occurs via the M^{161}IDHE^{165}NRKL motif [136], also present in the oncogenic virus SV-40. Intriguingly, this very motif is mutated in the *Dm-CK2-α* allele *Tik* (see Figure 1), and functional studies in Drosophila reveal that the CK2α-E^{165}D mutation elicits phenotypes that mimic overexpression of PP2A-Mts or its regulatory subunit PP2A-Widerborst [114,131]. These studies make it likely that the CK2-PP2A interaction serves to downregulate phosphatase activity. The remaining proteins fall into four classes; chromatin organization, RNA binding proteins, transcription factors, and others regulating signaling and the cytoskeleton. It will be of interest to determine if these proteins are targets of CK2 in vitro, and the consequences of phosphorylation during development.

Interactors of Dm-CK2-β and Dm-CK2-β′ are listed in Table 4, and are sorted by those that are unique to each subunit and those that overlap. In each case, the DPiM database includes several ribosomal proteins. Although these interactions may involve regulation of "*sentinel-like*" functions of ribosomal proteins [137], we have not considered this class of proteins as bona fide CK2 interactors because they often appear in large scale proteomic and yeast two-hybrid screens and can represent potential artefacts.

Table 4. Dm-CK2-β and Dm-CK2-β′ interactors in Drosophila S2-cells (DPiM).

Interacting Partners Unique to Dm-CK2-β

Protein	Function	Protein	Function
Dek (CK2-α)	Homeodomain	dMi-2 (Genetic)	Nucleosome binding
CG13800	Actin-Binding	Tango7	Neuron morphogenesis
Dre4 (CK2-α)	Chromatin Binding	CG3817	rRNA processing
Ssrp (CK2-α)	HMG Box Domain	CG1677	Zinc Finger Protein
eIF-3-S8	Translation Factor	CG5525	HSP60-family
CDK12	Protein Kinase	Xpc/mus210	Xeroderma pigmentosum-C
CG7033	HSP60-family	Cpb (CG17158)	Actin Capping Protein
CG8258	Unknown	Prp38	pre-mRNA processing
Arp14D	Actin related protein 2	D1 Chromosomal Protein	Satellite DNA-binding
Sop2	Actin related protein 2/3	CycK	Cyclin K
Cct5	T-complex Chaperonin 5	Hyd (Hyperplastic Disc)	E3-Ub-Ligase
Int6	Proto-oncogene	Scf/DCB-45 (CK2-α)	Chromatin Organization
Tcp1-ζ	HSP60-family	CG6724	WD40 repeats similar to Gβ
Arc-p34	Neuronal development	XNP	Neuronal development
Smg5	Nonsense mediated decay		

Interacting Partners Unique to Dm-CK2-β′

Protein	Function	Protein	Function
Porin	Mitochondrial OM channel	awd/abnormal wing discs	Nucleotide Kinase
Chd64	Juvenile Hormone Signaling	EB1	Myosin Binding
Fimbrin	Female meiosis	Smt3/SUMO	SUMO family
FK506-bp2	DNA Damage Response	Nlp/CRP1	Nucleoplasmin
Annexin B10	Annexin Family	PCNA/Mus209	DNA-Replication

Interacting Partners Common to Dm-CK2-β and Dm-CK2-β′

Protein	Function	Protein	Function
Fax	Axon connectivity	Nopp140	Cajal body protein
EloB/Elongin-B	Wing cell identity	Otefin	Germline stem cell renewal

Interactions shared with CK2-α in the DPiM database or those revealed by genetic studies are highlighted in red. Unnamed genes are indicated by their annotation symbol (CG#).

7.3. Interactors of Dm-CK2-β

Unique interactors of Dm-CK2-β encompass proteins involved in protein folding and turnover, chromatin structure and transcriptional control, cytoskeleton, cell cycle progression, RNA-processing, and neuronal development. Remarkably, only, dMi-2, a protein involved in nucleosome remodeling, has also been identified as a target for CK2 in genetic studies (see Tables 1 and 4). In contrast, four interactors of Dm-CK2-β, i.e., Dek, Dre-4, Ssrp and Scf, have also been isolated as interactors of Dm-CK2-α (see Table 3). It will be of interest to determine if these four proteins directly interact with Dm-CK2-α or Dm-CK2-β, or represent proteins that interact with the reconstituted holoenzyme in S2 cells. The remaining proteins interact exclusively with Dm-CK2-β, consistent with the view that some targets of CK2 such as Hairy [90], Raf [138], etc., can interact only through interaction with this regulatory subunit.

7.4. Interactors of Dm-CK2-β′

The interactors of Dm-CK2-β′ are not as extensive as those for Dm-CK2-β (Table 4), and include regulators of signaling, chromatin structure, DNA-replication/damage-response, etc. It is somewhat unexpected that proteins that interact with Dm-CK2-β and Dm-CK2-β′ do not overlap extensively. This preferential interaction partner specificity may underlie the ability of Dm-CK2-β′ to elicit dominant lethality upon ubiquitous expression (see above), whereby the inappropriate (spatial and/or temporal) presence of this subunit results in the formation of the CK2-β′-containing holoenzyme (α2β′2) due to competition for a common pool of CK2-α. Given the distinct "interactome", this alteration in the CK2 holoenzyme could diminish phosphorylation of proteins by the endogenous α2β2 holoenzyme or redirect activity to substrates incompatible with normal cellular and organismal viability.

7.5. Interactors Shared between Dm-CK2-β and -β′

Of the interacting proteins identified in the DPiM database, only four (Fax, Elongin-B, Otefin and Nopp140) are shared between Dm-CK2-β and -β′. Of interest is Nopp140 (see Table 4). Nopp140 is a highly conserved phosphoprotein that shuttles cargo between the nucleolus and the cytosol [139], and is thought to be critical in proliferative cells for Cajal body functions. While this protein has a native mass of ~70 kDa (as predicted from its gene structure), it appears as a 140 kDa polypeptide, primarily due to CK2-dependent phosphorylation. It has been estimated that Nopp140 may be phosphorylated at ≥70 sites within its C-terminal region, which is rich in Ser and Asp residues, and is conserved between Drosophila and mammals. These modifications, which confer a highly negative charge to the C-terminal domain, appear necessary for in vivo functioning of Nopp140, i.e., binding cargo proteins that contain nuclear localization signals (NLS). Interestingly, Nopp140 was not identified in the DPiM database as an interactor of Dm-CK2α (see Table 3), suggesting that CK2 targets this protein in a β/β′-dependent manner. Its identification as an interactor of both Dm-CK2-β and Dm-CK2-β′ strongly suggests that Nopp140 is modified by CK2 in all cells regardless of the expression patterns of these two CK2-β homologues, which would not be surprising given cell autonomous roles for this phospho-protein, and because loss of Nopp140 is cell lethal.

Together, the interactors of CK2 identified through combined biochemical/genetic approaches and the DPiM database reveal that our current knowledge of the Dm-CK2 "interactome" is, at best, partial, and the absence of developmentally important/relevant targets suggests that a case-by-case approach may still be required to identify its targets in Drosophila.

8. Roles of CK2 in Drosophila Eye Development

The functions of CK2 in other developmental programs have been inferred from tissue-specific and ectopic overexpression of the CK2-DN (Tik) mutant protein, RNAi against CK2 subunits in otherwise wild-type flies, or upon expression of CK2 target proteins harboring Ala/Asp mutations at known sites for phosphorylation. This has been achieved in large part due to the availability of the tissue-specific binary Gal4-UAS system [140–142], which enables genotype/phenotype relationships to be evaluated with mutants that would otherwise be dominantly lethal. Using this approach, it has been found that CK2 plays an important role in Notch signaling during development of two sensory organs (eye and bristle), through its targeting of the bHLH transcription factors E(spl)-M8, -M7, and -M5 [84], which are terminal effectors of this pathway [143–145]. In the following section, we review key findings on the roles of CK2 in eye development with an emphasis on its functions in early retinal neurogenesis, the potential implications on early neurogenesis in the mammalian retina, emerging data supporting the likelihood that this protein kinase plays additional roles in the developing eye, and conclude with a review of potentially new targets for this protein kinase.

Studies from our laboratory are revealing the importance of CK2 to the Notch signaling pathway during Drosophila eye development, with direct implications for a similar process in mammals, i.e., the specification of the Retinal Ganglion Cells (RGCs). Here, we focus on the Notch pathway in Drosophila, a preeminent genetic model that has been instrumental in the identification of the core components and regulators of this pathway, and has laid the foundations for our understanding of the mechanisms of Notch signaling [146–150], its importance to the development of other animals [148,151] and its association with disease states [152–156]. Although Notch signaling regulates diverse developmental programs, studies from our laboratory have primarily focused on its regulation by CK2 in early eye development.

The Drosophila eye has served as a model for understanding cell proliferation, cell signaling, polarity, specification and differentiation [157–159]. The compound eye of Drosophila is composed of ~750 units called ommatidia (also known as facets) which are patterned in a precise pseudo-crystalline array. Each facet is composed of eight photoreceptor neurons (Retinula cells, R1–R8), 12 accessory non-neuronal cells, and one sensory inter-ommatidial bristle (IOB). The precise hexagonal geometry of the adult eye and its constituent cell types are both essential for proper visual perception, reasons for which these features are highly conserved across all insects.

Eye development initiates during the third larval stage (see Figure 2), and involves progressive stages of cell specification and morphogenesis of a monolayer neuro-epithelium called the eye/antennal disc (eye anlagen). This onset of retinal neurogenesis is marked by the specification of the first photoreceptors, the R8 cells, and occurs in a wave of cell specification called the Morphogenetic Furrow (MF, see Figure 2A). In contrast to the specification of the R8 cells in the MF, recruitment of all secondary photoreceptors (R1–R7) occurs posterior to it. The MF therefore represents a 48-hour window of development that covers all retinal neurogenesis. For a more detailed description of R8 cell specification and roles in this sensory organ, see Reference [160]. In Drosophila, the bHLH transcription factor Atonal (Ato) specifies the R8 photoreceptors [161], which subsequently recruit all later retinal cell types' characteristic of the ommatidium (see above). The R8s are not clonally derived, and each is the outcome of inductive recruitment that occurs in a precise spatial/temporal manner. Hence, in the absence of Ato, no R8s or other retinal cells form, thus ablating the eye. Likewise, a defect in human *Atoh7* elicits blindness due to a loss of RGCs and the optic nerve [162], suggesting that lessons learned from fruit flies are applicable to mammals. R8/RGC patterning demands controlled repression of Ato/Atoh7 by the Enhancer of split (E(spl)) proteins (called Hes in vertebrates [163,164]), which also pattern other tissues and whose regulation by CK2 is now well understood (see below). Hence, the regulation of E(spl) activity during R8 patterning is broadly applicable and relevant to understanding Notch-dependent human developmental disorders.

During R8 ontogeny, Ato expression initiates as a stripe at the leading edge (stage-1) of the MF (Figure 2A). Cell-autonomous *ato* auto-activation [165] then produces pre-R8 cell clusters [166], the intermediate groups (IGs, see Figure 2A). Notch signaling through E(spl) proteins then acts to repress Ato (non-autonomously) at stage-2/3 in all but one cell from each IG [167]. That cell continues to maintain *senseless* (*sens*) expression and differentiates as an R8 [168,169]. The other cells of each IG remain in a non-neural (undifferentiated) state. This binary cell fate determination is termed lateral inhibition, and functions similarly during bristle patterning [170,171]. Repression of Ato by E(spl) proteins is therefore key to generating patterned R8s posterior to the MF (Figure 2A). One unusual aspect of Notch signaling during R8 ontogeny is that Notch is necessary for proper expression of the proneural protein Ato at stage-1, as well as that of the E(spl) repressors at stage-2/3 [172]. Given that the MF is a moving wave, cells at stage-1 are separated from those at stage-2/3 by ~5–10 min [173]. How Notch achieves these two mutually antagonistic functions within this short time frame remains unclear. In canonical Notch signaling, receptor activation elicits cleavage of the Notch intracellular domain (NICD) and its translocation to the nucleus to effect target gene activation [174]. It is difficult to envision how this mode of gene regulation rapidly switches from proneural to repressive modes. Our work (see below) suggests that CK2 plays a crucial role in enforcing a short temporal delay such that the repressive effects of Notch only manifest at stage-2/3 of the MF (Figure 2B). In a sense, CK2 may thus "decouple" these two phases of Notch signaling.

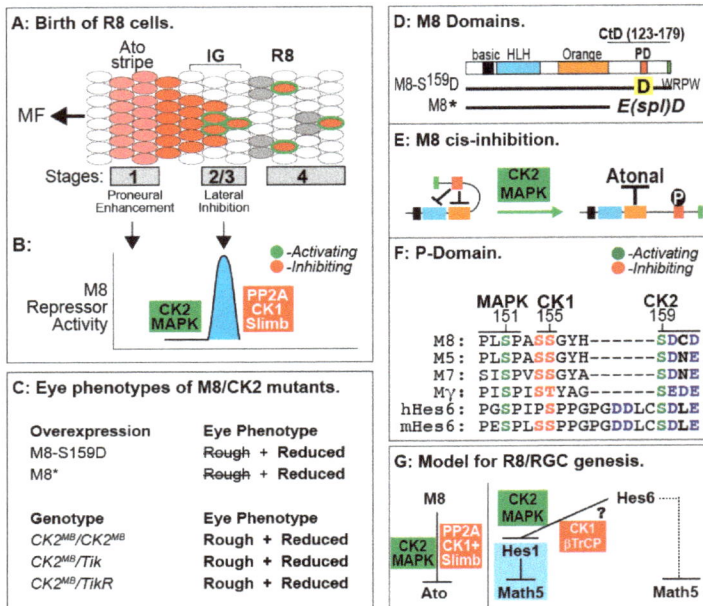

Figure 2. (**A**) R8 birth; Ato (pink/red), Sens (blue) and secondary R cells (grey); (**B**) CK2 and Mitogen Activated Protein Kinase (MAPK) activate M8 at stage-2/3 of the MF, and after R8 selection, PP2A and CK1 + Slimb mediate inactivation and/or destruction; (**C**) Eye phenotypes of CK2 and M8 mutants; (**D**) Functional domains in M8, and location of the phosphorylation domain (PD) in the C-terminal domain (CtD). The WRPW motif in M8 binds the essential co-repressor Groucho, and M8* (the product of the *E(spl)D* mutation) eliminates the CtD; (**E**) Regulation of cis-inhibited M8 by CK2 and MAPK. Note that in cis-inhibited M8, the PD blocks either HLH (blue) or Orange domains preventing interaction with Atonal; (**F**) Conservation of the PD in Drosophila M8/M5/M7/My and human/mouse Hes6; (**G**) Model for CK2 regulation of Drosophila M8 and mammalian Hes6. Dotted line denotes non-canonical mode of Hes6 action.

As mentioned above, E(spl) protein expression is necessary to resolve a single R8 from each IG. The *E(spl)Complex* encodes seven homologous and highly conserved bHLH repressors [144,145], of which M8, My and Mδ are expressed in the MF [175]. While loss of the *E(spl)C* elicits the abnormal specification of extra ("twinned") R8s from an IG [167], over-expression of M8/My/Mδ (at stage-2/3) does not dominantly repress Ato or the R8 fate [172,176,177]. The importance of M8 in Ato repression is highlighted by the *E(spl)D* mutation. This mutation, serendipitously identified in the 1950s [178,179], encodes M8* lacking its C-terminal domain (CtD, Figure 2C,D) and potently represses Ato, thus ablating R8s and the eye [177,180]. The mechanism underlying the hyperactivity of M8* remained an enigma, until we discovered that the E(spl) proteins are targeted by CK2 [84]. Specifically, CK2 interacts with and phosphorylates E(spl)-M8, -M7 and -M5; this modification targets a highly conserved phosphorylation domain (PD) located within the CtD (see Figure 2D,F). Remarkably, replacement of the CK2 phosphoacceptor of M8, Ser^{159}, with Asp (Figure 2D) results in a variant that ablates eye development via a mechanism virtually identical to that of M8* (Figure 2C, and see [84]). Phosphorylation displaces the autoinhibitory CtD, to expose the Orange domain and permit binding and repression of Ato (Figure 2E), a regulation that is circumvented by CtD deletion in M8* [181]. Consistent with a role in M8 repression of Ato, reduced CK2 activity elicits "twinned" R8s [182], as occurs upon excessive expression of Ato [183] or upon loss of *E(spl)C* [167]. These findings thus demonstrate that CK2 is a key participant of Notch signaling at the onset of eye development.

More recent studies are revealing that regulation of M8 activity involves multi-site PTM of the P-domain, and this involves activation of M8 by the kinases CK2 + MAPK [184], whereas inactivation involves the phosphatase PP2A, either alone or in combination with CK1 plus Slimb (βTrCP, see Figure 2B). Such a model posits that controlled activation and inactivation ensures that repressive effects of M8 occur in a spatially and/or temporally controlled manner. This mode of regulation could enable Notch to signal in a "pulsatile" manner, akin to that during genesis of somites. We believe that this mode of signal regulation may have direct implications on birth of RGCs in mammals, where Math5 (murine Ato homolog 5) expressivity is refined through Hes repressors (the homologues of fly E(spl) proteins). Specifically, previous studies have demonstrated that Hes6 (the homologue of fly M8) harbors a highly conserved P-domain that is targeted by CK2 and MAPK [185,186], and conserves sites for CK1 and βTrCP (Figure 2F). Furthermore, CK2 phosphorylation of mouse Hes6 also mediates its interaction with Hes1, the repressor of Math5/Atoh7 [187–190]. The role of Hes6 phosphorylation during RGC birth remains unknown; a possible model is discussed in the next section.

9. Lessons from Drosophila R8 Cells Applied to Birth of Mammalian RGCs

The striking parallels between the fly R8 and mammalian RGC [191], and the conserved P-domain (Figure 2F,G) begs the question of the role(s) of CK2, CK1 and βTrCP in the regulation of Hes6. Like the R8 cell, RGC patterning requires repression of Math5/Atoh7 by Hes1 [189,190,192–194]. This activity of Hes1 is, in turn, antagonized by Hes6 through protein–protein interactions, which (in cultured neuronal cells) requires phosphorylation of Hes6 by CK2 [187]. Post-translational regulation of Hes6 may have two distinct outcomes (Figure 2G). In the canonical mode (Figure 2G, blue box), CK2 would promote Hes6 inhibition of Hes1, thereby favoring Math5 activity and the RGC fate. In contrast, CK1 + βTrCP would promote Hes6 degradation, thereby permitting Hes1 to repress Math5 and the RGC fate. If so, the signaling circuit in the mammalian retina would be the inverse of that in flies. In a less likely alternative, Hes6 directly antagonizes Math5. If so, CK2 would promote Hes6 inhibition of Math5 and the RGC fate, while CK1 + βTrCP would promote, a mechanism akin to that in flies. However, this latter model would require that Hes6 has altered partner preference during RGC patterning. We predict that the expression of normal and mutant Hes6 (refractory to or mimicking CK2, MAPK, CK1 or βTrCP sites) in the early embryonic mouse retina may resolve the role and regulation of Hes6 during RGC birth and which of these two models is correct. In addition to the retina, post-translational regulation of Hes6 may occur elsewhere, given that Hes6 plays roles in late embryogenesis, myogenesis [195–197], and postnatal development [198,199], and its overexpression is linked to gliomas and breast and prostate cancer [200–202]. Our findings in Drosophila may aid efforts to answer similar questions in the more complex mouse model, and determine if mis-regulated Hes6 activity is linked to disease states.

10. Additional Roles of CK2 during Drosophila Eye Development

Unlike the role of CK2 during (Notch-dependent) birth of R8 cells, its roles later in eye development, i.e., the recruitment of R1–R7 photoreceptors have not been forthcoming. For example, after birth of R8s, Notch signaling is required in a reiterative manner for the specification of the R1–R7 cells, which are born in a precise order. These include, in order, the R2/R5, R3/R4, R1/R6 followed by the R7 cell. The hypomorphic allele of *Dm-CK2-α* called *CK2α-MB00477* (abbreviated as *CK2α^{MB}*, see Table 2) is the first mutation that directly implicates roles for CK2 at multiple stages of eye development. Importantly, this mutation provides "forward" genetic evidence, which is generally considered to be a benchmark in the field of Drosophila genetics. Our analyses of this mutation (Figure 1A) reveal that *CK2^{MB}* homozygous animals, or those that are trans-heterozygous with *Tik* or *TikR*, complete the third larval stage and die at the mid-pupal transition. As these animals are competent to transition through these two critical stages of development (relative to the onset of retinal neurogenesis, see Figure 1A), the compound eyes can be evaluated (for patterning and size) following their dissection from the pupal case. These animals display a highly perturbed eye, which is both rough in appearance and significantly (~50%) reduced in size (Figure 2C), and these defects are completely rescued by expression of a *tub-Dm-CK2-α* construct (Bandyopadhyay and Bidwai, in preparation). The former (rough eye) phenotype results from impaired lateral inhibition, i.e., the defective refinement of a single R8 from an IG. On its own, a defect in lateral inhibition cannot account for the reduced eye field, raising the likelihood that this phenotype may arise from defective recruitment of secondary photoreceptors due to defective (reduced) phosphorylation of additional CK2 targets in the developing eye.

11. Potential CK2 Targets Identified Via the Transcriptome of the Developing Eye

The complex eye defects of $CK2^{MB}/CK2^{MB}$ homozygous animals raise the prospect that CK2 plays additional roles in eye development, beyond that required for controlling R8 patterning through its regulation of E(spl)-M8 (see above). To reveal eye-specific proteins that may be regulated by CK2, we analyzed the "transcriptome" of the developing eye disc to identify additional targets of CK2. This sequence based prediction for high likelihood CK2 targets is facilitated by earlier studies that defined the substrate specificity of CK2, the consensus recognition, and the impact of amino acids vicinal to the phospho-acceptor (Ser/Thr). The following general principles have emerged for CK2; (1) it is an acidophilic protein kinase; (2) the substrate specificity is best described as S/T-E/D-x-D/E; (3) the presence of additional Asp/Glu residues either N- or C-terminal to the phosphoacceptor(s) further enhances phosphorylation of target proteins; (4) phosphorylation is negatively impacted by basic residues such as Arg/Lys since the presence of these residues within the consensus abrogates targeting by CK2; and (5) the presence of phospho-Ser/Thr (pSer/pThr) C-terminal to the primary phosphoacceptor augments targeting by CK2, revealing that this enzyme can participate in hierarchical phosphorylation either alone or in concert with other protein kinases. It should, however, be noted that some sites may be solvent exposed, but inaccessible in the tertiary structure, so this approach is, at best, predictive.

Eye disc specific gene expression patterns were identified from Flybase (flybase.org), and queried for proteins predicted to harbor CK2 consensus sites. Although protein abundance, regions of intrinsic disorder and stoichiometry appear to correlate with phospho-site conservation [203–205], we did not incorporate these principles into our analyses, because much of this information is still lacking for the proteome of the developing eye anlagen. The first round of analysis only included sequences from *D. melanogaster*, and this identified ~180 genes. Subsequently, homologous proteins were identified from 11 other fully sequenced and annotated Drosophila species (flybase.org) that encompass $~60 \times 10^6$ years of evolution [206,207], with the expectation that only high probability CK2 target sites with functional importance should be resilient through this time frame. The list of potential targets (Table 5) therefore only includes homologous proteins in which the CK2 site is conserved in all 12 species.

As is evident from Table 5, this list of high likelihood targets of CK2 includes 58 proteins regulating diverse aspects of eye development. Here, we review these proteins in accordance with their structural classification, biochemical functions and mutant phenotypes.

Table 5. Genes expressed in the developing eye with conserved CK2 sites.

Gene	WebLogo of CK2 Site(s)	Function
Acinus (Acn)		RNA splicing
Anterior Open (Aop)		Transcription Factor
Asteroid (Ast)		EGFR signaling
AXIN1 upregulated 1 (Axud1)		Cell proliferation
Cadherin 86C (Cad86C)		Cell adhesion/signaling
Cadherin N (CadN)		Cell adhesion/signaling
Capicua (Cic)		HMG family Transcription Factor
Claspin		ATR-Chk1 checkpoint pathway
Cubitus Interruptus (Ci)		Transcription Factor
Cullin 1 (Cul1)		Ubiquitin Ligase
Cullin 3 (Cul3)		Ubiquitin Ligase
Decapo (Dap)		CDK inhibitor
Daughter of Sevenless (Dos)		Sevenless RTK signaling
Decay		Regulator of apoptosis
Distal Antenna (Dan)		Transcription Factor
Distal antenna related (Danr)		Transcription Factor
Domino (Dom)		SNF2/RAD54 helicase family
Ebi		Chromatin binding
EGF-Receptor (EGFR)		RTK signaling
ELAV		Neurogenesis
Eyegone (Eyg)		Pax family transcription factor
Eyeless (Ey)		Transcription factor
Eyes Absent (Eya)		Transcription factor
Fat Facets (Faf)		Ubiquitin Ligase
Garnet (G)		Clathrin coatomer adaptor
Glass (Gl)		Transcription factor
Golden Goal (Gogo)		Axon guidance
GP150		Eye development
Head involution defective (Hid)		Cell death
Homeodomain interacting Kinase (HipK)		Eye development
IP3-Receptor		Inositol 1,4,5-tris-phosphate Receptor
Kismet (Kis)		Transcription factor
Klarsicht (Klar)		Kinesin binding
Klumpfuss (Klu)		Zinc finger protein
Liprin-γ		Sterile α motif
Liquid Facets (Lqf)		Ubiquitin binding and eye development
Neuralized (Neur)		E3 ubiquitin ligase
Osa		Transcription coactivator

Table 5. *Cont.*

Gene	WebLogo of CK2 Site(s)	Function
PDGF/VEGF related factor 1	SDND	Cell signaling
Pointed (Pnt)	TDPD	Transcription factor
Prickle (Pk)	SDDD TDEE	Regulates planar cell polarity
RapGAP1	TEHE TEEE TEGD	GTPase activating protein
Regulator of eph expression (Reph)	TESD SDGE	Ephrin signaling
Ret Oncogene (Ret)	TEAE	RTK signaling
Scribbler (Sbb)	TEPD	Transcription factor
Serrate (Ser)	TDID SEDD	Notch signaling
Seven in absentia (Sina)	TEHE	Regulation of R7 differentiation
Shaven (dPax2)	SEDD	D-Pax2 family transcription factor
Snf5-related 1 (Snr1)	TDAE	Chromatin structure
Sine Oculis (SO)	SDDD	Transcription factor
SoxNeuro (SoxN)	SEAE	Transcription factor
Spineless	SEAD	Regulates Rhodopsin expression
Spinster	SDSD	Regulates TGF-β/BMP signaling
Star	TEYD	EGF signaling and eye development
Sugarless	TEWD	Signaling in eye development
Target of wit (Twit)	SDHE	Eye development
Terribly reduced optic lobe (Trol)	TEGD	Cell polarity and signaling
Tolkin (Tok)	TDID	Negative regulator of gene expression
α-catenin	TDTE TEFE TEED	Actin binding

11.1. Transcription Factors

Of the ~60 interactors, >30% (21 out of 58) represent transcription factors or proteins that impact gene expression through modification of chromatin structure. Notably, two of these, e.g., Eyeless (Ey) and Eyegone (Eyg), are transcription factors that lie at the apex of the retinal neurogenesis hierarchy, a class of proteins called the "retinal determination" (RD) genes (for reviews, see [208–210]). This view reflects the remarkable findings from the laboratory of the late Walter Gehring (Basel) that ectopic expression of the Ey gene induces the formation of ectopic eyes in non-retinal tissues such as the wings, legs, and antenna [211]. This remarkable ability reflects the fact that Ey induces the transcription of additional RD-genes such as Sine Oculis (SO) and Eyes Absent (Eya) [212–214]. Both SO and Eya are predicted to be targets of CK2 (see Table 5), and studies from our laboratory have now confirmed this to be the case for SO (Majot and Bidwai, unpublished). The possibility that CK2 may regulate four critical eye-determination transcription factors (Ey, Eyg, SO and Eya) may underlie the complex eye defects of $CK2^{MB}/CK2^{MB}$ animals (Figure 2C). The potential targeting of Eyg is an excellent example for evaluating the emergence of orthologues. The Drosophila genome encodes two such genes, *Eyg* and *Twin of Eyegone* (*Toe*). Eyg harbors the CK2 consensus site DSDEEINV (bold residue is likely to be targeted by CK2), whereas the corresponding site on Toe is EEEEVINV. Because the D/E residues mimic Ser^{P04}, it raises the possibility that Eyg is CK2-regulated whereas Toe is CK2-independent. It will therefore be of interest to determine if Eyg is modified by CK2, identify the site(s) of phosphorylation, and determine the in vivo activities using its ability to elicit ectopic eye formation. Conversely, it would also be of interest to conduct domain swapping experiments to determine if Toe can be rendered CK2-dependent. Such studies could better illuminate the relevance of CK2 to these critical eye-specific TFs.

11.2. Signaling Pathways

Cell signaling is vital for most developmental programs. Two important and intersecting pathways are Notch and EGFR. While our previous work has revealed the centrality of CK2 to Notch pathway output in the developing eye and bristle (Section 8, see above), the role of this kinase in EGFR/Sevenless (Sev) signaling has not heretofore been suspect. While CK2 regulation of Raf, a mediator of EGFR/Sev signaling in flies is known [53] and shares many similarities to that in mammals, if/how Raf phosphorylation fine-tunes signaling has remained obscure. In addition to EGFR itself, CK2 consensus sites are conserved in several components regulating this pathway such as Asteroid, Daughter-of-Sevenless, Ret, and Sina, across ~60×10^6 years of Drosophila evolution. While Notch and EGFR have been generally thought to play opposing roles during development [215,216], our findings that EGFR/MAPK signaling is necessary for activity of the Notch effector E(spl)-M8 (Section 8, see above) make it likely that the former proposal is an oversimplification. If CK2 were to stimulate EGFR/MAPK signaling, it would place CK2 at the heart of the repressive effects of Notch signaling, without which R8 photoreceptors could not be patterned in the developing eye, which would perturb all subsequent steps of retinal neurogenesis, adult eye architecture, and vision. Given this possibility, a full and proper biochemical and genetic investigation of these RTK signaling components seems warranted.

11.3. Protein Turnover

Controlled protein turnover lies at the heart of eye development, wherein controlled degradation of transcription factors such as E(spl)-M8 seems necessary to allow timely termination of Notch signaling. We think that degradation, in principle, could be broadly applicable to all aspects of Notch signaling. Among the proteins identified as potential targets of CK2 are Neuralized (Neur), Fat-Facets (Faf), and Liquid-Facets (Lqf). Neur, a member of the RING family E3 ubiquitin ligase, is a key component of Notch signaling pathway, wherein it regulates activation of the Notch ligand via endocytosis [217,218]. In contrast, Faf is a de-ubiquitination (DUB) enzyme that negatively regulates RTK/Ras/MAPK signaling [219,220], whereas Lqf possesses Ubiquitin-interaction motifs [221]. Mutations in all three, Neur, Faf and Lqf, are associated with defects in eye development, and thus it will be of interest to determine how CK2 phosphorylation regulates these three proteins.

11.4. Regulators of the Cell Cycle, Cell Death, Cell Polarity and Cytoskeleton

Eye development hinges upon controlled proliferation of the eye anlagen, coordination of planar cell polarity that regulates photoreceptor positioning, cell death to remove excess non-specified and non-differentiated cells, and regulation of the cytoskeleton, which is necessary for formation of the MF, the apico-basal constriction that marks the initiation of retinal neurogenesis. Members controlling each of these aspects appear in the list of putative, highly conserved, targets for CK2. These include, proteins regulating the cell cycle such as the CDK inhibitor Decapo (Dap), the ATR-Chk1 checkpoint pathway component Claspin, and AXIN1 upregulated 1 (Axud1), and the well-known regulator of apoptosis Head involution defective (Hid). Other proteins regulating the cytoskeleton include Terribly reduced optic lobe (Trol), and Prickle, a key regulator of planar cell polarity in the developing eye.

Given the diverse array of potentially new targets of CK2 and the complex eye defects of $CK2^{MB}$ flies, a proper investigation of the proteome of the developing eye that is targeted by this kinase is warranted. Such studies will not only illuminate the extent to which CK2 regulates retinal neurogenesis in flies, but may also reveal new insights into its roles in mammalian eye development.

12. Summary and Future Perspectives

Many aspects of CK2 functions in Drosophila have emerged from studies from several laboratories. These include mutants, subunit diversity, functional non-redundancy of CK2-β homologues, interacting proteins and, importantly, the diverse roles played by this protein kinase during development. Many of these processes are likely to represent conserved features of animal development. The challenge before us is to decipher which roles are universally applicable, and which are specific to taxonomic groups. The availability of CK2 mutants with a perturbed eye now enables the application of phospho-proteomic studies, such as through the use of Phos-Tag to identify all phosphoproteins in the developing eye disc [222], rescue $CK2^{MB}/CK2^{MB}$ homozygous animals with a CK2α-Apex fusion [223,224] enabling direct identification of the CK2 "interactome", and finally through genome editing of individual CK2 target genes. Such studies, will, in due course, reveal the development-specific targets of DmCK2, and provide insights and routes to similar analysis in other vertebrate model organisms.

Acknowledgments: The work was supported, in part, by National Institutes of Health (NIH) grant (R01-EY015718) to Ashok P. Bidwai. No funds were received for covering the publication costs.

Author Contributions: M.B. and S.A. analyzed genome databases; M.B., C.P.B. and A.P.B. wrote the manuscript.

Conflicts of Interest: The authors declare no conflict of interest. The funding sponsors had no role in the design of the study; in the collection, analyses, or interpretation of data; in the writing of the manuscript, and in the decision to publish the results.

References

1. Burnett, G.; Kennedy, E.P. The enzymatic phosphorylation of proteins. *J. Biol. Chem.* **1954**, *211*, 969–980. [PubMed]
2. Krebs, E.G.; Graves, D.J.; Fischer, E.H. Factors affecting the activity of muscle phosphorylase b kinase. *J. Biol. Chem.* **1959**, *234*, 2867–2873. [PubMed]
3. Krebs, E.G. Protein phosphorylation and cellular regulation I (Nobel Lecture). *Angew. Chem.* **1993**, *32*, 1122–1129. [CrossRef]
4. Kennedy, E.P. Sailing to Byzantium. *Annu. Rev. Biochem.* **1992**, *61*, 1–28. [CrossRef] [PubMed]
5. Pinna, L.A. Protein kinase CK2: A challenge to canons. *J. Cell Sci.* **2002**, *115*, 3873–3878. [CrossRef] [PubMed]
6. Venerando, A.; Ruzzene, M.; Pinna, L.A. Casein kinase: The triple meaning of a misnomer. *Biochem. J.* **2014**, *460*, 141–156. [CrossRef] [PubMed]
7. Guerra, B.; Boldyreff, B.; Sarno, S.; Cesaro, L.; Issinger, O.G.; Pinna, L.A. CK2: A protein kinase in need of control. *Pharmacol. Ther.* **1999**, *82*, 303–313. [CrossRef]
8. Pinna, L.A. A historical view of protein kinase CK2. *Cell. Mol. Biol. Res.* **1994**, *40*, 383–390. [PubMed]
9. Filhol, O.; Martiel, J.L.; Cochet, C. Protein kinase CK2: A new view of an old molecular complex. *EMBO Rep.* **2004**, *5*, 351–355. [CrossRef] [PubMed]
10. Cozza, G.; Salvi, M.; Banerjee, S.; Tibaldi, E.; Tagliabracci, V.S.; Dixon, J.E.; Pinna, L.A. A new role for sphingosine: Up-regulation of Fam20C, the genuine casein kinase that phosphorylates secreted proteins. *Biochim. Biophys. Acta* **2015**, *1854*, 1718–1726. [CrossRef] [PubMed]
11. Tagliabracci, V.S.; Wiley, S.E.; Guo, X.; Kinch, L.N.; Durrant, E.; Wen, J.; Xiao, J.; Cui, J.; Nguyen, K.B.; Engel, J.L.; et al. A single kinase generates the majority of the secreted phosphoproteome. *Cell* **2015**, *161*, 1619–1632. [CrossRef] [PubMed]
12. Hathaway, G.M.; Traugh, J.A. Cyclic nucleotide-independant protein kinase from rabbit reticulocytes. Purification of casein kinases. *J. Biol. Chem.* **1979**, *254*, 762–768. [PubMed]
13. Hathaway, G.M.; Lubben, T.H.; Traugh, J.A. Inhibition of casein kinase II by heparin. *J. Biol. Chem.* **1980**, *255*, 8038–8041. [PubMed]
14. Hathaway, G.M.; Zoller, M.J.; Traugh, J.A. Identification of the catalytic subunit of casein kinase II by affinity labeling with 5′-p-fluorosulfonylbenzoyl adenosine. *J. Biol. Chem.* **1981**, *256*, 11442–11446. [PubMed]
15. Glover, C.V.C.; Shelton, E.R.; Brutlag, D.L. Purification and characterization of a type II casein kinase from *Drosophila melanogaster*. *J. Biol. Chem.* **1983**, *258*, 3258–3265. [PubMed]

16. Meggio, F.; Donella-Deana, A.; Brunati, A.M.; Pinna, L.A. Inhibition of rat liver cytosol casein kinases by heparin. *FEBS Lett.* **1982**, *141*, 257–262. [CrossRef]

17. Kuenzel, E.A.; Krebs, E.G. A synthetic substrate specific for casein kinase II. *Proc. Natl. Acad. Sci. USA* **1985**, *82*, 737–741. [CrossRef] [PubMed]

18. Kuenzel, E.A.; Mulligan, J.A.; Sommercorn, J.; Krebs, E.G. Substrate specificity determinants for casein kinase II as deduced from studies with synthetic peptides. *J. Biol. Chem.* **1987**, *262*, 9136–9140. [PubMed]

19. Meggio, F.; Marchiori, F.; Borin, G.; Chessa, G.; Pinna, L.A. Synthetic peptides including acidic clusters as substrates and inhibitors of rat liver casein kinase TS (type-2). *J. Biol. Chem.* **1984**, *259*, 14576–14579. [PubMed]

20. Marchiori, F.; Meggio, F.; Marin, O.; Borin, G.; Calderan, A.; Ruzza, P.; Pinna, L.A. Synthetic peptide substrates for casein kinase-2: Assessment of minimal structural requirements for phosphorylation. *Biochim. Biophys. Acta* **1988**, *971*, 332–338. [CrossRef]

21. Dahmus, M.E. Purification and properties of calf thymus casein kinase I and II. *J. Biol. Chem.* **1981**, *256*, 3319–3325. [PubMed]

22. Litchfield, D.W.; Lozeman, F.J.; Piening, C.; Sommercorn, J.; Takio, K.; Walsh, K.A.; Krebs, E.G. Subunit structure of casein kinase II from bovine testis. Demonstration that the α and α' subunits are distinct polypeptides. *J. Biol. Chem.* **1990**, *265*, 7638–7644. [PubMed]

23. Padmanabha, R.; Glover, C.V.C. Casein kinase II of yeast contains two distinct α polypeptides and an unusually large β subunit. *J. Biol. Chem.* **1987**, *262*, 1829–1835. [PubMed]

24. Bidwai, A.P.; Reed, J.C.; Glover, C.V.C. Casein kinase II of *Saccharomyces cerevisiae* contains two distinct regulatory subunits, β and β'. *Arch. Biochem. Biophys.* **1994**, *309*, 348–355. [CrossRef] [PubMed]

25. Boldyreff, B.; James, P.; Staudenmann, W.; Issinger, O.-G. Ser2 is the autophosphorylation site in the β subunit from bicistronically expressed human casein kinase-2 and from native rat liver casein kinase-2β. *Eur. J. Biochem.* **1993**, *218*, 515–521. [CrossRef] [PubMed]

26. Rigobello, M.P.; Jori, E.; Carignani, G.; Pinna, L.A. Isolation and characterization of a Type II casein kinase (casein kinase-TS) from *Saccharomyces cerevisiae*. *FEBS Lett.* **1982**, *144*, 354–358. [CrossRef]

27. Cochet, C.; Chambaz, E.M. Oligomeric structure and catalytic activity of G type casein kinase. *J. Biol. Chem.* **1983**, *258*, 1403–1406. [PubMed]

28. Fiege, J.J.; Cochet, C.; Pirollet, F.; Chambaz, E.M. Identification of the catalytic subunit of an oligomeric casein kinase (G type). *Biochemistry* **1983**, *22*, 1452–1459. [CrossRef]

29. Meggio, F.; Brunati, A.M.; Pinna, L.A. Autophosphorylation of type 2 casein kinase TS at both its α- and β-subunits. *FEBS Lett.* **1983**, *160*, 203–208. [CrossRef]

30. Dahmus, G.K.; Glover, C.V.C.; Brutlag, D.; Dahmus, M.E. Similarities in structure and function of calf thymus and *Drosophila* casein kinase II. *J. Biol. Chem.* **1984**, *259*, 9001–9006. [PubMed]

31. Saxena, A.; Padmanabha, R.; Glover, C.V.C. Isolation and sequencing of cDNA clones encoding α and β subunits of *Drosophila melanogaster* casein kinase II. *Mol. Cell. Biol.* **1987**, *7*, 3409–3417. [CrossRef] [PubMed]

32. Padmanabha, R.; Chen-Wu, J.L.P.; Hanna, D.E.; Glover, C.V.C. Isolation, sequencing, and disruption of the yeast *CKA2* gene: Casein kinase II is essential for viability in *Saccharomyces cerevisiae*. *Mol. Cell. Biol.* **1990**, *10*, 4089–4099. [CrossRef] [PubMed]

33. Chen-Wu, L.P.J.; Padmanabha, R.; Glover, C.V.C. Isolation, sequencing, and disruption of the *CKA1* gene encoding the alpha subunit of yeast casein kinase II. *Mol. Cell. Biol.* **1988**, *8*, 4981–4990. [CrossRef] [PubMed]

34. Roussou, I.; Dretta, G. The Schizosaccharomyces pombe casein kinase II alpha and beta subunits: Evolutionary conservation and positive role for the beta subunits. *Mol. Cell. Biol.* **1994**, *14*, 576–586. [CrossRef] [PubMed]

35. Hu, E.; Rubin, C. Casein kinase II from *Caenorhabditis elegans*. Cloning, characterization, and developmental regulation of the gene encoding the beta subunit. *J. Biol. Chem.* **1991**, *266*, 19796–19802. [PubMed]

36. Hu, E.; Rubin, C.S. Expression of wild-type and mutated forms of the catalytic (alpha) subunit of Caenorhabditis elegans casein kinase II in Escherichia coli. *J. Biol. Chem.* **1990**, *265*, 20609–20615. [PubMed]

37. Hu, E.; Rubin, C.S. Casein kinase II from Caenorhabditis elegans: Properties and developmental regulation of the enzyme; cloning and sequence analysis of cDNA and the gene for the catalytic subunit. *J. Biol. Chem.* **1990**, *265*, 5072–5080. [PubMed]

38. Dobrowlska, G.; Boldyreff, B.; Issinger, O.G. Cloning and sequencing of the casein kinase 2 alpha subunit from Zea mays. *Biochim. Biophys. Acta* **1991**, *1129*, 139–140. [CrossRef]

39. Jedlicki, A.; Hinrichs, M.V.; Allende, C.C.; Allende, J.E. The cDNAs coding for the alpha- and beta- subunits of *Xenopus* laevis casein kinase II. *FEBS Lett.* **1992**, *297*, 280–284. [CrossRef]

40. Meisner, H.; Heller Harrison, R.; Buxton, J.; Czech, M.P. Molecular cloning of the human casein kinase II alpha subunit: Evidence for two genes. *Biochemistry* **1989**, *28*, 4072–4076. [CrossRef] [PubMed]

41. Jakobi, R.; Voss, H.; Pyerin, W. Human phosvitin/casein kinase type II: Molecular cloning and sequencing of full-length cDNA encoding subunit beta. *Eur. J. Biochem.* **1989**, *183*, 227–233. [CrossRef] [PubMed]

42. Lozeman, F.J.; Litchfield, D.W.; Piening, C.; Takio, K.; Walsh, K.A.; Krebs, E.G. Isolation and characterization of human cDNA clones encoding the alpha and alpha′ subunits of casein kinase II. *Biochemistry* **1990**, *29*, 8436–8447. [CrossRef] [PubMed]

43. Takio, K.E.; Kuenzel, K.A.; Walsh, K.A.; Krebs, E.G. Amino acid sequence of the b subunit of bovine lung casein kinase II. *Proc. Natl. Acad. Sci. USA* **1987**, *84*, 4851–4855. [CrossRef] [PubMed]

44. Bidwai, A.P.; Reed, J.C.; Glover, C.V.C. The phosphorylation of Calmodulin by the catalytic subunit of casein kinase II is inhibited by the regulatory subunit. *Arch. Biochem. Biophys.* **1993**, *300*, 265–270. [CrossRef] [PubMed]

45. Bidwai, A.P.; Hanna, D.E.; Glover, C.V.C. The free catalytic subunit of casein kinase II is not toxic in vivo. *J. Biol. Chem.* **1992**, *267*, 18790–18796. [PubMed]

46. Birnbaum, M.J.; Wu, J.; O′Reilley, D.R.; Rivera-Marrero, C.A.; Hanna, D.E.; Miller, L.K.; Glover, C.V.C. Expression, purification and characterization of Drosophila casein kinase II using the baculovirus system. *Protein Expr. Purif.* **1992**, *3*, 142–150. [PubMed]

47. Rasmussen, T.; Skjøth, I.H.E.; Jensen, H.H.; Niefind, K.; Boldyreff, B.; Issinger, O.G. Biochemical characterization of the recombinant human Drosophila homologues Timekeeper and Andante involved in the Drosophila circadian oscillator. *Mol. Cell. Biochem.* **2005**, *274*, 151–161. [CrossRef] [PubMed]

48. Meggio, F.; Boldyreff, B.; Issinger, O.-G.; Pinna, L.A. Casein kinase 2 down regulation and activation by polybasic peptides are mediated by acidic residues in the 55–64 region of the b-subunit: A study with calmodulin as phosphorylatable substrate. *Biochemistry* **1994**, *33*, 4336–4342. [CrossRef] [PubMed]

49. Hathaway, G.M.; Traugh, J.A. Interaction of polyamines and magnesium with casein kinase II. *Arch. Biochem. Biophys.* **1984**, *233*, 133–138. [CrossRef]

50. Hathaway, G.M.; Traugh, J.A. Kinetics of activation of casein kinase II by polyamines and reversal of 2,3-bisphosphoglycerate inhibition. *J. Biol. Chem.* **1984**, *259*, 2850–2855. [PubMed]

51. Nuutinen, M.; Londesborough, J. The stimulation of casein kinase II from yeast by polyamines occurs with endogenous substrates at cytosolic salt concentrations. *Second Messengers Phosphoprot.* **1988**, *12*, 197–205.

52. Sarno, S.; Marin, O.; Meggio, F.; Pinna, L.A. Polyamines as negative regulators of casein kinase II: The phosphorylation of calmodulin triggered by polylysine and by the α-[66–86] peptide is prevented by spermine. *Biochem. Biophys. Res. Commun.* **1993**, *194*, 83–90. [CrossRef] [PubMed]

53. Stark, F.; Pfannstiel, J.; Klaiber, I.; Raabe, T. Protein kinase CK2 links polyamine metabolism to MAPK signalling in Drosophila. *Cell. Signal.* **2011**, *23*, 876–882. [CrossRef] [PubMed]

54. Sommercorn, J.; Krebs, E.G. Induction of casein kinase II during differentiation of 3T3-L1 cells. *J. Biol. Chem.* **1987**, *262*, 3839–3843. [PubMed]

55. Sommercorn, J.; Mulligan, J.A.; Lozeman, F.J.; Krebs, E.G. Activation of casein kinase II in response to insulin and to epidermal growth factor. *Proc. Natl. Acad. Sci. USA* **1987**, *84*, 8834–8838. [CrossRef] [PubMed]

56. Lemmon, M.A.; Schlessinger, J. Cell signaling by receptor tyrosine kinases. *Cell* **2010**, *141*, 1117–1134. [CrossRef] [PubMed]

57. Xu, C.; Kauffmann, R.C.; Zhang, J.; Kladny, S.; Carthew, R.W. Overlapping activators and repressors delimit transcriptional response to receptor tyrosine kinase signals in the Drosophila eye. *Cell* **2000**, *103*, 87–97. [CrossRef]

58. Yarden, Y.; Ullrich, A. Growth factor receptor tyrosine kinases. *Annu. Rev. Biochem.* **1988**, *57*, 443–478. [CrossRef] [PubMed]

59. Litchfield, D.W.; Dobrowolska, G.; Krebs, E.G. Regulation of casein kinase II by growth factors: A reevaluation. *Cell. Mol. Biol. Res.* **1994**, *40*, 373–381. [PubMed]

60. Ole-MoiYoi, O.K.; Brown, W.C.; Iams, K.P.; Nayar, A.; Tsukamoto, T.; Macklin, M.D. Evidence for the induction of casein kinase II in bovine lymphocytes transformed by the intracellular protozoan parasite *Theileria parva*. *EMBO J.* **1993**, *12*, 1621–1631. [PubMed]

61. Seldin, D.C.; Leder, P. Casein kinase II alpha transgene-induced murine lymphoma: Relation to *Theileriosis* in cattle. *Science* **1995**, *267*, 894–897. [CrossRef] [PubMed]

62. Glover, C.V.C. A filamentous form of *Drosophila* casein kinase II. *J. Biol. Chem.* **1986**, *261*, 14349–14354. [PubMed]

63. Lolli, G.; Pinna, L.A.; Battistutta, R. Structural determinants of protein kinase CK2 regulation by autoinhibitory polymerization. *ACS Chem. Biol.* **2012**, *7*, 1158–1163. [CrossRef] [PubMed]

64. Ackerman, P.; Glover, C.V.C.; Osheroff, N. Phosphorylation of DNA topoisomerase II by casein kinase II: Modulation of eukaryotic topoismerase II activity in vitro. *Proc. Natl. Acad. Sci. USA* **1985**, *82*, 3164–3168. [CrossRef] [PubMed]

65. Ackerman, P.; Glover, C.V.C.; Osheroff, N. Phosphorylation of DNA topoisomerase II in vivo and in total homogenates of *Drosophila* Kc cells: The role of casein kinase II. *J. Biol. Chem.* **1988**, *263*, 12653–12660. [PubMed]

66. Cardenas, M.E.; Gasser, S.M. Regulation of toposiomerase II by phosphorylation: A role for casein kinase II. *J. Cell Biol.* **1993**, *104*, 219–225.

67. Cardenas, M.E.; Walter, R.; Hanna, D.; Gasser, S.M. Casein kinase II copurifies with yeast DNA topoisomerase II and re-activates the dephosphorylated enzyme. *J. Cell Biol.* **1993**, *104*, 533–543.

68. Cardenas, M.; Dang, Q.; Glover, C.V.C.; Gasser, S.M. Casein kinase II phosphorylates the eukaryote-specific C-terminal domain of topoisomerase II in vivo. *EMBO J.* **1992**, *11*, 1785–1796. [PubMed]

69. Franchin, C.; Salvi, M.; Arrigoni, G.; Pinna, L.A. Proteomics perturbations promoted by the protein kinase CK2 inhibitor quinalizarin. *Biochim. Biophys. Acta* **2015**, *1854*, 1676–1686. [CrossRef] [PubMed]

70. Venerando, A.; Franchin, C.; Cant, N.; Cozza, G.; Pagano, M.A.; Tosoni, K.; Al-Zahrani, A.; Arrigoni, G.; Ford, R.C.; Mehta, A.; et al. Detection of phospho-sites generated by protein kinase CK2 in CFTR: Mechanistic aspects of Thr1471 phosphorylation. *PLoS ONE* **2013**, *8*, e74232. [CrossRef] [PubMed]

71. Giot, L.; Bader, J.S.; Brouwer, C.; Chaudhuri, A.; Kuang, B.; Li, Y.; Hao, Y.L.; Ooi, C.E.; Godwin, B.; Vitols, E.; et al. A protein interaction map of *Drosophila melanogaster*. *Science* **2003**, *302*, 1727–1736. [CrossRef] [PubMed]

72. Guruharsha, K.G.; Obar, R.A.; Mintseris, J.; Aishwarya, K.; Krishnan, R.T.; Vijayraghavan, K.; Artavanis-Tsakonas, S. Drosophila Protein interaction Map (DPiM): A paradigm for metazoan protein complex interactions. *Fly (Austin)* **2012**, *6*, 246–253. [CrossRef] [PubMed]

73. Guruharsha, K.G.; Rual, J.F.; Zhai, B.; Mintseris, J.; Vaidya, P.; Vaidya, N.; Beekman, C.; Wong, C.; Rhee, D.Y.; Cenaj, O.; et al. A Protein Complex Network of *Drosophila melanogaster*. *Cell* **2011**, *147*, 690–703. [CrossRef] [PubMed]

74. Horiuchi, J.; Jiang, W.; Zhou, H.; Wu, P.; Yin, J.C. Phosphorylation of conserved casein kinase sites regulates cAMP-response element-binding protein DNA binding in Drosophila. *J. Biol. Chem.* **2004**, *279*, 12117–12125. [CrossRef] [PubMed]

75. Zhao, W.; Bidwai, A.P.; Glover, C.V.C. Interaction of casein kinase II with ribosomal protein L22 of *Drosophila melanogaster*. *Biochem. Biophys. Res. Commun.* **2002**, *298*, 60–66. [CrossRef]

76. Bulat, V.; Rast, M.; Pielage, J. Presynaptic CK2 promotes synapse organization and stability by targeting Ankyrin2. *J. Cell Biol.* **2014**, *204*, 77–94. [CrossRef] [PubMed]

77. Jaffe, L.; Ryoo, H.-D.; Mann, R.S. A role for phosphorylation by casein kinase II in modulating Antennapedia activity in Drosophila. *Genes Dev.* **1997**, *11*, 1327–1340. [CrossRef] [PubMed]

78. Yanagawa, S.-I.; Matsuda, Y.; Lee, J.-S.; Matsubayashi, H.; Sese, S.; Kadowaki, T.; Ishimoto, A. Casein kinase I phosphorylates the Armadillo protein and induces its degradation in Drosophila. *EMBO J.* **2002**, *21*, 1733–1742. [CrossRef] [PubMed]

79. Packman, L.C.; Kubota, K.; Parker, J.; Gay, N.J. Casein kinase II phosphorylates Ser468 in the PEST domain of the Drosophila IkappaB homologue cactus. *FEBS Lett.* **1997**, *400*, 45–50. [CrossRef]

80. Szabo, A.; Papin, C.; Zorn, D.; Ponien, P.; Weber, F.; Raabe, T.; Rouyer, F. The CK2 kinase stabilizes CLOCK and represses its activity in the Drosophila circadian oscillator. *PLoS Biol.* **2013**, *11*, e1001645. [CrossRef] [PubMed]

81. Willert, K.; Brink, M.; Wodarz, A.; Varmus, H.; Nusse, R. Casein kinase 2 associates with and phosphorylates Disheveled. *EMBO J.* **1997**, *16*, 3089–3096. [CrossRef] [PubMed]

82. Bouazoune, K.; Brehm, A. dMi-2 chromatin binding and remodeling activities are regulated by dCK2 phosphorylation. *J. Biol. Chem.* **2005**, *280*, 41912–41920. [CrossRef] [PubMed]

83. Karandikar, U.; Trott, R.L.; Yin, J.; Bishop, C.P.; Bidwai, A.P. *Drosophila* CK2 regulates eye morphogenesis via phosphorylation of E(spl)M8. *Mech. Dev.* **2004**, *121*, 273–286. [CrossRef] [PubMed]

84. Trott, R.L.; Kalive, M.; Paroush, Z.; Bidwai, A.P. *Drosophila melanogaster* casein kinase II interacts with and phosphorylates the basic-helix-loop-helix (bHLH) proteins M5, M7, and M8 derived from the *Enhancer of split Complex*. *J. Biol. Chem.* **2001**, *276*, 2159–2167. [CrossRef] [PubMed]

85. Bourbon, H.M.; Martin-Blanco, E.; Rosen, D.; Kornberg, T.B. Phosphorylation of the Drosophila engrailed protein at a site outside its homeodomain enhances DNA binding. *J. Biol. Chem.* **1995**, *270*, 11130–11139. [CrossRef] [PubMed]

86. Gelsthorpe, M.E.; Tan, Z.; Phillips, A.; Eissenberg, J.C.; Miller, A.; Wallace, J.; Tsubota, S.I. Regulation of the *Drosophila melanogaster* protein, enhancer of rudimentary, by casein kinase II. *Genetics* **2006**, *174*, 265–270. [CrossRef] [PubMed]

87. Siomi, M.C.; Higashijima, K.; Ishizuka, A.; Siomi, H. Casein kinase II phosphorylates the fragile X mental retardation protein and modulates its biological properties. *Mol. Cell. Biol.* **2002**, *22*, 8438–8447. [CrossRef] [PubMed]

88. Bonet, C.; Fernandez, I.; Aran, X.; Bernues, J.; Giralt, E.; Azorin, F. The GAGA protein of Drosophila is phosphorylated by CK2. *J. Mol. Biol.* **2005**, *351*, 562–572. [CrossRef] [PubMed]

89. Kwong, P.N.; Chambers, M.; Vashisht, A.A.; Turki-Judeh, W.; Yau, T.Y.; Wohlschlegel, J.A.; Courey, A.J. The central region of the Drosophila co-repressor Groucho as a Regulatory Hub. *J. Biol. Chem.* **2015**, *290*, 30119–30130. [CrossRef] [PubMed]

90. Kahali, B.; Trott, R.; Paroush, Z.; Allada, R.; Bishop, C.P.; Bidwai, A.P. *Drosophila* CK2 phosphorylates Hairy and regulates its activity in vivo. *Biochem. Biophys. Res. Commun.* **2008**, *373*, 637–642. [CrossRef] [PubMed]

91. Zhao, T.; Eissenberg, J.C. Phosphorylation of heterochromatin protein 1 by casein kinase II is required for efficient heterochromatin binding in Drosophila. *J. Biol. Chem.* **1999**, *274*, 15095. [CrossRef] [PubMed]

92. Hovhanyan, A.; Herter, E.K.; Pfannstiel, J.; Gallant, P.; Raabe, T. Drosophila mbm is a nucleolar myc and casein kinase 2 target required for ribosome biogenesis and cell growth of central brain neuroblasts. *Mol. Cell. Biol.* **2014**, *34*, 1878–1891. [CrossRef] [PubMed]

93. Li, M.; Strand, D.; Krehan, A.; Pyerin, W.; Heid, H.; Neumann, B.; Mechler, B.M. Casein kinase 2 binds and phosphorylates the nucleosomal assembly protein-1 (NAP1) in *Drosophila melanogaster*. *J. Mol. Biol.* **1999**, *293*, 1067–1084. [CrossRef] [PubMed]

94. Goldstein, R.E.; Cook, O.; Dinur, T.; Pisante, A.; Karandikar, U.C.; Bidwai, A.; Paroush, Z. An EH1-like motif in odd-skipped mediates recruitment of groucho and repression in vivo. *Mol. Cell. Biol.* **2005**, *25*, 10711–10720. [CrossRef] [PubMed]

95. Wong, L.C.; Costa, A.; McLeod, I.; Sarkeshik, A.; Yates, J., III; Kyin, S.; Perlman, D.; Schedl, P. The functioning of the Drosophila CPEB protein Orb is regulated by phosphorylation and requires casein kinase 2 activity. *PLoS ONE* **2011**, *6*, e24355. [CrossRef] [PubMed]

96. Taliaferro, J.M.; Marwha, D.; Aspden, J.L.; Mavrici, D.; Cheng, N.E.; Kohlstaedt, L.A.; Rio, D.C. The Drosophila splicing factor PSI is phosphorylated by casein kinase II and tousled-like kinase. *PLoS ONE* **2013**, *8*, e56401. [CrossRef] [PubMed]

97. Akten, B.; Tangredi, M.M.; Jauch, E.; Roberts, M.A.; Ng, F.; Raabe, T.; Jackson, F.R. Ribosomal s6 kinase cooperates with casein kinase 2 to modulate the Drosophila circadian molecular oscillator. *J. Neurosci.* **2009**, *29*, 466–475. [CrossRef] [PubMed]

98. Jia, H.; Liu, Y.; Xia, R.; Tong, C.; Yue, T.; Jiang, J.; Jia, J. Casein kinase 2 promotes Hedgehog signaling by regulating both smoothened and Cubitus interruptus. *J. Biol. Chem.* **2010**, *285*, 37218–37226. [CrossRef] [PubMed]

99. Cartier, E.; Hamilton, P.J.; Belovich, A.N.; Shekar, A.; Campbell, N.G.; Saunders, C.; Andreassen, T.F.; Gether, U.; Veenstra-Vanderweele, J.; Sutcliffe, J.S.; et al. Rare autism-associated variants implicate syntaxin 1 (STX1 R26Q) phosphorylation and the dopamine transporter (hDAT R51W) in dopamine neurotransmission and behaviors. *EBioMedicine* **2015**, *2*, 135–146. [CrossRef] [PubMed]

100. Hu, L.; Huang, H.; Li, J.; Yin, M.X.; Lu, Y.; Wu, W.; Zeng, R.; Jiang, J.; Zhao, Y.; Zhang, L. Drosophila casein kinase 2 (CK2) promotes warts protein to suppress Yorkie protein activity for growth control. *J. Biol. Chem.* **2014**, *289*, 33598–33607. [CrossRef] [PubMed]

101. Trott, R.L.; Kalive, M.; Karandikar, U.; Rummer, R.; Bishop, C.P.; Bidwai, A.P. Identification and characterization of proteins that interact with *Drosophila melanogaster* protein kinase CK2. *Mol. Cell. Biochem.* **2001**, *227*, 91–98. [CrossRef] [PubMed]

102. Bidwai, A.P.; Saxena, A.; Zhao, W.; McCann, R.O.; Glover, C.V.C. Multiple, closely spaced alternative 5′ exons in the DmCKII-β gene of *Drosophila melanogaster*. *Mol. Cell Biol. Res. Commun.* **2000**, *3*, 283–291. [CrossRef] [PubMed]

103. Shevelyov, Y.Y. Copies of Stellate gene variants are located in the X heterochromatin of *Drosophila melanogaster* and are probably expressed. *Genetics* **1992**, *132*, 1033–1037. [PubMed]

104. Palumbo, G.; Bonaccorsi, S.; Robbins, L.G.; Pimpinelli, S. Genetic analysis of Stellate elements of *Drosophila melanogaster*. *Genetics* **1994**, *138*, 1181–1197. [PubMed]

105. Livak, K.J. Detailed structure of the *Drosophila melanogaster Stellate* genes and their transcripts. *Genetics* **1990**, *124*, 303–316. [PubMed]

106. Bidwai, A.P.; Zhao, W.F.; Glover, C.V.C. A gene located at 56F1–2 in *Drosophila melanogaster* encodes a novel metazoan β-like subunit of casein kinase II. *Mol. Cell Biol. Res. Commun.* **1999**, *1*, 21–28. [CrossRef] [PubMed]

107. Karandikar, U.; Anderson, S.; Mason, N.; Trott, R.L.; Bishop, C.P.; Bidwai, A.P. The *Drosophila SSL* gene is expressed in larvae, pupae, and adults, exhibits sexual dimorphism, and mimics properties of the β subunit of casein kinase II. *Biochem. Biophys. Res. Commun.* **2003**, *301*, 941–947. [CrossRef]

108. Kalmykova, A.I.; Shevelyov, Y.Y.; Polesskaya, O.O.; Dobritsa, A.A.; Evstafieva, A.G.; Boldyreff, B.; Issinger, O.-G.; Gvozdev, V.A. CK2βtes gene encodes a testis-specific isoform of the regulatory subunit of casein kinase 2 in *Drosophila melanogaster*. *Eur. J. Biochem.* **2002**, *269*, 1418–1427. [CrossRef] [PubMed]

109. Kalmykova, A.I.; Dobritsa, A.A.; Gvozdev, V.A. Su(Ste) diverged tandem repeats in a *Y Chromosome* of *Drosophila melanogaster* are transcribed and variously processed. *Genetics* **1998**, *148*, 243–249. [PubMed]

110. Kalmykova, A.I.; Shevelyov, Y.Y.; Dobritsa, A.A.; Gvozdev, V.A. Acquisition and amplification of a testis-expressed autosomal gene, SSL, by the Drosophila *Y Chromosome*. *Proc. Natl. Acad. Sci. USA* **1997**, *94*, 6297–6302. [CrossRef] [PubMed]

111. Jauch, E.; Wecklein, H.; Stark, F.; Jauch, M.; Raabe, T. The *Drosophila melanogaster* DmCK2β transcription unit encodes for functionally non-redundant protein isoforms. *Gene* **2006**, *374*, 142–152. [CrossRef] [PubMed]

112. Chantalat, L.; Leroy, D.; Filhol, O.; Nueda, A.; Benitez, M.J.; Chambaz, E.M.; Cochet, C.; Dideberg, O. Crystal structure of the human protein kinase CK2 regulatory subunit reveals its zinc finger-mediated dimerization. *EMBO J.* **1999**, *18*, 2930–2940. [CrossRef] [PubMed]

113. Lin, J.M.; Kilman, V.L.; Keegan, K.; Paddock, B.; Emery-Le, M.; Rosbash, M.; Allada, R. A role for casein kinase 2α in the Drosophila circadian clock. *Nature* **2002**, *420*, 816–820. [CrossRef] [PubMed]

114. Kunttas-Tatli, E.; Bose, A.; Kahali, B.; Bishop, C.P.; Bidwai, A.P. Functional dissection of *Timekeeper (Tik.)* implicates opposite roles for CK2 and PP2A during *Drosophila* neurogenesis. *Genesis* **2009**, *47*, 647–658. [CrossRef] [PubMed]

115. Niefind, K.; Guerra, B.; Ermakowa, I.; Issinger, O.G. Crystal structure of human protein kinase CK2: Insights into basic properties of the CK2 holoenzyme. *EMBO J.* **2001**, *20*, 5320–5331. [CrossRef] [PubMed]

116. Niefind, K.; Guerra, B.; Pinna, L.A.; Issinger, O.G.; Schomburg, D. Crystal structure of the catalytic subunit of protein kinase CK2 from Zea mays at 2.1 A resolution. *EMBO J.* **1998**, *17*, 2451–2462. [CrossRef] [PubMed]

117. Hanna, D.E.; Rethinaswamy, A.; Glover, C.V.C. Casein kinase II is required for cell cycle progression during G1 and G2/M in *Saccharomyces cerevisiae*. *J. Biol. Chem.* **1995**, *270*, 25905–25914. [CrossRef] [PubMed]

118. Kuntamalla, P.; Kunttas, E.; Karandikar, U.; Bishop, C.; Bidwai, A. *Drosophila* protein kinase CK2 is rendered temperature-sensitive by mutations of highly conserved residues flanking the activation segment. *Mol. Cell. Biochem.* **2009**, *323*, 49–60. [CrossRef] [PubMed]

119. Toth-Petroczy, A.; Palmedo, P.; Ingraham, J.; Hopf, T.A.; Berger, B.; Sander, C.; Marks, D.S. Structured states of disordered proteins from genomic sequences. *Cell* **2016**, *167*, 158–170. [CrossRef] [PubMed]

120. Konopka, R.J.; Smith, R.F.; Orr, D. Characterization of Andante, a new Drosophila clock mutant, and its interactions with other clock mutants. *J. Neurogenet.* **1991**, *7*, 103–114. [CrossRef] [PubMed]

121. Konopka, R.J.; Benzer, S. Clock mutants of *Drosophila melanogaster*. *Proc. Natl. Acad. Sci. USA* **1971**, *68*, 2112–2116. [CrossRef] [PubMed]

122. Akten, B.; Jauch, E.; Genova, G.K.; Kim, E.Y.; Edery, I.; Raabe, T.; Jackson, F.R. A role for CK2 in the Drosophila circadian oscillator. *Nat. Neurosc.* **2003**, *6*, 251–257. [CrossRef] [PubMed]

123. Buchou, T.; Vernet, M.; Blond, O.; Jensen, H.; Pointu, H.; Olsen, B.; Cochet, C.; Issinger, O.; Boldyreff, B. Disruption of the regulatory beta subunit of protein kinase CK2 in mice leads to a cell-autonomous defect and early embryonic lethality. *Mol. Cell. Biol.* **2003**, *23*, 908–915. [CrossRef] [PubMed]

124. Yang, X.; Coulombe-Huntington, J.; Kang, S.; Sheynkman, G.M.; Hao, T.; Richardson, A.; Sun, S.; Yang, F.; Shen, Y.A.; Murray, R.R.; et al. Widespread expansion of protein interaction capabilities by alternative splicing. *Cell* **2016**, *164*, 805–817. [CrossRef] [PubMed]

125. Kalive, M.; Trott, R.L.; Bidwai, A.P. A gene located at 72A in *Drosophila melanogaster* encodes a novel zinc-finger protein that interacts with protein kinase CK2. *Mol. Cell. Biochem.* **2001**, *227*, 99–105. [CrossRef] [PubMed]

126. Halabi, N.; Rivoire, O.; Leibler, S.; Ranganathan, R. Protein sectors: Evolutionary units of three-dimensional structure. *Cell* **2009**, *138*, 774–786. [CrossRef] [PubMed]

127. McLaughlin, R.N., Jr.; Poelwijk, F.J.; Raman, A.; Gosal, W.S.; Ranganathan, R. The spatial architecture of protein function and adaptation. *Nature* **2012**, *491*, 138–142. [CrossRef] [PubMed]

128. Mumby, M. PP2A: Unveiling a reluctant tumor suppressor. *Cell* **2007**, *130*, 21–24. [CrossRef] [PubMed]

129. Cho, U.S.; Morrone, S.; Sablina, A.A.; Arroyo, J.D.; Hahn, W.C.; Xu, W. Structural basis of PP2A inhibition by small t antigen. *PLoS Biol.* **2007**, *5*, e202. [CrossRef] [PubMed]

130. Arroyo, J.D.; Hahn, W.C. Involvement of PP2A in viral and cellular transformation. *Oncogene* **2005**, *24*, 7746–7755. [CrossRef] [PubMed]

131. Bose, A.; Majot, A.T.; Bidwai, A.P. The Ser/Thr Phosphatase PP2A regulatory subunit *Widerborst* inhibits Notch signaling. *PLoS ONE* **2014**, *9*, e101884. [CrossRef] [PubMed]

132. Jia, H.; Liu, Y.; Yan, W.; Jia, J. PP4 and PP2A regulate Hedgehog signaling by controlling Smo and Ci phosphorylation. *Development* **2009**, *136*, 307–316. [CrossRef] [PubMed]

133. Silverstein, A.M.; Barrow, C.A.; Davis, A.J.; Mumby, M.C. Actions of PP2A on the MAP kinase pathway and apoptosis are mediated by distinct regulatory subunits. *Proc. Natl. Acad. Sci. USA* **2002**, *99*, 4221–4226. [CrossRef] [PubMed]

134. Banreti, A.; Lukacsovich, T.; Csikos, G.; Erdelyi, M.; Sass, M. PP2A regulates autophagy in two alternative ways in Drosophila. *Autophagy* **2012**, *8*, 623–636. [CrossRef] [PubMed]

135. Margolis, S.S.; Perry, J.A.; Forester, C.M.; Nutt, L.K.; Guo, Y.; Jardim, M.J.; Thomenius, M.J.; Freel, C.D.; Darbandi, R.; Ahn, J.H.; et al. Role for the PP2A/B56delta phosphatase in regulating 14-3-3 release from Cdc25 to control mitosis. *Cell* **2006**, *127*, 759–773. [CrossRef] [PubMed]

136. Heriche, J.K.; Lebrin, F.; Rabilloud, T.; Leroy, D.; Chambaz, E.M.; Goldberg, Y. Regulation of protein phosphatase 2A by direct interaction with casein kinase 2alpha. *Science* **1997**, *276*, 952–955. [CrossRef] [PubMed]

137. Warner, J.R.; McIntosh, K.B. How common are extraribosomal functions of ribosomal proteins. *Mol. Cell* **2009**, *34*, 3–11. [CrossRef] [PubMed]

138. Boldyreff, B.; Issinger, O.G. A-Raf kinase is a new interacting partner of protein kinase CK2 beta subunit. *FEBS Lett.* **1997**, *403*, 197–199. [CrossRef]

139. Meier, U.T.; Blobel, G. Nopp 140 shuttles on tracks between nucleolus and cytoplasm. *Cell* **1992**, *70*, 127–138. [CrossRef]

140. Jenett, A.; Rubin, G.M.; Ngo, T.T.; Shepherd, D.; Murphy, C.; Dionne, H.; Pfeiffer, B.D.; Cavallaro, A.; Hall, D.; Jeter, J.; et al. A GAL4-driver line resource for Drosophila neurobiology. *Cell Rep.* **2012**, *2*, 991–1001. [CrossRef] [PubMed]

141. Elliott, D.A.; Brand, A.H. The GAL4 system: A versatile system for the expression of genes. *Methods Mol. Biol.* **2008**, *420*, 79–95. [PubMed]

142. Duffy, J.B. GAL4 system in Drosophila: A fly geneticist's Swiss army knife. *Genesis* **2002**, *34*, 1–15. [CrossRef] [PubMed]

143. Klambt, C.; Knust, E.; Tietze, K.; Campos-Ortega, J.A. Closely related transcripts encoded by the neurogenic gene complex Enhancer of split of *Drosophila melanogaster*. *EMBO J.* **1989**, *8*, 203–210. [PubMed]

144. Knust, E.; Schrons, H.; Grawe, F.; Campos-Ortega, J.A. Seven genes of the enhancer of split complex of *Drosophila melanogaster* encode helix-loop-helix proteins. *Genetics* **1992**, *132*, 505–518. [PubMed]

145. Delidakis, C.; Artavanis-Tsakonas, S. The enhancer of split [E(spl)] locus of Drosophila encodes seven independant helix-loop-helix proteins. *Proc. Natl. Acad. Sci. USA* **1991**, *89*, 8731–8735. [CrossRef]

146. Schweisguth, F.; Gho, M.; Lecourtois, M.; Morel, V. Signalling by Notch family receptors. *C. R. Seances Soc. Biol. Fil.* **1997**, *191*, 55–75. [PubMed]

147. Mumm, J.S.; Kopan, R. Notch signaling: From the outside in. *Dev. Biol.* **2000**, *228*, 151–165. [CrossRef] [PubMed]

148. Blaumuller, C.M.; Artavanis-Tsakonas, S. Comparative aspects of Notch signaling in lower and higher eukaryotes. *Perspect. Dev. Neurobiol.* **1997**, *4*, 325–343.

149. Tien, A.C.; Rajan, A.; Bellen, H.J. A Notch updated. *J. Cell Biol.* **2009**, *184*, 621–629. [CrossRef] [PubMed]

150. Ilagan, M.X.; Kopan, R. Notch signaling pathway. *Cell* **2007**, *128*, 1246. [CrossRef] [PubMed]

151. Louvi, A.; Artavanis-Tsakonas, S. Notch signalling in vertebrate neural development. *Nat. Rev. Neurosci.* **2006**, *7*, 93–102. [CrossRef] [PubMed]

152. Tao, J.; Jiang, M.M.; Jiang, L.; Salvo, J.S.; Zeng, H.C.; Dawson, B.; Bertin, T.K.; Rao, P.H.; Chen, R.; Donehower, L.A.; et al. Notch activation as a driver of osteogenic sarcoma. *Cancer Cell* **2014**, *26*, 390–401. [CrossRef] [PubMed]

153. Bajard, L.; Oates, A.C. Breathe in and straighten your back: Hypoxia, notch, and scoliosis. *Cell* **2012**, *149*, 255–256. [CrossRef] [PubMed]

154. De la Pompa, J.L.; Epstein, J.A. Coordinating tissue interactions: Notch signaling in cardiac development and disease. *Dev. Cell* **2012**, *22*, 244–254. [CrossRef] [PubMed]

155. Gridley, T. Notch signaling in the vasculature. *Curr. Top. Dev. Biol.* **2010**, *92*, 277–309. [PubMed]

156. Wu, M.N.; Raizen, D.M. Notch signaling: A role in sleep and stress. *Curr. Biol.* **2011**, R397–R398. [CrossRef] [PubMed]

157. Treisman, J.E. How to make an eye. *Development* **2004**, *131*, 3823–3827. [CrossRef] [PubMed]

158. Freeman, M. Cell determination strategies in the Drosophila eye. *Development* **1997**, *124*, 261–270. [PubMed]

159. Pichaud, F.; Treisman, J.; Desplan, C. Reinventing a common strategy for patterning the eye. *Cell* **2001**, *105*, 9–12. [CrossRef]

160. Majot, A.T.; Sizemore, T.S.; Bandyopadhyay, M.; Jozwick, L.M.; Bidwai, A.P. Protein kinase CK2: A window into the posttranslational regulation of the E(spl)/HES repressors from invertebrates and vertebrates. In *Protein Kinase CK2 Cellular Function in Normal and Disease States*; Ahmed, K., Issinger, O.-G., Szyska, R., Eds.; Springer: New York, NY, USA, 2015; Volume 12, pp. 81–108.

161. Jarman, A.P.; Grell, E.H.; Ackerman, L.; Jan, L.Y.; Jan, Y.N. *Atonal* is the proneural gene for Drosophila photoreceptors. *Nature* **1994**, *369*, 398–400. [CrossRef] [PubMed]

162. Ghiasvand, N.M.; Rudolph, D.D.; Mashayekhi, M.; Brzezinski, J.A.T.; Goldman, D.; Glaser, T. Deletion of a remote enhancer near ATOH7 disrupts retinal neurogenesis, causing NCRNA disease. *Nat. Neurosci.* **2011**, *14*, 578–586. [CrossRef] [PubMed]

163. Zhou, M.; Yan, J.; Ma, Z.; Zhou, Y.; Abbood, N.N.; Liu, J.; Su, L.; Jia, H.; Guo, A.Y. Comparative and evolutionary analysis of the HES/HEY gene family reveal exon/intron loss and teleost specific duplication events. *PLoS ONE* **2012**, *7*, e40649. [CrossRef] [PubMed]

164. Kageyama, R.; Ohtsuka, T.; Kobayashi, T. Roles of Hes genes in neural development. *Dev. Growth Differ.* **2008**, *50* (Suppl. 1), S97–S103. [CrossRef] [PubMed]

165. Sun, Y.; Jan, L.; Jan, Y. Transcriptional regulation of atonal during development of the Drosophila peripheral nervous system. *Development* **1998**, *125*, 3731–3740. [PubMed]

166. Powell, L.M.; Zur Lage, P.I.; Prentice, D.R.; Senthinathan, B.; Jarman, A.P. The proneural proteins Atonal and Scute regulate neural target genes through different E-box binding sites. *Mol. Cell. Biol.* **2004**, *24*, 9517–9526. [CrossRef] [PubMed]

167. Ligoxygakis, P.; Yu, S.Y.; Delidakis, C.; Baker, N.E. A subset of Notch functions during Drosophila eye development require Su(H) and E(spl) gene complex. *Development* **1998**, *125*, 2893–2900. [PubMed]

168. Nolo, R.; Abbott, L.A.; Bellen, H.J. Senseless, a Zn finger transcription factor, is necessary and sufficient for sensory organ development in Drosophila. *Cell* **2000**, *102*, 349–362. [CrossRef]

169. Pepple, K.L.; Atkins, M.; Venken, K.; Wellnitz, K.; Harding, M.; Frankfort, B.; Mardon, G. Two-step selection of a single R8 photoreceptor: A bistable loop between senseless and rough locks in R8 fate. *Development* **2008**, *135*, 4071–4079. [CrossRef] [PubMed]

170. Axelrod, J.D. Delivering the lateral inhibition punchline: It's all about the timing. *Sci. Signal.* **2010**, *3*, pe38. [CrossRef] [PubMed]

171. Simpson, P. Lateral inhibition and the development of the sensory bristles of the adult peripheral nervous system of Drosophila. *Development* **1990**, *109*, 509–519. [PubMed]

172. Ligoxygakis, P.; Bray, S.J.; Apidianakis, Y.; Delidakis, C. Ectopic expression of individual E(spl) genes has differential effects on different cell fate decisions and underscores the biphasic requirement for Notch activity in wing margin establishment in Drosophila. *Development* **1999**, *126*, 2205–2214. [PubMed]

173. Lubensky, D.K.; Pennington, M.W.; Shraiman, B.I.; Baker, N.E. A dynamical model of ommatidial crystal formation. *Proc. Natl. Acad. Sci. USA* **2011**, *108*, 11145–11150. [CrossRef] [PubMed]

174. Struhl, G.; Adachi, A. Nuclear access and action of Notch in vivo. *Cell* **1998**, *93*, 649–660. [CrossRef]

175. Nagel, A.C.; Preiss, A. Notchspl is deficient for inductive processes in the eye, and E(spl)D enhances split by interfering with proneural activity. *Dev. Biol.* **1999**, *208*, 406–415. [CrossRef] [PubMed]

176. Giebel, B.; Campos-Ortega, J.A. Functional dissection of the Drosophila enhancer of split protein, a suppressor of neurogenesis. *Proc. Natl. Acad. Sci. USA* **1997**, *94*, 6250–6254. [CrossRef] [PubMed]

177. Nagel, A.; Yu, Y.; Preiss, A. Enhancer of split [E(spl)D] is a gro-independent, hypermorphic mutation in Drosophila. *Dev. Genet.* **1999**, *25*, 168–179. [CrossRef]

178. Welshons, W.J. Dosage experiments with *split* mutations in the presense of an *enhancer of split*. *Drosoph. Inf. Serv.* **1956**, *30*, 157–158.

179. Welshons, W.J. Analysis of a gene in Drosophila. *Science* **1965**, *150*, 1122–1129. [CrossRef] [PubMed]

180. Knust, E.; Bremer, K.A.; Vassin, H.; Ziemer, A.; Tepass, U.; Campos-Ortega, J.A. The enhancer of split locus and neurogenesis in *Drosophila melanogaster*. *Dev. Biol.* **1987**, *122*, 262–273. [CrossRef]

181. Kahali, B.; Kim, J.; Karandikar, U.; Bishop, C.P.; Bidwai, A.P. Evidence that the C-terminal domain (CtD) autoinhibits neural repression by Drosophila E(spl)M8. *Genesis* **2010**, *48*, 44–55. [CrossRef] [PubMed]

182. Bose, A.; Kahali, B.; Zhang, S.; Lin, J.-M.; Allada, R.; Karandikar, U.; Bidwai, A. Drosophila CK2 regulates lateral-inhibition during eye and bristle development. *Mech. Dev.* **2006**, *123*, 649–664. [CrossRef] [PubMed]

183. White, N.; Jarman, A. Drosophila atonal controls photoreceptor R8-specific properties and modulates both receptor tyrosine kinase and Hedgehog signalling. *Development* **2000**, *127*, 1681–1689. [PubMed]

184. Bandyopadhyay, M.; Bishop, C.P.; Bidwai, A.P. The Conserved MAPK Site in E(spl)-M8, an effector of *Drosophila* Notch signaling, controls repressor activity during eye development. *PLoS ONE* **2016**, *11*, e0159508. [CrossRef] [PubMed]

185. Jhas, S.; Ciura, S.; Belanger-Jasmin, S.; Dong, Z.; Llamosas, E.; Theriault, F.M.; Joachim, K.; Tang, Y.; Liu, L.; Liu, J.; et al. Hes6 inhibits astrocyte differentiation and promotes neurogenesis through different mechanisms. *J. Neurosci.* **2006**, *26*, 11061–11071. [CrossRef] [PubMed]

186. Belanger-Jasmin, S.; Llamosas, E.; Tang, Y.; Joachim, K.; Osiceanu, A.M.; Jhas, S.; Stifani, S. Inhibition of cortical astrocyte differentiation by Hes6 requires amino- and carboxy-terminal motifs important for dimerization and phosphorylation. *J. Neurochem.* **2007**, *103*, 2022–2034. [CrossRef] [PubMed]

187. Gratton, M.-O.; Torban, E.; Jasmin, S.B.; Theriault, F.M.; German, M.S.; Stifani, S. Hes6 promotes cortical neurogenesis and inhibits Hes1 transcription repression activity by multiple mechanisms. *Mol. Cell. Biol.* **2003**, *23*, 6922–6935. [CrossRef] [PubMed]

188. Brown, N.L.; Dagenais, S.L.; Chen, C.M.; Glaser, T. Molecular characterization and mapping of ATOH7, a human atonal homolog with a predicted role in retinal ganglion cell development. *Mamm. Genome* **2002**, *13*, 95–101. [CrossRef] [PubMed]

189. Brown, N.L.; Kanekar, S.; Vetter, M.L.; Tucker, P.K.; Gemza, D.L.; Glaser, T. Math5 encodes a murine basic helix-loop-helix transcription factor expressed during early stages of retinal neurogenesis. *Development* **1998**, *125*, 4821–4833. [PubMed]

190. Brown, N.L.; Patel, S.; Brzezinski, J.; Glaser, T. Math5 is required for retinal ganglion cell and optic nerve formation. *Development* **2001**, *128*, 2497–2508. [PubMed]

191. Hsiung, F.; Moses, K. Retinal development in Drosophila: Specifying the first neuron. *Hum. Mol. Genet.* **2002**, *11*, 1207–1214. [CrossRef] [PubMed]

192. Wang, S.W.; Kim, B.S.; Ding, K.; Wang, H.; Sun, D.; Johnson, R.L.; Klein, W.H.; Gan, L. Requirement for math5 in the development of retinal ganglion cells. *Genes Dev.* **2001**, *15*, 24–29. [CrossRef] [PubMed]

193. Tomita, K.; Ishibashi, M.; Nakahara, K.; Ang, S.L.; Nakanishi, S.; Guillemot, F.; Kageyama, R. Mammalian hairy and Enhancer of split homolog 1 regulates differentiation of retinal neurons and is essential for eye morphogenesis. *Neuron* **1996**, *16*, 723–734. [CrossRef]

194. Wang, V.Y.; Hassan, B.A.; Bellen, H.J.; Zoghbi, H.Y. Drosophila atonal fully rescues the phenotype of Math1 null mice: New functions evolve in new cellular contexts. *Curr. Biol.* **2002**, *12*, 1611–1616. [CrossRef]

195. Malone, C.M.; Domaschenz, R.; Amagase, Y.; Dunham, I.; Murai, K.; Jones, P.H. Hes6 is required for actin cytoskeletal organization in differentiating C2C12 myoblasts. *Exp. Cell Res.* **2011**, *317*, 1590–1602. [CrossRef] [PubMed]

196. Cossins, J.; Vernon, A.E.; Zhang, Y.; Philpott, A.; Jones, P.H. Hes6 regulates myogenic differentiation. *Development* **2002**, *129*, 2195–2207. [CrossRef] [PubMed]

197. Murai, K.; Vernon, A.E.; Philpott, A.; Jones, P. Hes6 is required for MyoD induction during gastrulation. *Dev. Biol.* **2007**, *312*, 61–76. [CrossRef] [PubMed]

198. Pissarra, L.; Henrique, D.; Duarte, A. Expression of Hes6, a new member of the Hairy/Enhancer-of-split family, in mouse development. *Mech. Dev.* **2000**, *95*, 275–278. [CrossRef]

199. Bae, S.; Bessho, Y.; Hojo, M.; Kageyama, R. The bHLH gene Hes6, an inhibitor of Hes1, promotes neuronal differentiation. *Development* **2000**, *127*, 2933–2943. [PubMed]

200. Haapa-Paananen, S.; Kiviluoto, S.; Waltari, M.; Puputti, M.; Mpindi, J.P.; Kohonen, P.; Tynninen, O.; Haapasalo, H.; Joensuu, H.; Perala, M.; et al. HES6 gene is selectively overexpressed in glioma and represents an important transcriptional regulator of glioma proliferation. *Oncogene* **2012**, *31*, 1299–1310. [CrossRef] [PubMed]

201. Hartman, J.; Lam, E.W.; Gustafsson, J.A.; Strom, A. Hes-6, an inhibitor of Hes-1, is regulated by 17β-estradiol and promotes breast cancer cell proliferation. *Breast Cancer Res.* **2009**, *11*, R79. [CrossRef] [PubMed]

202. Carvalho, F.L.; Marchionni, L.; Gupta, A.; Kummangal, B.A.; Schaeffer, E.M.; Ross, A.E.; Berman, D.M. HES6 promotes prostate cancer aggressiveness independently of Notch signalling. *J. Cell. Mol. Med.* **2015**, *19*, 1624–1636. [CrossRef] [PubMed]

203. Beltrao, P.; Trinidad, J.C.; Fiedler, D.; Roguev, A.; Lim, W.A.; Shokat, K.M.; Burlingame, A.L.; Krogan, N.J. Evolution of phosphoregulation: Comparison of phosphorylation patterns across yeast species. *PLoS Biol.* **2009**, *7*, e1000134. [CrossRef]

204. Levy, E.D.; Michnick, S.W.; Landry, C.R. Protein abundance is key to distinguish promiscuous from functional phosphorylation based on evolutionary information. *Philos. Trans. R. Soc. Lond. B Biol. Sci.* **2012**, *367*, 2594–2606. [CrossRef] [PubMed]

205. Jin, J.; Pawson, T. Modular evolution of phosphorylation-based signalling systems. *Philos. Trans. R. Soc. Lond. B Biol. Sci.* **2012**, *367*, 2540–2555. [CrossRef] [PubMed]

206. Hedges, S.B.; Blair, J.E.; Venturi, M.L.; Shoe, J.L. A molecular timescale of eukaryote evolution and the rise of complex multicellular life. *BMC Evol. Biol.* **2004**, *4*, 2. [CrossRef] [PubMed]

207. Beverly, S.M.; Wilson, A.C. Molecular evolution in Drosophila and the higher Diptera II. A time scale for fly evolution. *J. Mol. Evol.* **1984**, *21*, 1–13. [CrossRef]

208. Baker, N.E.; Firth, L.C. Retinal determination genes function along with cell-cell signals to regulate Drosophila eye development: Examples of multi-layered regulation by master regulators. *Bioessays* **2011**, *33*, 538–546. [CrossRef] [PubMed]

209. Kumar, J.P. Retinal determination the beginning of eye development. *Curr. Top. Dev. Biol.* **2010**, *93*, 1–28. [PubMed]

210. Kumar, J.P. The molecular circuitry governing retinal determination. *Biochim. Biophys. Acta* **2009**, *1789*, 306–314. [CrossRef] [PubMed]

211. Halder, G.; Callerts, P.; Gehring, W.J. Induction of ectopic eyes by targeted expression of the eyeless gene in Drosophila. *Science* **1995**, *267*, 1788–1792. [CrossRef] [PubMed]

212. Nfonsam, L.E.; Cano, C.; Mudge, J.; Schilkey, F.D.; Curtiss, J. Analysis of the transcriptomes downstream of eyeless and the hedgehog, decapentaplegic and Notch signaling pathways in *Drosophila melanogaster*. *PLoS ONE* **2012**, *7*, e44583. [CrossRef] [PubMed]

213. Ostrin, E.J.; Li, Y.; Hoffman, K.; Liu, J.; Wang, K.; Zhang, L.; Mardon, G.; Chen, R. Genome-wide identification of direct targets of the Drosophila retinal determination protein Eyeless. *Genome Res.* **2006**, *16*, 466–476. [CrossRef] [PubMed]

214. Halder, G.; Callaerts, P.; Flister, S.; Walldorf, U.; Kloter, U.; Gehring, W.J. Eyeless initiates the expression of both sine oculis and eyes absent during Drosophila compound eye development. *Development* **1998**, *125*, 2181–2191. [PubMed]

215. Culi, J.; Martin-Blanco, E.; Modolell, J. The EGF receptor and N signalling pathways act antagonistically in Drosophila mesothorax bristle patterning. *Development* **2001**, *128*, 299–308. [PubMed]
216. Sundaram, M.V. The love-hate relationship between Ras and Notch. *Genes Dev.* **2005**, *19*, 1825–1839. [CrossRef] [PubMed]
217. Benhra, N.; Vignaux, F.; Dussert, A.; Schweisguth, F.; Le Borgne, R. Neuralized promotes basal to apical transcytosis of delta in epithelial cells. *Mol. Biol. Cell* **2010**, *21*, 2078–2086. [CrossRef] [PubMed]
218. Lai, E.C.; Rubin, G.M. Neuralized is essential for a subset of Notch pathway-dependent cell fate decisions during Drosophila eye development. *Proc. Natl. Acad. Sci. USA* **2001**, *98*, 5637–5642. [CrossRef] [PubMed]
219. Isaksson, A.; Peverali, F.A.; Kockel, L.; Mlodzik, M.; Bohmann, D. The deubiquitination enzyme fat facets negatively regulates RTK/Ras/MAPK signalling during Drosophila eye development. *Mech. Dev.* **1997**, *68*, 59–67. [CrossRef]
220. Huang, Y.; Fischer-Vize, J. Undifferentiated cells in the developing Drosophila eye influence facet assembly and require the Fat facets ubiquitin-specific protease. *Development* **1996**, *122*, 3207–3216. [PubMed]
221. Chen, X.; Zhang, B.; Fischer, J.A. A specific protein substrate for a deubiquitinating enzyme: Liquid facets is the substrate of Fat facets. *Genes Dev.* **2002**, *16*, 289–294. [CrossRef] [PubMed]
222. Kinoshita-Kikuta, E.; Yamada, A.; Inoue, C.; Kinoshita, E.; Koike, T. A novel phosphate-affinity bead with immobilized Phos-tag for separation and enrichment of phosphopeptides and phosphoproteins. *J. Integr. OMICS* **2011**, *1*, 157–169.
223. Sopko, R.; Foos, M.; Vinayagam, A.; Zhai, B.; Binari, R.; Hu, Y.; Randklev, S.; Perkins, L.A.; Gygi, S.P.; Perrimon, N. Combining genetic perturbations and proteomics to examine kinase-phosphatase networks in Drosophila embryos. *Dev. Cell* **2014**, *31*, 114–127. [CrossRef] [PubMed]
224. Chen, C.L.; Hu, Y.; Udeshi, N.D.; Lau, T.Y.; Wirtz-Peitz, F.; He, L.; Ting, A.Y.; Carr, S.A.; Perrimon, N. Proteomic mapping in live Drosophila tissues using an engineered ascorbate peroxidase. *Proc. Natl. Acad. Sci. USA* **2015**, *112*, 12093–12098. [CrossRef] [PubMed]

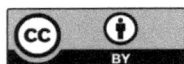

pharmaceuticals

MDPI

Review

The Link between Protein Kinase CK2 and Atypical Kinase Rio1

Konrad Kubiński * and Maciej Masłyk *

The John Paul II Catholic University of Lublin, ul. Konstantynów 1i, 20-708 Lublin, Poland
* Correspondence: kubin@kul.pl (K.K.); maciekm@kul.pl (M.M.); Tel.: +48-81-454-5451

Academic Editor: Lorenzo Pinna
Received: 30 November 2016; Accepted: 4 February 2017; Published: 7 February 2017

Abstract: The atypical kinase Rio1 is widespread in many organisms, ranging from Archaebacteria to humans, and is an essential factor in ribosome biogenesis. Little is known about the protein substrates of the enzyme and small-molecule inhibitors of the kinase. Protein kinase CK2 was the first interaction partner of Rio1, identified in yeast cells. The enzyme from various sources undergoes CK2-mediated phosphorylation at several sites and this modification regulates the activity of Rio1. The aim of this review is to present studies of the relationship between the two different kinases, with respect to CK2-mediated phosphorylation of Rio1, regulation of Rio1 activity, and similar susceptibility of the kinases to benzimidazole inhibitors.

Keywords: protein kinase CK2; protein kinase Rio1; phosphorylation; protein-protein interaction; benzimidazoles

1. Introduction

Protein kinases play important roles in key cellular processes, including the cell cycle, metabolism, and cell death [1,2]. The protein kinase superfamily with its 518 members comprises one of the largest protein superfamilies identified in the human genome [3]. In addition to their key roles in cell physiology, several protein kinases are linked to pathological states, including cancer [4,5]. This fact makes kinases attractive targets for therapeutic interventions.

The objective of the review article is to present a representative of the RIO family, namely the atypical protein kinase Rio1. The special intention is to emphasize the relationship of Rio1 from humans and yeast, with probably the most pleiotropic cellular kinase—CK2. Although the interaction between these two remarkably different kinases (Figure 1) has not been widely reported to date, we focus on some common aspects of their activity, namely protein-protein interaction, CK2-mediated Rio1 phosphorylation, and similar susceptibility to some benzimidazoles.

A

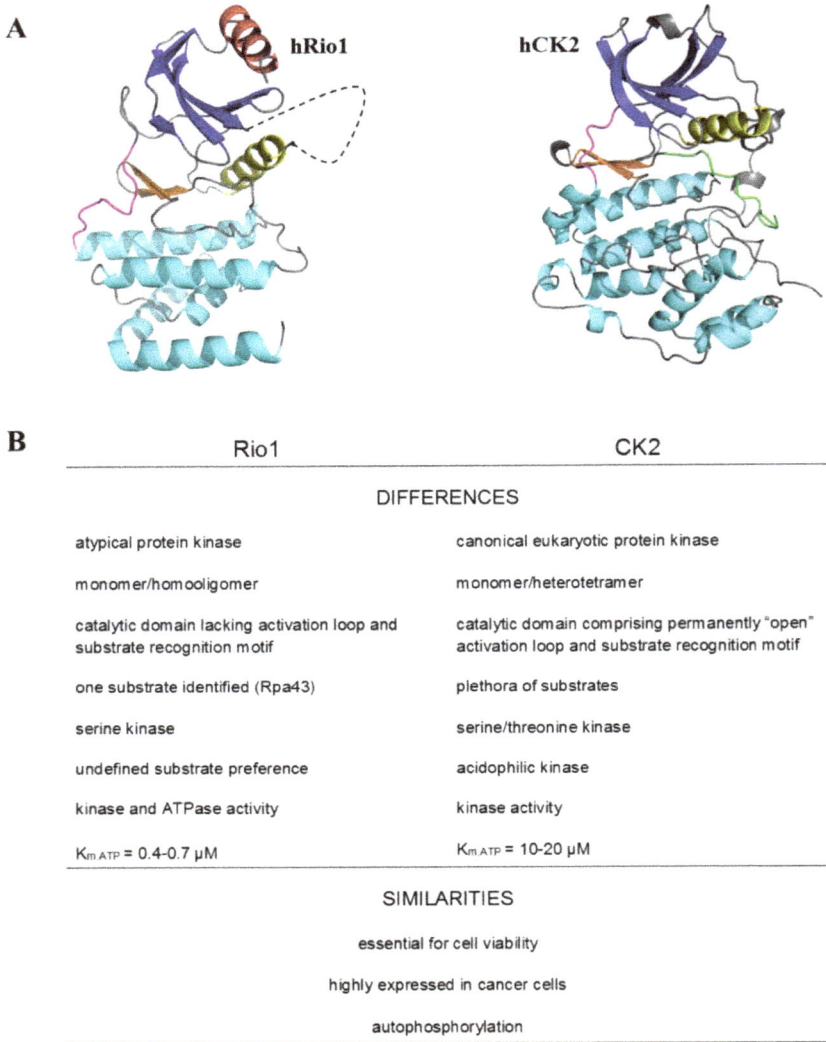

B

Rio1	CK2
DIFFERENCES	
atypical protein kinase	canonical eukaryotic protein kinase
monomer/homooligomer	monomer/heterotetramer
catalytic domain lacking activation loop and substrate recognition motif	catalytic domain comprising permanently "open" activation loop and substrate recognition motif
one substrate identified (Rpa43)	plethora of substrates
serine kinase	serine/threonine kinase
undefined substrate preference	acidophilic kinase
kinase and ATPase activity	kinase activity
$K_{m\,ATP}$ = 0.4-0.7 µM	$K_{m\,ATP}$ = 10-20 µM
SIMILARITIES	
essential for cell viability	
highly expressed in cancer cells	
autophosphorylation	

Figure 1. Differences and similarities between protein kinases Rio1 and CK2 [6–16]. (**A**) Comparison of the 3D structures of hRio1 and hCK2α visualised in PyMOL. The N-terminal β-sheets are coloured blue, the β-hairpin is coloured orange, the αC-helix is coloured yellow, the hinge is coloured magenta, the C-lobe α-helices are coloured cyan, the αR-helix is coloured red, the "flexible loop" is represented by blacked dashed line, and the activation loop is coloured green. (**B**) Comparison of other features of the two kinases.

2. Protein Kinase Rio1

RIO kinases comprise an atypical kinase family composed of four subfamilies: Rio1, Rio2, RioK3, and RioB. The members of the RIO family are evolutionarily conserved and are present in all three domains of life. RIO kinases exhibit a trimmed version of the domain present in the canonical eukaryotic protein kinases, which lack the activation loop and the substrate recognition region [7,17,18].

To date, only one crystal structure of human Rio1 has been developed (PDBID:4OTP). Like canonical eukaryotic kinases (ePKs) (including CK2), Rio1 consists of two main lobes called the N-terminal and C-terminal lobes. The N-terminal lobe consists of a 5-stranded antiparallel β-sheet (β1-5) and a single α-helix (αC), which is located between β3 and β4.

The N-terminal lobe is connected via a "hinge region" to a C-terminal lobe, containing three α-helices (αE, αF, and αG) and a β-hairpin (β6-7) [12]. In contrast to canonical ePKs, the N-terminal lobe of Rio1 contains a RIO-kinase-specific α-helix called αR. Another specific structural feature of Rio1 is the presence of a "flexible loop" located between β3, and the density of this region is not observed in the crystal structure of hRio1. Moreover the Rio1 structure lacks the activation or the "APE" loop and the substrate recognition motif located within subdomain VIII of the canonical ePKs C-terminal lobe [7,12,19] (Figure 1).

The enzyme is involved in processes critical for cellular proliferation, including ribosome biogenesis, cell cycle progression, and chromosome maintenance [12,20,21]. Both in yeast and in humans, Rio1 is required for the last cytoplasmic step of processing 20S pre-rRNA to mature 18S rRNA, i.e. the RNA component of the 40S ribosome subunit [12,22–24]. Depletion of Rio1 results in strong cytoplasmic accumulation of 20S pre-rRNA, a severe decrease in the 18S rRNA level, and finally cell cycle arrest [20]. Moreover, in humans, the kinase activity of the enzyme is essential for the recycling of endonuclease hNob1 and its binding partner hDim2 from cytoplasmic pre-40S and the translocation of the proteins into the nucleus [24]. As far as the process of ribosome biogenesis is concerned, Rio1 can act as a kinase as well as ATPase. Studies on yeast have revealed that Rio1's ATPase activity is required for late 40S biogenesis to regulate its dynamic association with pre-40S particles [12].

While the cytoplasmic functions of Rio1 are well characterized, little is known about its role in the nucleus, where it is also present. Recent studies have revealed that, Rio1 downregulates RNA polymerase I (Pol I) during anaphase by targeting its subunits Rpa43, thereby causing the polymerase to dissociate from rDNA; thus, Rio1 integrates rDNA replication and segregation with ribosome biogenesis [13].

Interestingly, the protein kinase Rio1 is characterized as an essential enzyme involved in cell viability; on the one hand; on the other hand only one physiological protein substrate (Rpa43) for this kinase is known. There are several proteins that undergo Rio1-mediated phosphorylation *in vitro*, namely, myelin basic protein, casein, histones H1 and H2A, enolase, Tomato mosaic virus MP, and the recently discovered subunit of RNA Pol I—Rpa43 [6,8,10,13,25].. The enzyme exhibits a capability of autophosphorylation at serine residues, but the physiological significance of the modification remains elusive [6,8]. It has been reported that autophosphorylation reduces oligomerization of Rio1 and promotes the most active monomeric form of the kinase [10].

3. Rio1 as an Interacting Partner and Target for CK2

There are 18 phosphorylated amino acids within the hRio1 sequence listed at PhosphoSitePlus (www.phosphosite.org). All the sites mentioned have been revealed by High Throughput Screening, but not confirmed by site-specific methods. Among all these phosphosites, there are three (S21, S22, and T509) located within two sequences that fulfil the minimal consensus for phosphorylation by protein kinase CK2 [11] (Figure 2). Another phosphoproteome analysis project (PHOSIDA) revealed that hRio1 undergoes phosphorylation within the sequence QFDDAD**S21S22**DSENRDL [26,27]. In turn our recent unpublished data have confirmed serines 21 and 22 as the only sites modified in vitro within the human kinase Rio1 by protein kinase CK2 (Figure 2).

Interestingly, protein kinase CK2 was the first interaction partner of Rio1, identified in yeast. By means of co-immunoprecipitation, Angermayr and coworkers revealed that Rio1 preferentially interacted with CK2α´, but not with the remaining yeast CK2 subunits: CK2α, CK2β, and CK2β´. Further mutagenesis studies have shown that the C-terminal domain of Rio1 is essential and sufficient for this interaction [28]. Moreover, with the use of mutant yeast strains, the authors showed Rio1 as a target of CK2 in vivo, which was phosphorylated mainly by a CK2 heterotetramer containing both

CK2α and CK2α′ subunits. In vitro kinase assays revealed a total of six clustered serine residues as the CK2 phosphorylation sites of yeast Rio1 (Figure 2) [28].

Although the physiologically important CK2-mediated phosphorylation of Rio1 affects the serine cluster, which is present exclusively in the yeast kinase (Figure 2) and has been proven to date in yeast cells only, it is the relevant starting point for further studies on regulation of the Rio1 via CK2-mediated phosphorylation.

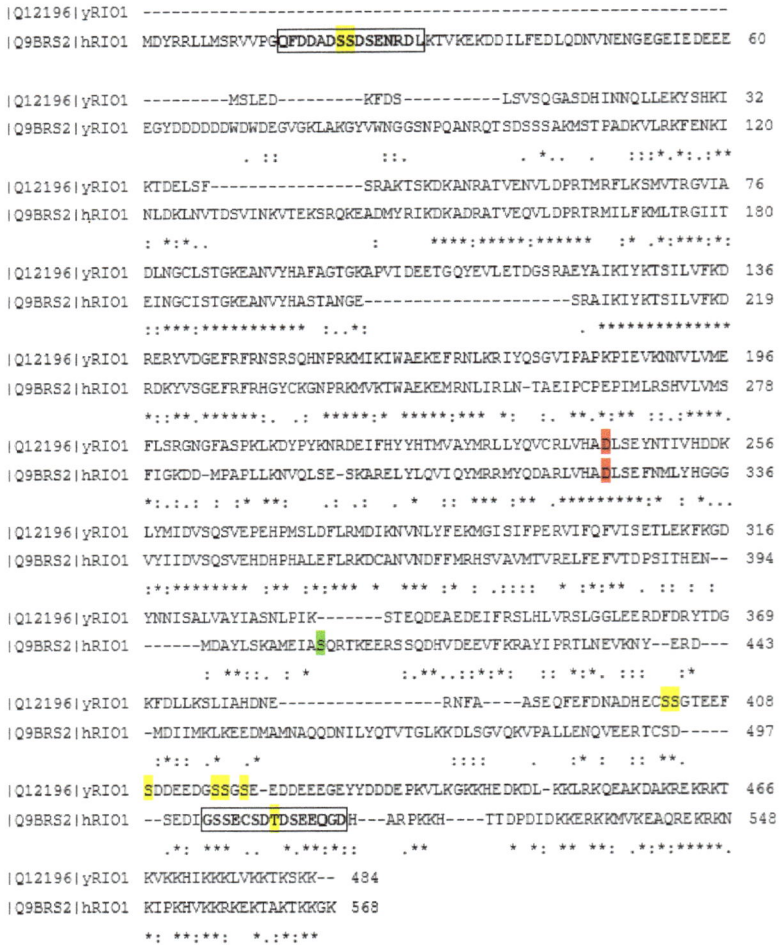

```
|Q12196|yRIO1  ------------------------------------------------------------
|Q9BRS2|hRIO1  MDYRRLLMSRVVPGQFDDADSSDSENRDLKTVKEKDDILFEDLQDNVNENGEGEIEDEEE  60


|Q12196|yRIO1  ---------MSLED---------KFDS----------LSVSQGASDHINNQLLEKYSHKI   32
|Q9BRS2|yRIO1  EGYDDDDDDWDWDEGVGKLAKGYVWNGGSNPQANRQTSDSSSAKMSTPADKVLRKFENKI  120
                       . ::          ::.          . *..  .   :::*.*:.:**
|Q12196|yRIO1  KTDELSF----------------SRAKTSKDKANRATVENVLDPRTMRFLKSMVTRGVIA   76
|Q9BRS2|hRIO1  NLDKLNVTDSVINKVTEKSRQKEADMYRIKDKADRATVEQVLDPRTRMILFKMLTRGIIT  180
                : *:*..            :       ****;*****:******  :* .*:***:*:
|Q12196|yRIO1  DLNGCLSTGKEANVYHAFAGTGKAPVIDEETGQYEVLETDGSRAEYAIKIYKTSILVFKD  136
|Q9BRS2|hRIO1  EINGCISTGKEANVYHASTANGE--------------------SRAIKIYKTSILVFKD  219
                ::***:*********** :..*:            . **************
|Q12196|yRIO1  RERYVDGEFRFRNSRSQHNPRKMIKIWAEKEFRNLKRIYQSGVIPAPKPIEVKNNVLVME  196
|Q9BRS2|hRIO1  RDKYVSGEFRFRHGYCKGNPRKMVKTWAEKEMRNLIRLN-TAEIPCPEPIMLRSHVLVMS  278
                *::**.******:.  .: *****:* *****:*** *:  :. **.*:** ::.:****.
|Q12196|yRIO1  FLSRGNGFASPKLKDYPYKNRDEIFHYYHTMVAYMRLLYQVCRLVHADLSEYNTIVHDDK  256
|Q9BRS2|hRIO1  FIGKDD-MPAPLLKNVQLSE-SKARELYLQVIQYMRRMYQDARLVHADLSEFNMLYHGGG  336
                *:.:.:  : :* **:  .: .:  .  *  :: *** :** .********:*  :  *...
|Q12196|yRIO1  LYMIDVSQSVEPEHPMSLDFLRMDIKNVNLYFEKMGISIFPPERVIFQFVISETLEKFKGD  316
|Q9BRS2|hRIO1  VYIIDVSQSVEHDHPHALEFLRKDCANVNDFFMRHSVAVMTVRELFEFVTDPSITHEN--  394
                :*;******** :** :*:*** *  *** :* :  .:::  * :*:** . :: : :
|Q12196|yRIO1  YNNISALVAYIASNLPIK-------STEQDEAEDEIFRSLHLVRSLGGLEERDFDRYTDG  369
|Q9BRS2|hRIO1  ------MDAYLSKAMEIASQRTKEERSSQDHVDEEVFKRAYIPRTLNEVKNY--ERD---  443
                : **::. : *      :.**..::*:*:  :: *:*. :::   :*
|Q12196|yRIO1  KFDLLKSLIAHDNE-----------------RNFA----ASEQFEFDNADHECSSGTEEF  408
|Q9BRS2|hRIO1  -MDIIMKLKEEDMAMNAQQDNILYQTVTGLKKDLSGVQKVPALLENQVEERTCSD-----  497
                :*:: .*  .*             ::::     . :* : :: **.
|Q12196|yRIO1  SDDEEDGSSGSE-EDDEEEGEYYDDDEPKVLKGKKHEDKDL-KKLRKQEAKDAKREKRKT  466
|Q9BRS2|hRIO1  --SEDIGSSECSDTDSEEQGDH---ARPKKH----TTDPDIDKKERKKMVKEAQREKRKN  548
                .*: *** .. *.**:*::  .**       * *: ** **: .*:*:*****.
|Q12196|yRIO1  KVKKHIKKKLVKKTKSKK--  484
|Q9BRS2|hRIO1  KIPKHVKKRKEKTAKTKKGK  568
                *: **:**: *.:*:**
```

Figure 2. Alignment of human (Q9BRS2) and yeast Rio1 (Q12196). The alignment was performed using a Clustal Omega tool on the uniprot.org website. CK2 phosphorylation sites are marked in yellow, catalytic amino acid residues are marked in red, and the autophosphorylation site is marked in green. Two putative CK2-phosphorylation sequences in hRio1 are marked with boxes. Identical amino acids are marked with asterisks, similar amino acids are marked with colons, and different amino acids are marked with dots.

4. Regulation of Rio1 via CK2-Mediated Phosphorylation in Yeast

Studies in yeast have revealed that CK2-mediated Rio1 phosphorylation can stimulate the activity of the atypical kinase in vitro. Six serines (S402, S403, S409, S416, S417, and S419) were identified as CK2 phosphorylation sites by means of site-directed mutagenesis. Consecutive mutation of the listed residues resulted in a decreased phosphorylation level, up to total abrogation of the signal in the case of mutation of all six serines. A Rio1 mutant mimicking the permanently phosphorylated enzyme, with the serines replaced with aspartic acids, showed approximately two fold higher phosphorylation activity toward histone H2B in comparison with the wild-type kinase and a Rio1 mutant lacking CK2-phosphorylated sites (S > A). In order to examine the possible biological importance of the in vitro studies, yeast cells harbouring a Rio1 mutant lacking serines modified by CK2 or a Rio1 mutant mimicking the state of permanent CK2-mediated phosphorylation were employed. The former yeast cells showed a significantly reduced growth rate, while the latter cells behaved indistinguishably from the wild-type yeast. The results show that phosphorylation of CK2-modified serines is essential for full activity of the kinase Rio1, and lack of the phosphorylation is disadvantageous for cell proliferation. Further, the authors revealed that the yeast cells harbouring the Rio1 mutant, which are not phosphorylated by CK2, had difficulties entering the S phase. Moreover, it has been shown that the S > A mutant shows low susceptibility to proteolytic degradation in contrast to the wild-type Rio1 and the S > D mutant [28].

In other studies, recombinant tobacco CK2-mediated phosphorylation of Rio1 from *Nicotiana tabacum* inhibited the interaction between Rio1 and the Movement Protein from *Tomato Mosaic Virus*. The authors suggest that phosphorylation occurs in the region of protein-protein interaction, and the process disrupts protein binding through changes in the protein conformation of Rio1 [25].

5. Collective Inhibition of CK2 and Rio1 by Benzimidazole Derivatives

Although the possible role of Rio1 in pathogenesis is not well established in comparison to many other kinases, it has been reported that the enzyme is upregulated in colon cancer, and there is a direct link between deregulation of ribosome biogenesis and tumor development [16]. In other studies, Read et al. showed that Rio1 and Rio2 were overexpressed in glioblastoma cells in an Akt-dependent manner and promoted tumorigenesis [29]. Taking this and the essential role of the Rio1 into consideration, the enzyme appears to be an attractive target in the fight against cancer. Therefore, selective and potent inhibitors of Rio1 are needed.

Currently there are not selective compounds targeting Rio1. The first small-molecule inhibitor of protein kinase Rio1 discovered is an antibiotic toyocamycin (TOYO). It is capable of inhibiting both ribosome biogenesis and kinase activity of Rio1 [10]. The antibiotic binds more tightly to Rio1 than ATP and exhibits mixed inhibition of the enzyme. Toyocamycin affects the kinase by stabilizing its less active oligomeric form. In other studies, a series of pyridine caffeic acid benzyl amides (CABA) were tested for their ability to inhibit the autophosphorylation activity of Rio1 [30]. Although three promising chemicals have been found, their activity starting from IC_{50} of 48 μM (AG490), at the ATP concentration of 1 μM which is optimal for Rio1, is rather low.

Derivatives of benzimidazoles are widely reported inhibitors of protein kinase CK2 from different sources, which show pro-apoptotic properties in tests on cancer cell lines and mouse xenografts [6,31–35]. While most benzimidazole chemicals show the highest potency against CK2, many of them can also affect other protein kinases, e.g., PIM, DYRK, or HIPK [31].

Our recent studies have revealed that Rio1 is inhibited in vitro by selected benzimidazoles with potency similar to that of CK2 (Table 1). The compounds with nanomolar activity against Rio1 appeared to be the most potent in vitro inhibitors of the kinase identified to date [9].

Interestingly, Rio1 has not been tested before with other kinases in studies on the selectivity of benzimidazole inhibitors of CK2. Our data have shown that the most potent compound, i.e., TIBI, can act as a strict ATP-competitive inhibitor of the atypical kinase. Since the first inhibitor of Rio1 discovered, i.e., toyocamycin was reported to stabilize the less catalytically active oligomer and to enhance the thermostability of the kinase, we attempted to verify if these phenomena are general properties of the ATP-competitive inhibitors of Rio1. The results obtained have shown that TIBI does not influence the ternary structure of Rio1 but enhances the thermostability of the kinase. Molecular docking calculations have revealed that TIBI binds to the ATP-binding pockets of both kinases in a similar manner (Figure 3).

Table 1. Inhibitors of protein kinase Rio1 [9,10,30].

TIBI	K92	DMAT	TBI	TBB	TCI	TOYO	AG490
Rio1, IC$_{50}$ [µM]							
0.09	0.19	0.19	0.33	1.74	1.9	3.66	47.88
CK2, IC$_{50}$ [µM]							
0.083	0.066	0.19	0.44	0.19	9.7	54.78	n.d. *

*n.d.—not determined.

Although the nanomolar activity of some benzimidazoles against Rio1 could be a promising starting point in designing novel inhibitors of the kinase, the fact that these compounds target also many other kinases creates a serious barrier to reaching reasonable selectivity. On the other hand, taking into consideration the activity of toyocamycin against Rio1 and its selectivity with respect to CK2, the derivatization of the antibiotic appears to be a more attractive approach in designing potent and selective Rio1 inhibitors.

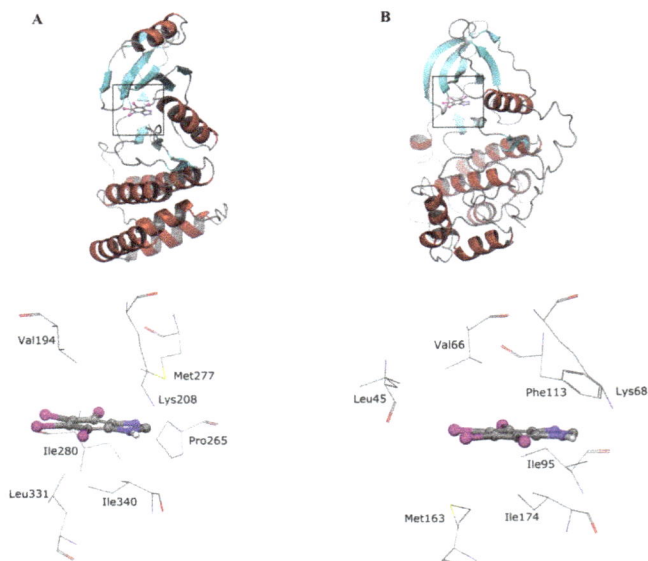

Figure 3. Docked binding modes obtained for TIBI in the ATP-binding pocket of (**A**) Rio1 and (**B**) CK2 [9].

6. Conclusions

Summing up, there are some relationships between Rio1 and CK2. The enzymes can interact with one another. Rio1 undergoes CK2-mediated phosphorylation and this modification can regulate Rio1 activity. Although the articles reviewed here clearly show the importance of CK2 activity in Rio1 regulation, further studies should be carried out, mainly on human cells, in order to elucidate this interaction. However, the most intriguing aspect of their relationship is the shared susceptibility to benzimidazole inhibitors. This issue should be taken into consideration when new benzimidazole-based biologically active chemicals are designed. Considering the limited selectivity of benzimidazoles, the chemicals are not promising candidates for selective Rio1 inhibitors. However, benzimidazoles targeting a variety of kinase overexpressed in some pathological states, are widely used as anti-kinases agents. The novel anti-Rio1 activity of benzimidazoles discovered recently should be taken into consideration whenever new compounds are tested against a panel of protein kinases, and in such a case the atypical protein kinase Rio1 cannot be disregarded.

Acknowledgments: This work was supported by the Polish Ministry of Science and Higher Education.

Conflicts of Interest: The authors declare no conflict of interest.

References

1. Hafen, E. Kinases and phosphatases—A marriage is consummated. *Science* **1998**, *280*, 1212–1213. [CrossRef] [PubMed]
2. Cohen, P. The origins of protein phosphorylation. *Nat. Cell Biol.* **2002**, *4*, E127–E130. [CrossRef] [PubMed]
3. Manning, G.; Whyte, D.B.; Martinez, R.; Hunter, T.; Sudarsanam, S. The protein kinase complement of the human genome. *Science* **2002**, *298*, 1912–1934. [CrossRef] [PubMed]
4. Blume-Jensen, P.; Hunter, T. Oncogenic kinase signalling. *Nature* **2001**, *411*, 355–365. [CrossRef] [PubMed]
5. Brognard, J.; Hunter, T. Protein kinase signaling networks in cancer. *Curr. Opin. Genet. Dev.* **2011**, *21*, 4–11. [CrossRef] [PubMed]
6. Angermayr, M.; Bandlow, W. Rio1, an extraordinary novel protein kinase. *FEBS Lett.* **2002**, *524*, 31–36. [CrossRef]
7. LaRonde-LeBlanc, N.; Wlodawer, A. A family portrait of the rio kinases. *J. Biol. Chem.* **2005**, *280*, 37297–37300. [CrossRef] [PubMed]
8. Laronde-Leblanc, N.; Guszczynski, T.; Copeland, T.; Wlodawer, A. Structure and activity of the atypical serine kinase rio1. *FEBS J.* **2005**, *272*, 3698–3713. [CrossRef] [PubMed]
9. Kubiński, K.; Masłyk, M.; Orzeszko, A. Benzimidazole inhibitors of protein kinase CK2 potently inhibit the activity of atypical protein kinase rio1. *Mol. Cell. Biochem.* **2017**, *426*, 195–203. [CrossRef] [PubMed]
10. Kiburu, I.N.; LaRonde-LeBlanc, N. Interaction of rio1 kinase with toyocamycin reveals a conformational switch that controls oligomeric state and catalytic activity. *PLoS ONE* **2012**, *7*, e37371. [CrossRef] [PubMed]
11. Meggio, F.; Pinna, L.A. One-thousand-and-one substrates of protein kinase CK2? *FASEB J.* **2003**, *17*, 349–368. [CrossRef] [PubMed]
12. Ferreira-Cerca, S.; Kiburu, I.; Thomson, E.; LaRonde, N.; Hurt, E. Dominant rio1 kinase/atpase catalytic mutant induces trapping of late pre-40s biogenesis factors in 80s-like ribosomes. *Nucleic Acids Res.* **2014**, *42*, 8635–8647. [CrossRef] [PubMed]
13. Iacovella, M.G.; Golfieri, C.; Massari, L.F.; Busnelli, S.; Pagliuca, C.; Dal Maschio, M.; Infantino, V.; Visintin, R.; Mechtler, K.; Ferreira-Cerca, S.; et al. Rio1 promotes rdna stability and downregulates rna polymerase i to ensure rdna segregation. *Nat. Commun.* **2015**, *6*, 6643. [CrossRef] [PubMed]
14. Filhol, O.; Cochet, C. Protein kinase CK2 in health and disease: Cellular functions of protein kinase ck2: A dynamic affair. *Cell. Mol. Life Sci* **2009**, *66*, 1830–1839. [CrossRef] [PubMed]
15. Litchfield, D.W. Protein kinase ck2: Structure, regulation and role in cellular decisions of life and death. *Biochem. J.* **2003**, *369*, 1–15. [CrossRef] [PubMed]
16. Ruggero, D.; Pandolfi, P.P. Does the ribosome translate cancer? *Nat. Rev. Cancer* **2003**, *3*, 179–192. [CrossRef] [PubMed]

17. Esser, D.; Siebers, B. Atypical protein kinases of the rio family in archaea. *Biochem. Soc. Trans.* **2013**, *41*, 399–404. [CrossRef] [PubMed]

18. LaRonde, N.A. The ancient microbial rio kinases. *J. Biol. Chem.* **2014**, *289*, 9488–9492. [CrossRef] [PubMed]

19. Hanks, S.K.; Quinn, A.M.; Hunter, T. The protein kinase family: Conserved features and deduced phylogeny of the catalytic domains. *Science* **1988**, *241*, 42–52. [CrossRef] [PubMed]

20. Vanrobays, E.; Gleizes, P.E.; Bousquet-Antonelli, C.; Noaillac-Depeyre, J.; Caizergues-Ferrer, M.; Gélugne, J.P. Processing of 20s pre-RNA to 18s ribosomal RNA in yeast requires rrp10p, an essential non-ribosomal cytoplasmic protein. *EMBO J.* **2001**, *20*, 4204–4213. [CrossRef] [PubMed]

21. LaRonde-LeBlanc, N.; Wlodawer, A. The rio kinases: An atypical protein kinase family required for ribosome biogenesis and cell cycle progression. *Biochim. Biophys. Acta* **2005**, *1754*, 14–24. [CrossRef] [PubMed]

22. Turowski, T.W.; Lebaron, S.; Zhang, E.; Peil, L.; Dudnakova, T.; Petfalski, E.; Granneman, S.; Rappsilber, J.; Tollervey, D. Rio1 mediates ATP-dependent final maturation of 40s ribosomal subunits. *Nucleic Acids Res.* **2014**, *42*, 12189–12199. [CrossRef] [PubMed]

23. Vanrobays, E.; Gelugne, J.P.; Gleizes, P.E.; Caizergues-Ferrer, M. Late cytoplasmic maturation of the small ribosomal subunit requires rio proteins in saccharomyces cerevisiae. *Mol. Cell. Biol* **2003**, *23*, 2083–2095. [CrossRef] [PubMed]

24. Widmann, B.; Wandrey, F.; Badertscher, L.; Wyler, E.; Pfannstiel, J.; Zemp, I.; Kutay, U. The kinase activity of human rio1 is required for final steps of cytoplasmic maturation of 40s subunits. *Mol. Biol. Cell.* **2012**, *23*, 22–35. [CrossRef] [PubMed]

25. Yoshioka, K.; Matsushita, Y.; Kasahara, M.; Konagaya, K.; Nyunoya, H. Interaction of tomato mosaic virus movement protein with tobacco rio kinase. *Mol. Cells* **2004**, *17*, 223–229. [PubMed]

26. Mayya, V.; Lundgren, D.H.; Hwang, S.I.; Rezaul, K.; Wu, L.; Eng, J.K.; Rodionov, V.; Han, D.K. Quantitative phosphoproteomic analysis of t cell receptor signaling reveals system-wide modulation of protein-protein interactions. *Sci. Signal.* **2009**, *2*, ra46. [CrossRef] [PubMed]

27. Gnad, F.; Gunawardena, J.; Mann, M. Phosida 2011: The posttranslational modification database. *Nucleic Acids Res.* **2011**, *39*, D253–D260. [CrossRef] [PubMed]

28. Angermayr, M.; Hochleitner, E.; Lottspeich, F.; Bandlow, W. Protein kinase CK2 activates the atypical rio1p kinase and promotes its cell-cycle phase-dependent degradation in yeast. *FEBS J.* **2007**, *274*, 4654–4667. [CrossRef] [PubMed]

29. Read, R.D.; Fenton, T.R.; Gomez, G.G.; Wykosky, J.; Vandenberg, S.R.; Babic, I.; Iwanami, A.; Yang, H.; Cavenee, W.K.; Mischel, P.S.; et al. A kinome-wide rnai screen in drosophila glia reveals that the rio kinases mediate cell proliferation and survival through TORC2-akt signaling in glioblastoma. *PLoS Genet.* **2013**, *9*, e1003253. [CrossRef] [PubMed]

30. Mielecki, M.; Krawiec, K.; Kiburu, I.; Grzelak, K.; Zagórski, W.; Kierdaszuk, B.; Kowa, K.; Fokt, I.; Szymanski, S.; Swierk, P.; et al. Development of novel molecular probes of the rio1 atypical protein kinase. *Biochim. Biophys. Acta* **2013**, *1834*, 1292–1301. [CrossRef] [PubMed]

31. Pagano, M.A.; Bain, J.; Kazimierczuk, Z.; Sarno, S.; Ruzzene, M.; Di Maira, G.; Elliott, M.; Orzeszko, A.; Cozza, G.; Meggio, F.; et al. The selectivity of inhibitors of protein kinase CK2: An update. *Biochem. J.* **2008**, *415*, 353–365. [CrossRef] [PubMed]

32. Pagano, M.A.; Andrzejewska, M.; Ruzzene, M.; Sarno, S.; Cesaro, L.; Bain, J.; Elliott, M.; Meggio, F.; Kazimierczuk, Z.; Pinna, L.A. Optimization of protein kinase CK2 inhibitors derived from 4,5,6,7-tetrabromobenzimidazole. *J. Med. Chem.* **2004**, *47*, 6239–6247. [CrossRef] [PubMed]

33. Hu, M.; Laronde-Leblanc, N.; Sternberg, P.W.; Gasser, R.B. Tv-rio1—An atypical protein kinase from the parasitic nematode trichostrongylus vitrinus. *Parasit. Vectors* **2008**, *1*, 34. [CrossRef] [PubMed]

34. Gianoncelli, A.; Cozza, G.; Orzeszko, A.; Meggio, F.; Kazimierczuk, Z.; Pinna, L.A. Tetraiodobenzimidazoles are potent inhibitors of protein kinase CK2. *Bioorg. Med. Chem.* **2009**, *17*, 7281–7289. [CrossRef]

35. Schneider, C.C.; Kartarius, S.; Montenarh, M.; Orzeszko, A.; Kazimierczuk, Z. Modified tetrahalogenated benzimidazoles with CK2 inhibitory activity are active against human prostate cancer cells LNCaP in vitro. *Bioorg. Med. Chem.* **2012**, *20*, 4390–4396. [CrossRef] [PubMed]

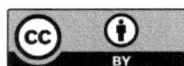

pharmaceuticals

MDPI

Article

The Phosphorylation of PDX-1 by Protein Kinase CK2 Is Crucial for Its Stability

Sabrina Klein [1], Rui Meng [1,2], Mathias Montenarh [1] and Claudia Götz [1,*]

[1] Medical Biochemistry and Molecular Biology, Saarland University, 66424 Homburg, Germany;
klein.sabrina@outlook.de (S.K.); mengruivip@163.com (R.M.); mathias.montenarh@uks.eu (M.M.)

[2] Cancer Center of Union Hospital, Tongji Medical College, Huazhong University of Science and Technology,
No. 156 Wujiadun, Hankou, Wuhan 430045, China

* Correspondence: claudia.goetz@uks.eu; Tel.: +49-6841-162-6502; Fax: +49-6841-162-6027

Academic Editor: Marc Le Borgne
Received: 24 November 2016; Accepted: 23 December 2016; Published: 28 December 2016

Abstract: The homeodomain protein PDX-1 is a critical regulator of pancreatic development and insulin production in pancreatic β-cells. We have recently shown that PDX-1 is a substrate of protein kinase CK2; a multifunctional protein kinase which is implicated in the regulation of various cellular aspects, such as differentiation, proliferation, and survival. The CK2 phosphorylation site of PDX-1 is located within the binding region of the E3 ubiquitin ligase adaptor protein PCIF1. To study the interaction between PDX-1 and PCIF1 we used immunofluorescence analysis, co-immunoprecipitation, GST-pull-down studies, and proximity ligation assay (PLA). For the analysis of the stability of PDX-1 we performed a cycloheximide chase. We used PDX-1 in its wild-type form as well as phosphomutants of the CK2 phosphorylation site. In pancreatic β-cells PDX-1 binds to PCIF1. The phosphorylation of PDX-1 by CK2 increases the ratio of PCIF1 bound to PDX-1. The stability of PDX-1 is extended in the absence of CK2 phosphorylation. Our results identified protein kinase CK2 as new important modulator of the stability of PDX-1.

Keywords: pancreatic and duodenal homeobox protein PDX-1; PDX-1 C-terminus interacting factor PCIF1; protein kinase CK2; protein stability

1. Introduction

Protein kinase CK2 is a multifunctional and pleiotropic protein kinase that plays critical roles in cell differentiation, proliferation, and survival [1–3]. CK2 is a multi-subunit protein kinase which is generated by the association of two catalytic α- and/or α'- subunits (38–42 kDa) with a dimer of the 27 kDa non-catalytic β-subunit. Up to now CK2 is known to phosphorylate more than 400 different proteins and the number is rapidly increasing [4]. CK2 phosphorylation of proteins can modulate the subcellular localization, change DNA binding and transcription factor activities, to mention but a few [4]. There are several reports that CK2 also affects the stability or break-down of proteins [5–10].

Recently, we identified the transcription factor PDX-1 as a new substrate for protein kinase CK2 [11]. The pancreatic duodenal homeobox 1 protein (PDX-1), also known as IPF-1, IDX-1, STF-1, GSF, and IUF-1, is expressed in the region of the developing foregut that later becomes the duodenum, distal stomach, and pancreas [12,13]. As development proceeds, PDX-1 expression gets restricted to mostly the hormone-producing β and δ cells of the endocrine pancreas. Murine PDX-1 is a 284 amino acid-long protein with a central homeodomain flanked by proline-rich N- and C-terminal domains. A transactivation domain maps to the N-terminus. The homeodomain contains the DNA binding domain as well as a nuclear localization signal [14,15]. Although the function of the C-terminus is poorly understood, there is some indication that the C-terminus has an inhibitory function whereas other data showed, that the C-terminus is required for full transactivation function [16–18]. PDX-1 is a phosphoprotein and a number of different kinases is known to phosphorylate PDX-1 (for review see [19]). Recently, we identified two phosphorylation sites for protein kinase CK2 in the C-terminus of PDX-1, namely threonine 231 and serine 232 [11] and found that the transcription factor activity of PDX-1 is modulated by the CK2 phosphorylation. Moreover, both phosphorylation sites are in the center of the binding domain for PCIF1 (PDX-1 C terminus interacting factor 1) [20], a protein which targets PDX-1 for ubiquitination and proteasomal degradation [21]. PCIF1, or the human homologue SPOP (Speckle type POZ (pox virus and zinc finger protein)), acts as E3 ubiquitin ligase adaptor which binds the Cullin moiety of the E3 ubiquitin ligase complex to their unique substrate binding adaptor proteins [22]. In the present study, we have analyzed whether the stability of PDX-1 and its interaction with PCIF1 might be affected by the phosphorylation of CK2 within the PCIF1 binding region.

2. Results

We have previously shown that PDX-1 is a substrate for protein kinase CK2 [11]. Phosphorylation sites were identified as threonine 231 and serine 232 of mouse PDX-1. We further showed that the transcription factor activity of PDX-1 is modulated by CK2 phosphorylation. Since the CK2 phosphorylation site of PDX-1 lies in the middle of the interaction domain with the E3 ubiquitin ligase adaptor protein PCIF1 we wanted to know whether the interaction with and the stability of PDX-1 might be affected by CK2 phosphorylation.

A prerequisite for a physical interaction is the co-localization of two proteins. In a first experiment we performed an in situ immunofluorescence analysis with PDX-1 and PCIF1 specific antibodies in mouse pancreatic MIN6 β-cells. Figure 1a shows the localization of PDX-1 (red) and the localization of PCIF1 (green). Merging both images (yellow color) revealed that PDX-1 and PCIF1 colocalize mostly in the nucleus. The fact that both proteins are present in the same place does not necessarily mean that they interact. In a further experiment we, therefore, performed a co-immunoprecipitation with a PDX-1 specific antibody. As there is a lower abundance of PCIF1 in β insulinoma cells ([20], and our observation), we transfected MIN6 cells with eukaryotic expression constructs for PDX-1 and PCIF1. After transfection, cell extracts were incubated with a PDX-1 specific antibody. Proteins of the immunocomplex were separated by SDS polyacrylamide gel electrophoresis and analyzed by immunoblot analysis with a PDX-1 specific and a FLAG-tag antibody against PCIF1. The result shown in Figure 1b demonstrates that both proteins were immunoprecipitated with the PDX-1 specific antibody (lane IP).

A more refined type of analysis to study the interaction of proteins in situ, is the proximity ligation assay PLA [23]. To analyze the role of a CK2 phosphorylation of PDX-1 we inhibited the CK2 activity with the at present most specific CK2 inhibitor CX-4945 [24]. By incubating MIN6 cells for four hours in the presence of 10 μM CX-4945, CK2 activity was reduced to 20% of the activity of untreated cells (−) (Figure 2b). As the transcription factor activity of PDX-1 is glucose responsive [25] and as the interaction with PCIF1 might also be affected by glucose we used glucose concentration of 5 and 25 mM. MIN6 cells were seeded on coverslips, glucose was withdrawn from the medium for 5 h and then added again in a concentration of 5 mM (normoglucose) or 25 mM (high glucose) to stimulate glucose-dependent processes. MIN6 cells were subjected to a PLA analysis with a PDX-1 and a PCIF1 specific antibody. A positive interaction was visualized by red fluorescent dots (Figure 2c). Counting the dots in three different independent areas demonstrated that glucose had no influence on the interaction (average 177 vs. 173 dots/50 cells). However, when cells were treated with the CK2 inhibitor, the mean value decreased to 150 dots/50 cells (85%) under normoglucose and even to 79 dots/50 cells (45%) under high glucose (Figure 2d). Thus, the interaction of both proteins is significantly reduced in the presence of the CK2 inhibitor; the reduction is most obvious under high glucose conditions.

a

b

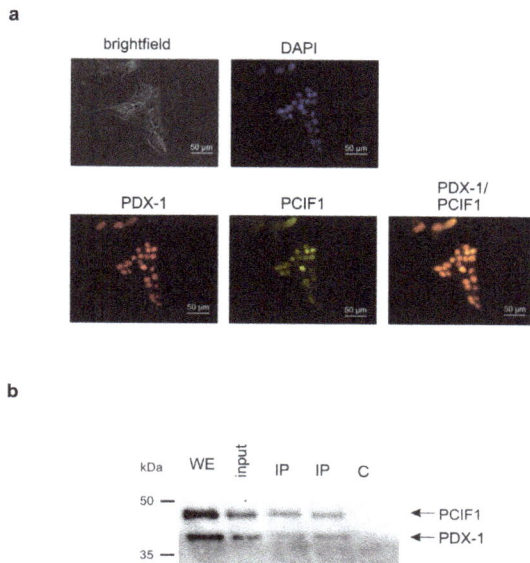

Figure 1. PDX-1 and PCIF1 interaction in MIN6 cells. (**a**) Immunofluorescence analysis of endogenous PDX-1 and PCIF1. MIN6 cells were cultured on coverslips and stained with a polyclonal rabbit antiserum against PDX-1, a goat polyclonal antiserum against PCIF1 (SPOP K-13) and DAPI for nuclei staining. As secondary antibodies, ALEXA-Fluor™488 or ALEXA-Fluor™594 were used. Immunofluorescence was analyzed using a Zeiss Axioskop fluorescence microscope (Zeiss, Jena, Germany). Magnification: 400×; and (**b**) co-immunoprecipitation of PDX-1 and PCIF1 from transfected MIN6 cell extracts. MIN6 cells were transfected with PDX-1 and FLAG-tagged PCIF1 for 24 h. Two mg of cell extract were precleared twice with a mixture of protein A sepharose beads and CL 4-B agarose beads over a period of 1 h. The supernatants were incubated with a rabbit PDX-1 antibody for 2 h. The immunoprecipitated proteins were separated by 12.5% SDS polyacrylamide gel electrophoresis, transferred to a polyvinylidenfluoride (PVDF) membrane and analyzed by Western blot with the mouse monoclonal M2 antibody against the FLAG-tag of PCIF1 and the polyclonal rabbit antiserum against PDX-1. WE: whole cell extract (20 μg), input: 10% of cell extracts used for immunoprecipitation, C: control without antibody, IP: immunoprecipitate, two independent precipitations.

To prove that the interaction of both proteins is phosphorylation-sensitive we performed a GST-pull-down assay with wild-type and phosphomutant proteins [26]. PCIF1 is not a known CK2 substrate; by in silico scanning of the polypeptide chain no sequence with the known consensus motif for CK2 (S/TxxD/E [27]) was found. Thus, we used in vitro translated [^{35}S]-methionine labeled PCIF1 in its wild-type form and incubated it with GST-tagged PDX-1 wild-type and the CK2-phosphodeficient (PDX-1$_{T231A/S232A}$) or the CK2-phosphomimicking (PDX-1$_{T231D/S232E}$) mutant. GST-tagged PDX-1 and bound PCIF1 were pulled-down with GSH sepharose, complexes were eluted and separated on an SDS polyacrylamide gel. Proteins were stained with Coomassie blue and subjected to autoradiography. The result is shown in Figure 3a. The Coomassie blue staining demonstrated that we used equal amounts of GST-PDX-1 forms. All PDX-1 variants bound to PCIF1, however, the phospho-mimicking mutant PDX-1$_{T231D/S232E}$ bound considerably more PCIF1. After evaluation of four independent experiments the binding capacity of the D/E mutant was calculated to be 1.5 fold better than for wild-type or the AA mutant (Figure 3b). Thus, we conclude that the CK2 phosphorylated form of PDX-1 binds better to the E3 ubiquitin ligase adaptor protein PCIF1.

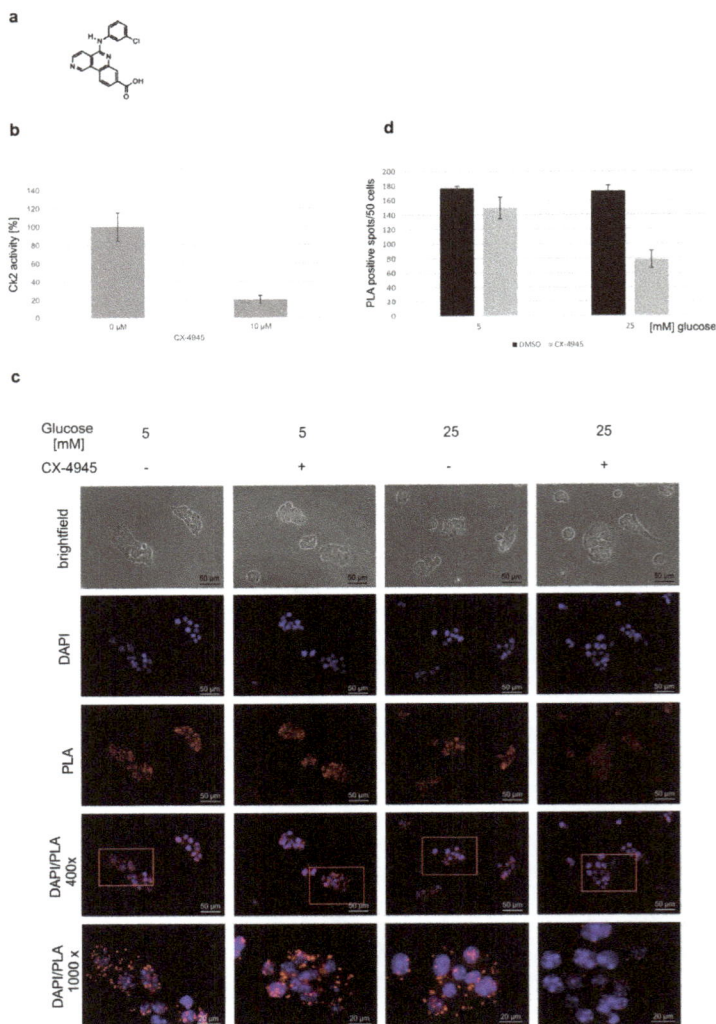

Figure 2. Influence of glucose and CK2 inhibitor CX-4945 on the interaction of PDX-1 and PCIF1. (**a**) Chemical structure of CX-4945 (Silmitasertib); (**b**) in vitro phosphorylation assay in the absence and presence of CX-4945. MIN6 were treated with DMSO as control (0 µM) or with 10 µM CX-4945 for 24 h. Kinase activity of CK2 in the cell extracts was measured with the synthetic CK2 specific peptide substrate, RRRDDDSDDD, in the presence of [^{32}P]γATP. Results from three individual experiments are shown; the activity in the control cells was set to 100%; (**c**) Duolink® in situ proximity ligation assay (PLA) of PDX-1 and PCIF1 in MIN6 cells. MIN6 cells were incubated with 5 mM or 25 mM glucose for 4 h after 5 h starvation and simultaneously with 10 µM CX-4945 (+) or an equal volume DMSO for control (−). Cells were subjected to Duolink® in situ proximity ligation assay using antibodies against PDX-1 (polyclonal rabbit antiserum) and PCIF1 (mouse monoclonal antibody SPOP B-8). Immunofluorescence was analyzed using a Zeiss Axioskop fluorescence microscope (Zeiss, Jena, Germany); and (**d**) quantification of the interaction. Single dots were counted in 50 cells of three different areas. Experiments in the absence of CX-4945 were used as reference (100%). The bar graph shows the median results of three independent counts.

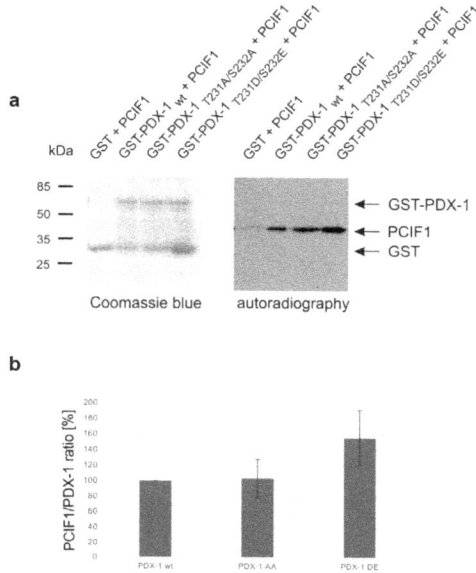

Figure 3. Interaction of PDX-1 and PCIF1 as a function of CK2 phosphorylation. (**a**) GST pull-down analysis of the PCIF1/PDX-1 interaction. About 10 μg GST-PDX-1$_{WT}$, GST-PDX-1$_{T231A/S232A}$, or GST-PDX-1$_{T231D/S232E}$ were incubated with 7.5 μL of in vitro translated and [^{35}S]-methionine labeled PCIF1 protein. The formed complex was coupled to GSH sepharose. Proteins eluted from the affinity resins were analyzed on a 12.5% SDS polyacrylamide gel, stained with Coomassie blue and afterwards subjected to autoradiography; and (**b**) after densitometric analysis of the PDX-1 and PCIF1 signals the PCIF1/PDX-1 ratio was calculated and the relative values were presented as bar graphs referred to the interaction of wild-type PDX-1 and PCIF1.

In the next step we asked whether binding of PDX-1 to PCIF1 might have an influence on the stability of PDX-1. To determine the stability of PDX-1 wild-type, as well as of the CK2 phosphorylation mutant PDX-1$_{T231A/S232A}$, MIN6 cells were transfected with PDX-1 constructs and 30 h after transfection cells were treated with cycloheximide for an inhibition of protein synthesis. Cells were either extracted immediately (0 h) or after 3, 6, 12, or 24 h of treatment. The cell extracts were analyzed on an SDS polyacrylamide gel followed by Western blot with an anti-FLAG-tag-antibody. As shown in Figure 4a, over a time course of 24 h, wild-type PDX-1 degraded more rapidly than the mutant PDX-1$_{T231A/S232A}$. The experiment was done in triplicate, the resulting bands for PDX-1 were scanned, quantified and normalized to the corresponding α-tubulin loading control. The mean ratios (PDX-1/ α-tubulin) +/- standard deviation of the densitometric quantification are shown in Figure 4b. The calculated half-life of wild-type PDX-1 was 12 h, which is in the range of published data [28,29] whereas, the half-life of mutant PDX-1$_{T231A/S232A}$ was about 24 h. Thus, PDX-1, which can no longer be phosphorylated by CK2, is much more stable than the corresponding wild-type form.

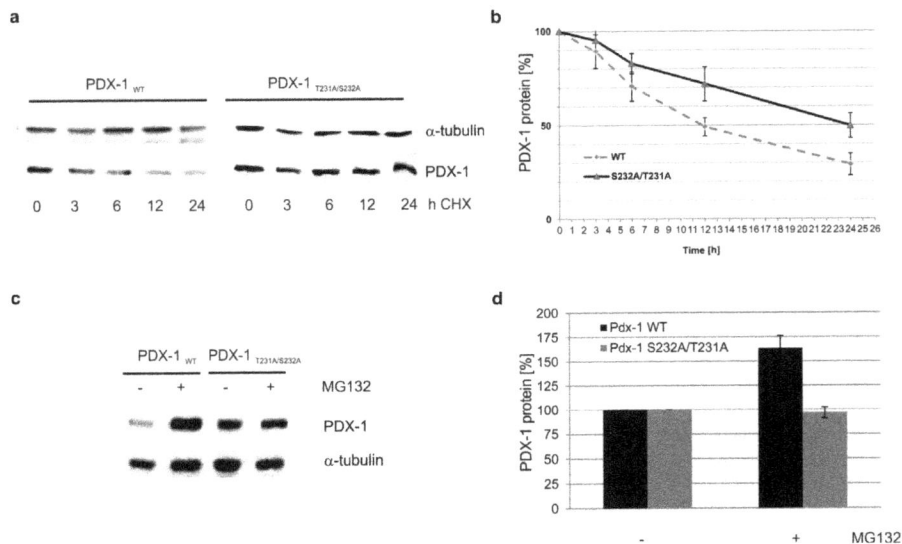

Figure 4. Stability of PDX-1$_{WT}$ and PDX-1$_{T231A/S232A}$ in MIN6 cells. (**a**) MIN6 cells were transfected with FLAG-PDX-1$_{WT}$ or the double mutant FLAG-PDX-1$_{T231A/S232A}$. Thirty hours post transfection, cells were treated with 100 µg/ml cycloheximide (CHX) to inhibit the protein synthesis. Cells were either extracted immediately (0 h) or after 3, 6, 12, and 24 h of treatment. The cell extract was analyzed on a 12.5% SDS polyacrylamide gel and transferred to a PVDF membrane followed by Western blotting with anti-FLAG tag- and anti-α-tubulin- antibodies. α-tubulin was used as a loading control. One representative blot out of three is shown; (**b**) densitometric quantification of the PDX-1 protein after normalization to the loading control at each time point. Mean ± S.D. stands for three independent experiments; (**c**) MIN6 cells transiently transfected with plasmids encoding FLAG-PDX-1$_{WT}$ or FLAG-PDX-1$_{S232A/T231A}$ were treated 48 h post transfection with (+) or without (−) 5 µM MG132 for 11 h. Cells were then lysed and the whole cell extracts were analyzed by Western blotting using anti FLAG-tag and anti-α-tubulin antibodies. α-tubulin was analyzed as a loading control. A quantification of the relative FLAG-PDX-1 protein level (FLAG-PDX-1/α-tubulin) is shown in (**d**). The results were the mean ± S.D. of three independent experiments.

It was shown that PCIF1 and Cullin 3 target PDX-1 for ubiquitination [21]. Therefore, we next tested whether the CK2 phosphorylation of PDX-1 might have an influence on its proteasomal degradation. MIN6 cells were transfected with FLAG-tagged wild-type PDX-1 or with mutant PDX-1$_{S232A/T231A}$ for 48 h. Cells were treated with or without 5 µM MG132, a proteasome inhibitor, for another 11 h and lysed. PDX-1 protein levels were analyzed on a 12.5% SDS polyacrylamide gel and transferred to a PVDF membrane followed by Western blotting using anti-FLAG tag and anti-α-tubulin antibodies. As shown in Figure 4c, treatment with MG132 led to a distinct accumulation of wild-type PDX-1 protein, whereas no significant change was observed in the PDX-1 double alanine mutant protein level. After quantification of the expression of both forms from three independent experiments the increase for the wild-type protein turned out to be more than 50% (Figure 4d). This observation meant that the phosphorylation mutant was less sensitive than wild-type PDX-1 to MG132 treatment, which indicated that the non-phosphorylated form was more resistant to proteasomal degradation whereas wild-type PDX-1 was targeted for degradation by the proteasome machinery.

From these various results we conclude that CK2 phosphorylation of PDX-1 has a massive influence on the stability of PDX-1 and this phosphorylation confers susceptibility of PDX-1 protein to proteasomal degradation.

3. Discussion

Protein kinase CK2 is classified as a serine/threonine kinase with more than 400 different substrates, which indicates the pleiotropic functions of CK2 [4]. We have recently identified PDX-1 as a substrate of CK2. PDX-1 is phosphorylated by CK2 at threonine 231 and serine 232 in the C-terminus [11]. By using CK2 inhibitors as well as by using PDX-1 where the threonine and the serine residues were mutated to alanine, it was shown that the CK2 phosphorylation of PDX-1 regulates its transcription factor activity. Here, we show that CK2 phosphorylation of PDX-1 regulates its stability. Furthermore, we demonstrated that CK2 phosphorylation influences the binding of PDX-1 and PCIF1, a factor which targets PDX-1 for proteasomal degradation. Our observations are summarized in Figure 5.

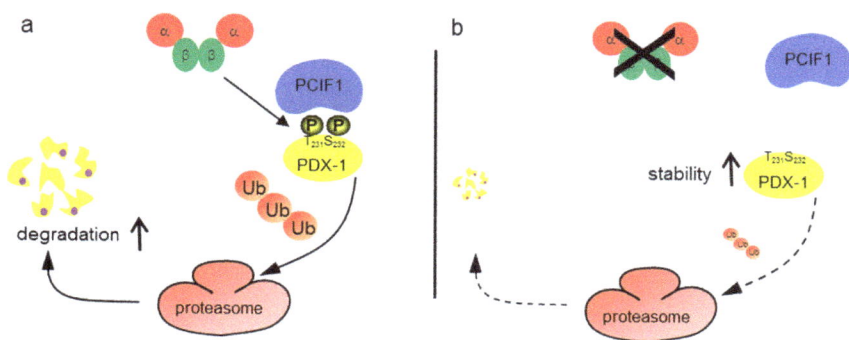

Figure 5. Model of the PDX-1-PCIF1 interaction (**a**) CK2 phosphorylates mouse PDX-1 at threonine 231 and serine 232. This site is located in the middle of a phosphodegron, which binds the E3 ubiquitin ligase protein PCIF1 in a phosphorylated form. PCIF1 targets PDX-1 to the proteasome where it is ubiquitinated and subsequently degraded; and (**b**) upon CK2 inhibition, T231 and S232 of PDX-1 are not phosphorylated. As these important residues of the phosphodegron are not phosphorylated, the interaction with PCIF1 is reduced and PDX-1 is more stable.

The stability of some proteins, such as myc [7], ataxin-3 [30], SAG-SCFE3 ubiquitin ligase [31], PML [8], PTEN [9], VHL [10], and NKX3.1 [32], is regulated by CK2 phosphorylation. Here, we show that the use of PDX-1, which could no more be phosphorylated by CK2 resulted in an elevated stability of PDX-1. There are some other reports showing that the stability of PDX-1 is regulated by phosphorylation. PDX-1 is phosphorylated in vivo on serine 61 and/or serine 66 by glycogen synthase kinase 3 (GSK3) in pancreatic β-cells [29]. This phosphorylation targets the protein for degradation by the proteasome, which results in a decreased half-life for the PDX-1 protein. In contrast, treatment of cells with a proteasome inhibitor led to distinct accumulation of GSK3 phosphorylated PDX-1 protein at serine 61/serine 66, whereas no significant change was observed for total PDX-1 protein. PDX-1 is also phosphorylated by the DNA-dependent protein kinase (DNA PK) and by the mammalian sterile 20-like kinase-1 (MST1) in the N-terminus at threonine 11 [33,34]. This phosphorylation resulted in the ubiquitination and degradation of PDX-1. It is of interest that under diabetic conditions, MST1 was strongly activated in β-cells of human and mouse islets. An et al. [35] recently reported that murine PDX-1 is phosphorylated at serine 269 by the homeodomain interacting protein kinase 2 (HIPK2). Treatment of β-cells with high glucose concentrations resulted in an enhanced phosphorylation at serine 269. It was further shown that HIPK2 phosphorylation at this site affected neither the stability of PDX-1 nor its transactivation potential. However, this phosphorylation affected the subcellular distribution of PDX-1 in MIN6 cells. The same site is also target of p38 MAPK phosphorylation [36]. p38 interacted with PDX-1 and phosphorylated the human protein at serine 268, which resulted in an increased expression and decreased ubiquitination of PDX-1. In βTC3 insulinoma cells this phosphorylation is induced upon a stimulus with glucagon like peptide GLP1 and acts as a positive regulator of PDX-1. In line with these observations we found that the PDX-1 stability was also affected by the CK2 phosphorylation of PDX-1 at threonine 231 and serine 232.

For the ubiquitination and subsequent proteasomal degradation of proteins a highly controlled orchestra of activating E1 enzymes, E2 conjugating enzymes and E3 ubiquitin ligase enzymes is necessary [36]. Targeting the substrates for ubiquitin-mediated degradation is the responsibility of adaptor proteins. Murine PCIF1, or its 100% human homologue SPOP, was identified as such an adaptor protein, which bridges the Cullin 3 moiety of an E3 ligase and its substrate [22]; PDX-1 was identified as one of these PCIF1-binding substrates [20]. Zhuang et al. [37] published a characteristic PCIF1 binding consensus motif which consists of Π-π-S-S/T-S/T (Π = nonpolar, π = polar). In SRC-3, another PCIF1-binding substrate, the binding region was defined as DVSST, where the polar and nonpolar residues occur in a reversed order [38]. For the interaction of PDX-1 and PCIF1, amino acids 210–238 of mouse PDX-1 are essential amino acids [20]. When checking this region (RSSGTPSGGGGGEEPEQDCAVTSGEELLA), we noticed the sequence $_{229}$AVTS$_{232}$ which is quite similar to the SRC-3 binding motif of PCIF1. The threonine and serine residue within this consensus motif are the phosphorylation sites for protein kinase CK2. We found that the binding of PDX-1 to PCIF1 was enhanced upon using phospho-mimicking mutants where T231 and S232 were exchanged by an acid residue; on the other hand, PDX-1 binds weaker to PCIF1 upon inhibition of CK2. There are several examples that binding of E3 ubiquitin ligases, like β-TRCP or FBW7, to their substrates is modulated by phosphorylation [39–41]. So-called phosphodegrons were also found for the PCIF1 substrates SRC-3 [38] and the ERG oncoprotein [42]; in both cases serine residues within the consensus motif are phosphorylated by CK1. The phosphorylation triggers the interaction between the E3 ligase adaptor protein PCIF1 and its substrate and thereby activates degradation.

PCIF1 is a nuclear protein with a speckled pattern of nuclear staining [20], PDX-1 and PCIF1 co-localize in the nucleus [20] and our observation). PCIF1 together with Cullin 3 mediates the ubiquitination of PDX-1 which was shown in ubiquitin overexpression systems [20,43]. Here, we have shown the influence of CK2 phosphorylation of PDX-1 upon its ubiquitination and proteasomal degradation by using the proteasome inhibitor MG132 [44]. We observed that the phosphorylation mutant of PDX-1 had a significant prolonged half-life (24 h) compared with the wild-type PDX-1 (12 h). Furthermore, the wild-type PDX-1, rather than the mutant form of PDX-1, accumulated in response to treatment with the proteasome inhibitor MG132 in β-cells. Thus, all these findings let us conclude that CK2-phosphorylated PDX-1 underwent rapid degradation in β- cells by the proteasomal pathway, further supporting the idea that modification by CK2 phosphorylation served as an important part to regulate the stability of the PDX-1 protein.

Some studies suggested a stimulatory effect of glucose on PDX-1 phosphorylation [16,22,32], whereas others showed that glucose stimulation of β-cells decreases PDX-1 phosphorylation [15]. Moreover, a decrease in C-terminal phosphorylation of PDX-1 was associated with an increase in protein stability. Here, we demonstrated a decrease in binding of PDX-1 to PCIF1 upon CK2 inhibition, which may be the reason for the enhanced stability of the phospho-deficient alanine mutant. The significance of phosphorylation of PDX-1 for the interaction is more obvious under high glucose conditions, a situation where the presence of a fully functional PDX-1 is extremely important for the regulation of insulin transcription, secretion and regulation of blood glucose homeostasis. Therefore, inhibition of CK2 seems to be an option to increase the stability of PDX-1 and subsequently, the level of insulin. A CK2 inhibitor is currently under clinical investigation for the treatment of cancer [24]. It may be an interesting question whether this inhibitor can also be used to treat *Diabetes mellitus*.

4. Materials and Methods

4.1. Cell Culture and Treatment

The mouse cell line MIN6 [45] was maintained in Dulbecco's modified Eagle's medium (Sigma-Aldrich, Munich, Germany) containing 5.5 mM D-glucose and 2 mM glutamine supplemented with 15% (v/i) fetal bovine serum and 100 µM β-mercaptoethanol in humidified 5% CO_2/95% air at 37 °C.

The CK2 inhibitor CX-4945 (SelleckChem, Munich, Germany) was dissolved in dimethyl sulfoxide (DMSO) to a 10 mM stock solution, which was used to treat the cells with the given final concentration. In control experiments we used the same volume of the solvent DMSO alone. To check the stability of the PDX-1 protein, MIN6 cells were transfected with FLAG-tagged PDX-1$_{WT}$ or with mutant PDX-1$_{T231A/S232A}$ and then further incubated for 30 h. The proteasome inhibitor MG132 (Calbiochem, Darmstadt, Germany) was dissolved as 10 mM stock solution in DMSO and applied on transfected cells 48 h post transfection in a final concentration of 5 µM for 11 h.

4.2. Plasmids

Full-length mouse PDX-1 was subcloned into the mammalian expression vector p3xFLAG/ CMV-7.1 (Sigma-Aldrich, Munich, Germany) using the BamH1 site. PDX-1 phosphorylation mutants were generated using a QuikChange site-directed mutagenesis kit (Stratagene, La Jolla, CA, USA) according to the manufacturer's protocol. As another eukaryotic expression vector we used pcDNA3.1-PDX-1$_{WT}$ [11]. PDX-1$_{WT}$ and mutants were also ligated with the bacterial expression vector pGEX-4T-1 (GE Healthcare, Freiburg, Germany) via its BamH1 site [11]. For mammalian expression of human PCIF1 we used pFLAG-CMV-2-SPOP, a kind gift of C. H. Chung, Seoul, South Korea [46]. The cDNA of human PCIF1 was also cloned into the BamH1/Xho1 sites of pET28a. All constructs generated by cloning and mutagenesis were verified by DNA sequencing.

4.3. Extraction of Cells and Western Blot Analysis

For harvesting, cells were scraped off the plate and sedimented by centrifugation (7 min, 4 °C, $400\times g$). Cells were washed with cold phosphate-buffered saline (PBS) and lysed with the double volume of RIPA buffer (50 mM Tris/HCl, pH 8.0, 150 mM NaCl, 0.5% sodium desoxycholate, 1% Triton X-100, 0.1% sodium dodecylsulfate) supplemented with the protease inhibitor cocktail complete^{TM} (Roche Diagnostics, Mannheim, Germany). After lysis, cell debris was removed by centrifugation. The protein content was determined according to a modified Bradford method (BioRad, Munich, Germany). SDS polyacrylamide gel electrophoresis and Western blot analysis was performed essentially as described [11]. PDX-1 was detected using a polyclonal antiserum from rabbit. The mouse monoclonal antibody FLAG M2 (F1804) and the mouse monoclonal antibody β-tubulin (clone DM1A) were from Sigma-Aldrich (Munich, Germany).

4.4. Co-Immunoprecipitation

For co-immunoprecipitation experiments, MIN6 cells were transfected with pcDNA3.1-PDX-1 and pFLAG-CMV-2-SPOP using Effectene^{TM} according to the provider (Qiagen, Hilden, Germany). 24 h after transfection, cells were extracted and 4 mg of total protein was subjected to immunoprecipitation. The cell lysates were pre-cleared twice with a mixture of protein A sepharose beads and CL 4-B sepharose beads (GE Healthcare, Freiburg, Germany) over a period of 1 h. The supernatant was incubated with a rabbit anti PDX-1 antibody for 2 h. Beads were washed four times with PBS (137 mM NaCl, 2.7 mM KCl, 8 mM Na_2HPO_4, 1.5 mM KH_2PO_4, pH 7.4). Bound proteins were eluted with SDS sample buffer (130 mM Tris-HCl, pH 6.8, 0.02% bromophenol blue (w/v), 10% β-mercaptoethanol, 20% glycerol (v/v), and 4% SDS), and analyzed by Western blot with the M2 FLAG-antibody for PCIF1 and the polyclonal rabbit antiserum against PDX-1. Proteins were visualized by the ECL Lumilight system of Roche Diagnostics (Mannheim, Germany).

4.5. Cycloheximide Chase

MIN6 cells were either transfected with FLAG-PDX-1$_{wt}$ or FLAG-PDX-1$_{T231A/S232A}$ mutant using Effectene™ (Qiagen, Hilden, Germany) as recommended by the manufacturer. Thirty hours after transfection, MIN6 cells were cultured in growth medium containing 100 µg/mL cycloheximide (Sigma-Aldrich GmbH, Munich, Germany) for 0, 3, 6, 12, or 24 h. Cells were harvested and lysed with RIPA buffer as described earlier and extracts were subjected to SDS polyacrylamide gel electrophoresis and Western blot analysis. The experiment was performed in triplicate. The PDX-1 signals were scanned and densitometrically quantified using the Quantity One (version 4.6.7.) software from BioRad (Munich, Germany). The values were normalized to an α-tubulin loading control which was analyzed on the same gel. The mean values +/- standard deviation of three independent experiments were represented in the corresponding graphs.

4.6. Immunofluorescence Analysis

MIN6 cells were seeded in a 6 cm plate on coverslips, cultured overnight, and immunofluorescence analysis was performed as described [47]. For identification of the PDX-1 protein, a rabbit polyclonal antiserum generated against the C-terminus of PDX-1 was used. PCIF1 was detected with a goat polyclonal antibody (SPOP K-13 from Santa Cruz Biotechnologies, Heidelberg, Germany). Secondary antibodies were goat anti rabbit AlexaFluor™594 and donkey anti goat AlexaFluor™488 (Invitrogen, Karlsruhe, Germany). Nuclei were visualized by 4,6-diamino-2-phenylindole (DAPI) staining. Analysis was carried out by fluorescence imaging performed on an Axioskop fluorescence microscope (Zeiss, Jena, Germany).

4.7. Duolink® in Situ Proximity Ligation Assay

For detection of the interaction between the PDX-1 protein and PCIF1, we used the Duolink® in situ Proximity Ligation Assay (PLA, Sigma-Aldrich GmbH, Munich, Germany) according to the manufacturer's protocol with MIN6 cells. PDX-1 was detected with the polyclonal rabbit antiserum, PCIF1 with a mouse monoclonal antibody (SPOP B-8, Santa Cruz Biotechnologies, Heidelberg, Germany). Detection of the interaction signals was carried out by fluorescence imaging performed on an Axioskop fluorescence microscope (Zeiss, Jena, Germany).

4.8. GST-Pull Down Assay

The pull-down assay was essentially done as described by Sun et al. [48]. Purified GST-tagged proteins (10 µg) were immobilized on GSH-sepharose and equilibrated with PBS-T binding buffer (PBS, pH 7.4, 1% Tween 20). Immobilized proteins were incubated for 2 h at 4 °C with 7.5 µL of PCIF1 product from an in vitro translation reaction. The translation from a pET28a-PCIF-1 plasmid was done as recommended by the manufacturer (Promega GmbH, Mannheim, Germany). After washing with cold PBS-T, bound proteins were eluted with SDS sample buffer (65 mM Tris-HCl, pH 6.8, 2% SDS, 5% β-mercaptoethanol, 10% glycerol, 0.01% bromophenol blue) and analyzed by SDS polyacrylamide gel electrophoresis, followed by protein staining with Coomassie blue and autoradiography.

4.9. In Vitro Phosphorylation

To determine the activity of CK2 after its inhibition, cells were treated with CX-4945 or left untreated, lysed, and the extracts were used in a kinase filter assay. In this assay we measured the incorporation rate of [^{32}P]-phosphate into the synthetic CK2 specific substrate peptide with the sequence RRRDDDSDDD [14]. Twenty microliter kinase buffer (50 mM Tris/HCl, pH 7.5, 100 mM NaCl, 10 mM MgCl$_2$, 1 mM dithiotreitol (DTT)) containing 30 µg protein were mixed with 30 µL CK2 mix (25 mM Tris/HCl, pH 8.5, 150 mM NaCl, 5 mM MgCl$_2$, 1 mM DTT, 50 µM ATP, 0.19 mM substrate peptide) containing 10 µCi/500 µl [^{32}P]γ ATP. The mixture was spotted onto a P81 ion exchange paper.

The paper was washed three times with 85 mM H_3PO_4. After treatment with ethanol, the paper was dried and the Čerenkov radiation was determined in a scintillation counter.

Acknowledgments: This work was supported by the Rolf M. Schwiete Stiftung, Mannheim, Germany (project Nr. 06/2015) to C.G. and M.M. We are grateful to C.H. Chung (NRL of Protein Biochemistry, School of Biological Sciences, Seoul National University, Korea [46]) for giving us pFLAG-CMV-2-SPOP. The authors thank Sarah Spohrer for performing the in vitro phosphorylation assays of MIN6 extracts.

Author Contributions: M.M. and C.G. conceived and designed the experiments; S.K., R.M. and C.G. performed the experiments and analyzed the data; M.M. and C.G. wrote the paper.

Conflicts of Interest: The authors declare no conflict of interest.

References

1. Litchfield, D.W. Protein kinase CK2: Structure, regulation and role in cellular decisions of life and death. *Biochem. J.* **2003**, *369*, 1–15. [CrossRef] [PubMed]
2. St-Denis, N.A.; Litchfield, D.W. From birth to death: The role of protein kinase CK2 in the regulation of cell proliferation and survival. *Cell Mol. Life Sci.* **2009**, *66*, 1817–1829. [CrossRef] [PubMed]
3. Trembley, J.H.; Wang, G.; Unger, G.; Slaton, J.; Ahmed, K. CK2: A key player in cancer biology. *Cell Mol. Life Sci.* **2009**, *66*, 1858–1867. [CrossRef] [PubMed]
4. Meggio, F.; Pinna, L.A. One-thousand-and-one substrates of protein kinase CK2? *FASEB J.* **2003**, *17*, 349–368. [CrossRef] [PubMed]
5. Desagher, S.; Osen-Sand, A.; Montessuit, S.; Magnenat, E.; Vilbois, F.; Hochmann, A.; Journot, L.; Antonsson, B.; Martinou, J.C. Phosphorylation of Bid by casein kinases I and II regulates its cleavage by caspase 8. *Mol. Cell* **2001**, *8*, 601–611. [CrossRef]
6. Krippner-Heidenreich, A.; Talanian, R.V.; Sekul, R.; Kraft, R.; Thole, H.; Ottleben, H.; Luscher, B. Targeting of the transcription factor Max during apoptosis: phosphorylation-regulated cleavage by caspase-5 at an unusual glutamic acid residue in position P1. *Biochem. J.* **2001**, *358*, 705–715. [CrossRef] [PubMed]
7. Channavajhala, P.; Seldin, D.C. Functional interaction of protein kinase CK2 and c-Myc in lymphomagenesis. *Oncogene* **2002**, *21*, 5280–5288. [CrossRef] [PubMed]
8. Scaglioni, P.P.; Yung, T.M.; Cai, L.F.; Erdjument-Bromage, H.; Kaufman, A.J.; Singh, B.; Teruya-Feldstein, J.; Tempst, P.; Pandolfi, P.P. A CK2-dependent mechanism for degradation of the PML tumor suppressor. *Cell* **2006**, *126*, 269–283. [CrossRef] [PubMed]
9. Vazquez, F.; Grossman, S.R.; Takahashi, Y.; Rokas, M.V.; Nakamura, N.; Sellers, W.R. Phosphorylation of the PTEN tail acts as an inhibitory switch by preventing its recruitment into a protein complex. *J. Biol. Chem.* **2001**, *276*, 48627–48630. [PubMed]
10. Ampofo, E.; Kietzmann, T.; Zimmer, A.; Jakupovic, M.; Montenarh, M.; Götz, C. Phosphorylation of the von Hippel-Lindau protein (VHL) by protein kinase CK2 reduces its protein stability and affects p53 and HIF-1α mediated transcription. *Int. J. Biochem. Cell Biol.* **2010**, *42*, 1729–1735. [CrossRef] [PubMed]
11. Meng, R.; Al-Quobaili, F.; Müller, I.; Götz, C.; Thiel, G.; Montenarh, M. CK2 phosphorylation of PDX-1 regulates its transcription factor activity. *Cell Mol. Life Sci.* **2010**, *67*, 2481–2489. [CrossRef] [PubMed]
12. Ashizawa, S.; Brunicardi, F.C.; Wang, X.P. PDX-1 and the pancreas. *Pancreas* **2004**, *28*, 109–120. [CrossRef] [PubMed]
13. Melloul, D. Transcription factors in islet development and physiology: Role of PDX-1 in beta-cell function. *Ann. N. Y. Acad. Sci.* **2004**, *1014*, 28–37. [CrossRef] [PubMed]
14. Moede, T.; Leibiger, B.; Pour, H.G.; Berggren, P.; Leibiger, I.B. Identification of a nuclear localization signal, RRMKWKK, in the homeodomain transcription factor PDX-1. *FEBS Lett.* **1999**, *461*, 229–234. [CrossRef]
15. Hessabi, B.; Ziegler, P.; Schmidt, I.; Hessabi, C.; Walther, R. The nuclear localization signal (NLS) of PDX-1 is part of the homeodomain and represents a novel type of NLS. *Eur. J. Biochem.* **1999**, *263*, 170–177. [CrossRef] [PubMed]
16. Hani, E.H.; Stoffers, D.A.; Chevre, J.C.; Durand, E.; Stanojevic, V.; Dina, C.; Habener, J.F.; Froguel, P. Defective mutations in the insulin promoter factor-1 (IPF-1) gene in late-onset type 2 diabetes mellitus. *J. Clin. Invest.* **1999**, *104*, R41–R48. [CrossRef] [PubMed]

17. Cockburn, B.N.; Bermano, G.; Boodram, L.L.; Teelucksingh, S.; Tsuchiya, T.; Mahabir, D.; Allan, A.B.; Stein, R.; Docherty, K.; et al. Insulin promoter factor-1 mutations and diabetes in Trinidad: Identification of a novel diabetes-associated mutation (E224K) in an Indo-Trinidadian family. *J. Clin. Endocrinol. Metab.* **2004**, *89*, 971–978. [CrossRef] [PubMed]
18. Lu, M.; Miller, C.; Habener, J.F. Functional regions of the homeodomain protein IDX-1 required for transactivation of the rat somatostatin gene. *Endocrinology* **1996**, *137*, 2959–2967. [PubMed]
19. Al-Quobaili, F.; Montenarh, M. Pancreatic duodenal homeobox factor-1 and diabetes mellitus type 2. *Int. J. Mol. Med.* **2008**, *21*, 399–404. [PubMed]
20. Liu, A.; Desai, B.M.; Stoffers, D.A. Identification of PCIF1, a POZ domain protein that inhibits PDX-1 (MODY4) transcriptional activity. *Mol. Cell Biol.* **2004**, *24*, 4372–4383. [CrossRef] [PubMed]
21. Claiborn, K.C.; Sachdeva, M.M.; Cannon, C.E.; Groff, D.N.; Singer, J.D.; Stoffers, D.A. PCIF1 modulates PDX1 protein stability and pancreatic beta cell function and survival in mice. *J. Clin. Invest.* **2010**, *120*, 3713–3721. [CrossRef] [PubMed]
22. Mani, R.S. The emerging role of speckle-type POZ protein (SPOP) in cancer development. *Drug Discov. Today* **2014**, *19*, 1498–1502. [CrossRef] [PubMed]
23. Söderberg, O.; Leuchowies, K.J.; Gullberg, M.; Janoius, M.; Weibrecht, O.; Larsson, L.G.; Landegren, U. Characterizing proteins and their interactions in cells and tissues using the in situ proximity ligation assay. *Methods* **2008**, *45*, 227–232. [CrossRef] [PubMed]
24. Siddiqui-Jain, A.; Drygin, D.; Streiner, N.; Chua, P.; Pierre, F.; O'Brien, S.E.; Bliesath, J.; Omori, M.; Huser, N.; Ho, C.; et al. CX-4945, an orally bioavailable selective inhibitor of protein kinase CK2, inhibits prosurvival and angiogenic signaling and exhibits antitumor efficacy. *Cancer Res.* **2010**, *70*, 10288–10298. [CrossRef] [PubMed]
25. Shao, S.; Fang, Z.; Yu, X.; Zhang, M. Transcription factors involved in glucose-stimulated insulin secretion of pancreatic beta cells. *Biochem. Biophys. Res. Commun.* **2009**, *384*, 401–404. [CrossRef] [PubMed]
26. Einarson, M.B.; Pugacheva, E.N.; Orlinick, J.R. GST Pull-down. *CSH Protoc.* **2007**. [CrossRef] [PubMed]
27. Meggio, F.; Marin, O.; Pinna, L.A. Substrate specificity of protein kinase CK2. *Cell Mol. Biol. Res.* **1994**, *40*, 401–409. [PubMed]
28. Humphrey, R.K.; Yu, S.M.; Flores, L.E.; Jhala, U.S. Glucose regulates steady-state levels of PDX1 via the reciprocal actions of GSK3 and AKT kinases. *J. Biol. Chem.* **2010**, *285*, 3406–3416. [CrossRef] [PubMed]
29. Boucher, M.J.; Selander, L.; Carlsson, L.; Edlund, H. Phosphorylation marks IPF1/PDX1 protein for degradation by glycogen synthase kinase 3-dependent mechanisms. *J. Biol. Chem.* **2006**, *281*, 6395–6403. [CrossRef] [PubMed]
30. Mueller, T.; Breuer, P.; Schmitt, I.; Walter, J.; Evert, B.O.; Wüllner, U. CK2-dependent phosphorylation determines cellular localization and stability of ataxin-3. *Hum. Mol. Genet.* **2009**, *18*, 3334–3343. [CrossRef] [PubMed]
31. He, H.; Tan, M.; Pamarthy, D.; Wang, G.; Ahmed, K.; Sun, Y. CK2 phosphorylation of SAG at Thr10 regulates SAG stability, but not its E3 ligase activity. *Mol. Cell Biochem.* **2007**, *295*, 179–188. [CrossRef] [PubMed]
32. Li, X.; Guan, B.; Maghami, S.; Bieberich, C.J. NKX3.1 is regulated by protein kinase CK2 in prostate tumor cells. *Mol. Cell Biol.* **2006**, *26*, 3008–3017. [CrossRef] [PubMed]
33. Lebrun, P.; Montminy, M.R.; Van, O.E. Regulation of the pancreatic duodenal homeobox-1 protein by DNA-dependent protein kinase. *J. Biol. Chem.* **2005**, *280*, 38203–38210. [CrossRef] [PubMed]
34. Ardestani, A.; Paroni, F.; Azizi, Z.; Kaur, S.; Khobragade, V.; Yuan, T.; Frogne, T.; Tao, W.; Oberholzer, J.; Pattou, F.; et al. MST1 is a key regulator of beta cell apoptosis and dysfunction in diabetes. *Nat. Med.* **2014**, *20*, 385–397. [CrossRef] [PubMed]
35. An, R.; da Silva Xavier, G.; Semplici, F.; Vakhshouri, S.; Hao, H.X.; Rutter, J.; Pagano, M.A.; Meggio, F.; Pinna, L.A.; Rutter, G.A. Pancreatic and duodenal homeobox 1 (PDX1) phosphorylation at serine-269 is HIPK2-dependent and affects PDX1 subnuclear localization. *Biochem. Biophys. Res. Commun.* **2010**, *399*, 155–161. [CrossRef] [PubMed]
36. Zhou, G.; Wang, H.; Liu, S.H.; Shahi, K.M.; Lin, X.; Wu, J.; Feng, X.H.; Qin, J.; Tan, T.H.; Brunicardi, F.C. p38 MAP kinase interacts with and stabilizes pancreatic and duodenal homeobox-1. *Curr. Mol. Med.* **2013**, *13*, 377–386. [CrossRef] [PubMed]

37. Zhuang, M.; Calabrese, M.F.; Liu, J.; Waddell, M.B.; Nourse, A.; Hammel, M.; Miller, D.J.; Walden, H.; Duda, D.M.; Seyedin, S.N.; et al. Structures of SPOP-substrate complexes: Insights into molecular architectures of BTB-Cul3 ubiquitin ligases. *Mol. Cell* **2009**, *36*, 39–50. [CrossRef] [PubMed]

38. Li, C.; Ao, J.; Fu, J.; Lee, D.F.; Xu, J.; Lonard, D.; O'Malley, B.W. Tumor-suppressor role for the SPOP ubiquitin ligase in signal-dependent proteolysis of the oncogenic co-activator SRC-3/AIB1. *Oncogene* **2011**, *30*, 4350–4364. [CrossRef] [PubMed]

39. Kumar, Y.; Shukla, N.; Thacker, G.; Kapoor, I.; Lochab, S.; Bhatt, M.L.; Chattopadhyay, N.; Sanyal, S.; Trivedi, A.K. Ubiquitin ligase, Fbw7, targets CDX2 for degradation via two phosphodegron motifs in a GSK3β-dependent manner. *Mol. Cancer Res.* **2016**, *14*, 1097–1109. [CrossRef] [PubMed]

40. Barbosa, S.; Carreira, S.; Bailey, D.; Abaitua, F.; O'Hare, P. Phosphorylation and SCF-mediated degradation regulate CREB-H transcription of metabolic targets. *Mol. Biol. Cell* **2015**, *26*, 2939–2954. [CrossRef] [PubMed]

41. Cheng, Y.; Gao, W.W.; Tang, H.M.; Deng, J.J.; Wong, C.M.; Chan, C.P.; Jin, D.Y. β-TrCP-mediated ubiquitination and degradation of liver-enriched transcription factor CREB-H. *Sci. Rep.* **2016**, *6*, 23938. [CrossRef] [PubMed]

42. Gan, W.; Dai, X.; Lunardi, A.; Li, Z.; Inuzuka, H.; Liu, P.; Varmeh, S.; Zhang, J.; Cheng, L.; Sun, Y.; et al. SPOP promotes ubiquitination and degradation of the ERG oncoprotein to suppress prostate cancer progression. *Mol. Cell* **2015**, *59*, 917–930. [CrossRef] [PubMed]

43. Bunce, M.W.; Boronenkov, I.V.; Anderson, R.A. Coordinated activation of the nuclear ubiquitin ligase Cul3-SPOP by the generation of phosphatidylinositol 5-phoshpate. *J. Biol. Chem.* **2008**, *283*, 8678–8686. [CrossRef] [PubMed]

44. Lee, D.H.; Goldberg, A.L. Proteasome inhibitors: Valuable new tools for cell biologists. *Trends Cell Biol.* **1998**, *8*, 397–403. [CrossRef]

45. Miyazaki, J.; Araki, K.; Yamato, E.; Ikegami, H.; Asano, T.; Shibasaki, Y.; Oka, Y.; Yamamura, K. Establishment of a pancreatic beta cell line that retains glucose-inducible insulin secretion: Special reference to expression of glucose transporter isoforms. *Endocrinology* **1990**, *127*, 126–132. [CrossRef] [PubMed]

46. Kwon, J.E.; La, M.; Oh, K.H.; Oh, Y.M.; Kim, G.R.; Seol, J.H.; Baek, S.H.; Chiba, T.; Tanaka, K.; Bang, O.S.; et al. BTB domain-containing speckle-type POZ protein (SPOP) serves as an adaptor of Daxx for ubiquitination by Cul3-based ubiquitin ligase. *J. Biol. Chem.* **2006**, *281*, 12664–12672. [CrossRef] [PubMed]

47. Faust, M.; Schuster, N.; Montenarh, M. Specific binding of protein kinase CK2 catalytic subunits to tubulin. *FEBS Lett.* **1999**, *462*, 51–56. [CrossRef]

48. Sun, Q.; Yu, X.; Degraff, D.J.; Matusik, R.J. Upstream stimulatory factor 2, a novel FoxA1-interacting protein, is involved in prostate-specific gene expression. *Mol. Endocrinol.* **2009**, *23*, 2038–2047. [CrossRef] [PubMed]

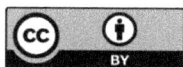

pharmaceuticals

MDPI

Article

Inhibition of Protein Kinase CK2 Prevents Adipogenic Differentiation of Mesenchymal Stem Cells Like C3H/10T1/2 Cells

Lisa Schwind *,†, Sarah Schetting † and Mathias Montenarh

Medical Biochemistry and Molecular Biology, Saarland University, Building 44, D-66424 Homburg, Germany; sasc23@gmx.de (S.S.); Mathias.Montenarh@uks.eu (M.M.)
* Correspondence: Lisa.Schwind@uks.eu; Tel.: +49-6841-16-26518
† These authors contributed equally to this work.

Academic Editor: Marc Le Borgne
Received: 29 November 2016; Accepted: 7 February 2017; Published: 9 February 2017

Abstract: Protein kinase CK2 as a holoenzyme is composed of two catalytic α- or α'-subunits and two non-catalytic β-subunits. Knock-out experiments revealed that CK2α and CK2β are required for embryonic development. Little is known about the role of CK2 during differentiation of stem cells. Mesenchymal stem cells (MSCs) are multipotent cells which can be differentiated into adipocytes in vitro. Thus, MSCs and in particular C3H/10T1/2 cells are excellent tools to study a possible role of CK2 in adipogenesis. We found downregulation of the CK2 catalytic subunits as well as a decrease in CK2 kinase activity with progression of differentiation. Inhibition of CK2 using the potent inhibitor CX-4945 impeded differentiation of C3H/10T1/2 cells into adipocytes. The inhibited cells lacked the observed decrease in CK2 expression, but showed a constant expression of all three CK2 subunits. Furthermore, inhibition of CK2 resulted in decreased cell proliferation in the early differentiation phase. Analysis of the main signaling cascade revealed an elevated expression of C/EBPβ and C/EBPδ and reduced expression of the adipogenic master regulators C/EBPα and PPARγ2. Thus, CK2 seems to be implicated in the regulation of different steps early in the adipogenic differentiation of MSC.

Keywords: adipogenesis; transcription factors; protein kinase; kinase inhibitor

---

1. Introduction

Mesenchymal stem cells (MSCs) are multipotent progenitor cells which can differentiate into adipocytes, chondrocytes, osteocytes, myocytes, and many other cell types [1]. Therefore, MSCs are promising therapeutic tools for tissue regeneration and repair. Understanding the molecular mechanisms underlying MSC differentiation seems to be important. Over the last few years, protein kinase CK2 turned out to play a key role in cell differentiation [2–5]. The serine/threonine kinase CK2 is implicated in a wide variety of different cellular processes including regulation of cell growth, cell proliferation, and apoptosis [6]. The cellular functions of CK2 are vital for proper cell function, organogenesis, embryogenesis, and organ homeostasis. In mammalian cells, CK2 is composed of two catalytic α- or α'-subunits and two non-catalytic β-subunits which form a tetrameric holoenzyme. In addition, there is increasing evidence for individual activities of the α- or β-subunits aside from the holoenzyme [7–9]. This notion is supported by the observation that various types of tissues express different levels of CK2α, CK2α', or CK2β [9,10].

In mice CK2α knock-out is lethal by embryonic day 11 [3,11]. Knock-out mice for CK2β die at embryonic day 6 [12], whereas knock-out mice for CK2α' are viable, but male mice are infertile due to a defective spermatozoa morphogenesis [13]. During mouse development, CK2 expression is high during organogenesis and considerably lower by birth [14]. Furthermore, earlier studies have shown a distinct role of CK2 during differentiation in several stem cell models for neuronal, osteogenic and hematopoietic differentiation [15–20]. Little is known about a role of CK2 in the differentiation of established mesenchymal stem cells to adipocytes [21].

The observation that the CK2 level and the CK2 kinase activity are elevated in cancer cells compared to normal, healthy cells has fuelled the search for specific inhibitors of the kinase activity in order to find tools for pharmacological treatment of cancer. There is a steadily increasing number of CK2 inhibitors published over the last 10 years, which can be classified as ATP analog, substrate analog, or compounds that inhibit the association of the CK2α and the CK2β subunit (for review see: [22,23]).

CX-4945 (5-(3-chlorophenyl)amino)benzo[c][2,6]naphthyridine-8-carboxylic acid), also known as Silmitasertib®, is a potent new-generation, orally available ATP-competitive inhibitor with a high specificity for CK2 [24,25]. CX-4945 has anti-proliferative activity in many cancer cell lines and is under clinical trials for cancer therapy [26,27].

Here, we have analyzed the effect of CX-4945 on the differentiation of the multipotent mesenchymal stem cell line C3H/10T1/2 into adipocytes. We conclude that CK2 positively affects adipogenesis in several ways early during differentiation.

2. Results

2.1. Characterization of CK2 and Adipogenic Transcription Factors during C3H/10T1/2 Differentiation

There is a limited number of models to study the differentiation of MSCs into adipocytes. One of the elegant model systems for this type of analysis is the MSC cell line C3H/10T1/2 [28]. To study adipogenesis in cell culture models like mouse embryo fibroblasts or the pre-adipocyte cell line 3T3-L1, a hormonal mixture—consisting of insulin, the glucocorticoid dexamethasone, and the phosphodiesterase inhibitor isobutyl-methyl-xanthine (IBMX)—is used. In order to set up the experimental conditions for the differentiation of C3H/10T1/2 cells, cells were treated with the same differentiation mix and monitored after a period of 12 days for the appearance of lipid droplets.

As shown in Figure 1a there were no signs of lipid droplets in untreated cells, whereas cells treated with the hormonal mix were full of droplets. These data show that the mixture of insulin, dexamethasone and IBMX is sufficient to induce differentiation of C3H/10T1/2 cells into adipocytes within 12 days. Next, we wondered whether there is an alteration in the expression of the CK2 subunits in the course of the differentiation process. Thus, differentiation was started as described above. Immediately before the start of differentiation (day 0) and then every two days, cells were lysed and the proteins in the cell extract were analyzed on a 12.5% SDS polyacrylamide gel followed by a transfer onto a PVDF membrane and Western blot with CK2α-, CK2α'-, and CK2β-specific antibodies. An antibody against GAPDH was used as a loading control. At day 4 there seems to be a slight increase in all three CK2 subunits, from day 6 on there was a continuous decrease in the level of CK2α and CK2β. CK2α' was even faster downregulated after day 4 until the end of differentiation at day 12 (Figure 1b). The protein bands for CK2α, CK2α', and CK2β were quantified from several experiments and the results are shown in Figure 1c. There was an increase for CK2α at days 4 and 6, whereas there was a continuous decrease in CK2α'. There was a slight increase in CK2β at day 6 followed by a decrease in the level of CK2β for the rest of the differentiation process. In order to analyze whether the decrease in the level of CK2 subunits might also correlate with a decrease in the protein kinase activity, we measured the CK2 kinase activity in the cell extract using the CK2 specific peptide substrate with the sequence RRRDDDSDDD [29]. As shown in Figure 1d, protein kinase activity at days 2 and 4 are mainly constant, whereas from day 6 onwards the kinase activity dropped to around 50% of the level in undifferentiated cells (day 0). Thus, in parallel to the decrease in the level of CK2α and CK2α' proteins, the CK2 kinase activity also decreased. These results indicate that CK2 seems to be dispensable at late stages of adipogenesis.

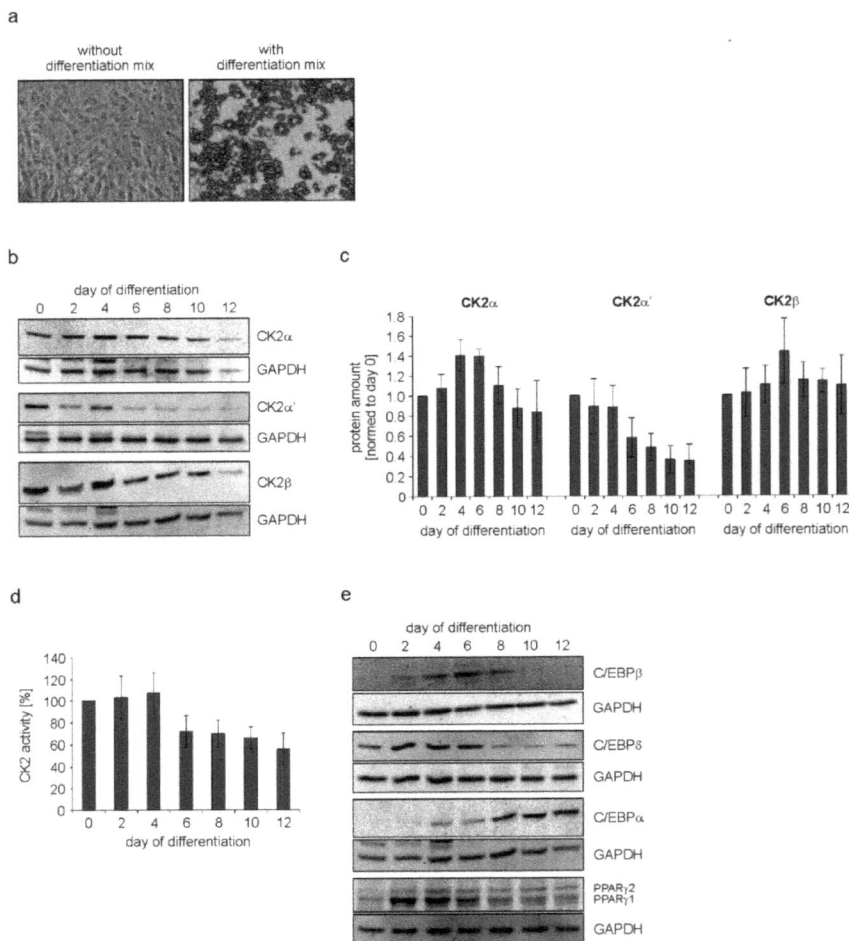

Figure 1. C3H/10T1/2 cells were differentiated for 12 days using IBMX, dexamethasone and insulin. (**a**) Bright field images showing the differentiation status at day 12 of differentiation. Control cells (without differentiation mix) were compared to cells differentiated with the mix. Lipid droplets were stained red with Oil Red O. Magnification 200×; (**b,e**) Cells were harvested at given time points during differentiation and protein expression was detected with specific antibodies using a Western Blot approach. GAPDH was used as loading control; (**c**) Quantification of the protein expression of CK2α, CK2α', and CK2β normalized to GAPDH; (**d**) CK2 activity during adipogenic differentiation of C3H/10T1/2 cells over time shown by the incorporation of $[^{32}P]$phosphate into the CK2 specific substrate peptide RRRDDDSDDD.

It is well-known that adipocyte differentiation is largely controlled by two families of transcription factors, namely the CCAAT/enhancer binding proteins (C/EBPs) and the peroxisome proliferator-activated receptors (PPARs) [30]. Adipogenesis is characterized by a cascade expression of C/EBPα, C/EBPβ, C/EBPδ, PPARγ1, and PPARγ2. In order to analyze the influence of the CK2 level and its enzyme activity on the expression of these different transcription factors, we repeated the experiment described above but in this case cell extracts were analyzed for the expression of C/EBPs and PPARγ. GAPDH expression was analyzed as a loading control. C/EBPδ and C/EBPβ were transiently expressed between day 2 and day 8 of the differentiation process (Figure 1e). C/EBPα showed a constant increase in the expression in the course of the differentiation process. The expression of PPARγ2 increased from day 2 on, whereas PPARγ1 showed a maximal expression between day 2 and day 6.

From these results, we conclude that CK2 expression is high at the beginning of differentiation. Moreover, a programmed expression of different transcription factors is initiated from early time points of differentiation.

2.2. Inhibition of CK2 Kinase Activity with CX-4945 Influences Differentiation, Proliferation, and CK2 Protein Expression

From the experiments described above, it is tempting to speculate that CK2 might be necessary at the beginning of the differentiation process, but not in the second part of the differentiation. To prove this hypothesis, we attempted to study the influence of the inhibition of CK2 on the differentiation. We chose the inhibitor CX-4945 because it is highly specific for CK2, orally available and in clinical trials for the treatment of cancer [26,31,32]. The optimal concentration of the CK2 inhibitor has to be tested for every cell line. Therefore, we incubated proliferating C3H/10T1/2 cells either with DMSO alone (which is the solvent for CX-4945) or with 5, 10, 15, or 20 μM CX-4945. Kinase activity was tested with the synthetic substrate peptide [29].

As shown in Figure 2a, there was a concentration-dependent reduction in the CK2 kinase activity ranging from 60% (5 μM CX-4945) up to 90% (20 μM CX-4945). For the following experiments we decided to use a concentration of 15 μM CX-4945, which resulted in a residual kinase activity of around 12%. To make sure, that CX-4945 was able to reduce the CK2 kinase activity during the whole differentiation process, we determined the activity from day 2 to day 12 of the differentiation. We found that the kinase activity was reduced by 75% to 85% in the presence of CX-4945 compared to cells without inhibitor over the whole period of differentiation (Figure 2b). In the next step, cells were incubated with the differentiation mix either in the presence or absence of 15 μM CX-4945 and the appearance of lipid droplets was monitored on day 12 of differentiation. As shown in Figure 2c, cells treated with the hormonal mix exhibited multiple lipid droplets, whereas in the presence of CX-4945 there were virtually no droplets. Thus, inhibition of CK2 by CX-4945 inhibits differentiation of the MSC cell line C3H/10T1/2 into adipocytes. Furthermore, cells looked healthy after treatment with CX-4945 and no morphological changes associated with apoptosis could be observed. This observation is in contrast to the effect of CX-4945 in many cancer cells [26,32].

It is known that 3T3-L1 pre-adipocytes respond to the treatment with the differentiation mix with mitotic clonal expansion (MCE) and that it is crucial for differentiation [33]. On the contrary, human MSC do not need MCE [34] and nothing is known about it in C3H/10T1/2 cells. Therefore, we asked whether CK2 inhibition might have an influence on the proliferation of C3H/10T1/2 cells. Cells were grown in the absence or presence of CX-4945 and counted at 0, 24, 48, and 72 h after the start of differentiation. The growth curve analysis, which is shown in Figure 2d, revealed a growth reduction in the presence of CX-4945. Thus, there seems to be an effect of CK2 inhibition on cell growth before the entrance into differentiation. A reduction in proliferation due to CX-4945 treatment could be the result of disturbances in cellular metabolism or apoptosis induction. So subsequently, we used an MTT assay to analyze metabolic activity 24 and 48 h after start of differentiation. As presented in Figure 2e, the metabolism of the cells was only marginally influenced by CX-4945-treatment compared to DMSO control. Apoptosis induction was examined by the detection of caspase-3 and one of its substrates poly [ADP-ribose] polymerase (PARP), which are cleaved in the event of apoptosis. Figure 2f shows that a part of caspase-3 and PARP full length proteins were cleaved 48 h after the start of differentiation, independently of the kind of treatment. Treating the cells with CX-4945 did not significantly enhance cleavage. From this experiment we conclude that the observed reduction of proliferation is not caused by metabolic disturbance or apoptosis, but by CK2 inhibition.

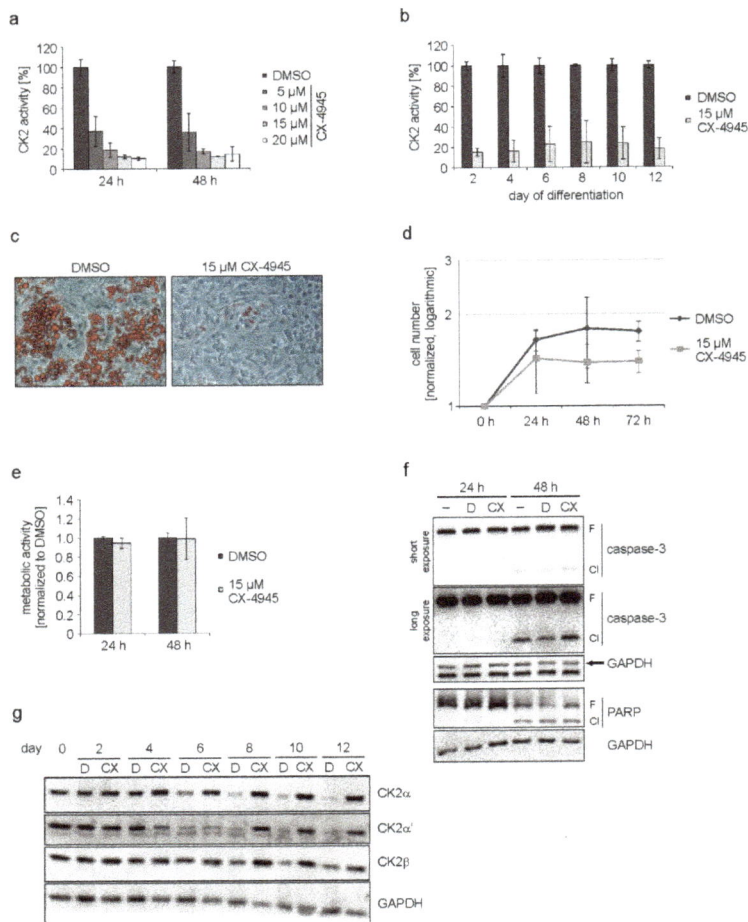

Figure 2. C3H/10T1/2 cells were differentiated in the presence of DMSO or CX-4945. (**a**) Proliferating C3H/10T1/2 cells were treated with 5, 10, 15, or 20 µM CX-4945 or DMSO as a control for 24 and 48 h. CK2 kinase activity was determined in an in vitro phosphorylation assay; (**b**) Cells were differentiated with differentiation mix containing DMSO or 15 µM CX-4945 and harvested at given time points. CK2 activity was determined in the protein extracts to confirm the inhibition over the complete differentiation process; (**c**) Differentiation status at day 12 of differentiation in cells treated with DMSO or 15 µM CX-4945. Lipid droplets were stained with Oil Red O and bright field images were recorded at 200× magnification; (**d**) Proliferation of DMSO- or 15 µM CX-4945-treated cells was determined at 0, 24, 48, and 72 h after the start of differentiation. Cell numbers were normalized to 0 h and are presented half-logarithmic; (**e**) Metabolic activity was examined in C3H/10T1/2 cells using MTT assay after differentiation of DMSO- or 15 µM CX-4945-treated cells for 24 or 48 h. Results were normalized to DMSO control values; (**f**) Differentiating cells were harvested 24 or 48 h after start of differentiation and cleavage of caspase-3 and PARP indicating apoptosis was examined using Western blot analysis −: untreated, D: DMSO-treated, CX: 15 µM CX-4945-treated, F: full length, Cl: cleavage product; (**g**) Western blot images of protein extracts from cells differentiated in the presence of DMSO (D) or 15 µM CX-4945 (CX) using specific antibodies for the CK2-subunits. GAPDH was used as loading control for all Western blots.

Since we have shown above that CK2 inhibition by CX-4945 resulted in impaired adipogenic differentiation, we wondered whether this had an influence on CK2 subunit expression. C3H/10T1/2 cells were treated with the hormonal mix to induce differentiation in the presence or absence of the CK2 inhibitor CX-4945. Proteins were extracted at different time points up to day 12 of differentiation and analyzed for CK2α, CK2α′, and CK2β subunits. The Western blot shown in Figure 2g shows that there is a reduction in CK2α, CK2α′, and CK2β expression during the differentiation, which is in agreement with the results shown in Figure 1b, whereas in the presence of the CK2 inhibitor (CX) no reduction could be observed. These results show that downregulation of CK2 subunits is accompanied with adipogenic differentiation. Inhibition of the kinase activity of CK2 prevents differentiation. In this case, the levels of the CK2 subunits remain constantly high.

2.3. Inhibition of CK2 Activity with CX-4945 Influences Expression of Important Adipogenic Transcription Factors

In Figure 1e, we have shown that differentiation of C3H/10T1/2 cells is accompanied by a specific expression of transcription factors. Therefore, in the next experiment we asked whether inhibition of CK2 with CX-4945 might influence the expression of these transcription factors. Thus, C3H/10T1/2 cells were incubated with the differentiation mix either in the presence or absence of CX-4945. Cells were harvested at different time points after the start of differentiation and proteins in the cell extracts were analyzed by SDS-polyacrylamide gel electrophoresis followed by Western blot with specific antibodies against C/EBPα, C/EBPβ, C/EBPδ, and PPARγ2. In this experiment, we focused on the PPARγ2 isoform, because this is the one responsible for adipogenesis [35,36].

As shown in Figure 3, in the presence of CX-4945, we observed an elevated and prolonged expression of C/EBPβ and C/EBPδ as well as a reduced expression of C/EBPα and PPARγ2 compared to the regular differentiation (DMSO). Thus, in addition to the influence on cell growth at early stages of differentiation, these results point to an influence of the CK2 kinase activity on the expression of the early transcription factors C/EBPβ and C/EBPδ, which then influence C/EBPα and PPARγ2 expression, leading finally to a block in differentiation.

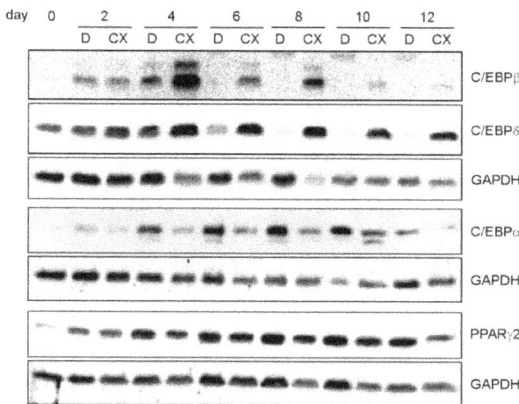

Figure 3. C3H/10T1/2 cells were differentiated in the presence of DMSO (D) or 15 μM CX-4945 (CX) and harvested at given time points during differentiation. Proteins were extracted and separated on a 12.5% SDS-polyacrylamide gel and transferred to a PVDF-membrane. C/EBPβ, C/EBPδ, C/EBPα, and PPARγ2 were detected with specific antibodies. GAPDH was used as a loading control.

3. Discussion

Obesity is a common health problem in industrialized countries, which is closely associated with other diseases such as hypertension, cancer, diabetes, and atherosclerosis just to mention a few. Therefore, there is an acute need for new and effective strategies to reduce obesity. Here, we have used the mouse embryo mesenchymal stem cell line C3H/10T1/2 which was first described in 1973 [28]. These cells behave in a manner similar to that of mesenchymal stem cells, making C3H/10T1/2 cells a useful model for cell differentiation. C3H/10T1/2 cells were stimulated either with BMP2 or with peptides derived from different regions of the bone morphogenetic protein receptor type Ia (BMPRIa) and then evaluated for their chondrogenic and osteogenic potential. The peptides were identified as inhibitors of the binding of CK2 to BMPRIa [16]. These peptides activate the BMP signaling in the absence of BMP [37]. Here, we have used a mix of dexamethasone, IBMX, and insulin to induce adipogenic differentiation. This process can be monitored by the appearance of lipid droplets which is more or less completed at day 12 after the start of differentiation. The differentiation process is governed by the regulated expression of several transcription factors such as C/EBPα, C/EBPβ, C/EBPδ, and PPARγ. In addition to the regulated expression of these transcription factors we also observed changing levels of the CK2 subunits. Interestingly, the catalytic CK2α' subunit was downregulated rapidly during differentiation whereas CK2α and CK2β initially increased and then slowly decreased. These results indicate that at least CK2α' is not necessary for differentiation. The reduction of the level of the CK2 subunits is accompanied by a decrease in the protein kinase activity. Therefore, we conclude that neither the CK2 subunits nor the enzymatic activity of CK2 is required towards the end of differentiation. The CK2 protein levels as well as the CK2 kinase activity are high at the beginning of differentiation. By immunohistochemistry and by in situ hybridization CK2 protein levels as well as mRNA levels for the individual subunits were found to be elevated in mouse embryogenesis [38]. Similar observations were made for rat, chicken, and *C. elegans* embryonic development [39–41]. An enhanced expression of CK2 goes along with an elevated CK2 kinase activity with a maximum at day 11 [14]. Knock-out experiments revealed that CK2α$^{-/-}$ as well as CK2β$^{-/-}$ mice are embryonically lethal [3,12]. The role of CK2 during differentiation of stem cells is less clear [17–19]. It was recently shown that in the pre-adipocyte cell line 3T3-L1 CK2 is necessary for early steps in differentiation which is in agreement with our present observation with C3H/10T1/2 cells [42]. An early step in differentiation of 3T3-L1 cells is one or two rounds of cell division prior to differentiation and it may well be that CK2 is necessary for this early step. Our present analysis of the cell growth properties showed that there is indeed an influence of CX-4945 on cell growth. This observation is compatible with the role of CK2 in proliferation. It is well known that the CK2 level and CK2 activity is high in rapidly proliferating cells such as tumour cells and low in healthy normal cells [43,44]. Over the last 10 years this particular observation has fuelled the search for specific inhibitors of the CK2 kinase activity in order to find a new therapeutic approach for the treatment of cancer. Among the numerous inhibitors now published for CK2 we have chosen CX-4945 because this inhibitor is bioavailable and used in clinical trials for the treatment of cancer [24,32]. As shown here, CX-4945 inhibits the differentiation of C3H/10T1/2 cells into adipocytes. This inhibition goes along with an early induction of the level of C/EBPδ and C/EBPβ. C/EBPδ interacts with C/EBPβ to induce C/EBPα and PPARγ2 expression during adipogenesis [45]. Our data, however, show that an elevated level of C/EBPβ and C/EBPδ is not sufficient to stimulate the expression of C/EBPα and PPARγ2, which are the master regulators of adipogenesis [35,46]. In contrast, there is a reduction in the level of C/EBPα and PPARγ2 in the presence of the CK2 inhibitor. One reason for this observation may be a missing CK2 phosphorylation of C/EBPδ and/or C/EBPβ. It was indeed recently shown that C/EBPδ is phosphorylated by CK2 [47]. Although the binding of C/EBPδ to C/EBPβ is not influenced by the CK2 phosphorylation of C/EBPδ, it was shown that the CK2 phosphorylated C/EBPδ transactivated the PPARγ2 promoter better than the non-phosphorylatable C/EBPδ mutant. This observation is in a good agreement with the results shown here and may explain them.

In summary, we would like to propose the model shown in Figure 4. CK2 seems to have a triple influence on early steps during the differentiation of mesenchymal stem cells. First, inhibition of the CK2 kinase activity reduced cell proliferation; second, CK2 inhibition increased the level of the two transcription factors C/EBPβ and C/EBPδ; and third, CK2 inhibition leads to a reduction in the expression of PPARγ2 and C/EBPα, two transcription factors, which are absolutely necessary for the differentiation into adipocytes.

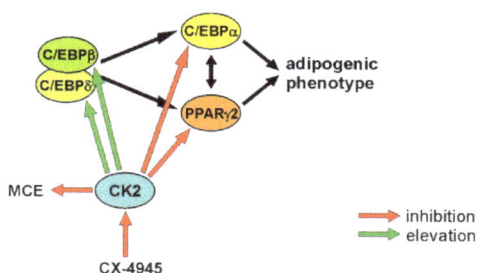

Figure 4. Schematic outline of the observations on adipogenic differentiation after inhibition of CK2 with CX-4945.

4. Materials and Methods

4.1. Cell Culture, Differentiation, and Treatment of Cells

The C3H/10T1/2 cell line (ATCC: CCL-226™) was isolated from a line of C3H mouse embryo cells [28]. This cell line was kindly provided by Angelika Barnekow, Münster. C3H/10T1/2 cells can be induced to terminally differentiate into adipocytes by the addition of different hormones or chemical agents. Cells are maintained in Dulbecco's modified Eagle's medium (DMEM; Thermo Fisher Scientific, St. Leon-Rot, Germany) supplemented with 10% (v/v) fetal calf serum (FCS) in a humidified atmosphere containing 5% CO_2 at 37 °C.

To differentiate C3H/10T1/2 cells into adipocytes, cells were seeded at a density of 2×10^4 cells/cm². When cells were two days post-confluent, medium was removed and substituted by the differentiation mix I (DMEM + 10% FCS, 0.5 mM IBMX, 0.25 μM dexamethasone, 5 μg/mL insulin) (corresponds to day 1 of the differentiation). After three days, mix I was replaced by fresh medium. From day six on, cells were incubated with differentiation mix II (DMEM + 10% FCS, 5 μg/mL insulin), which was replaced every three days.

The CK2 inhibitor CX-4945 (Selleckchemicals, Munich, Germany) was dissolved in dimethyl sulfoxide (DMSO; Merck, Darmstadt, Germany) to a 10 mM stock solution, which was used to treat the cells in a final concentration of 15 μM throughout the entire differentiation unless otherwise stated. In control experiments we used the same volume of the solvent DMSO alone.

4.2. Determination of Proliferation and Metabolic Activity

Cells were seeded in 24-well plates (5×10^4 cells/well). After three days, cells were differentiated in the presence of DMSO or 15 μM CX-4945. To determine proliferation, cells were counted in triplicates using a Neubauer chamber (factor: 10^4) at 0, 24, 48 and 72 h after start of differentiation. Cells were trypsinized and resuspended in a small amount of cell culture medium. A small amount of the cell suspension was mixed with an equal amount of the diazo dye trypan blue to stain dead cells. To determine the proliferation rate, only living cells were counted. The cell number determined for 0 h was set to 1.

To determine metabolic activity, cells were incubated for 1 h with 3-[4,5-dimethylthiazol-2-yl] 2,5-diphenyl tetrazolium bromide (MTT) reagent (1 mg/mL solved in PBS) at 24 and 48 h after start of differentiation. Subsequently, cells were lysed with solubilization solution (10% SDS, 0.6% acetic acid in DMSO) and absorption was measured at 595 nm. Results were normalized to DMSO.

4.3. Extraction of Proteins

Cells were washed with cold PBS, scraped off the plate, centrifuged ($250\times g$, 4 °C) and the pellet was extracted with RIPA-buffer (50 mM Tris-HCl, 160 mM NaCl, 0.5% sodium desoxycholate, 1% Triton X-100, 0.1% SDS, pH 8.0) in the presence of protease inhibitors (Complete™, Roche Diagnostics, Mannheim, Germany). After 30 min on ice, cells were sonicated (3×30 s). After lysing, the cell debris was removed by centrifugation at $13,000\times g$. The protein content was determined with the BioRad reagent dye (BioRad, Munich, Germany). Protein extracts were immediately used for Western Blot analysis or for in vitro phosphorylation.

4.4. SDS–Polyacrylamide Gel Electrophoresis and Western Blot Analysis

Proteins were analyzed by SDS-polyacrylamide gel electrophoresis according to the procedure of Laemmli [48]. Proteins dissolved in sample buffer (130 mM Tris-HCl, pH 6.8, 0.02% bromophenol blue, 10% β-mercaptoethanol, 20% glycerol, 4% SDS) were separated on a 12.5% SDS- polyacrylamide gel in electrophoresis buffer (25 mM Tris-HCl, pH 8.8, 192 mM glycine, 0.1% SDS) and transferred onto a PVDF membrane (Roche Diagnostics, Mannheim, Germany) in a buffer containing 20 mM Tris-HCl, 150 mM glycine, pH 8.3. The membrane was blocked with 5% dry milk in TBS-Tween 20 for one hour and then incubated with appropriate primary antibodies diluted in TBS-Tween 20 with 1% dry milk or 5% bovine serum albumin (BSA) according to the supplier's instructions. The membrane was washed twice with the incubation buffer and incubated with the peroxidase-coupled secondary antibody (anti-rabbit 1:30,000 or anti-mouse 1:10,000 in incubation buffer) for 1 h. Signals were visualized by the Lumilight system of Roche Diagnostics (Mannheim, Germany).

For the detection of protein kinase CK2 we used rabbit anti-peptide sera #26 (α-subunit), #30 (α'-subunit) and #32 (β-subunit) [49] and the mouse monoclonal antibody 6D5 (β-subunit) [50] or antibody 1A5 (α-subunit) [51]. C/EBPβ- (#3087), PPARγ- (#2430), caspase-3- (#9662), and PARP- (#9542) specific antibodies were from Cell Signalling Technology, the C/EBPδ-specific antibody (sc-151) was purchased from Santa Cruz Biotechnology Inc. (Heidelberg, Germany) and the C/EBPα- (ab40764) and PPARγ2- (ab45036) specific antibodies from Abcam (Cambridge, UK). Furthermore, we used a GAPDH specific antibody (sc-25778) from Santa Cruz Biotechnologies as loading control.

4.5. CK2 In Vitro Phosphorylation Assay

To determine the kinase activity of CK2, cells were lysed and the extracts were used in a kinase filter assay. In this assay, we measured the incorporation rate of $[^{32}P]$phosphate into the synthetic CK2 specific substrate peptide with the sequence RRRDDDSDDD [29]. Twenty μL kinase buffer (50 mM Tris-HCl, pH 7.5, 100 mM NaCl, 10 mM MgCl$_2$, 1 mM DTT) containing 30 μg proteins were mixed with 30 μL CK2 mix (25 mM Tris-HCl, pH 8.5, 150 mM NaCl, 5 mM MgCl$_2$, 1 mM dithiothreitol (DTT), 50 μM ATP, 0.19 mM substrate peptide) containing 10 μCi/500 μL $[^{32}P]$-γ-ATP. The mixture was spotted onto a P81 ion exchange paper. The paper was washed with 85 mM H$_3$PO$_4$ three times. After treatment with ethanol the paper was dried and the Čerenkov-radiation was determined in a scintillation counter.

4.6. Staining of Lipid Droplets in C3H/10T1/2 Cells

For staining lipids with Oil Red O (Sigma Aldrich, Munich, Germany), cells were grown in six-well plates and left untreated or differentiated into adipocytes as described above. After removing the medium and washing with PBS, cells were fixed in 3.7% formaldehyde in PBS for 2 min at room temperature and then washed three times with PBS. Oil Red O was dissolved in isopropanol (0.5 g/100·mL). A 60% solution of Oil Red O was prepared with bi-distilled water, incubated for 10 min at room temperature, and subsequently filtered through a folded filter (3MM, Whatman, UK).

Cells were incubated with Oil Red O (2 mL/well) for one hour at room temperature. After incubation, the Oil Red O was removed and cells were washed twice with distilled water. The staining of the lipid droplets was analyzed by phase contrast microscopy.

Author Contributions: M.M. conceived the experiments; L.S. and S.S. designed and performed the experiments and analyzed the data; M.M. and L.S. wrote the paper.

Conflicts of Interest: The authors declare no conflict of interest.

References

1. Cook, D.; Genever, P. Regulation of mesenchymal stem cell differentiation. *Adv. Exp. Med. Biol.* **2013**, *786*, 213–229.
2. Guerra, B.; Issinger, O.G. Protein kinase CK2 and its role in cellular proliferation, development and pathology. *Electrophoresis* **1999**, *20*, 391–408. [CrossRef]
3. Lou, D.Y.; Dominguez, I.; Toselli, P.; Landesman-Bollag, E.; O'Brien, C.; Seldin, D.C. The alpha catalytic subunit of protein kinase CK2 is required for mouse embryonic development. *Mol. Cell. Biol.* **2008**, *28*, 131–139. [CrossRef] [PubMed]
4. Mannowetz, N.; Kartarius, S.; Wennemuth, G.; Montenarh, M. Protein kinase CK2 and binding partners during spermatogenesis. *Cell Mol. Life Sci.* **2010**, *67*, 3905–3913. [CrossRef] [PubMed]
5. Dietz, K.N.; Miller, P.J.; Hollenbach, A.D. Phosphorylation of serine 205 by the protein kinase CK2 persists on Pax3-FOXO1, but not Pax3, throughout early myogenic differentiation. *Biochemistry* **2009**, *48*, 11786–11795. [CrossRef] [PubMed]
6. Filhol, O.; Cochet, C. Cellular functions of Protein kinase CK2: A dynamic affair. *Cell Mol. Life Sci.* **2009**, *66*, 1830–1839. [CrossRef] [PubMed]
7. Heriche, J.K.; Lebrin, F.; Rabilloud, T.; LeRoy, D.; Chambaz, E.M.; Goldberg, Y. Regulation of protein phosphatase 2A by direct interaction with casein kinase 2alpha. *Science* **1997**, *276*, 952–955. [CrossRef] [PubMed]
8. Lüscher, B.; Litchfield, D.W. Biosynthesis of casein kinase II in lymphoid cell lines. *Eur. J. Biochem.* **1994**, *220*, 521–526. [CrossRef] [PubMed]
9. Guerra, B.; Siemer, S.; Boldyreff, B.; Issinger, O.G. Protein kinase CK2: Evidence for a protein kinase CK2 subunit fraction, devoid of the catalytic CK2 subunit, in mouse brain and testicles. *FEBS Lett.* **1999**, *462*, 353–357. [CrossRef]
10. Stalter, G.; Siemer, S.; Becht, E.; Ziegler, M.; Remberger, K.; Issinger, O.-G. Asymmetric expression of protein kinase CK2 in human kidney tumors. *Biochem. Biophys. Res. Commun.* **1994**, *202*, 141–147. [CrossRef] [PubMed]
11. Dominguez, I.; Degano, I.R.; Chea, K.; Cha, J.; Toselli, P.; Seldin, D.C. CK2alpha is essential for embryonic morphogenesis. *Mol. Cell. Biochem.* **2011**, *356*, 209–216. [CrossRef] [PubMed]
12. Buchou, T.; Vernet, M.; Blond, O.; Jensen, H.H.; Pointu, H.; Olsen, B.B.; Cochet, C.; Issinger, O.G.; Boldyreff, B. Disruption of the regulatory subunit of protein kinase CK2 in mice leads to a cell-autonomous defect and early embryonic lethality. *Mol. Cell. Biol.* **2003**, *23*, 908–915. [CrossRef] [PubMed]
13. Xu, X.; Toselli, P.A.; Russell, L.D.; Seldin, D.C. Globozoospermia in mice lacking the casein kinase II' catalytic subunit. *Nat. Genet.* **1999**, *23*, 118–121. [PubMed]
14. Schneider, H.R.; Reichert, G.H.; Issinger, O.G. Enhanced casein kinase II activity during mouse embryogenesis. Identification of a 110-kDa phosphoprotein as the major phosphorylation product in mouse embryos and Krebs II mouse ascites tumor cells. *Eur. J. Biochem.* **1986**, *161*, 733–738. [CrossRef] [PubMed]
15. Bragdon, B.; Thinakaran, S.; Moseychuk, O.; King, D.; Young, K.; Litchfield, D.W.; Petersen, N.O.; Nohe, A. Casein kinase 2 beta-subunit is a regulator of bone morphogenetic protein 2 signaling. *Biophys. J.* **2010**, *99*, 897–904. [CrossRef] [PubMed]
16. Bragdon, B.; Thinakaran, S.; Moseychuk, O.; Gurski, L.; Bonor, J.; Price, C.; Wang, L.; Beamer, W.G.; Nohe, A. Casein kinase 2 regulates in vivo bone formation through its interaction with bone morphogenetic protein receptor type Ia. *Bone* **2011**, *49*, 944–954. [CrossRef] [PubMed]

17. Moseychuk, O.; Akkiraju, H.; Dutta, J.; D'Angelo, A.; Bragdon, B.; Duncan, R.L.; Nohe, A. Inhibition of CK2 binding to BMPRIa induces C2C12 differentiation into osteoblasts and adipocytes. *J. Cell Commun. Signal.* **2013**, *7*, 265–278. [CrossRef] [PubMed]

18. Cheng, P.; Kumar, V.; Liu, H.; Youn, J.I.; Fishman, M.; Sherman, S.; Gabrilovich, D. Effects of notch signaling on regulation of myeloid cell differentiation in cancer. *Cancer Res.* **2014**, *74*, 141–152. [CrossRef] [PubMed]

19. Dovat, S.; Song, C.; Payne, K.J.; Li, Z. Ikaros, CK2 kinase, and the road to leukemia. *Mol. Cell. Biochem.* **2011**, *356*, 201–207. [CrossRef] [PubMed]

20. Gratton, M.O.; Torban, E.; Jasmin, S.B.; Theriault, F.M.; German, M.S.; Stifani, S. Hes6 promotes cortical neurogenesis and inhibits Hes1 transcription repression activity by multiple mechanisms. *Mol. Cell. Biol.* **2003**, *23*, 6922–6935. [CrossRef] [PubMed]

21. Schwind, L.; Wilhelm, N.; Kartarius, S.; Montenarh, M.; Gorjup, E.; Götz, C. Protein kinase CK2 is necessary for the adipogenic differentiation of human mesenchymal stem cells. *Biochem. Biophys. Acta* **2014**, *1853*, 2207–2216. [CrossRef] [PubMed]

22. Cozza, G.; Bortolato, A.; Moro, S. How druggable is protein kinase CK2? *Med. Res. Rev.* **2009**, *30*, 419–462. [CrossRef] [PubMed]

23. Cozza, G.; Pinna, L.A.; Moro, S. Protein kinase CK2 inhibitors: A patent review. *Expert Opin. Ther. Pat.* **2012**, *22*, 1081–1097. [CrossRef] [PubMed]

24. Siddiqui-Jain, A.; Drygin, D.; Streiner, N.; Chua, P.; Pierre, F.; O'Brien, S.E.; Bliesath, J.; Omori, M.; Huser, N.; Ho, C.; et al. CX-4945, an Orally Bioavailable Selective Inhibitor of Protein Kinase CK2, Inhibits Prosurvival and Angiogenic Signaling and Exhibits Antitumor Efficacy. *Cancer Res.* **2010**, *70*, 10288–10298. [CrossRef] [PubMed]

25. Battistutta, R.; Cozza, G.; Pierre, F.; Papinutto, E.; Lolli, G.; Sarno, S.; O'Brien, S.E.; Siddiqui-Jain, A.; Haddach, M.; Anderes, K.; et al. Unprecedented selectivity and structural determinants of a new class of protein kinase CK2 inhibitors in clinical trials for the treatment of cancer. *Biochemistry* **2011**, *50*, 8478–8488. [CrossRef] [PubMed]

26. Pierre, F.; Chua, P.C.; O'Brien, S.E.; Siddiqui-Jain, A.; Bourbon, P.; Haddach, M.; Michaux, J.; Nagasawa, J.; Schwaebe, M.K.; Stefan, E.; et al. Pre-clinical characterization of CX-4945, a potent and selective small molecule inhibitor of CK2 for the treatment of cancer. *Mol. Cell Biochem.* **2011**, *356*, 37–43. [CrossRef] [PubMed]

27. Kim, J.; Kim, S.H. Druggability of the CK2 inhibitor CX-4945 as an anticancer drug and beyond. *Arch. Pharm. Res.* **2012**, *35*, 1293–1296. [CrossRef] [PubMed]

28. Reznikoff, C.A.; Brankow, D.W.; Heidelberger, C. Establishment and characterization of a cloned line of C3H mouse embryo cells sensitive to postconfluence inhibition of division. *Cancer Res.* **1973**, *33*, 3231–3238. [PubMed]

29. Kuenzel, E.A.; Krebs, E.G. A synthetic peptide substrate specific for casein kinase II. *Proc. Natl. Acad. Sci. USA* **1985**, *82*, 737–741. [CrossRef] [PubMed]

30. Gregoire, F.M.; Smas, C.M.; Sul, H.S. Understanding adipocyte differentiation. *Physiol. Rev.* **1998**, *78*, 783–809. [PubMed]

31. Pierre, F.; Chua, P.C.; O'Brien, S.E.; Siddiqui-Jain, A.; Bourbon, P.; Haddach, M.; Michaux, J.; Nagasawa, J.; Schwaebe, M.K.; Stefan, E.; et al. Discovery and SAR of 5-(3-chlorophenylamino)benzo[c][2,6]naphthyridine-8-carboxylic acid (CX-4945), the first clinical stage inhibitor of protein kinase CK2 for the treatment of cancer. *J. Med. Chem.* **2011**, *54*, 635–654. [CrossRef] [PubMed]

32. Chon, H.J.; Bae, K.J.; Lee, Y.; Kim, J. The casein kinase 2 inhibitor, CX-4945, as an anti-cancer drug in treatment of human hematological malignancies. *Front. Pharmacol.* **2015**, *6*, 70. [CrossRef] [PubMed]

33. Tang, Q.Q.; Otto, T.C.; Lane, M.D. Mitotic clonal expansion: A synchronous process required for adipogenesis. *Proc. Natl. Acad. Sci. USA* **2003**, *100*, 44–49. [CrossRef] [PubMed]

34. Janderova, L.; McNeil, M.; Murrell, A.N.; Mynatt, R.L.; Smith, S.R. Human mesenchymal stem cells as an in vitro model for human adipogenesis. *Obes. Res.* **2003**, *11*, 65–74. [CrossRef] [PubMed]

35. Rosen, E.D.; Sarraf, P.; Troy, A.E.; Bradwin, G.; Moore, K.; Milstone, D.S.; Spiegelman, B.M.; Mortensen, R.M. PPAR gamma is required for the differentiation of adipose tissue in vivo and in vitro. *Mol. Cell* **1999**, *4*, 611–617. [CrossRef]

Pharmaceuticals **2017**, *10*, 22

36. Ren, D.; Collingwood, T.N.; Rebar, E.J.; Wolffe, A.P.; Camp, H.S. PPARγ knockdown by engineered transcription factors: Exogenous PPARγ2 but not PPARγ1 reactivates adipogenesis. *Genes Dev.* **2002**, *16*, 27–32. [CrossRef] [PubMed]

37. Akkiraju, H.; Bonor, J.; Nohe, A. CK2.1, a novel peptide, induces articular cartilage formation in vivo. *J. Orthop. Res.* **2016**. [CrossRef] [PubMed]

38. Mestres, P.; Boldyreff, B.; Ebensperger, C.; Hameister, H.; Issinger, O.-G. Expression of casein kinase 2 during mouse embryogenesis. *Acta Anat.* **1994**, *149*, 13–20. [CrossRef] [PubMed]

39. Maridor, G.; Park, W.; Krek, W.; Nigg, E.A. Casein kinase II. cDNA sequences, developmental expression, and tissue distribution of mRNAs for alpha, alpha', and beta subunits of the chicken enzyme. *J. Biol. Chem.* **1991**, *266*, 2362–2368. [PubMed]

40. Hu, E.; Rubin, C.S. Casein kinase II from Caenorhabditis elegans. Cloning, characterization, and developmental regulation of the gene encoding the beta subunit. *J. Biol. Chem.* **1991**, *266*, 19796–19802. [PubMed]

41. Perez, M.; Grande, J.; Itarte, E. Developmental changes in rat hepatic casein kinases 1 and 2. *Eur. J. Biochem.* **1987**, *170*, 493–498. [CrossRef] [PubMed]

42. Wilhelm, N.; Kostelnik, K.; Götz, C.; Montenarh, M. Protein kinase CK2 is implicated in early steps of the differentiation of preadipocytes into adipocytes. *Mol. Cell Biochem.* **2012**, *365*, 37–45. [CrossRef] [PubMed]

43. Prowald, K.; Fischer, H.; Issinger, O.G. Enhanced casein kinase II activity in human tumour cell cultures. *FEBS Lett.* **1984**, *176*, 479–483. [CrossRef]

44. Faust, R.A.; Gapany, M.; Tristani, P.; Davis, A.; Adams, G.L.; Ahmed, K. Elevated protein kinase CK2 activity in chromatin of head and neck tumors: Association with malignant transformation. *Cancer Lett.* **1996**, *101*, 31–35. [CrossRef]

45. Wu, Z.; Bucher, N.L.; Farmer, S.R. Induction of peroxisome proliferator-activated receptor gamma during the conversion of 3T3 fibroblasts into adipocytes is mediated by C/EBPbeta, C/EBPdelta, and glucocorticoids. *Mol. Cell. Biol.* **1996**, *16*, 4128–4136. [CrossRef] [PubMed]

46. Lin, F.T.; Lane, M.D. Antisense CCAAT/enhancer-binding protein RNA suppresses coordinate gene expression and triglyceride accumulation during differentiation of 3T3-L1 preadipocytes. *Genes Dev.* **1992**, *6*, 533–544. [CrossRef] [PubMed]

47. Schwind, L.; Zimmer, A.; Götz, C.; Montenarh, M. CK2 phosphorylation of C/EBP regulates its transcription factor activity. *Int. J. Biochem. Cell Biol.* **2015**, *61*, 81–89. [CrossRef] [PubMed]

48. Laemmli, U.K. Cleavage of structural proteins during the assembly of the head of bacteriophage T 4. *Nature* **1970**, *227*, 680–682. [CrossRef] [PubMed]

49. Faust, M.; Schuster, N.; Montenarh, M. Specific binding of protein kinase CK2 catalytic subunits to tubulin. *FEBS Lett.* **1999**, *462*, 51–56. [CrossRef]

50. Nastainczyk, W.; Schmidt-Spaniol, I.; Boldyreff, B.; Issinger, O.-G. Isolation and characterization of a monoclonal anti-protein kinase CK2 -subunit antibody of the IgG class for the direct detection of CK2-subunit in tissue cultures of various mammalian species and human tumors. *Hybridoma* **1995**, *14*, 335–339. [CrossRef] [PubMed]

51. Nastainczyk, W.; Issinger, O.G.; Guerra, B. Epitope analysis of the MAb 1AD9 antibody detection site in human protein kinase CK2alpha-subunit. *Hybrid. Hybridomics* **2003**, *22*, 87–90. [CrossRef] [PubMed]

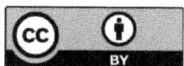

pharmaceuticals

MDPI

Article

Ablation of Protein Kinase CK2β in Skeletal Muscle Fibers Interferes with Their Oxidative Capacity

Nane Eiber [†], Luca Simeone [†] and Said Hashemolhosseini *

Institute of Biochemistry, Friedrich-Alexander University of Erlangen-Nuremberg, Fahrstrasse 17,
91054 Erlangen, Germany; nane.eib@web.de (N.E.); simeoneluca@gmail.com (L.S.)
* Correspondence: said.hashemolhosseini@fau.de; Tel.: +49-9131-85-24634
† Both authors contributed equally to this work.

Academic Editor: Mathias Montenarh
Received: 3 December 2016; Accepted: 14 January 2017; Published: 19 January 2017

Abstract: The tetrameric protein kinase CK2 was identified playing a role at neuromuscular junctions by studying CK2β-deficient muscle fibers in mice, and in cultured immortalized C2C12 muscle cells after individual knockdown of CK2α and CK2β subunits. In muscle cells, CK2 activity appeared to be at least required for regular aggregation of nicotinic acetylcholine receptors, which serves as a hallmark for the presence of a postsynaptic apparatus. Here, we set out to determine whether any other feature accompanies CK2β-deficient muscle fibers. Hind limb muscles gastrocnemius, plantaris, and soleus of adult wildtype and CK2β-deficient mice were dissected, cross-sectioned, and stained histochemically by Gomori trichrome and for nicotinamide adenine dinucleotide (NADH) dehydrogenase and succinate dehydrogenase (SDH) enzymatic activities. A reduction of oxidative enzymatic activity was determined for CK2β-deficient muscle fibers in comparison with wildtype controls. Importantly, the CK2β-deficient fibers, muscle fibers that typically exhibit high NADH dehydrogenase and SDH activities, like slow-type fibers, showed a marked reduction in these activities. Altogether, our data indicate additional impairments in the absence of CK2β in skeletal muscle fibers, pointing to an eventual mitochondrial myopathy.

Keywords: protein kinase CK2; skeletal muscle; C2C12; myopathy

1. Introduction

CK2 is a highly conserved, ubiquitously expressed serine/threonine kinase present in all eukaryotes [1,2]. It is involved in many biological processes, such as proliferation, apoptosis, differentiation, and tumorigenesis. The CK2 holoenzyme consists of a tetramer of two catalytic (α/α′) and two regulatory (β) subunits. Ablation studies have demonstrated the inability of CK2α to compensate for the loss of CK2α′ during mouse spermatogenesis [3,4], suggesting functional specialization. In mice, disruption of the gene encoding the CK2β subunit is lethal at a very early embryonic stage [5]. The precise mode of regulation of CK2 activity is poorly defined; i.e., as to whether CK2 is constitutively active or modulated in response to stimuli [1]. Recently, the involvement of CK2 in Wnt signaling, namely the canonical Wnt/β-catenin signaling pathway, has been reported [6,7]. Non-canonical Wnt signaling, like the planar-cell polarity pathway, is implicated in post-synaptic cytoskeletal reorganization. Members of Wnt signaling pathways, such as β-catenin, disheveled, and the tumor suppressor protein adenomatous polyposis coli, directly associate with proteins assembling the post-synaptic apparatus [8–10]. Canonical Wnt signaling is even active in adult skeletal muscle fibers [11]. Previously, CK2 was identified in mammalian skeletal muscle cells phosphorylating glycogen synthase from rabbit skeletal muscle [12]. Later, CK2 was reported being linked to the aggregation of nicotinic acetylcholine receptors and interacting with several components of the postsynaptic machinery, regardless whether in cultured immortalized C2C12 cells or in mice [13,14]. CK2β was shown to strongly interact with the phosphorylated intracellular domain of the muscle-specific receptor tyrosine kinase MuSK at the neuromuscular junction (NMJ) [13]. This interaction requires the entire intracellular MuSK domain with the exception of the C-terminal PDZ-binding motif, as well as the positive regulatory domain of CK2β [13]. Further, phosphorylation of serine residues within the kinase insert domain of MuSK by CK2 was demonstrated [13]. Importantly, phosphorylation of MuSK by CK2 prevents fragmentation of the NMJs [13]. Generation and characterization of myotube-specific CK2β knockout mice corroborated in vitro data and showed loss of muscle grip strength in an age-dependent fashion [13]. Later, at the NMJ CK2 was shown to additionally interact with the α and β subunits of the nicotinic acetylcholine receptors (AChR), disheveled, and strongly with Rapsyn, Rac1, 14-3-3γ, and Dok-7 [14]. It turned out that CK2 phosphorylates 14-3-3γ and Dok-7, but not Rapsyn or Rac1, at several serine residues [14]. Importantly, phosphomimetic Dok-7 mutants aggregate AChRs in C2C12 myotubes with a significantly higher frequency than wildtype Dok-7 [14]. In another report, 34 muscle biopsies of human patients with different muscle pathologies were analyzed regarding CK2 transcript amount and enzymatic activity. Interestingly, holoenzyme CK2 kinase activity was highly variable in limb girdle muscular dystrophy (LGMD) patients and appeared to be lower in mitochondrial myopathy patients [15].

Here, we set out to determine whether different histochemical stainings of hind limb muscle cross-sections of CK2β-deficient mice can enable us to gain more insight into potential extra-synaptic impairments of their skeletal muscle fibers. In comparison with wildtype controls, accumulated aggregates were detectable at the subsarcolemmal membrane of CK2β-deficient skeletal muscle fibers and accompanied by a lack of oxidative enzymatic activities of nicotinamide adenine dinucleotide (NADH) dehydrogenase and succinate dehydrogenase (SDH).

2. Results

CK2 is ubiquitously expressed and was reported to be further accumulated at the postsynaptic apparatus of skeletal muscle fibers [13,14]. We wondered about the subcellular localization of extra-synaptic CK2 within muscle fibers. After transfection of protein fusions of individual CK2 subunits with GFP into primary cultured muscle cells and their differentiation to myotubes, the GFP fluorophore was detected all along the myotubes, indicating that CK2 might be also necessary at extra-synaptic sites (data not shown). To look for extra-synaptic changes, mutant hind limb muscle fiber cryosections of adult (>6–8 months) wildtype and mutant mice were stained with hematoxylin and eosin. Gastrocnemius, plantaris, and soleus muscle cross sections possessed fibers of smaller and variable diameters, containing a significantly higher number of central nuclei and partly subsarcolemmal aggregations (data not shown). We set out to determine whether other types of histochemical stainings might elucidate potential changes comparing wildtype and CK2β-deficient muscles. We decided to choose the hind limb muscles, gastrocnemius, plantaris, and soleus, which represent examples of both glycolytic and oxidative skeletal muscles. While gastrocnemius is mostly composed of glycolytic fibers, plantaris contains some oxidative fibers. The soleus muscle in mice is mainly composed of glycolytic and oxidative fibers in a similar ratio. Low-resolution images of different histochemical stainings demonstrated subsarcolemmal aggregates on cryosections from mutant, but not wildtype muscles (Figure 1). Further, a high number of tiny little speckles were visible on mutant sections and not on the wild types, especially at high-resolution (Figures 1–3). We proceeded to examine histochemical stainings of the hind limb muscles by high-resolution microscopy and densitometrical quantifications of staining patterns (Figures 2 and 3).

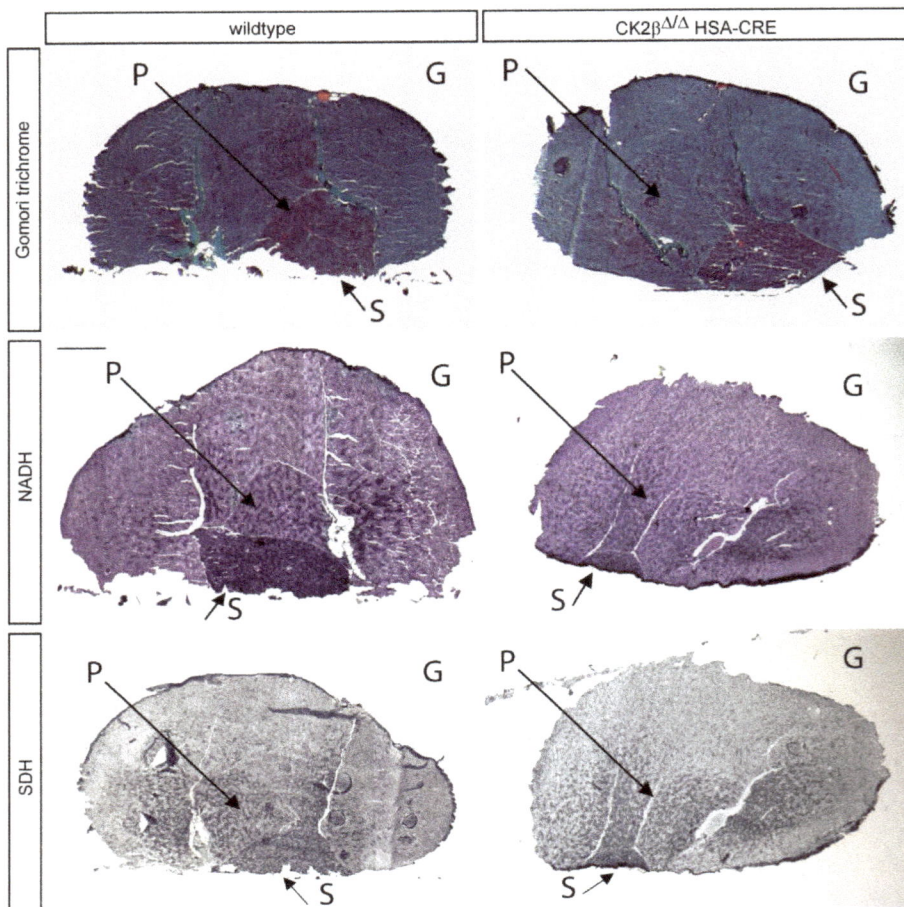

Figure 1. Typical images of full size hind limb cross sections after application of different types of histochemical stainings show gastrocnemius (G), plantaris (P), and soleus (S) of wildtype and CK2β-deficient (CK2$^{\Delta/\Delta}$ HSA-Cre) muscles of mice. Histochemical stainings by Gomori trichrome and for detection of NADH dehydrogenase and SDH enzyme activities are indicated.

2.1. Gomori Trichrome Staining Revealed Impairments in CK2β-Deficient Muscle Fibers

Gomori trichrome is a staining procedure that combines the plasma and connective fiber stain in a phosphotungstic acid solution to which glacial acetic acid has been added [16]. It is commonly used to identify potential metabolic impairments in human muscle pathologies, likely indicating mitochondrial myopathies. Skeletal muscle fibers containing structurally abnormal mitochondria below the sarcolemmal membrane and within the fiber itself that stain red with Gomori trichrome staining are occasionally seen in mitochondrial myopathies and in other myopathy disorders. Cross sections of plantaris and soleus muscle from adult wildtype and CK2β-deficient mice were stained with Gomori trichrome and imaged by high-resolution microscopy (Figures 2 and 3). Interestingly, muscles from CK2β-deficient mice in comparison with wildtype controls contained red-colored subsarcolemmal aggregates within their muscle fibers (Figures 2 and 3). Most likely, these aggregates indicate abnormal mitochondria which accumulated at the subsarcolemmal membrane (Figures 2 and 3).

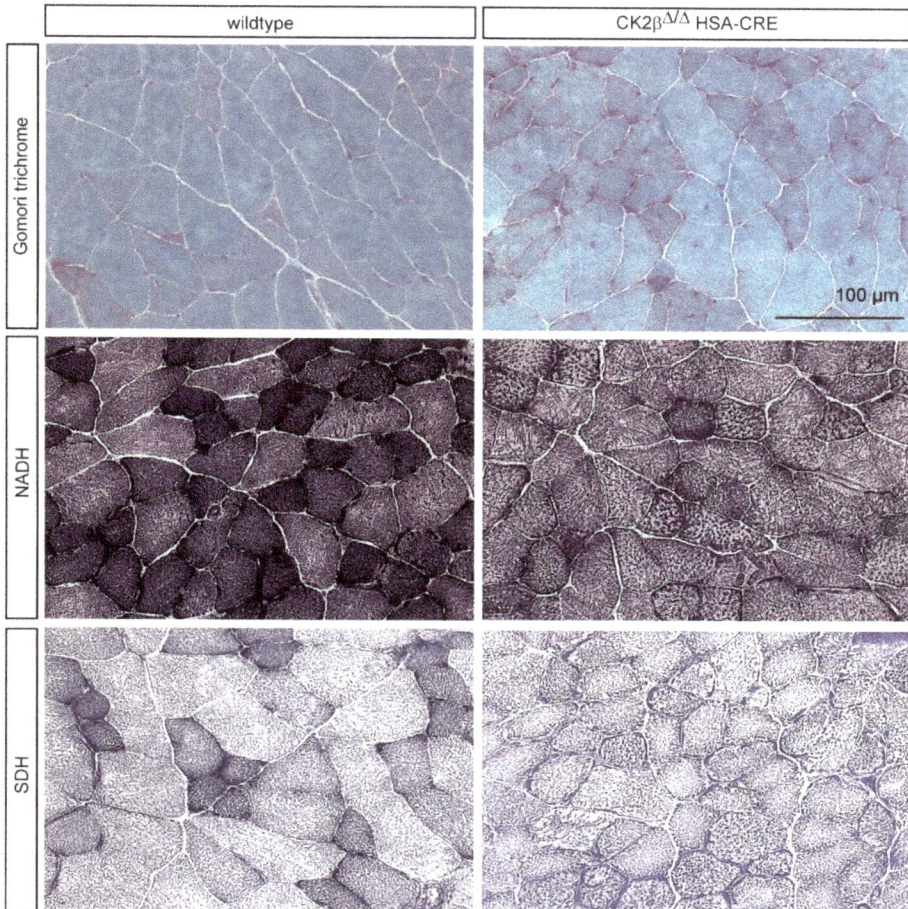

Figure 2. Typical images of hind limb cross sections after different histochemical stainings show plantaris muscles of wildtype and CK2β-deficient mice at high resolution. Note that mitochondria appear accumulated at the subsarcolemmal membrane of CK2β-deficient muscle fibers (red-colored in Gomori trichrome-stained muscle sections), while after NADH dehydrogenase and SDH stainings dark-colored slow type muscle fibers in wildtype cross sections are less dark-colored in CK2β-deficient muscle fibers. Further, in comparison with wildtype muscles fiber diameters are significantly reduced on mutant muscle cross sections. The scale bar shown is representative for all images of muscle cross-sections in this figure.

2.2. Nicotinamide Adenine Dinucleotide (NADH) Dehydrogenase Staining Detected a Diminished Enzymatic Activity in CK2β-Deficient Muscle Fibers

NADH tetrazolium reductases are flavoprotein enzymes that have the property of transferring hydrogen from a reduced nicotinamide adenine dinucleotide (NADH) to various dyes. Usually, tetrazolium compounds function as the hydrogen acceptor when these reductases are being demonstrated histochemically, and the product of the reduction is the water-insoluble purple-blue formazan pigment marking the site of enzyme activity [17]. Accordingly, this staining detects the activity of the enzyme NADH dehydrogenase, which is also called NADH/coenzyme

Q-Oxidoreductase; or briefly NADH reductase. Here, we will use the term NADH dehydrogenase or NADH dehydrogenase staining. We continued investigating cross sections of plantaris and soleus muscle from adult wildtype and CK2β-deficient mice by NADH dehydrogenase staining (Figures 2 and 3). By Gomori trichrome staining, we observed that muscles from CK2β-deficient mice appear to be accompanied by abnormal mitochondria (Figures 2 and 3). We wondered whether changes in the oxidative capacity of CK2β-deficient skeletal muscle fibers were reflected in NADH dehydrogenase staining. We detected a significant number of dark-colored fibers in wildtype muscle cross sections, pointing to slow fiber types known to contain a high number of mitochondria (Figures 2 and 3). In comparison, CK2β-deficient skeletal muscle fibers did not possess these dark-colored NADH dehydrogenase stained fibers. Instead, CK2β-deficient muscles contained fibers which were only slightly more colored compared to neighboring fast fibers (Figures 2 and 3). The loss of color intensity of slow type fibers was densitometrically examined and compared between wildtype and CK2β-deficient skeletal muscle fibers (Figures 2 and 3). CK2β-deficient slow type muscle fibers were 0.74-fold less dark-colored in plantaris and 0.76-fold less dark-colored in soleus muscles in comparison with wildtype controls (Table 1).

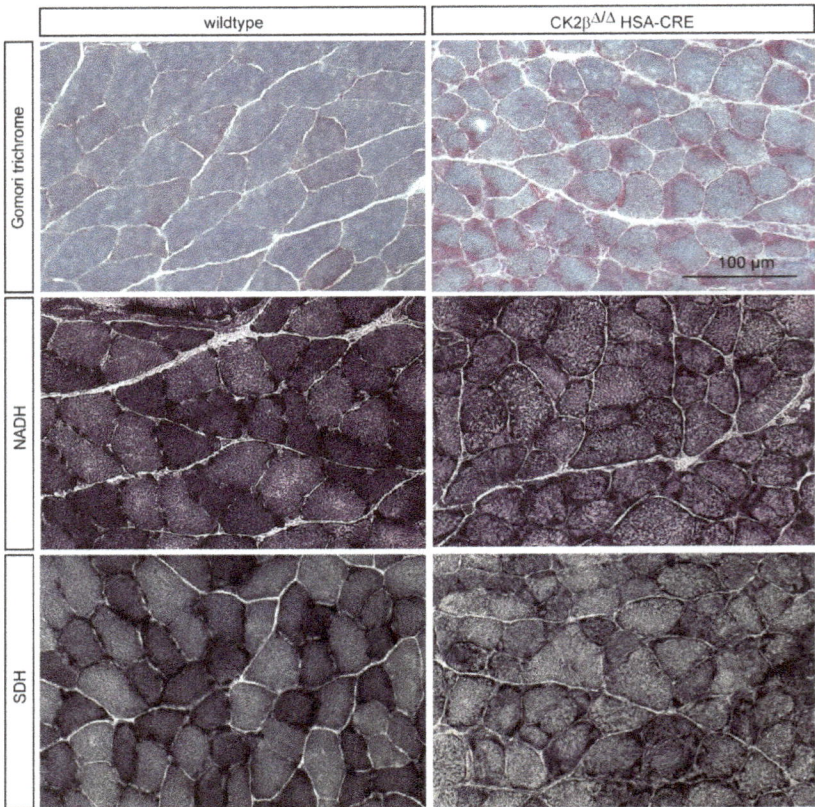

Figure 3. High-resolution images of hind limb cross sections after different histochemical stainings show soleus muscles of wildtype and CK2β-deficient mice. Note that, in comparison with wildtype controls, cross sections of CK2β-deficient muscle fibers are of more granular appearance after NADH dehydrogenase and SDH staining, and there are a significant number of fibers with lower diameter. The scale bar shown is representative for all images of muscle cross-sections.

Table 1. Densitometry measurement of NADH dehydrogenase and SDH staining intensities in slow type fibers of plantaris and soleus muscle of wildtype and CK2β-deficient mice.

Densitometry	Wildtype	CK2β$^{\Delta/\Delta}$ HSA-Cre
	Plantaris	
NADH dehydrogenase	221.6 ± 1.37, N = 43	165.9 ± 2.97, N = 46
SDH	186.4 ± 2.24, N = 50	109.8 ± 1.88, N = 46
	Soleus	
NADH dehydrogenase	221.4 ± 0.87, N = 37	169.5 ± 2.46, N = 47
SDH	193.8 ± 1.30, N = 35	141.0 ± 2.90, N = 42

2.3. Succinate Dehydrogenase Activity Is Reduced in CK2β-Deficient Muscle Fibers

Succinic dehydrogenase (SDH) catalyzes the oxidation of succinic acid to fumaric acid. The histochemical activity of this enzyme is detectable as a change in color of muscle fibers after incubation of muscle tissue sections with a succinate substrate in the presence of a tetrazolium compound, a water-soluble compound employed in histochemistry as a redox indicator [17]. The rest of this staining chemistry is comparable to the NADH dehydrogenase staining procedure [17]. Cross sections of adult muscles from wildtype and CK2β-deficient mice were made and stained to reveal SDH activity and determine oxidative capacity of respective skeletal muscle fibers. Importantly, slow fiber types of CK2β-deficient muscles were significantly less intensively dark-colored compared to slow fiber types of wildtype muscles. The change in oxidative capacity of slow type fibers of CK2β-deficient muscles was quantified densitometrically and turned out to be 1.37-fold higher in wildtype, in comparison with CK2β-deficient soleus, and 1.69-fold in comparison with CK2β-deficient plantaris muscle fibers (Table 1).

3. Discussion

Up to now, protein kinase CK2 was shown in muscle cells most likely responsible for the maintenance, rather than the formation, of NMJs [13,14]. Interestingly, analyzing CK2 transcript distribution and enzyme activity in human skeletal muscle biopsies from patients suffering either from LGMD of unknown classification, mitochondrial myopathy, or neurogenic muscular atrophy, and normal controls, no significant changes were observed [15]. However, a high variation of CK2 activity was detected in biopsies from LGMD patients [15]. In the case of the mitochondrial myopathy patients, in three out of four biopsies, a decrease of CK2 activity was detected [15]. Here, we examined hind limb muscle cross sections of wildtype and CK2β-deficient mice and looked for additional extra-synaptic impairments by different type of histochemical stainings. By regular hematoxylin and eosin staining, we detected smaller and variable fiber diameters and central nuclei on CK2β-deficient muscle cross sections in comparison with wildtype controls (data not shown). These findings encouraged us to investigate in more detail potential changes between CK2β-deficient and wildtype muscles by applying Gomori trichrome staining and stainings that allow for the measurement of the oxidative capacity of CK2β-deficient muscle fibers by detecting the activities of NADH dehydrogenase and SDH (Figures 2 and 3). It turned out that, by Gomori trichrome, NADH dehydrogenase, and SDH stainings (Figures 2 and 3), mutant fibers were on average reduced in diameter, as detected by hematoxylin and eosin stainings (data not shown). Importantly, Gomori trichrome staining detected accumulations at the subsarcolemmal membrane, most likely pointing to mitochondria and indicating changes in the oxidative capacity of the CK2-deficient skeletal muscle fibers (Figures 1–3). During development, several weeks after birth muscle fibers gradually mature into adult muscle fibers. Slow type fibers are known to possess more mitochondria and a higher oxidative capacity. They become dark-colored after NADH dehydrogenase and SDH staining. In this study, we investigated gastrocnemius, plantaris, and soleus muscles by histochemical stainings and detected the oxidative fibers of CK2β-deficient muscle fibers less intensely stained in comparison with wildtype controls (Figures 1–3). These less colored fibers in CK2β-deficient muscles appear to be the remains of previously dark-colored oxidative fibers (Figures 2 and 3).

Our data indicate a potential role of the protein kinase CK2 regarding oxidative metabolism in adult skeletal muscle fibers. Further experiments are required to identify the molecular mechanism and understand the potential impact of CK2 regarding human myopathies.

4. Materials and Methods

4.1. Mice Mating and Genotyping

Mice mating and genotyping were performed as described previously [5,13,18]. Mouse experiments were performed in accordance with animal welfare laws and approved by the responsible local committees (animal protection officer, Sachgebiet Tierschutzangelegenheiten, FAU Erlangen-Nuremberg, AZ: I/39/EE006 and TS-07/11) and government bodies (Regierung von Unterfranken). Mice were housed in cages that were maintained in a room with temperature $22 \pm 1\,°C$ and relative humidity 50%–60% on a 12 h light/dark cycle. Water and food were provided ad libitum.

4.2. Dissecting of Skeletal Muscles and Tissue Sections

Hind limb muscles were dissected and then quick-frozen in prechilled isopentane as described [13]. Muscles were cryotome-sectioned (10 μm). Cryotome sections were used for histochemical stainings. Sections were embedded in DPX or mowiol (Sigma-Aldrich Chemie GmbH, München, Germany) as earlier described [11,19].

4.3. Histochemical Stainings, Immunohistochemistry, Imaging, and Data Analysis

Modified Gomori trichrome staining was perfomed by incubation of muscle sections in Shandon hematoxylin (Fisher Scientific GmbH, Schwerte, Germany) for 15 min, followed by a 15 min wash in tap water and 45 min incubation in Gomori solution (Sigma-Aldrich Chemie GmbH), washed in tap water, and incubated in 100% ethanol.

For nicotinamide adenine dinucleotide (NADH) dehydrogenase staining, sections were incubated for 30 min at 37 °C in a solution containing NBT (Sigma-Aldrich Chemie GmbH), 50 mM Tris/HCl, and NADH (Sigma-Aldrich Chemie GmbH), then washed in distilled water.

For succinate dehydrogenase (SDH) staining sections were incubated for 45 min at 37 °C in a solution containing Tris 0.2 M pH 7.2, cobalt (II)-chloride, MTT (methylthiazolyldiphenyl-tetrazolium bromide), and NADH. Afterwards, sections were incubated for 30 min in 4% PFA and washed in H_2O.

Stained cryosections were analyzed and documented using a Zeiss Axio Examiner Z1 microscope equipped with an AxioCam MRm camera and ZEISS AxioVision Release 4.8 (Carl Zeiss MicroImaging, Göttingen, Germany). Densitometric quantifications were done using ImageJ [20].

4.4. Statistical Analysis

Data are presented as the mean values, and the error bars indicate $\pm$ standard deviation. The number of biological replicates per experimental variable (n) is usually $n > 5$ or as indicated in the figure legends. The significance was calculated by an unpaired two-tailed t test, or as indicated by the figure legends, and are provided as real p-values that are believed to be categorized for different significance levels. *** $p < 0.001$, ** $p < 0.01$, or * $p < 0.05$.

Acknowledgments: This work was supported by the Deutsche Forschungsgemeinschaft (HA 3309/1-3), Interdisciplinary Centre for Clinical Research at the University Hospital of the University of Erlangen-Nuremberg (IZKF E2, E17), and the Johannes und Frieda Marohn-Stiftung to Said Hashemolhosseini.

Author Contributions: Nane Eiber, Luca Simeone, and Said Hashemolhosseini conceived and designed the experiments; Nane Eiber and Luca Simeone performed the experiments; Nane Eiber and Said Hashemolhosseini analyzed the data; Said Hashemolhosseini wrote the paper.

Conflicts of Interest: The authors declare no conflict of interest.

References

1. Olsten, M.E.; Litchfield, D.W. Order or chaos? An evaluation of the regulation of protein kinase ck2. *Biochem. Cell Biol.* **2004**, *82*, 681–693. [CrossRef] [PubMed]
2. Meggio, F.; Pinna, L.A. One-thousand-and-one substrates of protein kinase ck2? *FASEB J.* **2003**, *17*, 349–368. [CrossRef] [PubMed]
3. Escalier, D.; Silvius, D.; Xu, X. Spermatogenesis of mice lacking ck2α′: Failure of germ cell survival and characteristic modifications of the spermatid nucleus. *Mol. Reprod. Dev.* **2003**, *66*, 190–201. [CrossRef] [PubMed]
4. Xu, X.; Toselli, P.A.; Russell, L.D.; Seldin, D.C. Globozoospermia in mice lacking the casein kinase II α′ catalytic subunit. *Nat. Genet.* **1999**, *23*, 118–121. [PubMed]
5. Buchou, T.; Vernet, M.; Blond, O.; Jensen, H.H.; Pointu, H.; Olsen, B.B.; Cochet, C.; Issinger, O.G.; Boldyreff, B. Disruption of the regulatory beta subunit of protein kinase ck2 in mice leads to a cell-autonomous defect and early embryonic lethality. *Mol. Cell. Biol.* **2003**, *23*, 908–915. [CrossRef] [PubMed]
6. Song, D.H.; Dominguez, I.; Mizuno, J.; Kaut, M.; Mohr, S.C.; Seldin, D.C. Ck2 phosphorylation of the armadillo repeat region of beta-catenin potentiates wnt signaling. *J. Biol. Chem.* **2003**, *278*, 24018–24025. [CrossRef] [PubMed]
7. Abicht, A.; Stucka, R.; Schmidt, C.; Briguet, A.; Hopfner, S.; Song, I.H.; Pongratz, D.; Muller-Felber, W.; Ruegg, M.A.; Lochmuller, H. A newly identified chromosomal microdeletion and an n-box mutation of the achr epsilon gene cause a congenital myasthenic syndrome. *Brain* **2002**, *125*, 1005–1013. [CrossRef] [PubMed]
8. Luo, Z.G.; Wang, Q.; Zhou, J.Z.; Wang, J.; Luo, Z.; Liu, M.; He, X.; Wynshaw-Boris, A.; Xiong, W.C.; Lu, B.; et al. Regulation of achr clustering by dishevelled interacting with musk and pak1. *Neuron* **2002**, *35*, 489–505. [CrossRef]
9. Wang, J.; Jing, Z.; Zhang, L.; Zhou, G.; Braun, J.; Yao, Y.; Wang, Z.Z. Regulation of acetylcholine receptor clustering by the tumor suppressor APC. *Nat. Neurosci.* **2003**, *6*, 1017–1018. [CrossRef] [PubMed]
10. Zou, Y. Wnt signaling in axon guidance. *Trends Neurosci.* **2004**, *27*, 528–532. [CrossRef] [PubMed]
11. Huraskin, D.; Eiber, N.; Reichel, M.; Zidek, L.M.; Kravic, B.; Bernkopf, D.; von Maltzahn, J.; Behrens, J.; Hashemolhosseini, S. Wnt/beta-catenin signaling via axin2 is required for myogenesis and, together with yap/taz and tead1, active in iia/iix muscle fibers. *Development* **2016**, *143*, 3128–3142. [CrossRef] [PubMed]
12. Picton, C.; Woodgett, J.; Hemmings, B.; Cohen, P. Multisite phosphorylation of glycogen synthase from rabbit skeletal muscle. Phosphorylation of site 5 by glycogen synthase kinase-5 (casein kinase-ii) is a prerequisite for phosphorylation of sites 3 by glycogen synthase kinase-3. *FEBS Lett.* **1982**, *150*, 191–196. [CrossRef]
13. Cheusova, T.; Khan, M.A.; Schubert, S.W.; Gavin, A.C.; Buchou, T.; Jacob, G.; Sticht, H.; Allende, J.; Boldyreff, B.; Brenner, H.R.; et al. Casein kinase 2-dependent serine phosphorylation of musk regulates acetylcholine receptor aggregation at the neuromuscular junction. *Genes Dev.* **2006**, *20*, 1800–1816. [CrossRef] [PubMed]
14. Herrmann, D.; Straubinger, M.; Hashemolhosseini, S. Protein kinase ck2 interacts at the neuromuscular synapse with rapsyn, rac1, 14-3-3gamma, and dok-7 proteins and phosphorylates the latter two. *J. Biol. Chem.* **2015**, *290*, 22370–22384. [CrossRef] [PubMed]
15. Heuss, D.; Klascinski, J.; Schubert, S.W.; Moriabadi, T.; Lochmuller, H.; Hashemolhosseini, S. Examination of transcript amounts and activity of protein kinase ck2 in muscle lysates of different types of human muscle pathologies. *Mol. Cell Biochem.* **2008**, *316*, 135–140. [CrossRef] [PubMed]
16. Thompson, S.W. *Selected Histochemical and Histopathological Methods*; C.C. Thomas: Springfield, IL, USA, 1966.
17. Sheehan, D.C.; Hrapchak, B.B. *Theory and Practice of Histotechnology*, 2nd ed.; Battelle Press: Columbus, OH, USA, 1987.
18. Kravic, B.; Huraskin, D.; Frick, A.D.; Jung, J.; Redai, V.; Palmisano, R.; Marchetto, S.; Borg, J.P.; Mei, L.; Hashemolhosseini, S. LAP proteins are localized at the post-synaptic membrane of neuromuscular junctions and appear to modulate synaptic morphology and transmission. *J. Neurochem.* **2016**, *139*, 381–395. [CrossRef] [PubMed]

Pharmaceuticals **2017**, *10*, 13

19. Simeone, L.; Straubinger, M.; Khan, M.A.; Nalleweg, N.; Cheusova, T.; Hashemolhosseini, S. Identification of erbin interlinking musk and erbb2 and its impact on acetylcholine receptor aggregation at the neuromuscular junction. *J. Neurosci.* **2010**, *30*, 6620–6634. [CrossRef] [PubMed]
20. Schindelin, J.; Rueden, C.T.; Hiner, M.C.; Eliceiri, K.W. The imagej ecosystem: An open platform for biomedical image analysis. *Mol. Reprod. Dev.* **2015**, *82*, 518–529. [CrossRef] [PubMed]

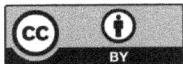

MDPI AG

St. Alban-Anlage 66

4052 Basel, Switzerland

Tel. +41 61 683 77 34

Fax +41 61 302 89 18

http://www.mdpi.com

Pharmaceuticals Editorial Office

E-mail: pharmaceuticals@mdpi.com

http://www.mdpi.com/journal/pharmaceuticals

www.ingramcontent.com/pod-product-compliance
Lightning Source LLC
Chambersburg PA
CBHW051715210326
41597CB00032B/5483